W9-BKI-813

EDITION

6

The Human Body in Health and Illness

Barbara Herlihy, BSN, MA, PhD (Physiology), RN
Professor of Biology
University of the Incarnate Word
School of Mathematics, Science, and Engineering
San Antonio, Texas

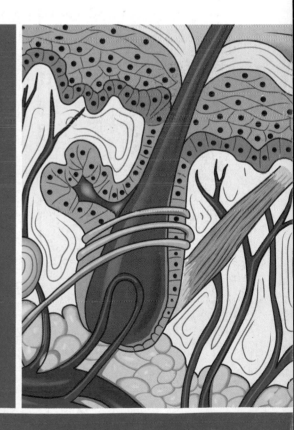

ELSEVIER

ELSEVIER

3251 Riverport Lane
St. Louis, Missouri 63043

THE HUMAN BODY IN HEALTH AND ILLNESS, SIXTH EDITION   ISBN: 978-0-323-49844-9

Copyright © 2018, Elsevier Inc.
Previous editions copyrighted 2014, 2011, 2007, 2003, 2000

All rights reserved. No part of this publication may be reproduced or transmitted in any form or by any means, electronic or mechanical, including photocopying, recording, or any information storage and retrieval system, without permission in writing from the Publisher. Details on how to seek permission, further information about the Publisher's permissions policies, and our arrangements with organizations such as the Copyright Clearance Center and the Copyright Licensing Agency can be found at our website: www.elsevier.com/permissions.

This book and the individual contributions contained in it are protected under copyright by the Publisher (other than as may be noted herein).

Notice

Practitioners and researchers must always rely on their own experience and knowledge in evaluating and using any information, methods, compounds or experiments described herein. Because of rapid advances in the medical sciences, in particular, independent verification of diagnoses and drug dosages should be made. To the fullest extent of the law, no responsibility is assumed by Elsevier, authors, editors or contributors for any injury and/or damage to persons or property as a matter of products liability, negligence or otherwise, or from any use or operation of any methods, products, instructions, or ideas contained in the material herein.

Library of Congress Cataloging-in-Publication Data

Names: Herlihy, Barbara L., author.
Title: The human body in health and illness / Barbara Herlihy.
Description: Sixth edition. | St. Louis, Missouri : Elsevier, [2018] |
    Includes bibliographical references and index.
Identifiers: LCCN 2017031809 | ISBN 9780323498449 (paperback : alk. paper)
Subjects: | MESH: Physiological Phenomena | Pathologic Processes | Health
Classification: LCC QP34.5 | NLM QT 104 | DDC 612--dc23 LC record available at
    https://lccn.loc.gov/2017031809

Executive Content Strategist: Kellie White
Senior Content Development Manager: Laurie Gower
Associate Content Development Specialist: Elizabeth Kilgore
Publishing Services Manager: Jeff Patterson
Senior Project Manager: Anne Konopka
Design Direction: Renee Duenow

Printed in Canada

Last digit is the print number: 9   8   7   6   5   4   3   2

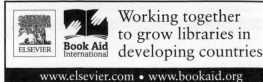

Working together
to grow libraries in
developing countries

www.elsevier.com • www.bookaid.org

evolve

ELSEVIER

YOU'VE JUST PURCHASED
MORE THAN
A TEXTBOOK!

Evolve Student Resources for Herlihy: *The Human Body in Health and Illness*, Sixth Edition, offer the following features:

- **Animations from the Elsevier Animation Collection**
  Visualize complex biological processes with detailed animations for further review and reinforcement.

- **Audio Glossary**
  Not sure how to say it? To help improve your vocabulary comprehension, we have definitions and audio pronunciations of more than 1000 terms.

- **Body Spectrum Electronic Anatomy Coloring Book**
  More than 80 illustrations to color online or offline offer a fun and effective way to reinforce elements from the textbook.

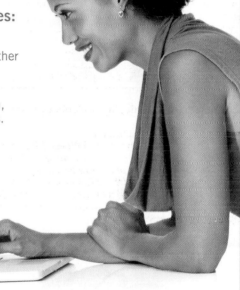

- **Flashcards**
  Mix up how you study by quizzing yourself with interactive flashcards.

- **Practice Chapter Exam**
  Lessen the pop-quiz anxiety with 20-question multiple-choice and matching tests.

- **Word-Part Multiple-Choice Questions**
  Make medical terminology easy to study with fun multiple-choice questions organized by chapter.

- **Topic-by-Topic**
  Missed something in class? Or just missed class? Topic-by-Topic is designed to take you step by step through each chapter with questions as you read, review, or both!

Activate the complete learning experience that comes with each textbook purchase by registering at

http://evolve.elsevier.com/Herlihy

REGISTER TODAY!

You can now purchase Elsevier products on Evolve!
Go to evolve.elsevier.com/html/shop-promo.html to search and browse for products.

To all who live compassionately, seeing the divine in each other, our fur friends, and Mother Earth. We are all connected in life.
Love,

Barbara

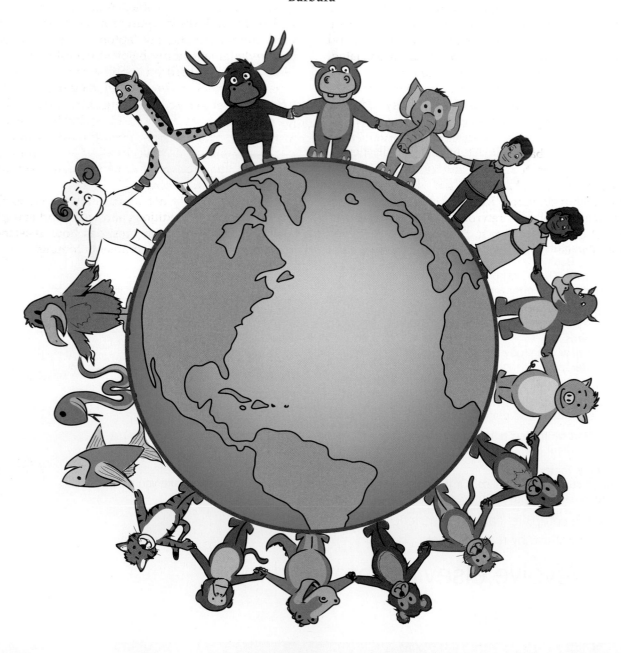

Acknowledgments

The publishing and republishing of an anatomy and physiology text require the combined efforts of various persons with diverse talents. I have been blessed to work with many generous and talented individuals at Elsevier and offer my grateful thanks, especially to Elizabeth Kilgore, Kellie White, and Anne Konopka. Liz, your patience, kindness, organizational skills, and motivational "encouragements" are much appreciated.

Many thanks also to my students and friends at the University of the Incarnate Word. They have graciously supported me through all six editions. A special thanks to Dr. Bonnie McCormick, the wisest and kindest of "bosses" at the University of the Incarnate Word. Thanks to my husband, Jerry; he has contributed much to this text by constructing tables, proofreading, and offering many helpful hints; he, too, is a physiologist. Thanks to my daughter Kellie, a clinical nurse specialist, who proofread, rewrote, and photocopied in the midst of being a mom to three adorable toddlers. Whew! Thanks to my children, grandchildren, and racquetball buddies for their insistence on leisure and play; they are in charge of my mental health. I highly recommend "grannyhood"; it is beyond joy and gets better!

Thanks to my fur babies Annie and Lucy (woof and woof) and Minky (purr) for the hours they hovered around me and my laptop. As usual, a special acknowledgment to my beloved dachshund, Pretzyl, who labored so hard on the first two editions. Four other furry helpers—Julia, Kenner, Cajun, and Zeke— are missed but certainly not forgotten. A well-fed feral cat population has been added, and with the completion of this edition, I will reward myself with a "rescue" dachshund...or two. To all of you who humor me about my pet collection and devotion, many, many thanks for understanding.

Last but certainly not least, many thanks to those who used previous editions and were kind enough to forward comments and suggestions. Your assistance is so appreciated. Keep the comments coming!

To the Instructor

Here she is…the sixth edition of *The Human Body in Health and Illness*…older, wiser, still smiling and eager to walk with you on your journey into the health professions. It's an exciting journey for all, and we wish you all the best.

The Human Body in Health and Illness tells the story of the human body with all its parts and the way these parts work together. It is a story that we have told many times in our classes. It is also a story that gets better with each telling as the body continues to reveal its mysteries and how marvelously it has been created. I hope that you enjoy telling the story as much as I do.

The Human Body in Health and Illness is a basic anatomy and physiology text addressed to the student preparing for a career in the health professions. It is written for students with minimal preparation in the sciences; no prior knowledge of biology, chemistry, or physics is required. The text provides all the background science information needed for an understanding of anatomy and physiology.

The basic principles of chemistry and biochemistry are presented in Chapters 2 and 4, and they set the stage for an understanding of cellular function, fluid and electrolyte balance, endocrine function, and digestion. Chapter 5, Microbiology Basics, presents clinically relevant microbiological topics. Check out the stories "Rick, Nick, and the Sick Tick" and "Dr. Semmelweis Screams: 'Wash Those Mitts!'" The latter is an amusing presentation of a sad tale in the history of medicine and corresponds to the current emphasis on hand hygiene and health care–associated infection.

The anatomy and physiology content is presented in a traditional order, from simple to complex. The text begins with a description of a single cell and progresses through the various organ systems. There are two key themes that run throughout the text: (1) the relationship between structure and function—the student must understand that an organ is anatomically designed to perform a specific physiological function, and (2) homeostasis—the role that each organ system plays in sustaining life and what happens when that delicate balance is disturbed.

The text addresses two concerns about the selection of content. The first has to do with the amount of content. The field of anatomy and physiology is huge; therefore there must be a selection of content that can be mastered in the short period of time that a semester (or even two) allows. This text focuses on the physiology that is basic and most clinically relevant. Pathophysiology is introduced primarily to clarify physiological function. For instance, the different types of anemias illustrate the various steps in the making of the red blood cell. A second concern has to do with the recognition that we are not preparing physiologists; instead, we want the student to be able to use the physiology to understand clinically relevant content such as pathophysiology, physical assessment, diagnostics, and pharmacology. An understanding of physiology is crucial for advancement in the medically related sciences.

TEXTBOOK STRENGTHS

- Anatomy and physiology are clearly and simply explained. A meticulously prepared set of **illustrations**—complete with amusing cartoons—supports the text. In fact, the story of the body is told as much through the art as through the written word.
- The text **truly integrates pathophysiology;** it is not merely boxed in or tacked on at the end. The integrated pathophysiology is used primarily to amplify the normal anatomy and physiology. The expanded **Medical Terminology and Disorders** tables and frequent references to common medical terminology allow the text to be used for an introductory course in pathophysiology and medical terminology.
- In addition to the pathophysiology, other topics are liberally integrated throughout the text. These include **common diagnostic procedures** such as blood count, lumbar puncture, urinalysis, and electrocardiography. **Pharmacological topics** are also introduced and, like the pathophysiology, are used to amplify the normal anatomy and physiology. For instance, the discussion of the neuromuscular junction is enhanced by a description of the effects of the neuromuscular blocking agents. Because of the effort of the text to make clinical correlations, it sets the stage for the more advanced health science courses, including pharmacology and medical-surgical nursing.
- **Re-Think** boxes are liberally distributed throughout each chapter and encourage students to master that content before progressing through the chapter. **Ramp It Up!** boxes develop selected clinically relevant topics that are simply too advanced to be included in the text as basic information. These boxed

features contain new or advanced content commonly used in the clinical setting and allow instructors to scale their coverage in a manner appropriate to the course. They offer students the chance to make further connections between the text and their future careers. *(See the To the Student preface on page ix for descriptions and examples of each of the chapter features.)*

- **Medical terminology** is introduced, defined, and used throughout the text. Common clinical terms such as *hyperkalemia, vasodilation, hypertension*, and *diagnosis* are defined and reused so that the student gradually builds up a substantial medical vocabulary. The expanded **Medical Terminology and Disorders** tables were deliberately constructed to maximize the use of common medical terms and disorders. To help foster a broader understanding of medical terminology, word parts and their meanings are included for nearly every term presented. Repetition of these helps students gain greater ground in understanding the very specific medical language they will be learning to use for a future in the health professions. A description is also provided, which gives the definition or other pertinent information on the topic.
- The **Review Your Knowledge** section has been expanded to include questions that require an analytical response. The **Go Figure** questions are based on the story told by the artwork. The questions can only be answered by analyzing the art and/or the information presented in the tables. This exercise encourages the student to see beyond the "pretty pictures" and realize that a picture is truly worth a thousand words. I would encourage you to assist your students to see that the art and the text are conveying the same message.
- The text is supported by many activities, exercises, puzzles, and games (e.g., Body Bingo) on **Evolve** (http://evolve.elsevier.com/Herlihy). These activities emphasize the focus of this text—clinically relevant anatomy and physiology.
- Last, the text incorporates many **amusing anecdotes** from the history of medicine. Although the human body is perfectly logical and predictable, we humans think, do, and say some strange things. Tales from the medical crypt provide some good laughs and much humility.

CLASSROOM RESOURCES

Materials from the **Study Guide** and **Evolve Instructor Learning Resources** can be used to:
1. Remediate students who are having difficulty in grasping the content.
2. Remediate students who have missed class(es).
3. Provide review for students engaged in pathophysiology and pharmacology whose memories need to be refreshed in the physiology.

STUDY GUIDE

The Study Guide for *The Human Body in Health and Illness* offers something for students at all levels of learning and is a ready-made resource for instructors looking for homework assignments. Each chapter includes two parts: Part I, Mastering the Basics, with matching, labeling, and coloring exercises; and Part II, Putting It All Together, containing multiple-choice questions, case studies, and word puzzles. Textbook page references are included with the questions, and the answer key is available on the Evolve website, only to instructors.

EVOLVE INSTRUCTOR LEARNING RESOURCES

The Evolve website for *The Human Body in Health and Illness* (http://evolve.elsevier.com/Herlihy) includes all of the Student Resources, as well as the following Instructor Resources:
- Answer Key for the Study Guide, Audience Response System questions, Image Collection, and ExamView Test Banks that include over 2300 questions!
- Instructor's Chapter Exams, Classroom Activities—including Bingo, Line 'Em Up, Sorting, and Word Puzzles—and the TEACH Instructor Resource.

TEACH Instructor Resource on Evolve

Instructors who adopt the textbook will also receive access to the TEACH Instructor Resource, which links all parts of the Herlihy educational package with customizable **Lesson Plans** based on objectives drawn from the text. The TEACH Lesson Plans are based on the chapter-by-chapter organization of *The Human Body in Health and Illness* and can be modified or combined to meet your curriculum's scheduling and teaching needs.

TEACH has been completely updated and revised for this edition. The TEACH Lesson Plans help instructors prepare for class and make full use of the rich array of ancillaries and resources that come with the textbook. The content covered in each textbook chapter is divided across one or more lesson plans, each designed to occupy 50 minutes of class time. Lesson plans are organized into easily understandable sections that are each tied to the chapter learning objectives:
- **Instructor Preparation** This section provides a checklist of all the things you need to do to prepare for class, including a list of all the items you need to bring to class to perform any activity or demonstration included in the lesson plan.
- **Student Preparation** Textbook readings, study guide exercises, online activities, and other applicable homework assignments for each lesson are provided here, along with an overall estimated completion time.
- **The 50-Minute Lesson Plan** A lecture outline that reflects the chapter lecture slides that come as part

of TEACH is included, as well as classroom activities and online activities, one or more critical thinking questions, and time estimates for the classroom lecture and activities.

- **Assessment Plan** To ensure that your students have mastered all the objectives, the TEACH Instructor Resource includes a separate Assessment Plan section. An easy-to-use table maps each assessment tool to the lesson plans and chapter objectives so that you can see all your assessment options—by chapter, by lesson, and by objective—and choose accordingly.

To the Student

This book will take you on an amazing journey through the human body. You will learn many body parts and, more importantly, how they work in an integrated manner to keep you going. You will use this information in your clinical practice when patients become ill with disorders of those structures. The following special features were created to help make learning enjoyable and fun.

TEXTBOOK FEATURES

KEY TERMS

Key terms are listed at the beginning of each chapter, along with a page reference. Each is (1) presented in the text in blue print, (2) accompanied by a pronunciation guide, (3) thoroughly explained within the chapter, and (4) defined in the glossary.

OBJECTIVES

Numbered objectives identify the goals for each chapter.

ILLUSTRATIONS

Original illustrations and full-color cartoons help you make sense of anatomy and physiology using humor, clarity, and insight.

 ### DO YOU KNOW...

Most of these boxed vignettes refer to clinical situations; others relate to interesting and amusing historical events related to anatomy and physiology.

 ### RAMP IT UP!

These features challenge you with more advanced anatomy and physiology topics.

 ### RE-THINK

These questions are liberally placed throughout the chapter to help reinforce important concepts.

 ### AS YOU AGE

These boxed features contain numbered lists describing how the aging process affects human anatomy and physiology.

 ### SUM IT UP!

These features appear regularly throughout the chapters and help you synthesize key concepts.

MEDICAL TERMINOLOGY AND DISORDERS TABLES

These tables describe medical terms and specific disorders related to individual body systems, with a focus on developing a strong working medical vocabulary, which is necessary for a career in the health professions.

END-OF-CHAPTER FEATURES

Summary Outline

A detailed outline at the end of each chapter summarizes key concepts and serves as an excellent review of the chapter content. Use it as a study tool to review your reading and prepare for exams.

Review Your Knowledge

The matching and multiple-choice questions in this section cover the major points of the chapter and allow you to test your comprehension.

Go Figure

This review section asks you to interpret the figures in the chapter and reinforces the importance of the concepts presented.

ANSWERS TO REVIEW YOUR KNOWLEDGE AND GO FIGURE QUESTIONS

The **Appendix** contains answers to all Review Your Knowledge and Go Figure questions found in the textbook.

GLOSSARY

The glossary includes a pronunciation guide and a brief definition of all key terms and many other words in the text.

STUDY GUIDE

Enhance your learning of the textbook content with the accompanying **Study Guide for *The Human Body in Health and Illness*.** The Study Guide has something to offer students at all levels of learning, from labeling and coloring exercises to multiple-choice practice tests and case studies.

Contents

Introduction to the Human Body

http://evolve.elsevier.com/Herlihy

Objectives

1. Define the terms anatomy and physiology.
2. List the levels of organization of the human body.
3. Describe the 12 major organ systems.
4. Define homeostasis.
5. Describe the anatomical position.
6. List common terms used for relative positions of the body.
7. Describe the three major planes of the body.
8. List anatomical terms for quadrants and regions of the body.
9. Describe the major cavities of the body.

Key Terms

abdominopelvic cavity (p. 10)
anatomical position (p. 6)
anatomy (p. 1)
cranial cavity (p. 10)
dorsal cavity (p. 9)
frontal plane (p. 7)
homeostasis (p. 6)

mediastinum (p. 10)
organs (p. 2)
pericardial cavity (p. 10)
physiology (p. 1)
pleural cavities (p. 10)
quadrants (p. 10)
sagittal plane (p. 7)

spinal (vertebral) cavity (p. 10)
thoracic cavity (p. 10)
transverse plane (p. 7)
ventral cavity (p. 9)
viscera (p. 9)

The human body is a wonderful creation. Millions of microscopic parts work together in a coordinated fashion to keep you going for about 75 years. Most of us are curious about our bodies—how they work, why they do not work, what makes us tick, and what makes us sick. As you learn more about the body, you will sometimes feel like this cartoon character: "What is this? Why do I need it? How does it work? Why don't I have one?" As you study anatomy and physiology, you will learn the answers to these questions.

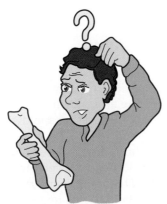

ANATOMY AND PHYSIOLOGY: WHAT THEY ARE

WHAT'S IT MEAN?

Anatomy (ah-NAT-o-mee) is the branch of science that studies the structure of the body. For example, anatomy describes what the heart looks like, how big it is, what it is made of, how it is organized, and where it is located. The word *anatomy* comes from the Greek word meaning to dissect. The science of anatomy arose from observations made by scientists centuries ago as they dissected bodies that were usually stolen from the local graveyard.

Physiology (fiz-ee-OL-o-jee) is the branch of science that describes how the body functions. For example, physiology describes how the heart pumps blood and why the pumping of blood is essential for life. Pathophysiology (path-o-fiz-ee-OL-o-jee) is the branch of science that describes the consequences of the improper functioning of the body—that is, how a body part functions when a person has a disease. Pathophysiology describes what happens during a heart attack and when the heart functions poorly or not at all.

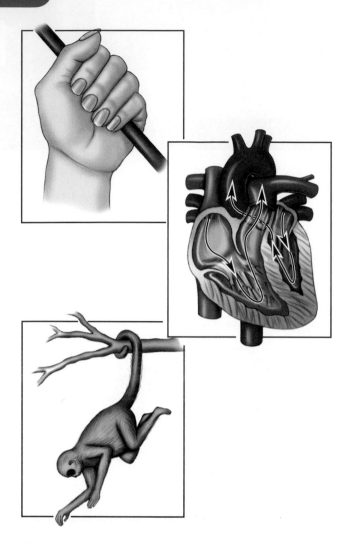

FIG. 1.1 Structure and function are closely related.

WHY DO I NEED TO KNOW THIS?

Why study anatomy and physiology as part of your professional curriculum? Unless you gain a good understanding of normal anatomy and physiology, you cannot understand the diseases and disorders experienced by your patients, nor can you understand the basis for the various forms of treatment, such as drug therapy and surgical procedures. You want to give your patients the best possible care, so you must have a sound understanding of the human body.

Anatomy and physiology are closely related. Structure and function go together. When you examine the anatomy of a body part, ask yourself how its structure relates to its function. For example, the structure of the hand is related to its function: its ability to grasp an object (Fig. 1.1). The heart pumps blood, and the long, strong, flexible tail of the monkey allows it to hang from the tree. Structure and function are related.

? Re-Think

1. What is the difference between anatomy and physiology?
2. Using any household item, explain what is meant by "structure and function are related."

 Do You Know...

Why This Grave Is Being Robbed, and Why the Grave Robber Is in Big, Big Trouble?

Dissection of the human body during medieval times was not allowed. Thus, the only way that early anatomists were able to obtain human bodies for dissection was to rob graves. Medieval scientists hired people to rob graves. Punishment for robbing graves was swift and severe. This lad will be in big, big trouble if he is caught, and it looks as if he will be. Surprisingly, grave robbing was common early in this century and in this country. Many a medical student who enrolled in the most prestigious medical schools had to "get" his own cadaver.

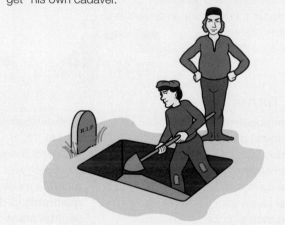

THE BODY'S LEVELS OF ORGANIZATION

The body is organized from the very simple to the complex, from the microscopic atom to the complex human organism. Note the progression from simple to complex in Fig. 1.2. Tiny atoms form molecules. These, in turn, form larger molecules. The larger molecules are eventually organized into *cells*, the basic unit of life. Specialized groups of cells form *tissues*. Tissues are then arranged into **organs**, such as the heart, stomach, and kidney. Groups of organs, in turn, create *organ systems*. Each organ system has a function, such as digestion, excretion, or reproduction. All the organ systems together form the human organism. From simple to complex, the body is built from the tiny atom to the human being.

MAJOR ORGAN SYSTEMS

Twelve major organ systems make up the human body. Each performs specific functions that enable the human body to operate as a coordinated whole. Refer to Fig. 1.3 and identify the location and distribution of the organs of each system.

- The integumentary (in-teg-yoo-MEN-tar-ee) system consists of the skin and related structures, such as hair and nails. The integumentary system forms a covering for the body, helps regulate body temperature, and contains some of the structures necessary for sensation.

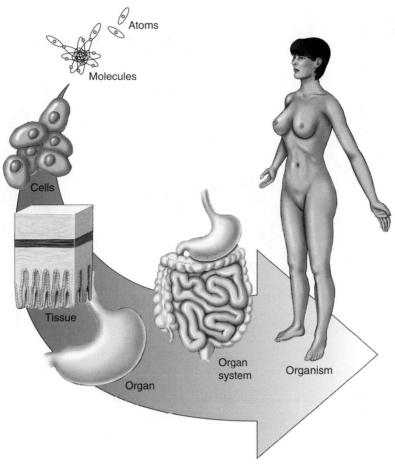

FIG. 1.2 Levels of organization, from atoms to human organism.

- The skeletal system forms the basic framework of the body. It consists primarily of bones, joints, and cartilage. The skeleton protects and supports body organs and enables us to move around.
- The muscular system has three types of muscles. *Skeletal muscles* attach to the bones and are responsible for movement of the skeleton and the maintenance of body posture. *Smooth* and *cardiac muscles* are found in various organs and tubes; contraction and relaxation of these muscles help the organ systems carry out their functions.
- The nervous system is made up of the brain, spinal cord, nerves, and sense organs. Sensory nerves receive information from the environment and bring it to the spinal cord and brain, where it is interpreted. Decisions made by the brain and spinal cord are transmitted along motor nerves to various body structures.
- The endocrine (EN-doh-krin) system contains numerous glands that secrete hormones and chemical substances that regulate body activities such as growth, reproduction, metabolism, and water balance.
- The circulatory (SER-kyoo-lah-tor-ee) system consists of the blood, heart, and blood vessels. This system pumps (heart) and transports (blood vessels) blood throughout the body. Blood carries nutrients and oxygen to all the body's cells and also carries the waste away from the cells to the organs of excretion.
- The lymphatic (lim-FAT-ik) system is made up of the lymph nodes, lymphatic vessels, lymph, and other lymphatic organs. Lymph and lymphatic structures play an important role in fluid balance and in the defense of the body against pathogens and other foreign material.
- The immune system is an elaborate defense system that protects the body not only from pathogens, but also from allergens, such as pollens, bee venom, and some of our own cells that have gone awry (cancer cells). The immune system is widely distributed throughout the body (it is not shown in Fig. 1.3).
- The respiratory system contains the lungs and other structures that conduct air to and from the lungs. Oxygen-rich air moves into the lungs; the oxygen is picked up by the blood and distributed throughout the body. Carbon dioxide–rich air moves out of the lungs, thereby ridding the body of waste.
- The digestive system is comprised of organs designed to ingest food and break it down into substances that can be absorbed by the body. Food that is not absorbed is eliminated as waste.
- The urinary system contains the kidneys and other structures that help excrete waste products from the body through the urine. More importantly, the

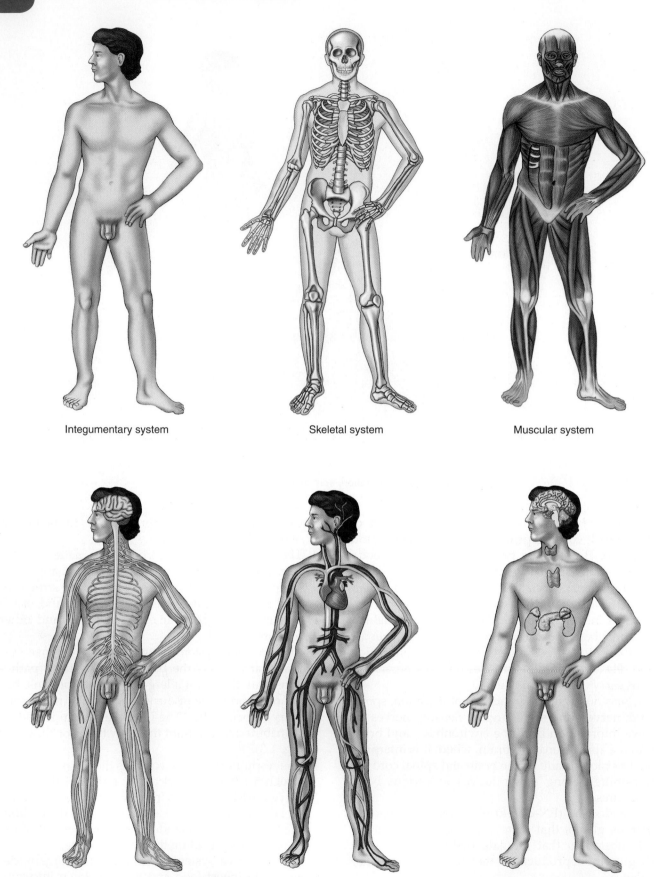

Integumentary system

Skeletal system

Muscular system

Nervous system

Circulatory system

Endocrine system

FIG. 1.3 **Major organ systems of the body.**

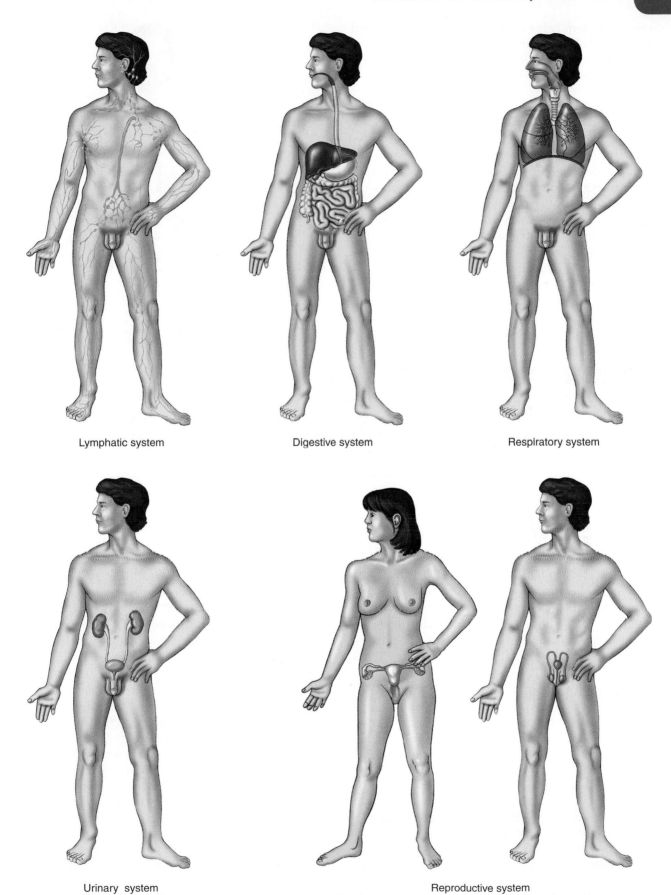

Lymphatic system   Digestive system   Respiratory system

Urinary system   Reproductive system

FIG. 1.3, cont'd

urinary system helps control water, electrolyte, and acid–base balance in the body.

- The reproductive system is made up of organs and structures that enable humans to reproduce.

HOMEOSTASIS: STAYING THE SAME

Homeostasis (ho-me-o-STAY-sis) literally means staying *(stasis)* the same *(homeo)*. The term refers to the body's ability to maintain a stable internal environment in response to a changing environment. For example, in a healthy person, body temperature stays around 98.6°F (37°C), even when room temperature increases to 100°F or decreases to 60°F. The amount of water in your cells stays the same whether you drink 2, 3, or 4 liters (L) of water per day. Your blood sugar remains within normal limits whether you have just eaten a turkey dinner or have fasted for 6 hours. Mechanisms that help maintain homeostasis are called *homeostatic mechanisms*. Homeostatic imbalance results in disease or dysfunction.

◎ Sum It Up!

Anatomy and physiology describe the structure and function of the body. The body is constructed from simple to complex (atoms to molecules to cells to tissues to organs to organ systems to the human organism). The 12 major organ systems are shown in Fig. 1.3. Homeostatic mechanisms enable the body to "stay the same" despite changing internal and external environments.

ANATOMICAL TERMS: TALKING ABOUT THE BODY

Special terms describe the location, position, and regions of body parts. Because these terms are used frequently, you should become familiar with them now. People in the medical field are often accused of speaking their own language. Indeed, we do! We always use these terms as if the body were standing in its anatomical position.

ANATOMICAL POSITION

In its **anatomical position**, the body is standing erect, with the face forward, the arms at the sides, and the toes and palms of the hands directed forward (Fig. 1.4).

RELATIVE POSITIONS

Specific terms describe the position of one body part in relation to another body part. These are directional terms. They are like the more familiar directions of north, south, east, and west; however, whereas describing Canada as being located north of the United States would be correct, describing the head as "north of the chest" would sound strange. Therefore, in locating body parts, we use other terminology. The terms come in pairs. Note that the two terms in each pair are

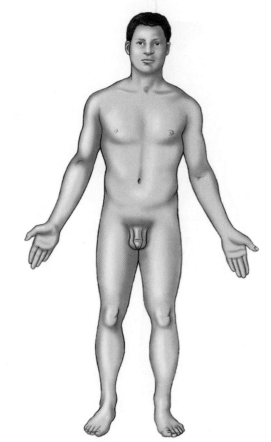

FIG. 1.4 **Anatomical position.**

generally opposites. Remember, the references are valid only for the body in its anatomical position.

- *Superior* and *inferior. Superior* means that a part is above another part or is closer to the head. For example, the head is superior to the chest. *Inferior* means that a part is located below another part or is closer to the feet. The chest, for example, is inferior to the head.
- *Anterior* and *posterior. Anterior* means toward the front surface (the belly surface). *Posterior* means toward the back surface. For example, the heart is anterior to the spinal cord, but the heart is posterior to the breastbone. Another word for anterior is *ventral*, and another word for posterior is *dorsal*. Consider the dorsal fin of a fish. It is the dorsal part of the shark that can be seen moving effortlessly and very quickly toward your surfboard!
- *Medial* and *lateral.* Imagine a line drawn through the middle of your body, dividing it into right and left halves. This is the midline. *Medial* means toward the midline of the body. The nose, for example, is medial to the ears. *Lateral* means away from the midline of the body. For example, the ears are lateral to the nose. In the anatomical position, the hand is closer to the lateral thigh than to the medial thigh.
- *Proximal* and *distal. Proximal* means that the structure is nearer to the point of attachment, often the trunk of the body. Because the elbow is closer to the point of attachment than is the wrist, the elbow is described as proximal to the wrist. The wrist is proximal to the

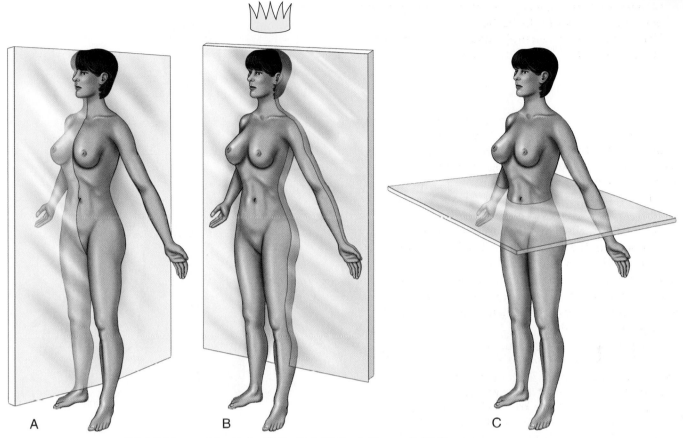

FIG. 1.5 Planes of the body. (A) Sagittal. (B) Frontal (coronal). (C) Transverse.

fingers, meaning that the wrist is closer to the trunk than are the fingers. *Distal* means that a part is farther away from the point of attachment than another part. For example, the wrist is distal to the elbow, and the fingers are distal to the wrist.

- *Superficial* and *deep*. *Superficial* means that a part is located on or near the surface of the body. The skin is superficial to the muscles. *Deep* means that the body part is away from the surface of the body. The bones, for example, are deep to the skin.
- *Central* and *peripheral*. *Central* means that the part is located in the center. *Peripheral* means away from the center. The heart, for example, is located centrally, whereas the blood vessels are located peripherally (away from the center and extending toward the limbs). The brain and spinal cord are called the central nervous system, and the nerves are called the peripheral nervous system.

? Re-Think

1. Use the terms *proximal* and *distal* to describe the relationship of the wrist to the elbow.
2. Use the terms *proximal* and *distal* to describe the relationship of the fingers to the wrist.
3. Use the terms *medial* and *lateral* to describe the parts of the thigh. Do the same with the eye.

PLANES OF THE BODY

When we refer to the left side of the body, the top half of the body, or the front of the body, we are referring to the planes of the body. Each plane divides the body with an imaginary line in one direction. Fig. 1.5 shows the following three important planes:

1. Sagittal plane (see Fig. 1.5A). The **sagittal plane** divides the body lengthwise into right and left portions. If the cut is made exactly down the midline of the body, the right and left halves of the body are equal. This division is a midsagittal section.
2. Frontal plane (see Fig. 1.5B). The **frontal plane** divides the body into anterior (ventral) and posterior (dorsal) portions. This plane creates the front part of the body and the back part of the body. The frontal plane is also called the *coronal plane*. Coronal means "crown," so the imaginary line for the coronal plane is made across the part of the head where a crown would sit and then downward through the body.
3. Transverse plane (see Fig. 1.5C). The **transverse plane** divides the body horizontally, creating an upper (superior) and a lower (inferior) body. When the body or an organ is cut horizontally or transversely, it is called a cross section.

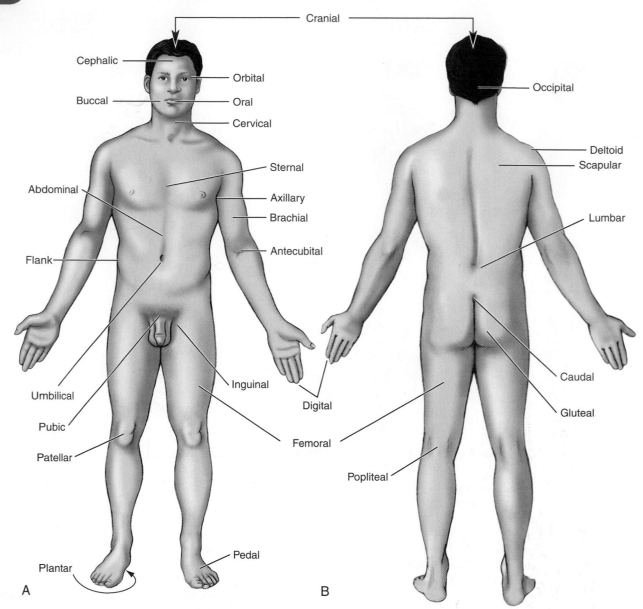

FIG. 1.6 Regional terms. (A) Anterior view. (B) Posterior view.

REGIONAL TERMS

Specific terms describe the different regions or areas of the body. Fig. 1.6 illustrates the terms used to identify the regions on the anterior and posterior surfaces of the body.

On the anterior surface, identify the following regions:

Abdominal: anterior trunk just below the ribs
Antecubital: area in front of the elbow
Axillary: armpit
Brachial: arm
Buccal: cheek area; cavity between the gum and cheek
Cephalic: head
Cervical: neck region
Cranial: nearer to the head
Digital: fingers, toes
Femoral: thigh area

Flank: fleshy area along each side between the lower ribs and the top of the hip bones
Inguinal: area where the thigh meets the trunk of the body; often called the groin
Oral: mouth
Orbital: area around the eye
Patellar: front of the knee over the kneecap
Pedal: foot
Plantar: sole of the foot
Pubic: genital area
Sternal: middle of the chest (over the breastbone area)
Umbilical: navel
On the posterior surface, identify the following regions:
Caudal: near to the lower region of the spinal column (near the tailbone)
Deltoid: rounded area of the shoulder closest to the arm
Gluteal: buttocks

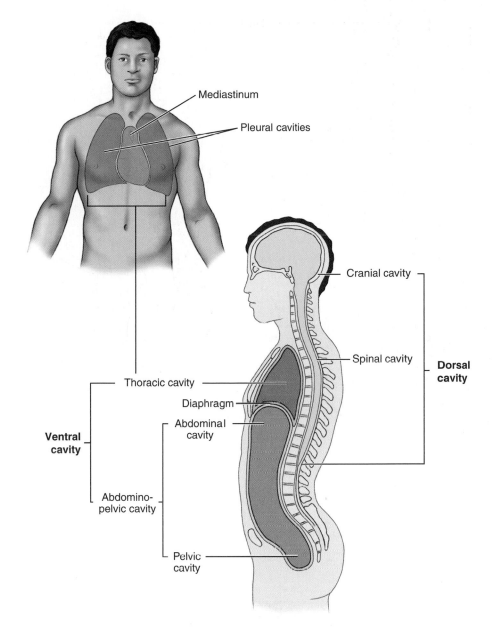

FIG. 1.7 **Major body cavities.**

Lumbar: area of the back between the ribs and the hips
Occipital: back of the head
Popliteal: behind, or back of, the knee area
Scapular: shoulder blade area

Sum It Up!

Specific terms describe the relative positions of one body part to the other. The terms are paired as opposites and include superior and inferior, anterior (ventral) and posterior (dorsal), medial and lateral, proximal and distal, superficial and deep, and central and peripheral. The body can be cut into three planes: sagittal (right and left), frontal or coronal (front and back), and transverse (top and bottom) planes. Common terms are used to identify specific areas of the anterior and posterior surface areas.

? Re-Think

1. A sagittal plane yields right and left halves of the body. Compare this with frontal and transverse planes.
2. Of the following terms, which can be seen only on the posterior view of the body: umbilical, antecubital, gluteal, lumbar, sternal, patellar, and popliteal?

CAVITIES OF THE BODY

The organs, called **viscera** (VISS-er-ah), are located within the cavities of the body. Cavities are large internal spaces. The body contains two major cavities: the **dorsal cavity** and the **ventral cavity** (Fig. 1.7).

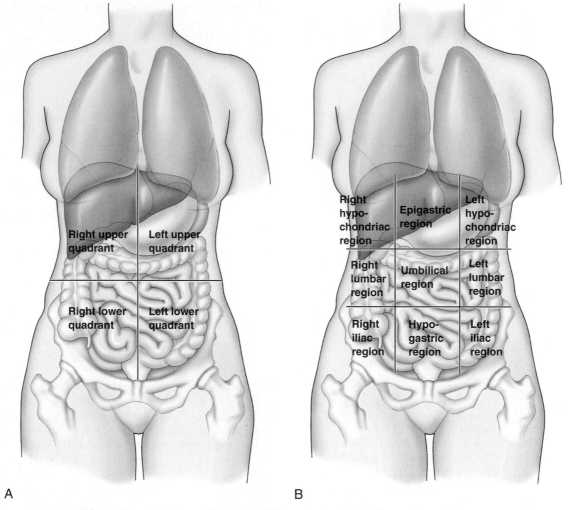

FIG. 1.8 The abdominopelvic cavity. (A) Four quadrants. (B) Nine regions.

DORSAL CAVITY

The dorsal cavity is located toward the back of the body and has two divisions, the **cranial cavity** and the **spinal (vertebral) cavity**.

The cranial cavity is located within the skull and contains the brain. The spinal, or vertebral, cavity extends downward from the cranial cavity and is surrounded by bony vertebrae; it contains the spinal cord. The cranial and spinal cavities form one continuous space.

VENTRAL CAVITY

The larger ventral cavity is located toward the front of the body and has two divisions, the **thoracic** (thoh-RASS-ik) **cavity** and the **abdominopelvic** (ab-DOM-i-no-PEL-vik) **cavity**.

THORACIC CAVITY

The thoracic cavity is located above the diaphragm and is surrounded by the rib cage. The thoracic cavity is divided into two compartments by the **mediastinum** (MEE-dee-ass-TI-num), a space that contains the

heart, thymus gland, and parts of the esophagus, trachea, and large blood vessels attached to the heart. The **pericardial** (pair-i-KAR-dee-al) **cavity** (not shown) is located within the mediastinum and contains the heart. The right and left lungs are located on either side of the mediastinum in the **pleural cavities**. The lungs occupy most of the space within the thoracic cavity.

ABDOMINOPELVIC CAVITY

The abdominopelvic cavity is located below the diaphragm. The upper portion of this cavity is the abdominal cavity. It contains the stomach, most of the intestines, and the liver, gallbladder, pancreas, spleen, and kidneys. The lower portion of the abdominopelvic cavity is called the *pelvic cavity*. It extends downward from the level of the hips and includes the remainder of the intestines, the rectum, the urinary bladder, and the internal parts of the reproductive system.

Because the abdominopelvic cavity is so large, it is subdivided into smaller areas for study. **Quadrants** and regions divide the abdominopelvic cavity. Note the organs located in each quadrant or region, as shown in Fig. 1.8.

Division into Quadrants

The abdominopelvic cavity can be divided into four quadrants (see Fig. 1.8A). The quadrants are named for their positions: right upper quadrant (RUQ), left upper quadrant (LUQ), right lower quadrant (RLQ), and left lower quadrant (LLQ).

Quadrant terms are used frequently in the clinical setting. For example, a patient in the emergency room who has acute pain in the RLQ may be diagnosed with appendicitis. Note that the RLQ appears to be on your left. This is similar to looking in a mirror. Keep this in mind when you are studying the diagrams in the text. Here's an easy way to remember this: Lower your right arm. It will be lateral to the RUQ and RLQ.

Division into Regions

A second system divides the abdominopelvic cavity into nine separate regions that resemble the squares for tic-tac-toe (see Fig. 1.8B). The three central regions (from top to bottom) are the epigastric, umbilical, and hypogastric regions. The epigastric region is located below the breastbone. Epigastric literally means upon *(epi)* the stomach *(gastric)*. The umbilical region is the centermost region and surrounds the umbilicus, or navel (belly button). The hypogastric region is located just below the umbilical region. Hypogastric literally means below *(hypo)* the stomach *(gastric)*.

Six regions are located on either side of the central regions. They include the hypochondriac, lumbar, and iliac regions. The right and left hypochondriac regions are located on either side of the epigastric region and overlie the lower ribs. The word *hypochondriac* literally means below *(hypo)* the cartilage *(chondro)* and refers to the composition of the ribs (cartilage). The right and left lumbar regions are located on either side of the umbilical region and are inferior to the hypochondriac regions. The right and left iliac regions, also called the right and left inguinal regions, are located on either side of the hypogastric region. Knowledge of these regions helps you understand terms such as *epigastric pain* and *umbilical hernia*. Remember that quadrants and regions refer only to the abdominopelvic cavity and not to the thoracic cavity.

Other Cavities

Four smaller cavities are located in the head. They include the oral cavity, nasal cavities, orbital cavities, and middle ear cavities. (These cavities are described in later chapters.)

 Re-Think

1. What structure separates the thoracic cavity from the abdominopelvic cavity?
2. Of the following terms, determine which pertain to the ventral cavity: thoracic cavity, brain, vertebral cavity, abdominopelvic cavity, pleural cavity, dorsal cavity, mediastinum, stomach, heart, and spinal cord.

 Sum It Up!

The organs or viscera are located within body cavities. The two major cavities are the dorsal cavity, located toward the back of the body, and the larger ventral cavity, located in the front of the body. The dorsal cavity is subdivided into the cranial cavity and the spinal cavity. The ventral cavity is divided by the diaphragm into the thoracic cavity (including the mediastinum, pericardial cavity, and pleural cavities) and the abdominopelvic cavity. The abdominopelvic cavity is divided into quadrants and regions.

📖 **Medical Terminology and Disorders**   **Introduction to Medical Terminology**

The medical profession has its own language, called **medical terminology.** In general, there are four main types or kinds of word parts. By learning these and how they can be put together, you can often "translate" many long and challenging medical words by breaking them up into their word parts.

- A **word root** is *the core of the word* and provides the basic meaning or "subject" of the word. The other word parts, such as suffixes and prefixes, modify the word root so that it takes on a new meaning. For example, in the word **hepatitis,** the word root is **hepat-,** meaning *liver.*
- A **suffix** is *a word part attached to the end of the word root;* it modifies the word root. If we add **-itis,** which is a suffix that means *inflammation,* to the word root for liver, **hepat-,** we get **hepatitis,** which means *inflammation of the liver.*
- A **prefix** is a word part attached to the beginning of the word root; it modifies the word root. For example, the word **nutrition** refers to a normal and healthy food intake. By adding the prefix **mal-** (French for *bad*), as in **malnutrition,** the word root has been modified to mean *poor or bad nutrition.*
- **Combining vowels** are *word parts used to ease the pronunciation,* as in *angioplasty* (angi/o/plasty). Angi- means *blood vessel,* and **-plasty** means *repair of.* The **-o-** joining the word parts eases the pronunciation; it does not modify the meaning of the word. When you see **angi/o-,** you are seeing the word root and its combining vowel.

In the Medical Terminology and Disorders tables you will see many terms with which you are probably familiar, but what you may not be familiar with is what their individual word parts are and how they are put together to make up many of the words you use every day. For instance, consider **-ectomy,** which means *excision* or *removal of.* Think of all the terms that have **-ectomy** at the end—such as lob**ectomy,** vas**ectomy,** hyster**ectomy,** append**ectomy,** tonsill**ectomy**—and you will see how valuable knowing what this one word part is.

Continued

Medical Terminology and Disorders   Introduction to Medical Terminology—cont'd

MEDICAL TERM	WORD PARTS	WORD PART MEANING OR DERIVATION	DESCRIPTION
anatomy	ana-	up or apart	**Anatomy** is *the branch of science that describes the structure of a body, especially as revealed by dissection.* For example, the heart has four chambers.
	-tomy	incision; to cut	
antecubital	ante-	before; in front of	**Antecubital space** is *the area of the arm anterior to the elbow.* A sample of blood is commonly drawn from a vein in the antecubital space.
	-cubital	From the Latin word *cubitum,* meaning "elbow"	
biology	bio-	life	**Biology** is *the study of life and living organisms.*
	-logy	study of	
diagnosis	dia-	apart	**Diagnosis** is *the process of identifying the nature and cause of a disease or injury through an analysis of data, such as the patient's symptoms and laboratory studies.*
	-gnos/o-	knowing	
	-osis	condition or increase	
pathologist	path/o-	pertaining to disease	A **pathologist** examines tissue for evidence of disease.
	-logist	one who specializes in	
homeostasis	home/o-	sameness	**Homeostasis** refers to *the relative constancy of the internal environment of the body despite many challenges to upset the balance.*
	-stasis	stand still	
transverse	trans-	across	A **transverse** plane cuts across the body; an upper and lower body is created.
	-verse	From the Latin word *vertere,* meaning "to turn"	
midepigastric	mid-	middle	*Related to the middle of the epigastric region of the abdomen.* A person may complain of midepigastric discomfort.
	-epi	above or upon	
	-gastr/o-	Stomach	
	-ic	pertaining to	
Prognosis	pro-	before	*Refers to a likely course or outcome of a disease.* For example, the prognosis of a person who seeks early treatment of a basal cell carcinoma (skin cancer) is excellent; the prognosis of a person with metastatic cancer is less favorable.
	-gnos/o-	knowing	
	-osis	condition or increase	
quadrant	quadr/i-	four	The abdominopelvic cavity is divided into four equal areas called **quadrants**.
	-ant	performing/promoting..	

Get Ready for Exams!

Summary Outline

Anatomy is the study of structure; physiology is the study of function. Structure (anatomy) and function (physiology) are related.

I.   **The Body's Levels of Organization**
   A. From simple to complex: atoms to molecules to cells to tissues to organs to organ systems to human organism
   B. Major organ systems (12)
     1. Integumentary system
     2. Skeletal system
     3. Muscular system
     4. Nervous system
     5. Endocrine system
     6. Heart and circulatory system
     7. Lymphatic system

     8. Immune system
     9. Respiratory system
    10. Digestive system
    11. Urinary system
    12. Reproductive system
   C. Homeostasis: the body's ability to maintain a stable internal environment in response to various internal and external challenges.

II. **Anatomical Terms: Talking About the Body**
   A. Anatomical position: the body standing erect, arms by the side, with palms and toes facing forward
   B. Relative positions: superior–inferior, anterior–posterior, medial–lateral, proximal–distal, superficial–deep, central–peripheral
   C. Planes (three): sagittal, frontal (coronal), and transverse planes

D. Regional terms: listed in Fig. 1.6
E. Cavities of the body
  1. Dorsal cavity
    a. Cranial cavity: contains the brain
    b. Spinal (vertebral) cavity: contains the spinal cord
  2. Ventral cavity
    a. Thoracic cavity: superior to the diaphragm; contains the pleural cavities (lungs), mediastinum, and pericardial cavity
    b. Abdominopelvic cavity: located inferior to the diaphragm
    c. Abdominal cavity: upper part that contains the stomach, most of the intestines, and the liver, spleen, and kidneys
    d. Pelvic cavity: lower part that contains the reproductive organs, urinary bladder, and lower part of the intestines
    e. For reference: the abdominopelvic cavity is divided into four quadrants and nine regions.

Review Your Knowledge

Matching: Directions of the Body
Directions: Match the following words with their descriptions. Some words may be used more than once or not at all.
a. posterior
b. distal
c. medial
d. anterior
e. proximal
f. superior
g. deep

1. ___ Toward the midline of the body; opposite of *lateral*
2. ___ Structure that is nearer to the trunk than another part; opposite of *distal*
3. ___ Part of the radius (forearm bone) that is closer to the wrist than to the elbow
4. ___ The lungs are located above the diaphragm; their position relative to the diaphragm is described as being above
5. ___ Toward the front (the belly surface); another word is *ventral*

Matching: Regional Terms
Directions: Match the following words with their descriptions.
a. inguinal
b. oral
c. lumbar
d. axillary
e. buccal
f. patellar
g. flank
h. antecubital
i. sternal
j. scapular

1. ___ Armpit
2. ___ Kneecap area
3. ___ Breastbone area
4. ___ Front part of the elbow area
5. ___ Fleshy area along the side between the ribs and hip bone
6. ___ Pertaining to the mouth
7. ___ Lower back area extending from the chest to the hips
8. ___ Pertains to the space between the cheek and gum
9. ___ Groin region
10. ___ Shoulder blade area

Multiple Choice
1. This part of the humerus (arm bone) is closer to the elbow than to the axillary region.
  a. Anterior
  b. Superior
  c. Distal
  d. Proximal
2. Describe the relationship of the mediastinum to the diaphragm.
  a. Distal
  b. Deep
  c. Anterior
  d. Superior
3. The umbilical region is located
  a. inferior to the inguinal region.
  b. superior to the RUQ.
  c. inferior to the diaphragm.
  d. within the midepigastric region.
4. The sternal area is
  a. the groin.
  b. referred to as the breastbone area.
  c. located within the RLQ.
  d. observed only on the posterior view of the body.
5. Which of the following is not descriptive of the mediastinum?
  a. Thoracic cavity
  b. Dorsal cavity
  c. Ventral cavity
  d. Superior to the diaphragm
6. The frontal plane
  a. splits the body into right- and left-half sections.
  b. is also the coronal plane.
  c. splits the body into a top and a bottom section.
  d. creates a transverse cross section.
7. Which of the following terms best describes when a person sweats in order to decrease body temperature?
  a. Pathophysiology
  b. Evisceration
  c. Homeostasis
  d. Midsagittal
8. Which of the following is true of these terms: sternal, umbilical, patellar, and antecubital?
  a. All are superior to the inguinal area.
  b. All lie within the ventral cavity.
  c. All can be viewed on the anterior body.
  d. All lie within the dorsal cavity.
9. These structures are located within the pleural cavities, the thoracic cavity, and the ventral cavity.
  a. Heart and great vessels
  b. Lungs
  c. Brain and spinal cord
  d. Intestines
10. These structures are located within the pericardial cavity, the mediastinum, and the thoracic cavity.
  a. Heart and great vessels
  b. Liver and stomach
  c. Lungs
  d. Intestines

11. The common element of the words pathology, pathogen, and pathophysiology is that they all refer to
 a. persons who dissect bodies.
 b. homeostatic mechanisms.
 c. disease.
 d. drugs that are used to treat diseases.

Go Figure

1. Which of the following is correct according to Fig. 1.1?
 a. The heart is the most important part of the body.
 b. All three illustrations indicate the importance of homeostasis.
 c. Anatomical structure and physiologic function are closely related.
 d. The relationship of structure and function can only be applied to the heart.

2. According to Fig. 1.4, which of the following characterizes the anatomical position?
 a. The knees are bent as in kneeling.
 b. The head is turned to the left.
 c. The arms and hands are positioned so that the thumbs are touching the thighs.
 d. The hands are open, and the little-finger side of the hand is nearest the thighs.

3. Refer to Fig. 1.5. A midsagittal section yields half of a body. Which body regions are preserved in this half-body section?
 a. The patellar (right and left), flank (right and left), and brachial (right and left) are preserved.
 b. Neither the right nor left patellar areas and neither the right nor left antecubital areas are preserved.
 c. The head and two arms are preserved.
 d. A left or right inguinal, pedal, and axillary area is preserved.

4. Which of the following is correct according to Fig. 1.6?
 a. The brachial, lumbar, and antecubital areas can only be identified on the posterior view of the body.
 b. The inguinal and flank areas are the same.
 c. The gluteal, lumbar, and scapular areas are inferior to the umbilicus.
 d. The femoral, popliteal, and patellar areas are located in the lower extremities.

5. Which of the following is correct according to Fig. 1.7?
 a. The thoracic cavity is a ventral cavity that includes the mediastinum and pleural cavities.
 b. The diaphragm separates the two pleural cavities.
 c. The dorsal cavity includes the pleural cavities and the mediastinum.
 d. All structures in the dorsal cavity are superior to the diaphragm.

6. Which of the following is correct according to Fig. 1.8?
 a. The ventral cavity is divided into quadrants.
 b. The dorsal cavity is divided into regions.
 c. RUQ, LUQ, RLQ, and LLQ describe only the abdominal cavity.
 d. RUQ, LUQ, RLQ, and LLQ are quadrants that define the abdominopelvic cavity.

7. Which of the following is correct according to Fig. 1.8?
 a. The left iliac region is located within the LUQ.
 b. The hypogastric region is located within the RUQ.
 c. The umbilical region surrounds the navel or belly button.
 d. The right lung is located within the RUQ.

Basic Chemistry

Objectives

1. Define the terms *matter*, *element*, and *atom*, and do the following:
   - List the four elements that comprise 96% of body weight.
   - Describe the three components of an atom.
   - Describe the role of electrons in the formation of chemical bonds.
2. Differentiate among ionic, covalent, and hydrogen bonds.
3. Explain ions, including the differences among electrolytes, cations, and anions.

4. Explain the difference between a molecule and a compound, and list five reasons why water is essential to life.
5. Explain the role of catalysts and enzymes.
6. Differentiate between an acid and a base, and define pH.
7. List the six forms of energy and describe the role of adenosine triphosphate (ATP) in energy transfer.
8. Differentiate among a mixture, solution, suspension, colloidal suspension, and precipitate.

Key Terms

acid (p. 23)
adenosine triphosphate (ATP) (p. 25)
anion (p. 20)
aqueous solution (p. 26)
atom (p. 16)
atomic mass (p. 17)
atomic number (p. 16)
base (p. 23)
catalyst (p. 22)
cation (p. 20)
colloid (p. 27)

compound (p. 21)
covalent bond (p. 18)
electrolyte (p. 20)
element (p. 16)
energy (p. 24)
enzyme (p. 22)
hydrogen bond (p. 18)
ion (p. 20)
ionic bond (p. 18)
ionization (p. 20)
isotope (p. 17)

matter (p. 15)
mixture (p. 26)
molecule (p. 21)
neutralization (p. 23)
pH (p. 23)
polar molecule (p. 19)
precipitate (p. 27)
radioactivity (p. 17)
solute (p. 26)
solution (p. 26)
suspension (p. 26)

Why a chapter on chemistry? Because our bodies are made of different chemicals. The food we eat, the water we drink, and the air we breathe are all chemical substances. We digest our food, move our bodies, experience emotions, and think great thoughts because of chemical reactions. To understand the body, we must understand some general chemical principles.

MATTER, ELEMENTS, AND ATOMS

MATTER

Chemistry is the study of matter. **Matter** is anything that occupies space and has weight. Anything that you see as you look around is matter.

Matter exists in three states: solid, liquid, and gas. Solid matter—such as skin, bones, and teeth—has a definite shape and volume. Liquid matter—such as blood, saliva, and digestive juices—takes the shape of the container that holds it. A gas, or gaseous matter—such as the air we breathe—has neither shape nor volume.

Matter can undergo both physical and chemical changes. The logs in a fireplace illustrate the difference between a physical and a chemical change (Fig. 2.1). The logs can undergo a physical change by being chopped into smaller chips of wood with a hatchet. The wood chips are smaller than the log, but they are still wood. The matter (wood) has not essentially changed; only the physical appearance has changed. A chemical change occurs when the wood is burned. When burned, the wood ceases to be wood. The chemical composition of the ashes is essentially different from that of wood.

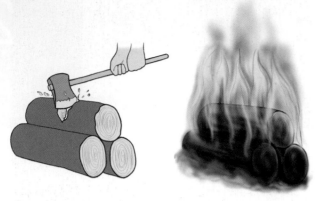

FIG. 2.1 **Changes in matter: physical change (wood chips) and chemical change (ashes).**

The body contains many examples of physical and chemical changes. For example, digestion involves physical and chemical changes. Chewing breaks the food into smaller pieces; this is a physical change. Potent chemicals digest or change the food into simpler substances; this is a chemical change.

ELEMENTS

All matter, living or dead, is composed of elements. An **element** is matter that is composed of atoms that have the same number of positive charges in their nuclei. Even a very small amount of an element such as sodium contains millions and millions of sodium atoms. The same name is used for both the element and the atom. Although more than 100 elements exist, only about 25 elements are required by living organisms.

 Do You Know...

Why Children Should Not Be Allowed to Play in Traffic and Chew on Old Paint?

Aside from the obvious safety issues, old paint and emissions from motor vehicles contain high amounts of lead. Exposure to high levels of lead causes lead poisoning, a serious condition that damages the major organs, including the brain, liver, kidney, and bone marrow. The old name for chronic lead poisoning is plumbism, from the Latin word for lead (*plumbum*). The chemical symbol for lead is Pb. (By the way, a plumber is called a plumber because ancient water pipes were made of *plumbum*, or lead.) Why does plumbism have such a great history? Lead was used to make pipes that carried water and was used to make pottery, particularly drinking vessels. This practice killed many of the rich and famous—those wealthy enough to afford leaded wine goblets. Because of the toxic nature of lead, pipes and pottery in the United States are no longer made of lead, gasoline and paint are now lead-free by law, and the disposal of acid lead batteries is regulated. Is the lead problem a done deal? No! Children are still huffing lead fumes from car emissions, playing with toys laced with lead paint, wearing clothing impregnated with lead, and more recently, drinking lead-laced water. Go figure!

The most abundant elements found in the body are listed in Table 2.1. Four elements—carbon, hydrogen, oxygen, and nitrogen—make up 96% of the body weight. The trace elements are present in tiny amounts, but despite the small amounts required, the trace elements are essential for life. (Not all the trace elements appear in Table 2.1.)

Each of the elements included in Table 2.1 is represented by a symbol, and the first letter of the symbol is always capitalized. For example, the symbol O is for oxygen, N is for nitrogen, Na is for sodium, K is for potassium, and C is for carbon. These symbols are used frequently, so you should memorize the symbols of the major elements.

ATOMS

ATOMIC STRUCTURE

Elements are composed of atoms, the basic units of matter. An **atom** is the smallest unit of an element with that element's chemical characteristics. An atom is composed of three subatomic particles: protons, neutrons, and electrons. The arrangement of the subatomic particles resembles the sun and planets (Fig. 2.2A), with the sun in the center and the planets constantly moving around the sun in orbits, or circular paths. The atom is composed of a nucleus (the sun) and shells, or orbits, that surround the nucleus (see Fig. 2.2B).

Where are the subatomic particles located? The protons and the neutrons are located in the nucleus (see Fig. 2.2C). Protons carry a positive (+) electrical charge; neutrons carry no electrical charge. The electrons are located in the shells, or orbits, surrounding the nucleus like planets. Electrons carry a negative (−) electrical charge. In each atom, the number of protons (+) is equal to the number of electrons (−). The atom is therefore electrically neutral; it carries no net electrical charge.

All protons are alike, all neutrons are alike, and all electrons are alike. So what makes one atom different from another atom? The difference is primarily in the numbers of protons and electrons in each atom. For example, hydrogen is the simplest and smallest atom. It has one proton and one electron. Helium has two protons and two electrons. Lithium has three protons and three electrons. Hydrogen, helium, and lithium are different atoms because of the different numbers of protons and electrons.

 Re-Think

1. How does the structure of an atom resemble the solar system (sun and planets)?
2. What electrical charge is carried by the proton, electron, and neutron?
3. Identify the locations of the proton, neutron, and electron.

OTHER CHARACTERISTICS OF ATOMS

Two terms describe individual atoms. The **atomic number** is the number of protons in the nucleus. Thus, hydrogen has an atomic number of 1, helium has an

Table **2.1**	Common Elements in the Human Body	
ELEMENT	**SYMBOL**	**PERCENTAGE OF BODY WEIGHT**
Oxygen	O	65.0
Carbon	C	18.5
Hydrogen	H	9.5
Nitrogen	N	3.2
Calcium	Ca	
Phosphorus	P	
Potassium	K	
Sulfur	S	
Sodium	Na	
Chlorine	Cl	
Magnesium	Mg	
Iron	Fe	
Iodine*	I	
Chromium*	Cr	
Cobalt*	Co	
Copper*	Cu	
Fluorine*	F	
Selenium*	Se	
Zinc*	Zn	

*Trace elements.

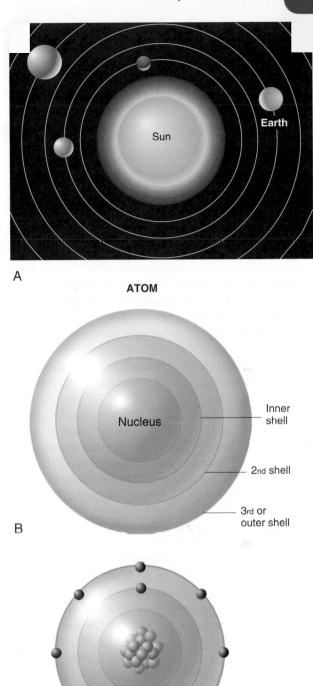

A

ATOM

B

C

Electron (−)
Proton (+)
Neutron (o)

FIG. 2.2 Structure of the atom. (A) Subatomic particles arranged like the sun and the planets. (B) Nucleus and electron shells. (C) Protons and neutrons located in the nucleus and electrons encircling the nucleus in orbits.

atomic number of 2, and lithium has an atomic number of 3. The **atomic mass** of an atom is determined by adding the numbers of protons and neutrons in the nucleus. Thus, the atomic mass of hydrogen is also 1 because the hydrogen nucleus contains one proton and no neutrons. The atomic mass of helium is 4 because the nucleus contains two protons and two neutrons. (The atomic mass is roughly equivalent to the atomic weight.)

An **isotope** (EYE-so-tohp) is a different form of the same atom. For example, hydrogen has different forms. Hydrogen has an atomic number of 1 and an atomic mass of 1; it has one proton and no neutrons in the nucleus. A second and less common form of hydrogen is called *heavy hydrogen*. It has one proton and one neutron in its nucleus; thus, its atomic number is 1, but its atomic mass is 2. Because its atomic number is 1, it is still a hydrogen atom. The additional neutron in the nucleus, however, makes it heavy and changes its atomic mass. Heavy hydrogen is an isotope of hydrogen. Remember! An isotope has the same atomic number as an atom but a different atomic mass.

Isotopes are often unstable and their nuclei break down, or decay, giving off energy. In doing so, the unstable nuclei become more stable. Unstable isotopes are called *radioisotopes*. The process of spontaneous breakdown (decay) is called **radioactivity**. Radioisotopes are damaging to tissue and are used clinically to destroy cells. For example, radioactive iodine is used to destroy excess thyroid tissue. Other radioisotopes are used to destroy cancer cells, and radioisotopes can

also be used diagnostically. For example, radioactive iodine (^{131}I) is normally taken up by the thyroid gland at a certain rate. Alterations in the rate of ^{131}I uptake can indicate thyroid dysfunction. A radioactive blast from the past! Bathing in radioactive water at radium spas was popular in the United States in the early 20th century. Accompanying this health craze was the ingestion of radioactive tonics, a practice that quickly died out as mortality rate from radiation toxicity was documented.

 Re-Think

1. What is the difference between the atomic number and atomic mass?
2. What is an isotope? A radioisotope?

ELECTRON SHELLS

Electrons surround the nucleus in orbits called *energy levels* or *electron shells* (see Fig. 2.2C). The number of shells varies from one atom to the next. Some atoms, such as hydrogen, have only one shell; other atoms, such as sodium, have three shells. Each shell can hold a specific number of electrons. The inner shell closest to the nucleus can hold only two electrons. The second and third shells can each hold eight electrons.

The only electrons that are important for chemical bonding are the electrons in the outermost shell. If it is not filled with its proper number of electrons, the outer shell becomes unstable. It then tries to give up electrons to empty the shell, acquire electrons to fill the shell, or share electrons so that each participating atom acquires the proper number of electrons in its outer shells. The tendency of the outer shell to want to become stable forms the basis of chemical bonding.

CHEMICAL BONDS

Atoms are attracted to each other because they want to achieve a stable outer electron shell. In other words, they want to fill or empty the outer electron shell. The force of attraction between the atoms is similar to the force of two magnets. When you try to separate the magnets, you can feel the pull. The electrical attraction between atoms is a chemical bond. The three types of chemical bonds are ionic bonds, covalent bonds, and hydrogen bonds.

IONIC BONDS

An **ionic** (eye-ON-ik) **bond** is caused by a transfer of electrons between atoms. The interaction of the sodium and chlorine atoms illustrates an ionic bond (Fig. 2.3A). The sodium atom has 11 protons in the nucleus and 11 electrons in the shells. Two electrons are in the inner shell, eight in the second shell, and only one in the outer shell. This single electron makes the outer shell unstable. To become more stable, the sodium atom would like to donate the single electron. Donating an electron forms a bond between the two atoms.

Sodium often bonds with chlorine. The chlorine (Cl) atom has 17 protons in the nucleus and 17 electrons orbiting in its shells. The electrons are positioned as follows: two electrons in the inner shell, eight in the

second shell, and seven in the outer shell. The seven electrons make the outer shell unstable. The chlorine atom would like to add a single electron. The electrical attraction occurs between the outer shells of the sodium and chlorine atoms. The single electron in the outer shell of the sodium (Na) atom is attracted to the seven electrons in the outer shell of the chlorine atom. Thus, the sodium atom and chlorine atom bond ionically to form sodium chloride (NaCl), or table salt.

COVALENT BONDS

A second type of chemical bond is the **covalent** (ko-VAYL-ent) **bond.** Covalent bonding involves a sharing of electrons by the outer shells of the atoms. Covalent bonding is like joining hands (see Fig. 2.3B). The formation of water from hydrogen and oxygen atoms illustrates covalent bonding. Oxygen has eight electrons, two in the inner shell and only six in the outer shell. An oxygen atom needs two electrons to complete the outer shell. Hydrogen has only one electron and requires one electron to complete its inner shell.

Water is formed when two hydrogen atoms, each with one electron, share those electrons with one oxygen atom. By sharing the electrons of the oxygen, each of the two hydrogen atoms has completed the inner shells (capacity is two electrons). By sharing the electrons of two hydrogen atoms, the outer shell of the oxygen is completed, with eight electrons. Water is represented as H_2O (two hydrogen atoms and one oxygen atom).

Carbon atoms always form covalent bonds. A carbon atom has four electrons in the outer shell. Carbon, one of the major elements in the body, most commonly bonds with hydrogen, oxygen, nitrogen, and other carbon atoms. Covalent bonding of carbon with hydrogen, oxygen, and nitrogen forms complex molecules such as proteins and carbohydrates. Covalent bonds are strong and do not break apart in an aqueous (water) solution. The strength of these bonds is important because the protein produced by the body must not fall apart when exposed to water.

Many proteins, such as hormones, are transported around the body by blood, which is mostly water. If the covalent bonds of the protein broke apart in water, the hormones would be unable to accomplish their tasks. So many chemical reactions in the body involve carbon that a separate branch of chemistry—organic chemistry—studies only carbon-containing substances. In contrast, inorganic chemistry studies non–carbon-containing substances.

HYDROGEN BONDS

A third type of bond is a **hydrogen bond** (see Fig. 2.3C). It differs from the ionic and covalent bonds in that the hydrogen bond is not caused by the transfer or sharing of electrons of the outer shells of atoms. A hydrogen bond is best illustrated by the weak attraction between

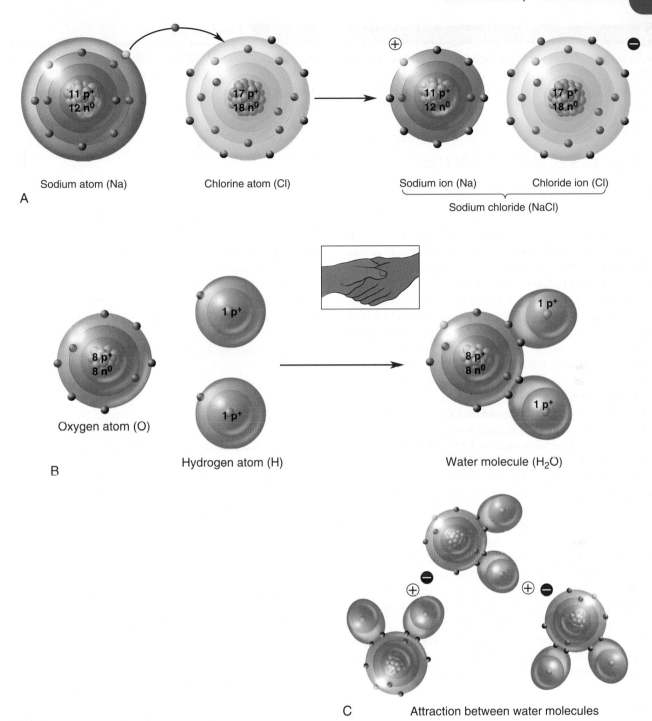

FIG. 2.3 Chemical bonds. (A) Ionic bond. (B) Covalent bond. (C) Hydrogen bond.

water molecules. Water is composed of hydrogen and oxygen. The weak positive charge around the hydrogen of one water molecule is attracted to the weak negative charge of the oxygen in a second water molecule. Because the bond occurs between two molecules, it is called an *intermolecular bond*.

POLARITY

Water engages in hydrogen bonding because it is a **polar molecule**. What makes water a polar molecule?

Because of the uneven sharing of electrons within a water molecule, there is a slight positive charge around the hydrogen end of the water and a slight negative charge around the oxygen end. Note how lopsided the water molecule appears in Fig. 2.3C; more importantly, the *charges* are lopsided. A polar molecule is defined as a molecule that has a lopsided charge—a positive end and a negative end. The lopsided charge means that the positive end—hydrogen—of one water molecule is attracted to the negative end—oxygen—of a second water molecule.

? Re-Think

1. Explain the role of the outer electron shell to ionic and covalent bonding.
2. Explain why water is described as a polar molecule.

IONS

CATIONS, ANIONS, AND ELECTROLYTES

Several other terms are related to the activity of the electrons in the outer shells of the atoms. If the negatively charged electrons are lost from or gained by the outer shell of an atom, the electrical charge of the atom changes. In other words, the electrical charge of the atom changes from a neutral charge (i.e., no charge) to a positive (+) charge or negative (−) charge. Atoms that carry an electrical charge are called **ions**. If the ion is positively charged (+), it is a **cation** (CAT-eye-on). If the ion is negatively charged (−), it is an **anion** (AN-eye-on).

An **electrolyte** (eh-LECK-tro-LITE) is a substance that forms ions when it is dissolved in water. Electrolytes, as the name implies, are capable of conducting an electrical current. For example, the electrocardiogram (ECG) and the electroencephalogram (EEG) record electrical events in the heart and brain.

ION FORMATION

Ions are formed when electrons in the outer shell are lost or gained. For example, the sodium atom has 11 protons (positive charge) and 11 electrons (negative charge). If a single electron is donated, the sodium is left with 11 positive (+) charges and only 10 negative (−) charges. Sodium is said to carry a net charge of +1. The sodium ion, represented as Na^+, is therefore a cation.

The chlorine atom has 17 protons (positive charge) and 17 electrons (negative charge). If an electron is gained, the chlorine then contains 17 (+) charges and 18 (−) charges. Chlorine is said to carry a net charge of −1 and is considered an anion. The chlorine anion is called *chloride* and is represented as Cl^-. Some atoms may give up more than one electron and have a stronger positive charge. Calcium, for example, gives up two electrons. It is represented as Ca^{2+}. Table 2.2 presents other important ions. Note that combinations of atoms, such as bicarbonate (HCO_3^-), can also carry an electrical charge and are therefore ions.

IONIZATION

When an electrolyte splits, or breaks apart in solution, the electrolyte is said to dissociate (Fig. 2.4). For example, NaCl is an electrolyte. In the solid state, it appears as tiny white granules. When dissolved in

Table 2.2	Common Ions	
NAME	**SYMBOL**	**FUNCTION**
Cations		
Sodium	Na^+	Fluid balance (chief extracellular cation), nerve and muscle function
Calcium	Ca^{2+}	Component of bones and teeth, blood clotting, muscle contraction
Iron	Fe^{2+}	Component of hemoglobin (oxygen transport)
Hydrogen	H^+	Important in acid–base balance. Its concentration determines the pH of a solution.
Potassium	K^+	Nerve and muscle function, chief intracellular cation
Ammonium	NH_4^+	Important in acid–base regulation
Anions		
Chloride	Cl^-	Chief extracellular anion
Bicarbonate	HCO_3^-	Important in acid–base regulation
Phosphate	PO_4^{3-}	Component of bones and teeth, component of ATP (energy)

ATP, Adenosine triphosphate.

water, however, the table salt dissociates. What is happening?

$$NaCl \rightarrow Na^+ + Cl^-$$
salt   sodium ion   chloride ion
(cation)   (anion)

When the salt is placed in water, the ionic bonds holding the sodium and chlorine together weaken. The solid NaCl then splits into Na^+ (sodium ion) and Cl^- (chloride ion). In other words, the NaCl dissociates. Because the products of this dissociation are ions, this dissociation process is referred to as **ionization** (EYE-on-eye-zay-shin). Only electrolytes ionize.

 Do You Know...

What the Patient's "Lytes" Are?

This is medical jargon for electrolytes. One of the most important clinical tools is the assessment of the patient's electrolytes. Actually, the "lytes" are really ions such as Na^+ (sodium), K^+ (potassium), Cl^- (chloride), Mg^{2+} (magnesium), and HCO_3^- (bicarbonate). The terms *electrolytes* and *ions* are used interchangeably in the clinical setting.

 Re-Think

1. Using table salt (NaCl) as an example, explain the difference between an electrolyte, ion, cation, and anion.
2. Define ionization using table salt as an example. What ions are produced?

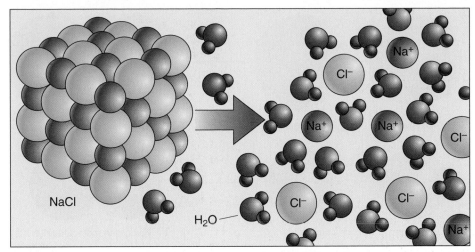

FIG. 2.4 Ionization—dissociation of NaCl → Na+ + Cl- in water.

MOLECULES AND COMPOUNDS

MOLECULES

When two or more atoms bond, they form a **molecule**. Two identical atoms may bond. For example, one atom of oxygen may bond with another atom of oxygen to form a molecule of oxygen, which is designated O_2. The same bonding is true for nitrogen (N_2) and hydrogen (H_2) (Fig. 2.5). A molecule can also be formed when atoms of different elements combine. For example, when two atoms of hydrogen combine with one atom of oxygen, a molecule of water (H_2O) is formed.

COMPOUNDS

A substance that contains molecules formed by two or more different atoms is called a **compound**. For example, if two atoms of hydrogen combine with one atom of oxygen, water is formed. Water is considered both a molecule and a compound.

SOME IMPORTANT COMPOUNDS AND MOLECULES

WATER

Water is the most abundant compound in the body. It constitutes approximately two-thirds of an adult's body weight and even more of a child's body weight. Water is essential for life. Although we can last for many weeks without food, we can last only a few days without water. What makes water so special?

- *Water as the universal solvent.* Water is called the universal solvent because most substances dissolve in water. Its use as a solvent is one of the most important characteristics of water. The ability to dissolve substances is largely because of the polar structure of water (positive charge on one end, negative charge on the other end). For example, the plasma protein albumin carries a negative (−) charge. It is attracted to the positive (+) end of the water molecule. The attraction

of the electrical charges allows albumin to dissolve in water. Many nutrients, waste products, and hormones dissolve in water for transport throughout the body.
- *Water as temperature regulator.* Water has the ability to absorb large amounts of heat without the temperature of the water itself increasing dramatically. This ability means that heat can be removed from heat-producing tissue, like exercising muscle, while the body maintains a normal temperature. Also, when water evaporates from the skin surface, it carries with it a considerable amount of heat. Water, therefore, plays an important role in the body's temperature regulation.
- *Water as an ideal lubricant.* Water is a major component of mucus and other lubricating fluids. Lubricating fluids decrease friction as two structures slide past each other, thereby minimizing wear and tear.
- *Water in chemical reactions.* Water plays a crucial role in many chemical reactions. For example, water is necessary to break down carbohydrates during digestion.
- *Water as a protective device.* Water may also be used to protect an important structure. For example, the cerebrospinal fluid surrounds and cushions the delicate brain and spinal cord. Similarly, amniotic fluid surrounds and cushions the developing infant in the mother's womb.

 Re-Think

1. Physiologically, why is water so important?
2. Why do so many substances dissolve in water?

OXYGEN

Oxygen (O_2), a molecule composed of two oxygen atoms, exists in nature as a gas. The air we breathe contains 21% oxygen. Oxygen is essential for life; without a continuous supply, we would quickly die. The oxygen we inhale is used by cells to liberate the energy from the food we eat. This energy powers the body; like an engine, if the body has no energy, it stops running. The importance of oxygen accounts for the urgency

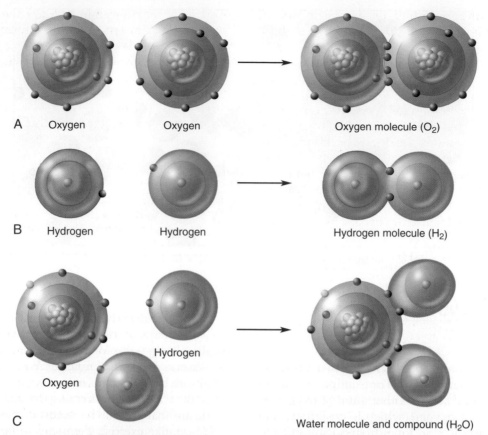

FIG. 2.5 Molecules and compounds. (A) Oxygen (O_2). (B) Hydrogen (H_2). (C) Water (H_2O).

associated with cardiopulmonary resuscitation (CPR). If the heart stops beating, the delivery of oxygen to the tissue ceases, and the brain dies.

CARBON DIOXIDE

Carbon dioxide (CO_2) is a compound that consists of one carbon atom and two oxygen atoms—hence the name carbon dioxide (*di-* means "two"). CO_2 is a waste product, so it must be eliminated from the body. It is made when food is chemically broken down for energy.

◎ Sum It Up!

Chemistry is the study of matter. Matter is composed of elements such as hydrogen, oxygen, carbon, and nitrogen. Each element is composed of millions of the same atoms. Atoms are composed of subatomic particles called protons, neutrons, and electrons. Two characteristics of atoms are the atomic number (number of protons) and the atomic mass (number of protons and neutrons). Chemical bonds are formed through the interaction of one atom with another. The three chemical bonds are ionic, covalent, and hydrogen bonds. The transfer of electrons is responsible for the formation of ions (cations and anions). Cations are positively charged ions, whereas anions are negatively charged ions. Molecules and compounds are formed when atoms interact in a particular fashion. Water (H_2O), oxygen (O_2), and carbon dioxide (CO_2) are examples of important molecules and compounds. Water is the most abundant compound in the body and has numerous characteristics that make it essential to life.

CHEMICAL REACTIONS

A chemical reaction is a process whereby the atoms of molecules or compounds interact to form new chemical combinations. For example, glucose interacts with oxygen to form carbon dioxide, water, and energy. This chemical interaction is characterized by the breaking of the chemical bonds of glucose and oxygen and the making of new bonds as carbon dioxide and water are formed. The reaction is represented as follows:

$$\underset{\text{glucose}}{C_6H_{12}O_6} + \underset{\text{oxygen}}{O_2} \rightarrow \underset{\text{carbon dioxide}}{CO_2} + \underset{\text{water}}{H_2O} + \text{energy}$$

The rates of chemical reactions (how fast they occur) are important. Chemical substances called **catalysts** (KAT-ah-lists) speed up the rate of a chemical reaction. When proteins perform the role of catalysts, they are called **enzymes** (EN-zymes). Most chemical reactions require a catalyst.

ACIDS AND BASES

A normally functioning body requires a balance between substances classified as acids and as bases. Acid–base balance is important because the chemical reactions in the body occur only when these substances are in balance. Imbalances of acids and bases are common and cause life-threatening clinical problems. An understanding of the chemistry of acids and bases is crucial to understanding acid–base balance.

ACIDS

We all recognize the sour taste of an acid. Grapefruit juice, lemon juice, and vinegar are acids. In addition to a sour taste, very strong acids, such as hydrochloric acid (HCl), can cause severe burns. Acid splashed in your eye, for example, can damage the eye tissue to the point of blindness. An **acid** is an electrolyte that dissociates into a hydrogen ion (H$^+$) and an anion. Its dissociation is represented as follows:

$$\underset{\text{hydrochloric acid}}{HCl} \rightarrow \underset{\text{hydrogen ion}}{H^+} + \underset{\text{chloride ion}}{Cl^-}$$

In this reaction, HCl dissociates into H$^+$ and the chloride ion (Cl$^-$). For our purposes, the most important component is the H$^+$. The amount of H$^+$ in a solution determines its acidity.

A strong acid dissociates (breaks apart) completely into H$^+$ and an anion. HCl, found within the stomach, is a strong acid; it yields many hydrogen ions. A weak acid does not dissociate completely. Vinegar, or acetic acid, is a weak acid. Vinegar dissociates slightly into H$^+$. Most of the vinegar remains in its undissociated form, and its dissociation is represented as follows:

$$vinegar \rightleftharpoons H^+ + acetate^-$$

The heavy arrow pointing to the left indicates that the vinegar remains as vinegar, forming very little H$^+$. Because the number of hydrogen ions (H$^+$) determines the acidity of a solution, vinegar is classified as a weak acid. This weakness is the reason that vinegar does not burn your hand. HCl is so strong that it can actually burn a hole through your hand.

BASES

A **base** has a bitter taste and is slippery like soap. Bases are substances that combine with H$^+$. Bases often contain the hydroxyl ion (OH$^-$), such as sodium hydroxide (NaOH). NaOH dissociates into sodium ion (Na$^+$) and the hydroxyl ion (OH$^-$) as follows:

$$NaOH \rightarrow Na^+ + OH^-$$

OH$^-$ is a hydrogen ion eliminator. In other words, the OH$^-$ soaks up a hydrogen ion. The addition of a base makes a solution less acidic.

NEUTRALIZATION OF ACIDS AND BASES

When an acid is mixed with a base, as in the following example, the H$^+$ of the acid combines with the OH$^-$ of the base to form water. In addition, the Na$^+$ and the Cl$^-$ combine to form a salt, NaCl. The reaction is important because the H$^+$ is converted to water. In other words, the acid has been **neutralized** or eliminated. It is no longer an acid. This chemical reaction is represented as follows:

$$\underset{\text{acid}}{HCl} + \underset{\text{base}}{NaOH} \rightarrow \underset{\text{water}}{H_2O} + \underset{\text{salt}}{NaCl}$$

? Re-Think

1. What makes an acid an acid?
2. What makes a base a base?
3. Describe how an acid like HCl is neutralized by a base such as NaOH?

MEASUREMENT: THE pH SCALE

One unit of measurement, **pH**, indicates how many H$^+$ ions are in a solution. The pH scale ranges from 0 to 14 (Fig. 2.6). At the midpoint of the scale, pH 7, the number of H$^+$ ions in pure water is equal to the number of OH$^-$ ions. Therefore, the solution is neutral. A pH that measures less than 7 on the scale indicates that the solution has more H$^+$ than OH$^-$. The solution is then said to be acidic. The pH of stomach contents ranges between 1 and 4—very acidic.

A pH measuring more than 7 indicates fewer H$^+$ ions than OH$^-$ ions. These substances are bases, and the solution is said to be basic, or alkaline (AL-kah-lin). The pH scale measures the degree of acidity or alkalinity. A pH of 0 is most acidic, whereas a pH of 14 is most alkaline.

Note the color change in Fig. 2.6 as the pH changes from blue (alkaline) to pink (acidic).

READING THE pH SCALE

Each pH unit represents a 10-fold change in H$^+$ concentration. For example, a change in 1 pH unit (from 7 to 6) represents a 10-fold increase in H$^+$, whereas a change in 2 pH units (from 7 to 5) represents a 100-fold increase in H$^+$ concentration. The important point is that very small changes in the pH reading indicate very large changes in the H$^+$ concentration.

pH OF BODY FLUIDS

Note the pH of some of the body fluids (see Fig. 2.6). The stomach contents are very acidic, with a pH of 1 to 4. The pH of urine is normally acidic, with a pH range of 5 to 8, although a number of conditions, including diet, can change urinary pH. The intestinal secretions are alkaline, with a pH range of 8 to 10.

Blood pH is maintained within a narrow range of 7.35 to 7.45, a slightly alkaline pH. Because the blood

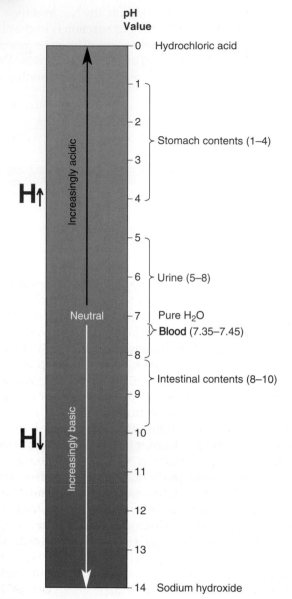

FIG. 2.6 **The pH scale. The scale indicates the H⁺ concentration. Pink indicates the acidic range, and blue indicates the basic, or alkaline, range.**

pH is normally slightly alkaline (called the alkaline reserve), a blood pH of less than 7.35 is more acidic than normal, and the patient is said to be acidotic. If the patient's blood pH is higher than 7.45, the patient is said to be alkalotic. Because all of the body's enzymes work best at a normal blood pH, both acidosis and alkalosis cause serious clinical problems and must be corrected. The need to maintain the body's normal alkaline state is the reason for monitoring blood pH closely during the course of a patient's illness.

The blood pH is regulated on a minute-by-minute basis by three means: a buffer system, the lungs, and the kidneys. (These processes of regulation are described in Chapters 24 and 25.)

 Do You Know...

Why Antacids Are Used?

Patients with ulcers often have excess stomach acid. The stomach acid (HCl) can be neutralized with a drug that contains a base. Because these drugs oppose acids, they are called *antacids*. One of the most commonly used antacids contains aluminum hydroxide. The hydroxyl ion (OH⁻) of the drug combines with the H⁺ of the stomach acid, thereby neutralizing the acid.

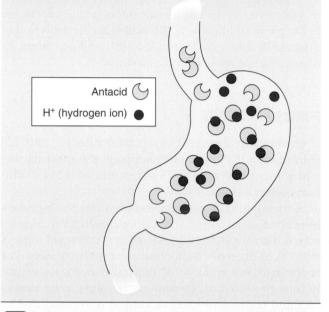

 Sum It Up!

Chemical reactions are processes whereby one chemical substance is converted into a different chemical substance. The rate of a chemical reaction can be increased by a catalyst, or enzyme. A normally functioning body requires a balance between acids and bases. Hydrogen ion concentration is measured by pH. As H⁺ increases, pH decreases; as H⁺ decreases, pH increases. Normal blood pH is 7.35 to 7.45 and is therefore slightly alkaline. When pH falls below 7.35, the person is said to be acidotic; when pH rises above 7.45, the person is said to be alkalotic. Blood pH is regulated within normal limits by three mechanisms: buffers, lungs, and kidneys.

? Re-Think

1. What does pH measure?
2. Why is it important to monitor the patient's blood pH?
3. What blood pH is indicative of acidosis? Of alkalosis?

ENERGY

Energy is the ability to perform work. The body depends on a continuous supply of energy. Even at rest, the body is continuously working and using up energy. Heart muscle, for example, is contracting and forcing blood throughout a large network of blood vessels. The cells of the pancreas are continuously making enzymes so that we can digest our food. Without energy, the body ceases to function.

Table 2.3	Forms of Energy		
FORM OF ENERGY	**DESCRIPTION**		**EXAMPLE**
Mechanical	Energy that causes movement		Movement of legs in running, walking; contraction of heart muscle, causing movement of blood
Chemical	Energy stored in chemical bonds		Fuel to do work, such as running
Electrical	Energy released from the movement of charged particles		Electrical signal involved in transmission of information along nerves
Radiant	Energy that travels in waves		Light stimulates the eyes for vision; ultraviolet radiation from the sun causes tanning
Thermal	Energy transferred because of a temperature difference		Responsible for body temperature
Nuclear	Energy released during the decay of radioactive substances such as isotopes		Not useful physiologically

FORMS OF ENERGY

There are six forms of energy, summarized in Table 2.3. Mechanical energy is expressed as movement. For example, when the leg muscles contract, you are able to walk. Chemical energy is stored within the chemical bonds holding the atoms together. When the chemical bonds are broken, chemical energy is released. The released energy can then be used to perform other types of work, such as digesting food. This process is similar to the running of a car's engine; the energy released from the burning, or breakdown, of the gas is used to turn the engine, and the running engine then moves your car.

CONVERSION OF ENERGY

Energy is easily converted from one form to another. For example, when a log burns, the chemical energy stored in it is converted to heat (thermal energy) and light (radiant energy). In a similar way, the chemical energy stored in the muscle is converted into mechanical energy when the muscle contracts and moves your leg.

The conversion of energy in the body is generally accompanied by the release of heat. For example, when muscles contract during strenuous exercise, chemical energy is converted into both mechanical energy and heat (thermal) energy. Consider how hot you get while exercising. (Body temperature is further described in Chapter 7.)

ENERGY TRANSFER: THE ROLE OF ADENOSINE TRIPHOSPHATE

The energy used to power the body comes from the food we eat (Fig. 2.7A). As the food is broken down, energy is released. This energy, however, cannot be used directly by the cells of the body. The energy must first be transferred to another substance, called **adenosine triphosphate (ATP)**. ATP is an energy transfer molecule.

ATP is composed of three parts: a base, a sugar, and three phosphate groups (see Fig. 2.7B). Note the phosphate groups of the ATP molecule; they have unique chemical bonds. The squiggly lines connecting the second and third phosphate groups indicate that these bonds are high-energy bonds. When these bonds are broken, a large amount of energy is released. More importantly, the energy released from ATP can be used directly by the cell to perform its tasks.

The energy stored within the high-energy bonds is similar to the energy stored in a loaded mousetrap (see Fig. 2.7C). Energy is stored in the trap when you set the metal bar in its loaded position. When the trap is set off by the mouse, the metal bar snaps back into its original position, thereby releasing the stored energy. Similarly, when energy is needed by the body, ATP is split. The energy that was stored in ATP is released. In other words, the bond that holds the end phosphate group is broken, and energy is released. With the release of energy, the splitting of ATP also yields adenosine diphosphate (ADP) and phosphate (P). This process can be shown as follows:

$$ATP \rightarrow energy + ADP + P$$

ADP is almost identical to ATP, but the molecule now has one less phosphate group. ATP is replenished when energy, obtained from burning food, reattaches the end phosphate to ADP, as follows:

$$ADP + P + energy \rightarrow ATP$$

 Re-Think

1. What is meant by the conversion of energy?
2. Explain why ATP is an energy transfer molecule rather than an energy storage molecule.

MIXTURES, SOLUTIONS, SUSPENSIONS, AND PRECIPITATES

You will encounter several other chemical terms in clinical situations.

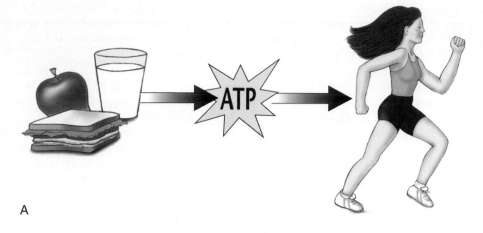

A

Structure of ATP:

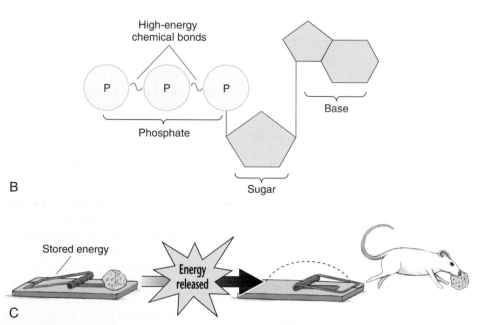

B

C

FIG. 2.7 Energy. (A) Source of energy. (B) Storage of energy within the high-energy bonds of adenosine triphosphate (ATP). (C) Release of energy.

MIXTURES

Mixtures are combinations of two or more substances that can be separated by ordinary physical means. When separated, the substances retain their original properties. For example, imagine that you have a mixture of sugar and little bits of iron. A magnet is then moved close to this sugar–iron mixture. The magnet pulls all the iron away from the sugar, thereby separating the two substances. Note that the two substances have retained their original properties. The sugar is still sugar, and the iron is still iron.

SOLUTIONS

Solutions are mixtures. In a solution, the particles that are mixed together remain evenly distributed. Salt water is an example of a solution. A solution has two parts, a solvent and a solute. The solute is the substance present in the smaller amount; it is the substance being dissolved. The salt in the salt water is the solute. The solute can be solid, liquid, or gas.

The solvent is the part of the solution present in the greater amount; it does the dissolving and is usually liquid or gas. Water is the solvent in salt water. If water is the solvent, the solution is referred to as an aqueous solution. If alcohol is the solvent, the solution is referred to as a *tincture*. A solution is always clear, and the solute does not settle to the bottom.

SUSPENSIONS

Suspensions are mixtures. In a suspension, the particles are relatively large and tend to settle to the bottom unless the mixture is shaken continuously. For example, if sand and water are shaken together and then allowed to sit undisturbed, the sand gradually settles to the bottom.

In a colloidal suspension, the particles do not dissolve, but they are so small that they remain suspended within the liquid, even when not being shaken. A **colloid** (KOL-oyd) is a gel-like substance that resembles egg whites. The body contains many colloidal suspensions. Blood plasma is a colloidal suspension because the proteins remain suspended within the plasma. Other examples of colloidal suspensions include mayonnaise and jelly.

PRECIPITATES

A precipitation reaction is the formation of a solid in a solution during a chemical reaction. The solid is called the **precipitate**. The formation of precipitates has several clinical consequences. For example, kidney stones are precipitates of salts in the urine and form especially when the salts are highly concentrated—hence, the direction to "drink plenty of fluids" as a preventive measure. Similarly, cholesterol-laden bile forms precipitates called *gallstones;* dietary teaching regarding cholesterol intake is provided in hopes of decreasing gallstone formation. Finally, you will be mixing medications; some combinations of drugs form precipitates that, if administered intravenously, act as emboli (such as moving blood clots) that could kill a patient. Clinically, precipitates are very important.

 Sum It Up!

Energy is the ability to do work. Without an adequate supply of energy, the body cannot work, and it dies. Energy is derived from food and transferred to high-energy bonds in ATP. When needed, the energy is released from ATP and used to power the body. Other chemical terms include mixtures, solutions, suspensions, and precipitates.

? **Re-Think**

1. Normal saline (0.9% NaCl) is a salt solution. Explain why it is a solution and not a colloid. What is the solute, and what is the solvent?
2. What is meant by a precipitate?

Get Ready for Exams!

Summary Outline

Our bodies are made of different chemicals. To understand the body, you need to understand some general chemical principles.

I. Matter, Elements, and Atoms
  A. Matter
  1. Anything that occupies space and has weight
  2. Exists in three states: solid, liquid, and gas
  3. Undergoes physical and chemical changes
  B. Elements
  1. Composed of atoms that have the same positive charge in their nuclei (same atomic number)
  2. Four elements (carbon, hydrogen, oxygen, and nitrogen) make up 96% of body weight.
  C. Atoms
  1. Composed of three subatomic particles: neutrons, protons, and electrons
  2. Atomic number: number of protons
  3. Atomic mass: number of neutrons and protons
  4. Isotope: atom with the same atomic number but a different atomic mass
  5. Radioisotope: an unstable isotope

II. Chemical Bonds
  A. Ionic bond: involves donation and acceptance of electrons
  B. Covalent bond: shares electrons of interacting atoms
  C. Hydrogen bond: an example, intermolecular bonds formed by polar molecules

III. Ions
  A. Ion: atom that carries an electrical charge
  1. Cation: positively charged ion
  2. Anion: negatively charged ion
  B. Electrolyte: substance that forms ions (ionization) when dissolved in water

IV. Molecules and Compounds
  A. Molecule: substance formed by two or more atoms (e.g., O_2, H_2O)
  B. Compound: substance that forms when two or more different atoms bond (e.g., H_2O)
  C. Important molecules and compounds: include water, oxygen, and carbon dioxide

V. Acids and Bases
  A. Acid: electrolyte that dissociates into hydrogen ion (H^+)
  B. Base: substance such as OH^- that combines with and eliminates H^+
  C. Neutralization reaction: acid and a base chemically react to form a salt and water
  D. pH scale: measures acidity and alkalinity. A pH of 7 is neutral. A pH less than 7 is acidic and a pH higher than 7 is basic, or alkaline.
  E. Normal pH of the blood: 7.35 to 7.45. A person with a pH less than 7.35 is acidotic, and a person with a pH higher than 7.45 is alkalotic.
  F. Regulation of blood pH: buffers, respiratory system, and kidneys

VI. Energy
  A. Definition: ability to do work
  B. Forms of energy
  1. Six forms of energy: see Table 2.3
  2. Most energy released as heat
  C. Role of adenosine triphosphate (ATP)
  1. ATP: energy transfer molecule
  2. Energy stored in high-energy phosphate bonds

VII. Mixtures, Solutions, Suspensions, and Precipitates
  A. Mixture: blend of two or more substances that can be separated by ordinary physical means
  B. Solutions, suspensions, and colloidal suspensions: types of mixtures
  C. Precipitate: solid formed during a chemical reaction

Review Your Knowledge

Matching: Atoms and Elements
Directions: Match the following words or symbols with their descriptions below.

a. atom
b. K
c. matter
d. Na
e. ion

1. ___ Composed of three particles: protons, neutrons, and electrons
2. ___ Symbol for potassium
3. ___ Symbol for sodium
4. ___ Exists in three states: liquid, solid, and gas
5. ___ Formed when sodium loses an electron

Matching: Structure of the Atom
Directions: Match the following words with their descriptions. Some words may be used more than once, but others may not be used at all.

a. atomic mass
b. isotope
c. protons
d. electrons
e. neutrons
f. atomic number

1. ___ Number of protons in the nucleus
2. ___ Sum of number of protons and neutrons
3. ___ Same atomic number but different atomic mass
4. ___ Number of these in each atom equal to number of protons
5. ___ Circulate in orbits around the nucleus

Matching: Ions and Electrolytes
Directions: Match the following words with their descriptions.

a. cation
b. ions
c. electrolyte
d. anion
e. ionization

1. ___ Classification of KCl
2. ___ Classification of K^+ and Cl^-
3. ___ K^+ is an ion classified as this
4. ___ Cl^- is an ion classified as this
5. ___ Dissociation of KCl → K^+ + Cl^-

Matching: Acids and Bases
Directions: Match the following words or symbols with their descriptions. Some words may be used more than once, but others may not be used at all.

a. alkalosis
b. pH
c. H^+
d. base
e. acid
f. acidosis

1. ___ Electrolyte that dissociates into H^+ and an anion
2. ___ Ion that makes a solution acidic
3. ___ Measurement of hydrogen ion concentration $[H^+]$
4. ___ Condition characterized by pH lower than 7.35
5. ___ Condition caused by excess H^+

Multiple Choice

1. The ionization of salt (NaCl)
   a. is called a neutralization reaction.
   b. lowers pH.
   c. produces a cation (Na^+) and an anion (Cl^-).
   d. causes acidosis.
2. Which of the following is true of iodine and radioactive iodine?
   a. Both have the same atomic numbers.
   b. Both have the same atomic mass.
   c. Neither have electrons in their orbitals.
   d. Both create radiation hazards.
3. Which of the following is not true of Na^+?
   a. It is called the sodium ion.
   b. It has more protons than electrons.
   c. It is called a cation.
   d. It is measured by pH.
4. Which of the following is true of water?
   a. It is a molecule.
   b. It is an aqueous solvent.
   c. It is a compound.
   d. All of the above are true.
5. Which of the following best describes ATP?
   a. It is a buffer, removing H^+ from solution.
   b. It is an energy transfer molecule.
   c. It is a radioactive isotope of phosphate.
   d. It ionizes to H^+, thereby lowering pH.
6. Which of the following has donated an electron?
   a. H_2O
   b. Cl^-
   c. Na^+
   d. HCO_3^-
7. Which of the following is least descriptive of the nucleus of the atom?
   a. Its contents determine the atomic number.
   b. Its contents determine the atomic mass.
   c. It is the "home" of the electrons.
   d. It is the "home" of the protons.
8. Which of the following is descriptive of the patient with a blood pH of 7.28?
   a. The patient has a deficiency of H^+.
   b. The pH is within normal limits.
   c. The patient is acidotic.
   d. The patient is dehydrated.

Go Figure

1. Which of the following is true according to Fig. 2.2?
   a. Panel A: the planets represent the "home" of the protons and neutrons.
   b. Panel B: all electrons occupy the outer shell.
   c. Panel C: the protons and neutrons are located within the nucleus.
   d. Panel A and C: the electrons are represented by the sun.
2. Which of the following is true according to Fig. 2.3?
   a. The stable inner shell of an atom contains eight electrons.
   b. The chloride ion has more electrons than protons.
   c. The sodium ion has more electrons than protons.
   d. Sodium and chlorine bond covalently.
3. Which of the following is true according to Fig. 2.3?
   a. Hydrogen and oxygen bond ionically to form water.
   b. The oxygen atom has an unstable outer electron shell.
   c. The ionic bonding of sodium and chlorine changes the atomic number of the sodium and chlorine.
   d. The ionic bonding of sodium and chlorine changes the atomic mass of the sodium and chlorine.
4. Which of the following is true according to Fig. 2.4?
   a. Ionization refers to the splitting of NaCl into Na^+ and Cl^-.
   b. Ionization refers to the formation of table salt from the sodium ion and chloride ion.
   c. NaCl cannot ionize in water.
   d. All of the above are true.

5. Which of the following is true according to Fig. 2.5?
   a. The covalent bonding of two oxygen atoms yields an oxygen compound.
   b. Two hydrogen atoms bond ionically with one oxygen atom, yielding water.
   c. Water is formed as two hydrogen atoms share their electrons with one oxygen atom.
   d. A hydrogen atom can react with an oxygen atom but cannot react with another hydrogen atom.

6. Which of the following is true according to Fig. 2.6?
   a. As [H$^+$] decreases, the strip in the diagram becomes a deeper pink.
   b. As pH increases, the strip in the diagram becomes a deeper pink.
   c. The normal blood pH is slightly alkaline.
   d. All of the above are true.

7. Which of the following is true according to Fig. 2.7?
   a. ATP means "all the power."
   b. The setting of the mousetrap represents the storage of energy in ATP.
   c. The release of the mousetrap is summarized as ADP + P + energy → ATP.
   d. The lucky mouse represents the source of the stored energy.

Objectives

1. Label a diagram of the main parts of a typical cell, and do the following:
   - Explain the role of the nucleus.
   - Describe the functions of the main organelles of the cell.
   - Identify the components of the cell membrane.
2. Do the following regarding transport mechanisms:
   - Describe the active and passive movements of substances across a cell membrane.
   - Define tonicity and compare isotonic, hypotonic, and hypertonic solutions.
3. Describe the phases of the cell cycle, including mitosis.
4. Explain what is meant by cell differentiation.
5. Explain the processes and consequences of uncontrolled and disorganized cell growth and apoptosis.

Key Terms

active transport (p. 36)
apoptosis (p. 44)
cell (p. 30)
cell cycle (p. 41)
cell membrane (p. 31)
cytoplasm (p. 32)
differentiation (p. 43)
diffusion (p. 36)
endocytosis (p. 40)
endoplasmic reticulum (ER) (p. 34)

equilibrium (p. 38)
exocytosis (p. 40)
facilitated diffusion (p. 38)
filtration (p. 39)
Golgi apparatus (p. 34)
lysosomes (p. 35)
mitochondria (p. 34)
mitosis (p. 41)
nucleus (p. 31)
organelles (p. 34)

osmosis (p. 38)
passive transport (p. 36)
permeable (p. 31)
phagocytosis (p. 35)
pinocytosis (p. 40)
ribosomes (p. 34)
stem cells (p. 43)
tonicity (p. 39)

What do this monk and a cell have in common? While looking at a piece of cork under a microscope in the 1600s, Robert Hooke saw cubelike structures that resembled the rooms, or cells, occupied by monks in a monastery. Hooke thus called his structures "cells." The study of cellular structure and function is called *cytology*.

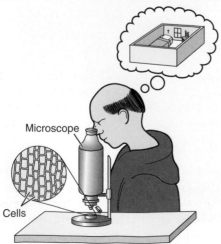

Microscope

Cells

The **cell** is the structural and functional unit of all living matter. Cells vary considerably in size, shape, and function. A red blood cell (RBC), for example, is tiny, whereas a single nerve cell may measure 4 feet in length (Fig. 3.1). The shapes and structures of the cells are also very different. The RBC is shaped like a Frisbee and is able to bend. The shape allows it to squeeze through tiny blood vessels and deliver oxygen and other nutrients throughout the body. Some nerve cells are very long, and many resemble bushes or trees. Their shapes enable them to conduct electrical signals quickly over long distances. Cell structure and function are closely related.

TYPICAL CELL

Despite the differences, cells have many similarities. Fig. 3.2 is a typical cell with all known cellular components. Each specialized cell, such as a nerve cell, possesses some or all of the properties of the typical cell. Table 3.1 lists and summarizes the functions of the cellular components.

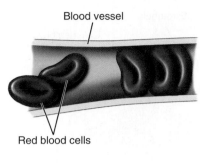

Blood vessel

Red blood cells

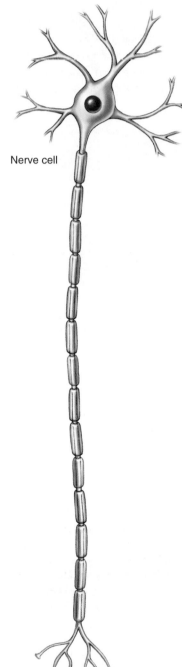

Nerve cell

FIG. 3.1 Cells come in all shapes and sizes.

CELL MEMBRANE

The cell is encased by a **cell membrane**, also called the *plasma membrane*. The cell membrane separates intracellular (inside the cell) material from extracellular (outside the cell) material. In addition to physically holding the cell together, the cell membrane performs other important functions. One of its chief functions is the selection of substances allowed to enter or leave the cell. Because the membrane chooses the substances allowed to cross it, the membrane is said to be selectively **permeable**, or semipermeable.

What makes up a cell membrane? The cell membrane is composed primarily of phospholipids and protein, as well as a small amount of carbohydrates (Fig. 3.3). The phospholipids are arranged in two layers. The protein molecules in the membrane perform several important functions; they provide structural support for the membrane, act as binding sites for hormones, and poke holes, or pores, through the lipid membrane. These pores form channels through which water and dissolved substances flow.

Substances move across the semipermeable membrane in two ways. They can dissolve in the lipid portion of the membrane, as do oxygen and carbon dioxide (lipid-soluble substances). Substances can also cross the membrane by flowing through the pores. Water and electrically charged substances such as sodium and chloride cannot penetrate the lipid membrane and must use the pores. These are called water-soluble substances. The size of the pores also helps select which substances cross the membrane. Substances larger than the pores cannot cross the membrane, whereas smaller substances such as sodium and chloride flow through easily. The solubility characteristics of the membrane also play an important role in pharmacology. Drugs are classified as lipid (fat) soluble or water soluble. Drug solubility determines its distribution throughout the body

 Re-Think

1. What is meant by a semipermeable membrane?
2. How does a fat-soluble substance cross the cell membrane? How does a water-soluble substance cross the cell membrane?

INSIDE THE CELL

The inside of the cell is divided into two compartments: the nucleus and the cytoplasm. The inside of the cell resembles the inside of a raw egg; the "yellow yolk" is the nucleus, and the "white" is the cytoplasm.

NUCLEUS

The **nucleus** is the control center of the cell (see Fig. 3.2). In particular, the nucleus contains the genetic information and controls all protein synthesis. Most adult cells have one nucleus; only mature RBCs have

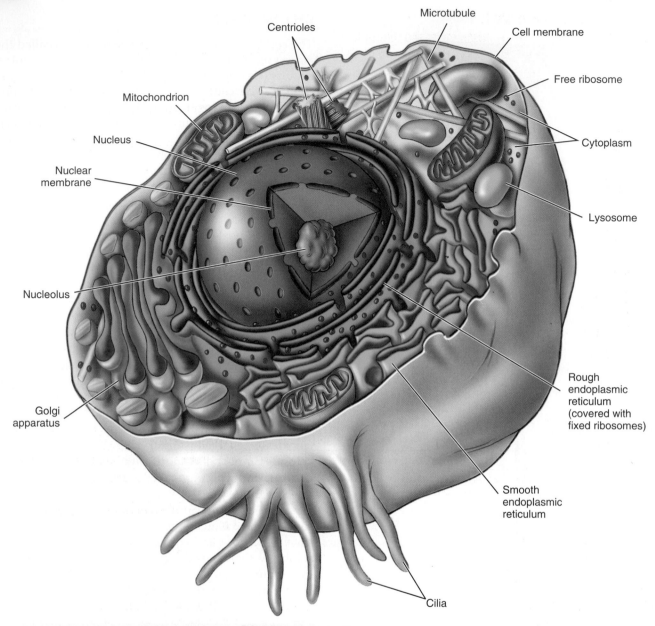

FIG. 3.2   **A typical cell.**

no nucleus. Surrounding the nucleus is a double-layered nuclear membrane. The nuclear membrane contains large pores that allow the free movement of certain substances between the nucleus and cytoplasm.

The nucleus is filled with a fluid substance called *nucleoplasm*. Within the nucleoplasm are two other structures: the nucleolus and chromatin. The nucleolus, or little nucleus, synthesizes ribosomes that move through nuclear pores into the cytoplasm, where they play a role in protein synthesis. The nucleolus also produces a nucleotide necessary for protein synthesis.

Chromatin is composed mainly of strands of DNA (deoxyribonucleic acid), the carriers of the genetic code. In nondividing cells, chromatin appears as a tangled array of fine filaments. In dividing cells, however, chromatin strands coil tightly, forming

DNA-containing structures called *chromosomes*. The genetic code and protein synthesis are described more fully in Chapter 4.

 Re-Think

Why is the nucleus called the control center of the cell?

CYTOPLASM

Cytoplasmic Gel

The **cytoplasm**, or the "gel in the cell," is found inside the cell but outside the nucleus (like the white of a raw egg). The cytoplasm contains the cytosol and organelles. The cytosol is the intracellular fluid and is composed primarily of water, electrolytes, proteins, and nutrients. The cytosol also contains inclusion bodies, insoluble materials such as glycogen granules and

Table 3.1   Cell Structure and Function

CELL STRUCTURE	DESCRIPTION AND FUNCTION
Cell Membrane	Contains the cellular contents; selects what enters and leaves the cell
Cilia	Hairlike projections that move substances across surface of cell membrane
Flagellum	Single long hair for swimming movement of the sperm
Microvilli	Accordion-like folds in the membrane; increase transport of water and dissolved solute
Nucleus	Control center of the cell; stores genetic information
Chromatin	Threadlike structures in the nondividing cell that contain DNA; chromatin threads form chromosomes in a dividing cell
Nucleolus	Synthesizes RNA and ribosomes
Nucleoplasm	Gel in the nucleus
Nuclear membrane	Separates the nucleoplasm from the cytoplasm
Cytoplasm	Gel located inside the cell but outside the nucleus
Cytosol	Medium composed of water and dissolved solute; organelles suspended in the cytosol
Organelles	Tiny organs suspended in the cytosol
Mitochondria	Site of ATP production; "power plants" of the cell

Endoplasmic reticulum (ER)
  Rough ER…
  Smooth ER…
	Membranes that form channels for the flow of cellular substances such as proteins
	Contains ribosomes where protein is synthesized
	Site of lipid and steroid synthesis; synthesis of glycogen in liver and skeletal muscle

Golgi apparatus	Finishes and packages protein for export

Ribosomes
  Free
  Fixed
	Site of protein synthesis
	Ribosomes that float within the cytosol; make protein used within the cell.
	Ribosomes fixed to the ER, making it appear rough; concerned with the synthesis of protein that is exported

Lysosomes	Intracellular house cleaning, phagocytosis, removal of damaged organelles
Cytoskeleton	Microfilaments and microtubules that provide for intracellular shape, support, and movement
Centrioles	Paired, short, rod-shaped microtubules that form spindles and help separate the chromosomes during mitosis
Inclusion bodies	Temporary insoluble material such as glycogen granules and pigments such as melanin

ATP, Adenosine triphosphate.

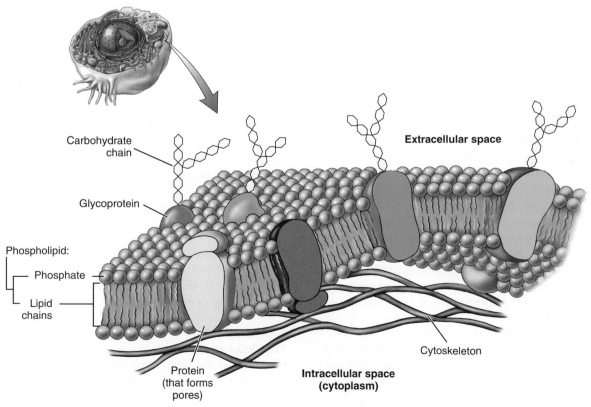

FIG. 3.3   **Structure of the cell membrane: phospholipid bilayer and protein.**

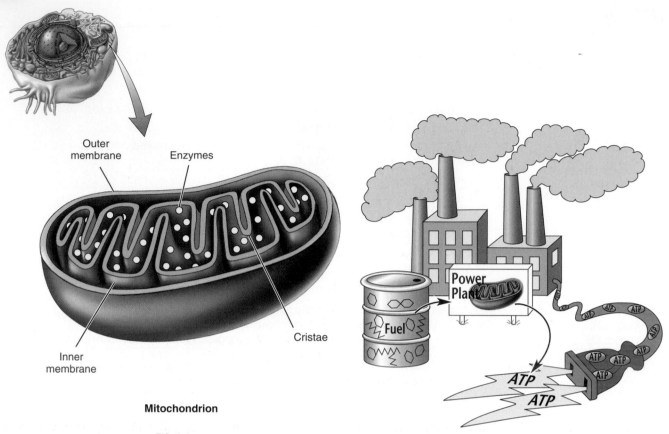

Outer
membrane   Enzymes

Cristae

Inner
membrane

Mitochondrion

FIG. 3.4   Mitochondria are the "power plants" of the cells.

pigments such as melanin. The **organelles**, or "little or-gans,"
are dispersed throughout the cytoplasm; each
organelle has a specific role. Locate the organelles in
Fig. 3.2 and Table 3.1.

CYTOPLASMIC ORGANELLES

Mitochondria

The **mitochondria** are tiny, slipper-shaped organelles.
The number of mitochondria per cell varies, depend-ing
on the metabolic activity of the cell (how hard the
cell works). The more metabolically active the cell,
the greater the number of mitochondria. The liver, for
example, is very active and therefore has many mito-chondria
per cell. Bone cells are less active metaboli-cally
and have fewer mitochondria.

The mitochondrial membrane has two layers (Fig.
3.4); the outer layer is smooth, whereas the inner layer
has many folds, referred to as *cristae*. The enzymes as-sociated
with ATP production are located along the cris-tae.
Because the mitochondria produce most of the ener-gy
(ATP) in the body, they are referred to as the "power
plants" of the cell. (See Chapter 2 for an explanation of
ATP and Chapter 4 for a description of ATP production.)

Ribosomes

Ribosomes are cytoplasmic organelles involved in
protein synthesis. Some ribosomes are attached to the
endoplasmic reticulum and are called *fixed ribosomes*.

Fixed ribosomes are largely concerned with the syn-thesis
of exportable protein—that is, protein secreted
by the cell for use elsewhere in the body. Other ribo-somes,
called *free ribosomes,* float freely within the cyto-plasm
and generally synthesize proteins that are used
within the cell.

Endoplasmic Reticulum

The **endoplasmic reticulum (ER)** is a network of mem-branes
within the cytoplasm (see Fig. 3.2). These long,
folded membranes form channels through which sub-stances,
especially newly synthesized protein, move.
The two types of ER include the type containing ribo-somes
along its surface; it is called *rough endoplasmic re-ticulum
(RER)* because of its rough, sandpaper-like ap-pearance.
The RER is primarily concerned with protein
synthesis. Protein synthesized along the RER is trans-ported
through the channels and delivered to the Golgi
apparatus for further processing. The ER that does not
contain ribosomes on its surface appears smooth; it is
called *smooth endoplasmic reticulum (SER)*. SER is primar-ily
involved in the synthesis of lipids, steroids, glycer-ides,
and glycogen in skeletal muscle and liver cells.

Golgi Apparatus

The **Golgi apparatus** is a series of flattened membra-nous
sacs (Fig. 3.5). Proteins synthesized along the
RER are transported to the Golgi apparatus through

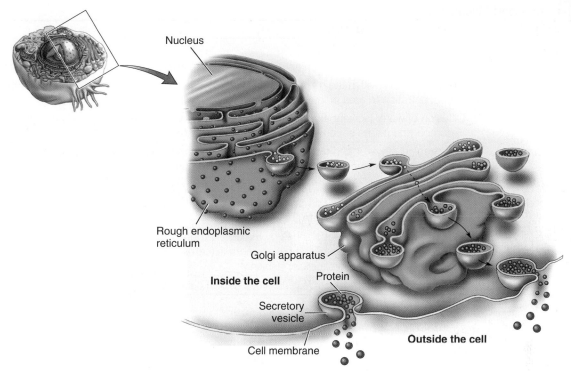

Nucleus

Rough endoplasmic reticulum

Golgi apparatus

Inside the cell

Protein

Secretory vesicle

Outside the cell

Cell membrane

FIG. 3.5   The Golgi apparatus: packages the protein for export.

channels formed by the ER. The Golgi apparatus puts the finishing touches on the protein. For example, a glucose molecule may be attached to a protein within the Golgi apparatus. A segment of the Golgi membrane then wraps itself around the protein and pinches itself off to form a secretory vesicle. In this way, the Golgi apparatus packages the protein. Note that many of the organelles, particularly the ribosomes, ER, and Golgi apparatus, are involved in protein synthesis. (Protein synthesis is described in Chapter 4.)

Lysosomes

Lysosomes are membranous sacs containing powerful enzymes. Lysosomal enzymes break down intracellular waste and debris, including damaged organelles, and thus help "clean house." Lysosomal enzymes perform several other functions. They participate in the destruction of ingested bacteria, a process called **phagocytosis**. Lysosomes also break down the contractile proteins of inactive muscles, as occurs in retired athletes and chronically bedridden persons.

Cytoskeleton

The cytoskeleton is composed of threadlike structures called *microfilaments* and *microtubules*. The cytoskeleton helps maintain the shape of the cell and assists the cell in various forms of cellular movement. Cellular movement is particularly evident in muscle cells, which contain large numbers of microfilaments. Microtubules are the primary component of the cytoskeleton. In addition to making the cell strong and rigid, the microtubules anchor the position of the organelles within

the cytoplasm. Microtubules also play a key role in cell division; they form the spindle apparatus that helps distribute the chromosomes to opposite ends of the dividing cell. (Cell division is explained in Chapter 4.)

Centrioles

Centrioles are paired, rod-shaped, and short microtubular structures that form the spindle apparatus in a dividing cell. Cells that have no centrioles are incapable of cell division; these include neurons, mature RBCs, skeletal muscle cells, and cardiac muscle cells. The cytoplasm surrounding the centrioles is called the *centrosome*. Microtubules of the cytoskeleton begin at the centrosome and spread throughout the cytoplasm.

 Re-Think

1. What is the primary function of the mitochondria?
2. What is the difference between fixed and free ribosomes?
3. What is the difference between the rough and smooth ER?

ON THE CELL MEMBRANE

MICROVILLI

For cells that are particularly involved with the movement of large amounts of water and its dissolved solutes, the membrane forms accordion-like folds called *microvilli* (sing., microvillus). The folding of the cell membrane increases surface area, thereby increasing the amount of fluid absorbed. For example, some of the cells in the digestive tract have millions of foldings, called microvilli, to absorb water and the end products of digested food.

Table 3.2   Transport Mechanisms

MECHANISM	DESCRIPTION AND FUNCTION
Passive	
Diffusion	Movement of a substance from an area of high concentration to an area of low concentration
Facilitated diffusion	Helper molecule within the membrane assists movement of substances from area of high concentration to area of low concentration
Osmosis	Diffusion of water (solvent) from an area with more water to an area with less water; the water compartments are separated by a semipermeable membrane
Filtration	The pushing of water and dissolved substances from an area of high pressure to an area of low pressure; the water and dissolved substances are pushed
Active	
Active transport pump	Moves a substance uphill (from an area of low concentration to an area of high concentration); requires an input of energy (ATP)
Endocytosis	Taking in or ingestion of substances by the cell membrane
Phagocytosis	Engulfing of solid particles by the cell membrane (cellular eating)
Pinocytosis	Engulfing of liquid droplets (cellular drinking)
Exocytosis	Secretion of cellular products (e.g., protein, debris) out of the cell

ATP, Adenosine triphosphate.

CILIA

Cilia are short, hairlike projections on the outer surface of the cell membrane. Cilia use wavelike motions to move substances across the surface of the cell. For example, cilia are abundant on the cells that line the respiratory passages. The cilia help move mucus and trapped dust and dirt toward the throat, away from the lungs. Once in the throat, the mucus can be removed by coughing or swallowing. The cilia therefore help clear the respiratory passages. Cigarette smoking damages the cilia and thus deprives the smoker of this benefit.

FLAGELLA

Flagella (meaning "whiplike") are similar to cilia in that both are hairlike projections of the cell membrane. Flagella, however, are thicker, longer, and fewer in number; they help move the cell. The tail of the sperm is an example of a flagellum; the tail enables the sperm to swim.

◎ Sum It Up!

The cell is the structural and functional unit of all living matter. Although cells differ considerably, they also share many similarities. The "typical cell" illustrates these similarities. The cell is surrounded by a cell membrane. The inside of the cell is divided into the nucleus, the control center, and the cytoplasm, which contains the cytosol and many little organs, or organelles, each of which has a special task to perform. Table 3.1 lists the organelles and their functions.

MOVEMENT ACROSS THE CELL MEMBRANE

Cells are bathed in an extracellular fluid that is rich in nutrients such as oxygen, glucose, and amino acids. These nutrients are needed in the cell and must therefore be able to cross the cell membrane. The cell's waste, which accumulates within the cell, must also be able to cross the cell membrane. Wastes are eventually eliminated from the body.

A number of mechanisms assist in the movement of water and dissolved substances across the cell membrane. The transport mechanisms can be divided into two groups: **passive transport** and **active transport** mechanisms. Table 3.2 summarizes both types of transport.

The passive transport mechanisms require no additional energy in the form of ATP. Passive transport is something like the downward movement of a ball (Fig. 3.6A). The ball is at the top of the hill. Once released, the ball rolls downhill. The ball does not need to be pushed; it moves passively, without any input of energy. Passive transport mechanisms cause water and dissolved substances to move without additional energy, like a ball rolling downhill.

Active transport mechanisms require an input of energy in the form of ATP. Active transport is like the upward movement of a ball (see Fig. 3.6B). For the ball to move uphill, it must be pushed, therefore requiring an input of energy.

PASSIVE TRANSPORT MECHANISMS

The passive mechanisms that move substances across the membrane include diffusion, facilitated diffusion, osmosis, and filtration.

DIFFUSION

Diffusion is the most common transport mechanism. Diffusion is the movement of a substance from an area of higher concentration to an area of lower concentration. For example, a tablet of red dye is placed in a glass of water (Fig. 3.7A). The tablet dissolves, and the dye moves from an area where it is most concentrated

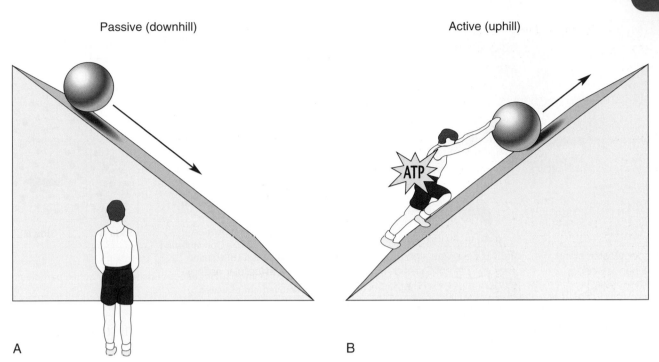

Passive (downhill)   Active (uphill)

A   B

FIG. 3.6   Transport mechanisms. (A) Passive transport mechanism. The ball rolls downhill on its own. (B) Active transport mechanism. The ball must be pushed uphill using adenosine triphosphate (ATP).

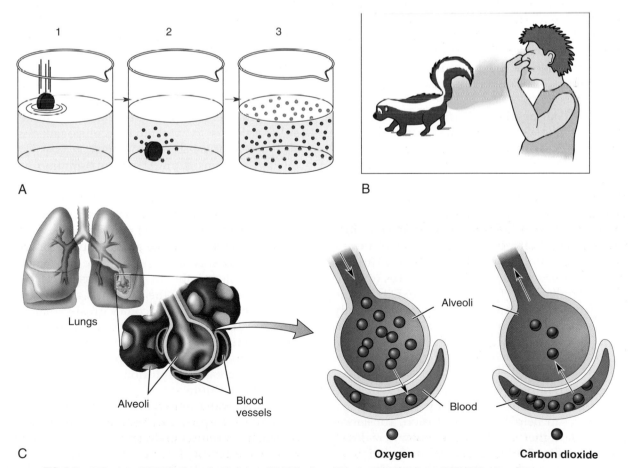

FIG. 3.7   Diffusion. (A) Diffusion of a red dye. (B) Diffusion of Perfume's "perfume." (C) Diffusion of oxygen and carbon dioxide across the alveolar cell membrane in the lung.

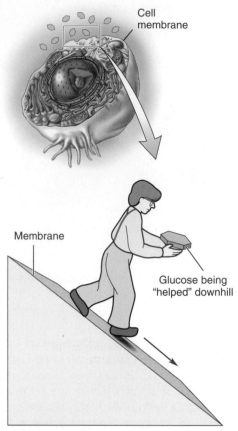

FIG. 3.8   Facilitated diffusion.

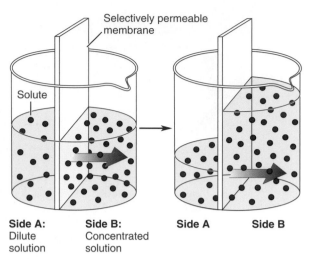

FIG. 3.9   Osmosis. The effect of osmotically active particles on the movement of water.

(glass 1) to an area where it is less concentrated (glasses 2 and 3). Diffusion continues until the dye is evenly distributed throughout the glass. The point at which no further net diffusion occurs (glass 3) is called **equilibrium**.

The scent of our pet skunk, Perfume, also illustrates diffusion (see Fig. 3.7B). Perfume's scent does not take long to permeate the area! Diffusion is involved in many physiological events. For example, diffusion causes oxygen to move across the membrane of an alveolus of the lung into the blood (see Fig. 3.7C). Oxygen diffuses from the alveolus because the concentration of oxygen is higher within the alveolus than within the blood. Conversely, carbon dioxide, a waste product that accumulates within the blood, diffuses in the opposite direction (carbon dioxide moves from the blood into the alveolus). The lungs then exhale the carbon dioxide, thereby eliminating waste from the body. Thus, the process of diffusion moves oxygen into the blood and carbon dioxide out of the blood.

FACILITATED DIFFUSION

Facilitated diffusion is a form of diffusion that is responsible for the transport of many substances (*facilitate* means "to help"). As in diffusion, substances move from a higher concentration toward a lower concentration (Fig. 3.8). In facilitated diffusion, however, the substance is helped across the membrane by a molecule within the membrane. The helper molecule increases the rate of diffusion. The transport of glucose by facilitated diffusion is illustrated in Fig. 3.8 by a boy carrying the glucose. Note that he is moving downhill, indicating that facilitated diffusion is a passive transport process.

OSMOSIS

Osmosis is a special case of diffusion. Osmosis is the diffusion of water through a selectively permeable membrane. A selectively permeable—or semipermeable—membrane allows the passage of some substances while restricting the passage of others. During osmosis, the water diffuses from an area with more water to one with less. The dissolved substances, however, do not move.

Two different solutions in the glass illustrate osmosis. The glass is divided into two compartments (A and B) by a semipermeable membrane (Fig. 3.9). Compartment A contains a dilute glucose solution, whereas compartment B contains a more concentrated glucose solution. The membrane is permeable only to water. The glucose cannot cross the membrane and is therefore confined to its compartment.

During osmosis, the water moves from compartment A to compartment B (from the area where there is more water to the area with less). The following two effects occur: (1) the amount, or volume, of water in compartment B becomes greater than the volume in compartment A; and (2) the concentrations of the solutions in both compartments change. The solution in compartment A becomes more concentrated, whereas the solution in compartment B becomes more dilute.

Because water moves toward the more concentrated solution, it appears to be "pulled" in that direction. Sometimes osmosis is described as a "pulling" pressure. For example, Na^+ is said to pull or hold water. More correctly stated, water diffuses into the more concentrated saline solution.

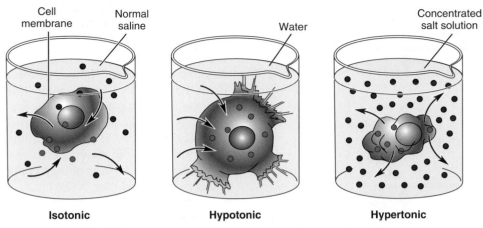

FIG. 3.10   Tonicity : isotonic, hypotonic, and hypertonic solutions.

Because osmosis causes water to move into a compartment, it can cause swelling. For example, tissue injury causes leakage and accumulation of proteins within the tissue space. The confined proteins act osmotically. Water diffuses toward the protein, causing the tissues to swell, a condition called *edema*.

 Re-Think

What are the driving forces for diffusion, facilitated diffusion, and osmosis?

TONICITY

Tonicity is the ability of a solution to affect the volume and pressure within a cell. Note what happens when a cell is placed in solutions of different concentrations (Fig. 3.10). The following three terms are used to illustrate tonicity: *isotonic, hypotonic,* and *hypertonic.*

Isotonic Solution

An isotonic solution has the same concentration as intracellular fluid (*iso* means "same"). Consider an RBC placed in an isotonic solution. Because the solution is isotonic, no net movement of water occurs; the cell neither gains nor loses water.

Hypotonic Solution

If an RBC is placed in pure water (a solution containing no solute), then water moves into the cell by osmosis (from where there is more water to where there is less water). The pure water, being more dilute than the inside of the cell, is said to be hypotonic. Hypotonic solutions cause RBCs to burst, or lyse, in a process referred to as *hemolysis.* Because of hemolysis, pure water is not administered intravenously.

 Do You Know...

Why a Blood Clot May Continue to "Grow," Even When the Bleeding Stops?

The components of the blood clot are osmotically active particles. Water therefore diffuses into the blood clot, causing it to enlarge. If the expanding blood clot is located within the brain, it presses on the brain tissue, causing a variety of life-threatening neurological deficits.

Hypertonic Solutions

If an RBC is placed within a very concentrated salt solution, water diffuses out of the RBC into the bathing solution, causing the RBC to shrink, or crenate. The salt solution is referred to as a *hypertonic solution.*

Why is the tonicity of a solution important? If the cell gains water, the RBC membrane bursts. If the RBC loses water, the cell shrinks. In both cases, RBC function is impaired. Isotonic solutions do not cause cells to swell or shrink. While the RBC was used to explain tonicity, other cells respond in the same way. Clinically, isotonic solutions are frequently administered intravenously. Commonly used isotonic solutions include normal saline (0.9% NaCl), 5% D/W (5% dextrose or glucose in water, or D_5W), and Ringer's solution. Under special conditions, hypotonic or hypertonic solutions may be administered intravenously.

 Re-Think

1. Why does the exposure of an RBC to a hypotonic environment cause hemolysis?
2. What is the advantage of administering an isotonic IV solution?

 Do You Know...

How to Shrink a Swollen Brain?

This can be done by administering a hypertonic solution (e.g., mannitol) intravenously. Because a hypertonic solution contains more solute than what is present in the interstitial or tissue fluid of the brain, water leaves the brain tissue in response to osmosis and moves into the blood. As the blood is carried away from the brain, brain swelling (cerebral edema) decreases.

FILTRATION

With diffusion and osmosis, water and dissolved substances move across the membrane in response to a difference in concentrations. With **filtration**, water and dissolved substances cross the membrane in response to differences in pressures. In other words, pressure pushes substances across the membrane.

A syringe can illustrate filtration (Fig. 3.11). Syringe 1 is filled with water. If a force is applied to the

Syringe #1

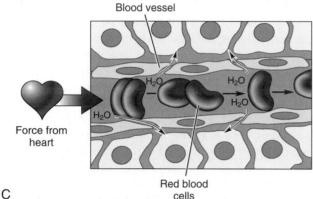

Force on
plunger   H₂O

A

Syringe #2

H₂O

Force on
plunger   H₂O   H₂O

B

Blood vessel

Force from
heart

Red blood
cells

C

FIG. 3.11   Filtration. (A) Water is forced through the needle.
(B) Water (H₂O) is forced through the holes in the barrel of the
syringe. (C) Water is forced out of the capillary through holes, or
pores.

plunger, the water is pushed out through the needle. The water moves in response to a pressure difference, with greater pressure at the plunger than at the tip of the needle. In the second syringe, tiny holes are made in the sides of the barrel. When force is applied to the plunger, water squirts out the sides of the syringe and out the tip of the needle.

Where does filtration occur in the body? The movement of fluid across the capillary wall can be compared with the movement of water in the syringe with holes in its side (syringe 2). A capillary is a tiny vessel that contains blood. The capillary wall is composed of a thin layer of cells with many little pores. The pressure in the capillary pushes water and dissolved substances out of the blood and through the pores in the capillary wall into the tissue spaces. This process is *filtration*; it is movement caused by pushing. (Capillary filtration is further explained in Chapter 19.)

ACTIVE TRANSPORT MECHANISMS

The active transport mechanisms include active transport pumps, endocytosis, and exocytosis.

ACTIVE TRANSPORT PUMPS

Active transport refers to a transport mechanism that requires an input of energy (ATP) to achieve its goal. It is necessary to pump certain substances because the amount of some substances in the cell is already so great that the only way to move additional substances into the cell is to pump them in. For example, the cell normally contains a large amount of potassium ions (K⁺). The only way to move additional K⁺ into the cell is to pump it in. To move the K⁺ from an area of low concentration to an area of high concentration (uphill), energy is invested (Fig. 3.12A).

ENDOCYTOSIS

Endocytosis is a transport mechanism that involves the intake of food or liquid by the cell membrane (see Fig. 3.12B). In endocytosis, the particle is too large to move across the membrane by diffusion. Instead, the particle is surrounded by the cell membrane, which engulfs it and takes it into the cell. There are two forms of endocytosis. If the endocytosis involves a solid particle, it is called *phago-cytosis* (fag-oh-sye-TOH-sis) (*phago-* means "eating"). For example, white blood cells eat, or phagocytose, bacteria, thereby helping the body defend itself against infection. If the cell ingests a water droplet, the endocytosis is called **pinocytosis** (pin-oh-sye-TOH-sis), or "cellular drinking."

EXOCYTOSIS

Whereas endocytosis brings substances into the cells, **exocytosis** (EX-oh-sigh-toe-sis) moves substances out of the cells (see Fig. 3.12C). For example, the cells of the pancreas make proteins for use outside the pancreas. The pancreatic cells synthesize the protein and wrap it in a membrane. This membrane-bound vesicle moves toward and fuses with the cell membrane. The protein is then expelled from the vesicle into the surrounding space.

 Sum It Up!

Water and dissolved substances must be able to move across cell membranes. This is achieved through passive and active transport mechanisms. Passive transport mechanisms require no investment of energy (ATP) and include diffusion, facilitated diffusion, osmosis, and filtration. Concentrations of solutions are expressed as tonicity: isotonic, hypotonic, and hypertonic. The active transport mechanisms require an input of ATP and include the active transport pumps, endocytosis (phagocytosis and pinocytosis), and exocytosis.

? **Re-Think**

Why does an active transport pump require an input of energy?

CELL DIVISION

Cell division is necessary for the body's growth, repair, and reproduction. The frequency of cell division varies considerably from one tissue to the next. Some cells reproduce very frequently, whereas other cells

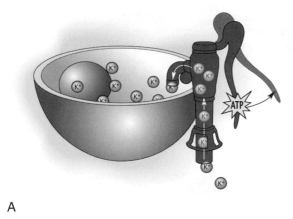

A

Endocytosis

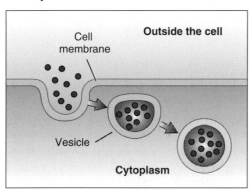

B

Exocytosis

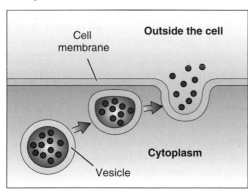

C

FIG. 3.12 Active transport. (A) The active pumping of potassium ions (K⁺) into the cell. (B) Endocytosis. (C) Exocytosis.

reproduce very slowly or not at all. For example, the cells that line the digestive tract are replaced every few days, and more than 2 million RBCs are replaced every second. Certain nerve cells in the brain and spinal cord, however, do not reproduce at all.

Two types of cell division are mitosis and meiosis. Meiosis occurs only in sex cells and will be discussed in Chapter 26. **Mitosis**, which is involved in bodily growth and repair, is the splitting of one mother cell into two

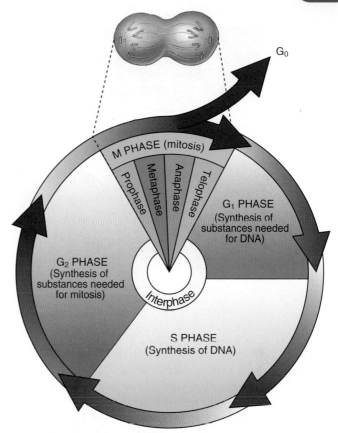

FIG. 3.13 Cell cycle: interphase and mitosis.

identical "daughter cells." The key word is *identical*. In other words, an exact copy of genetic information, stored within the chromosomes, must be passed from the mother cell to the two daughter cells. Mitosis is described in more detail in the next section ("Cell Cycle").

Do You Know...

Some Good News About the Aging Older Brain?

Neurons in the brain do not undergo mitosis and therefore do not replicate. Therefore, we have always assumed that there are no "new" brain neurons. Recently, however, new neurons in the brain have been identified, even in older brains. The neurons arise from newly discovered stem cells located in the brain. Brain cell replacement in the aging brain does happen!

CELL CYCLE

The **cell cycle** is the sequence of events that the cell goes through from one mitotic division to the next. The cell cycle is divided into two major phases: interphase and mitosis (Fig. 3.13).

INTERPHASE

During interphase, the cell carries on with its normal functions and gets ready for mitosis through growth and DNA replication. Interphase is divided into three phases: first gap phase (G_1), phase (S), and second gap phase (G_2).

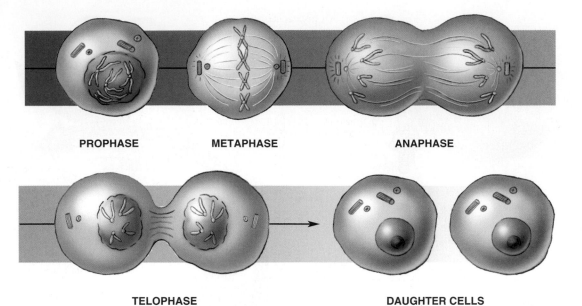

PROPHASE   **METAPHASE**   **ANAPHASE**

TELOPHASE   **DAUGHTER CELLS**

FIG. 3.14   Stages of mitosis.

- First gap phase (G_1)—During this phase, the cell carries on its normal activities and begins to make the DNA and other substances necessary for cell division.
- Phase S—During the S phase, the cell duplicates its chromosomes, thereby making enough DNA for two identical cells.
- Second gap phase (G_2)—This phase is the final preparatory phase for cell division (mitosis); it includes the synthesis of enzymes and other proteins needed for mitosis. At the end of G_2, the cell enters the mitotic (M) phase.

MITOSIS

During the mitotic (M) phase, the cell divides into two cells in such a way that the nuclei of both cells contain identical genetic information. Mitosis consists of four phases: prophase, metaphase, anaphase, and telophase (Fig. 3.14).

- During prophase, the chromosomes coil so tightly that they become visible under a light microscope. Each chromosome pair is composed of two identical strands of DNA called *chromatids;* each chromatid is attached at a point called the *centromere.* At the same time, two pairs of centrioles move to opposite poles of the nucleus. Late in prophase, the nuclear membrane disappears.
- During metaphase, the chromatids are aligned in a narrow central zone; spindle fibers connect the chromatids and centrioles.
- Anaphase begins when the centromere splits and the chromatids are pulled to opposite poles (end of anaphase).
- During telophase, each new cell reverts to the interphase state; the nuclear membrane reforms, the chromosomes uncoil, and the chromatin strands reappear. Telophase and cytokinesis mark the end

of mitosis. Cytokinesis (sye-toh-kin-EE-sis), which begins in late anaphase, is the pinching of the cell membrane to split the cytoplasm into two distinct cells.

Repeat! Mitosis is a type of cell division that produces two genetically identical daughter cells. How can you remember the stages of mitosis? Think of "*Play Me A Tune*": *p*rophase, *m*etaphase, *a*naphase, *t*elophase.

At the end of mitosis, the daughter cells have two choices. They can enter G_1 and repeat the cycle (and divide again) or they can enter another phase, called *G zero* (G_0) (see Fig. 3.13). Cells in G_0 "drop out" of the cell cycle and rest; they do not undergo mitosis. Cells may re-enter the cell cycle after days, weeks, or years. The inability to stop cycling and enter G_0 is characteristic of cancer cells. Cancer cells constantly divide and proliferate. Anticancer drugs are more active against cells that are cycling than against cells resting in G_0. Thus, tumors that contain many cycling cells respond best to chemotherapy.

Anticancer drugs are classified according to the cell cycle phases that they affect. Some anticancer drugs are called *cell cycle phase–specific.* These drugs affect the cell when it is in a particular phase. With the use of this terminology, the anticancer drug methotrexate is considered cell cycle S phase–specific. Other drugs are cell cycle M phase–specific and cell cycle G_2 phase–specific. Some anticancer drugs can act at any phase of the cell cycle and are called *cell cycle phase–nonspecific.* By knowing the cell cycle terminology, you can understand anticancer drugs better.

 Re-Think

1. Explain how interphase prepares the cell for mitosis.
2. What are the phases of mitosis, and what is the major accomplishment of each phase?

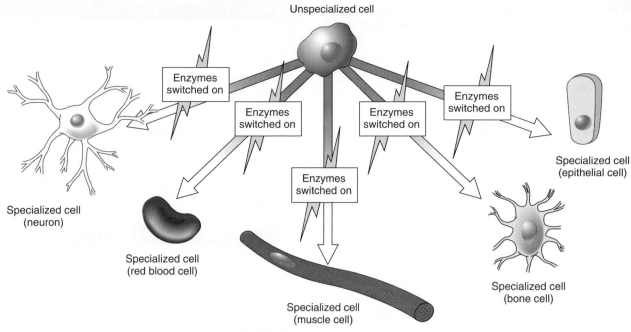

Unspecialized cell

Enzymes switched on

Enzymes switched on

Enzymes switched on

Enzymes switched on

Enzymes switched on

Specialized cell (neuron)

Specialized cell (red blood cell)

Specialized cell (muscle cell)

Specialized cell (bone cell)

Specialized cell (epithelial cell)

FIG. 3.15 Cell differentiation.

CELL DIFFERENTIATION

Mitosis assures us that the division of one cell produces two identical cells. How do we account for the differences in cells such as muscle cells, RBCs, and bone cells? In other words, how do cells differentiate or develop different characteristics?

An embryo begins life as a single cell, the fertilized ovum. Through mitosis, the single cell divides many times into identical cells. Then, at some time during their development, the cells start to specialize, or **differentiate** (Fig. 3.15). One cell, for example, may switch on enzymes that produce RBCs. Other enzymes are switched on and produce bone cells. Regardless of the mechanism, you started life as a single adorable cell and ended up as billions of specialized cells!

What does it mean when a tissue biopsy (surgical removal of tissue for examination) shows many poorly differentiated cells? It means that the tissue cells have failed to differentiate or specialize. In other words, the poorly differentiated cells of a liver tumor do not resemble normal liver cells. Failure to differentiate is characteristic of cancer cells.

STEM CELLS

Stem cells are relatively undifferentiated or unspecialized cells whose only function is the production of additional unspecialized cells. Each time a stem cell divides, one of its daughter cells differentiates while the other daughter cell prepares for further stem cell division. The rate of stem cell division varies with the tissue type; the stem cells within the bone marrow and skin are capable of dividing more than once a day, whereas the stem cells in adult cartilage may remain inactive

for years. Stem cell research is of particular interest because of the possibility of replacing damaged tissue and growing new organs. How amazing it would be if newly discovered stem cells could be used to repair a damaged spinal cord or restore the dopamine-secreting cells in the brains of persons with Parkinson's disease. Another advance in stem cell research is the development of a new technique that coaxes adult cells to regress to an embryonic state. These undifferentiated cells are called *induced pluripotent stem cells* (iPS cells). The iPS cells can then be induced to specialize into the desired cell type, such as bone, muscle, or blood cells. A major hurdle in stem cell research has been the use of embryos as stem cell donors. This technique required the destruction of the embryo, thereby creating an ethical dilemma for many. The development of iPS cells eliminates this issue and hopefully will hasten stem cell research.

? Re-Think

1. Explain why Fig. 3.15 illustrates cell differentiation.
2. What is the relationship between stem cells and cellular differentiation?

ORDER, DISORDER, AND DEATH

Most cell growth is orderly. Cells normally reproduce at the proper rate and align themselves in the correct positions. At times, however, cell growth becomes uncontrolled and disorganized. Too many cells are produced. This process is experienced by the patient as a lump or tumor (*tumor* means "swelling").

Tumors may be classified as benign (noncancerous) or malignant (cancerous). Cancer cells are appropriately named. *Cancer* means "crab"; cancer cells, like a crab, send out clawlike extensions that invade surrounding tissue. Cancer cells also detach from the original tumor (primary site) and spread throughout the body (secondary sites). Widespread invasion of the body by cancer cells often causes death. The spreading of cancer cells is referred to as *metastasis*.

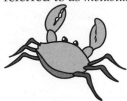

There is also a programmed sequence of events that leads to cell death called **apoptosis**, or cell suicide. Apoptosis helps rid the body of old, unnecessary, and unhealthy cells. Because the body replaces a million cells per second, the elimination of some cells by apoptosis is necessary. Apoptosis, however, can go into overdrive, causing excessive cellular death and disease.

A Pap smear is a diagnostic procedure used to detect cancer. A sample of cells (a smear) is obtained, usually from around the cervix. The smear is then examined under a microscope for changes that could indicate cancer. A positive Pap smear can indicate cancer in its early stages. Early detection is associated with a very high cure rate.

Sometimes cells are injured so severely that they die, or necrose (from the Greek word *necros*, meaning "death"). For example, the cells may be deprived of oxygen for too long a period, be poisoned, be damaged by bacterial toxins, or suffer the damaging effects of radiation.

 Sum It Up!

The union of the sperm and egg forms a single cell that divides by mitosis into billions of identical cells. The cell cycle is the sequence of events that the cell goes through from one mitotic division to the next. The cell cycle is divided into two phases: the interphase and the mitotic phase. Mitosis splits a cell into two genetically identical cells. There are four stages of mitosis: prophase, metaphase, anaphase, and telophase. The cells then specialize, or differentiate, into many different types of cells, all of which are needed to perform a wide variety of functions. Most cells grow in an orderly way. Cells can, however, grow abnormally. The result is sometimes a tumor, which may be benign or malignant (cancerous).

As You Age

1. All cells show changes as they age. The cells become larger, and their capacity to divide and reproduce tends to decrease.
2. Normal cells have built-in mechanisms to repair minor damage; this ability to carry out repair declines in aging cells.
3. When DNA is damaged, changes in membranes and enzymes occur in the cell. Changes in the transport of ions and nutrients occur at the cell membrane. The chromosomes in the nucleus undergo such changes as clumping, shrinkage, and fragmentation.
4. Certain genetic disorders, such as Down syndrome, are more common in children born to older women.
5. Organelles such as mitochondria and lysosomes are present in reduced numbers as a person ages. In addition, cells function less efficiently.

Note: The Medical Terminology and Disorders table appears in Chapter 4

Get Ready for Exams!

Summary Outline

The cell is the structural and functional unit of all living matter.

I. A Typical Cell
  A. Cell membrane (plasma membrane)
    1. Composition: phospholipid bilayer and protein
    2. Semipermeable: selection of nutrients and waste that cross the membrane
    3. Structures on cell membrane: cilia, flagella, microvilli
  B. Structures inside the cell
    1. Nucleus: control center of the cell; stores genetic information and contains chromatin and the nucleolus
    2. Cytoplasm: gel-like substance inside the cell membrane but outside the nucleus; cytosol and organelles
    3. Organelles: in the cytoplasm
    4. Mitochondria: "power plants" of the cell
    5. Ribosomes (free and fixed): involved in protein synthesis

  6. Endoplasmic reticulum (two types): rough endoplasmic reticulum (RER) and smooth endoplasmic reticulum (SER)
  7. Golgi apparatus: packages and puts the finishing touches on newly synthesized protein
  8. Lysosomes: intracellular "housekeepers"
  9. Cytoskeleton: (microfilaments and microtubules) provides shape and support to the cell
  10. Centrioles: play a role in cell reproduction
II. Movement Across the Cell Membrane: Passive and Active Mechanisms
  A. Passive transport mechanisms
    1. Passive transport mechanisms: require no input of energy (ATP)
    2. Diffusion: causes a substance to move from an area of greater concentration to an area of lesser concentration
    3. Facilitated diffusion: same as diffusion but uses a helper molecule to increase the rate of diffusion

4. Osmosis: a special case of diffusion using a semi-permeable membrane; involves diffusion of water from an area with more water to an area of less water
5. Concentrations of a solution are expressed as tonicity; solutions are isotonic, hypotonic, or hypertonic.
6. Filtration: movement of water and dissolved substances from an area of high pressure to an area of low pressure

B. Active transport mechanisms
1. Active transport: requires an input of energy (ATP)
2. Active transport pumps: move substances from an area of low concentration to an area of high concentration
3. Endocytosis: moves substances into a cell; pinocytosis: cellular "drinking"; phagocytosis: cellular "eating"
4. Exocytosis: moves substances out of a cell

III. Cell Division
A. Mitosis: produces two identical cells
B. Meiosis: occurs only in sex cells

IV. Cell Cycle
A. Interphase (G_1, S, and G_2 phases)
B. Mitosis (M phase)
1. The splitting of one mother cell into two identical daughter cells
2. Four phases of mitosis: prophase, metaphase, anaphase, and telophase
3. A cell can exit from the cell cycle and enter G_0 (resting).
C. Cell cycle phase–specific and phase-nonspecific drugs
1. Some drugs aim at a specific phase of cell cycle.
2. Some drugs are cell cycle phase–nonspecific.

V. Cell Differentiation: From Stem Cells to Specialized Cells

VI. Order, Disorder, and Death

Review Your Knowledge

Matching: Cell Structure
Directions: Match the following words with their descriptions.

a. mitochondria
b. endoplasmic reticulum
c. ribosomes
d. cilia
e. lysosomes
f. nucleus
g. cytoplasm

1. ___ Control center of the cell; contains the DNA
2. ___ Short, hairlike projections on the outer surface of the cell
3. ___ "Power plants" of the cell; most ATP made here
4. ___ Classified as rough and smooth
5. ___ Organelles attached to the endoplasmic reticulum; involved in protein synthesis
6. ___ Digestive organelles that engage in phagocytosis; intracellular "house cleaning"
7. ___ "Gel in the cell" (outside the nucleus)

Matching: Transport and Tonicity
Directions: Match the following words with their descriptions. Some words may be used more than once.

a. hypotonic
b. diffusion
c. pinocytosis
d. isotonic
e. hypertonic
f. osmosis
g. filtration
h. facilitated diffusion
i. exocytosis

1. ___ Pressure gradient is the driving force for this type of passive transport.
2. ___ Passive transport mechanism whereby glucose is "helped" across the membrane by a helper molecule within the membrane
3. ___ Protein-containing vesicle within a cell fuses with the cell membrane and ejects the protein
4. ___ Called "cellular drinking"
5. ___ An example of this transport mechanism is the swelling of a blood clot as water is pulled into the clot.
6. ___ Describes a solution that is more concentrated than the inside of a cell
7. ___ Solution that causes a red blood cell to swell with water and burst
8. ___ Solution that has the same concentration as the inside of a red blood cell
9. ___ Drop of red dye is added to a beaker of water; in 2 hours, the beaker of water is uniformly colored red.
10. ___ Because of its salt concentration, normal saline is considered this.

Multiple Choice
1. The selectively permeable membrane
   a. permits filtration but not diffusion or osmosis.
   b. determines which substances enter and leave the cell.
   c. allows for the unrestricted movement of water and electrolytes across the cell membrane.
   d. permits diffusion but not osmosis.
2. Which of the following is *not* true of the mitochondria?
   a. Numbers of mitochondria reflect the metabolic activity of the cell.
   b. Mitochondria are the organelles that make most of the body's ATP.
   c. Mitochondria are located in the cytoplasm.
   d. Mitochondria are the sites of protein synthesis.
3. This semipermeable phospholipid bilayer controls what enters and leaves the cell.
   a. Mitochondria
   b. Cell membrane
   c. Lysosome
   d. Rough endoplasmic reticulum

4. Most of the DNA and genetic information is stored within the
   a. nucleus.
   b. Golgi apparatus.
   c. lysosomes.
   d. centrioles.

5. Which of the following is common to the RER, ribosomes, and Golgi apparatus?
   a. ATP-producing organelles
   b. "house cleaning" by proteolytic enzymes
   c. Ammonia-producing organelles
   d. Protein-producing organelles

6. Which of the following is an *incorrect* statement regarding the cellular organelles?
   a. Most ATP is produced in the mitochondria.
   b. Lysosomes contain potent enzymes that digest cellular waste and debris.
   c. Most DNA is located within the Golgi apparatus.
   d. The RER is involved in protein synthesis.

7. The words *rough* and *smooth* refer to the
   a. ribosomes.
   b. endoplasmic reticulum.
   c. Golgi apparatus.
   d. cell membrane.

8. A stem cell develops into a muscle cell. Which of the following most accurately describes this process?
   a. Apoptosis
   b. Necrosis
   c. Neoplastic
   d. Differentiation

9. A beaker contains two compartments. Compartment A contains a 20% glucose solution, and compartment B contains a 5% glucose solution. The membrane is permeable to water but impermeable to glucose. Which statement is true at equilibrium?
   a. The volume in A is greater than the volume in B.
   b. The volume in A is less than the volume in B.
   c. The volume remains the same in both compartments.
   d. Glucose diffuses from A to B.

10. With regard to the cell cycle, which of the following is correct?
    a. The M phase is the same as interphase.
    b. Cells cannot enter phase G_0 when they complete the cycle.
    c. Cell division occurs during the M phase.
    d. Prophase, metaphase, anaphase, and telophase occur during phase G_1.

11. Blood pressure forces water and dissolved solutes out of the capillaries and into the tissue space. This process is called
    a. osmosis.
    b. active transport.
    c. pinocytosis.
    d. filtration.

12. Cytology is
    a. synonymous with *physiology*.
    b. the type of metabolism that most cells use to extract energy from food.
    c. the study of genetics.
    d. the study of cell structure and function.

13. What might happen if pure water were administered intravenously (directly into the blood via the veins)?
    a. The patient would become dehydrated.
    b. The red blood cells would undergo hemolysis.
    c. The red blood cells would lose volume and shrink.
    d. The water would dilute the blood; water would be "pulled" into the capillaries from the tissue spaces.

Go Figure

1. Which of the following is true according to Figs. 3.1 and 3.2?
   a. All cells look like the "typical cell."
   b. The ER and Golgi apparatus are membranous cytoplasmic organelles.
   c. All ribosomes are attached to the ER and are concerned with protein synthesis.
   d. All cells look like red blood cells.

2. Which of the following is true according to Fig. 3.2 and Table 3.1?
   a. The mitochondria and lysosomes are organelles that are located within the nucleus.
   b. The rough endoplasmic reticulum is rough because it is populated with ribosomes.
   c. Cilia, flagella, and microvilli populate the endoplasmic reticulum, giving it a rough appearance.
   d. The ribosomes are characterized as either rough or smooth.

3. Which of the following is true according to Fig. 3.3?
   a. The cell membrane is a phospholipid, thereby making the entire membrane permeable to water.
   b. The cell membrane separates cytoplasmic contents from nuclear contents.
   c. Proteins embedded within the cell membrane create pores through which water and dissolved solutes pass.
   d. The cell membrane is designed as an impermeable and unchanging structure.

4. Which of the following is true according to Fig. 3.4?
   a. The inner mitochondrial membrane is called the Golgi apparatus.
   b. The mitochondria consume most of the energy of the cell.
   c. The mitochondria are the "power plants" of the cells.
   d. Each cell has only one mitochondrion.

5. Which of the following is true according to Fig. 3.5 and Table 3.1?
   a. The Golgi apparatus forms the inner membrane of the mitochondrion.
   b. The Golgi apparatus delivers amino acids to the rough endoplasmic reticulum.
   c. The Golgi apparatus assembles amino acids into proteins.
   d. The secretory vesicle fuses with the cell membrane so as to eject exportable protein from the cell.

6. Which of the following is true according to Fig. 3.6 and Table 3.2?
   a. Diffusion and osmosis require an input of energy.
   b. The driving force for filtration is a concentration gradient.
   c. The driving force for diffusion is a pressure gradient.
   d. The active transport pump requires an input of energy.

7. Which of the following is true according to Fig. 3.7?
   a. Equilibrium is achieved in beaker A-2.
   b. The mechanism by which the red dye achieves equilibrium is similar to that of Perfume's contribution to room air.
   c. Fig. 3.7C indicates that oxygen diffuses into the alveoli of the lung from the blood, whereas carbon dioxide osmoses from the lung into the blood.
   d. Diffusion cannot occur across a membrane.

8. Which of the following is true according to Fig. 3.8?
   a. The boy represents the helper molecule in the membrane during facilitated diffusion.
   b. Facilitated diffusion is an active transport mechanism.
   c. The boy represents the active transport pump in a membrane.
   d. The boy represents the pressure gradient that causes filtration.

9. Which of the following is true according to Fig. 3.9?
   a. Water diffuses from side B to A.
   b. Solute diffuses from side B to A.
   c. Neither solute nor solvent diffuses.
   d. Water diffuses from side A to B.

10. Which of the following is true according to Fig. 3.10?
    a. Placing an RBC in a hypertonic solution causes the cell to swell and burst.
    b. Because It Is Isotonic, normal saline causes no change in the volume of the RBC.
    c. Placing a cell in a hypotonic solution causes water to leave the cell.
    d. The rigid cell wall of the RBC prevents any change in cell volume when the RBC is placed in distilled water.

11. Which of the following is true according to Fig. 3.11?
    a. Water is filtered into the tissue spaces in response to a pressure gradient.
    b. Water diffuses out of the venous end of the capillary into the tissue spaces.
    c. Red blood cells are filtered along the entire length of the capillary.
    d. Water can not cross the capillary wall.

12. The transport in Fig. 3.12
    a. occurs in a manner that is consistent with Fig. 3.6A.
    b. is the same as the transport mechanism described in Fig. 3.8.
    c. only involves the movement of a substance into the cell.
    d. can move a solute against its gradient.

13. Which of the following is true according to Fig. 3.13?
    a. The cell rests when it enters interphase.
    b. The M phase consists of the G_1 phase, S phase, and G_2 phase.
    c. The cell divides during the M phase.
    d. The cell is most active during the G_0 phase.

14. Which of the following is true according to Fig. 3.14?
    a. Cytokinesis is most prominent during telophase.
    b. Prophase, metaphase, anaphase, and telophase are stages of the M phase of the cell cycle.
    c. The chromatids are aligned in a narrow central zone during metaphase.
    d. All of the above are true.

Cell Metabolism

Objectives

1. Define metabolism, anabolism, and catabolism.
2. Explain the use of carbohydrates in the body, and differentiate between the anaerobic and aerobic metabolism of carbohydrates.
3. Explain the use of fats in the body.
4. Explain the use of proteins in the body.
5. Describe the roles of DNA and RNA in protein synthesis, the structure of a nucleotide, and the steps in protein synthesis.

Key Terms

aerobic catabolism (p. 50)
amino acids (p. 54)
ammonia (p. 56)
anabolism (p. 48)
anaerobic catabolism (p. 50)
base pairing (p. 56)
base sequencing (p. 57)
carbohydrates (p. 48)
catabolism (p. 48)
cholesterol (p. 52)

deoxyribonucleic acid (DNA) (p. 56)
disaccharides (p. 49)
fatty acids (p. 52)
genetic code (p. 57)
gluconeogenesis (p. 51)
glucose (p. 48)
glycerol (p. 52)
glycogen (p. 50)
glycolysis (p. 50)
lipids (p. 52)

metabolism (p. 48)
monosaccharides (p. 48)
peptide bond (p. 54)
polysaccharides (p. 49)
proteins (p. 54)
ribonucleic acid (RNA) (p. 57)
transcription (p. 58)
translation (p. 58)
urea (p. 55)

To carry on its function, the cell, like a factory, must bring in and use raw material. The raw material comes from the food we eat and includes carbohydrates, protein, and fat. Once inside the cell, the raw materials undergo thousands of chemical reactions. The cellular processing of the raw materials is called *metabolism*.

METABOLISM

Metabolism can be divided into two parts: anabolism and catabolism (Fig. 4.1).

Anabolism (ah-NAB-oh-liz-em) includes reactions that build larger, more complex substances from simpler substances, such as the building of a large protein from individual amino acids. The process is similar to the building of a brick wall from individual bricks. Anabolic reactions generally require an input of energy in the form of adenosine triphosphate (ATP).

Catabolism (kah-TAB-oh-liz-em) includes reactions that break down larger, more complex substances into simpler substances, such as the breakdown of a large protein into individual amino acids. This process is similar to the knocking down of a brick wall. Catabolism releases energy that is converted into ATP and used to "run" the body.

CARBOHYDRATES

We have all eaten sugars and starchy food. Bread, potatoes, rice, pasta, and jelly beans are some of our favorite foods. These are all carbohydrates. **Carbohydrates** are organic compounds composed of carbon (C), hydrogen (H), and oxygen (O). Carbohydrates are classified according to size (Fig. 4.2). **Monosaccharides** (mon-oh-SAK-ah-rides) are single (mono) sugar (saccharide) compounds. *Disaccharides* (dye-SAK-ah-rides) are double (di) sugars, and *polysaccharides* (pahl-ee-SAK-ah-rides) are many (poly) sugar compounds. The shorter monosaccharides and disaccharides are called *sugars*, and the longer chain polysaccharides are called *starches*. The carbohydrates are listed in Table 4.1.

MONOSACCHARIDES

Monosaccharides are sugars containing three to six carbons. The six-carbon simple sugars include glucose, fructose, and galactose. **Glucose** is the most important of the three and is used by the cells as an immediate source of energy.

There are also five-carbon monosaccharides; they include ribose and deoxyribose. These sugars are used in the synthesis of ribonucleic acid (RNA) and deoxyribonucleic acid (DNA).

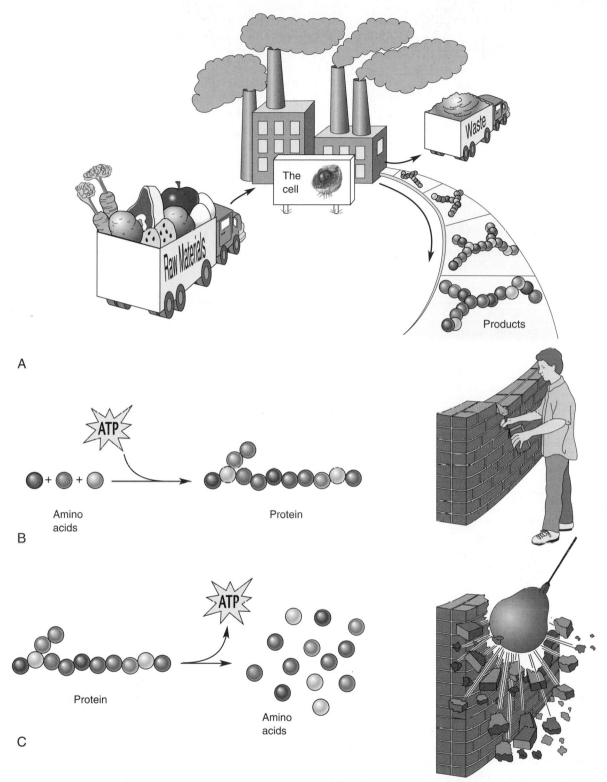

A

ATP

Amino
acids

Protein

B

Protein

ATP

Amino
acids

C

FIG. 4.1 Metabolism. (A) Raw materials to run the factory. (B) Anabolism. (C) Catabolism.

DISACCHARIDES

Disaccharides are double sugars and are made when two monosaccharides are linked together. The disaccharides include sucrose (table sugar), maltose, and lactose; they are present in the food we eat. They must be digested, or broken down, into monosaccharides before they can be absorbed across the walls of the digestive tract and used by the cells.

POLYSACCHARIDES

Polysaccharides are made of many glucose molecules linked together. Some are linked together in straight

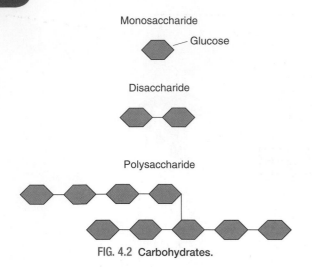

FIG. 4.2 Carbohydrates.

Table **4.1**   Carbohydrates

NAME	FUNCTION
Monosaccharides (Simple Sugars)	
Glucose	Most important energy source
Fructose	Converted to glucose
Galactose	Converted to glucose
Deoxyribose	Sugar in DNA
Ribose	Sugar in RNA
Disaccharides (Double Sugars)	
Sucrose	Splits into monosaccharides (glucose + fructose)
Maltose	Splits into monosaccharides (glucose + glucose)
Lactose	Splits into monosaccharides (glucose + galactose)
Polysaccharides (Many Sugars)	
Starches	Found in plant foods; digested to monosaccharides
Glycogen	Animal starch; excess glucose stored in liver and skeletal muscle
Cellulose	Nondigestible by humans; forms dietary fiber or roughage

DNA, Deoxyribonucleic acid; *RNA*, ribonucleic acid.

chains, and others in branched chains. The three polysaccharides of interest to us are plant starch, animal starch (glycogen), and cellulose.

Starch is the storage polysaccharide in plants. It is a series of glucose molecules linked together in a branched pattern. Starchy foods such as potatoes, peas, grains, and pasta contain this type of starch and are part of our healthy diet.

Glycogen (GLYE-koh-jen) is also called *animal starch* and is a highly branched polysaccharide. Glycogen is the form in which humans store glucose; these glucose molecules are joined together in long branched chains called *glycogen*. Glycogen is stored primarily in the liver and skeletal muscle. Glycogen performs

two important roles. First, glycogen stores help regulate blood sugar. When blood sugar levels become low, the glycogen in the liver is converted to glucose and released into the blood, where it restores normal blood sugar levels. When blood glucose increases after a meal, the excess glucose is converted in the liver to glycogen for storage. Second, glycogen acts as storage energy in skeletal muscle. When muscle contractile activity increases, as in running, glycogen is converted to glucose and burned as fuel.

Cellulose is a straight-chain polysaccharide found in plants. Although humans do not have the enzymes to digest cellulose as a source of nutrients, this polysaccharide plays an important role in our digestive process. The cellulose provides the fiber in our diet and improves digestive function.

[?] Re-Think

1. What is the relationship between glucose and glycogen?
2. Where is most glycogen stored?
3. Explain how glycogen helps in the regulation of blood glucose levels.

USES OF GLUCOSE

What about that mound of jelly beans, those oval globs of sugar that you just ate? The jelly beans are eaten, digested, and absorbed. Then what? Glucose is used by the body in three ways: (1) it can be burned immediately as fuel for energy, (2) it can be stored as glycogen and burned as fuel at a later time, and (3) it can be stored as fat and burned as fuel at a later time. The "stored as fat" phrase is the most distressing, from a weight-gain perspective!

THE BREAKDOWN OF GLUCOSE

Glucose is broken down under the following two conditions: (1) in the absence of oxygen (this process is called **anaerobic catabolism**) and (2) in the presence of oxygen (this process is called **aerobic catabolism**). In the absence of oxygen, glucose is broken down through a series of chemical reactions, first into pyruvic acid and then into lactic acid. This anaerobic process occurs in the cytoplasm and is called **glycolysis** (glye-KOHL-i-sis) (Fig. 4.3A). Because most of the energy is still locked up in the lactic acid molecule, glycolysis produces only a small amount of ATP.

If oxygen is available, glucose is completely broken down to form carbon dioxide, water, and ATP (see Fig. 4.3B). The glucose is first broken down to pyruvic acid in the cytoplasm. The pyruvic acid molecules then move into the mitochondria—the "power plants" of the cell. In the presence of oxygen and special enzymes in the mitochondria, the pyruvic acid

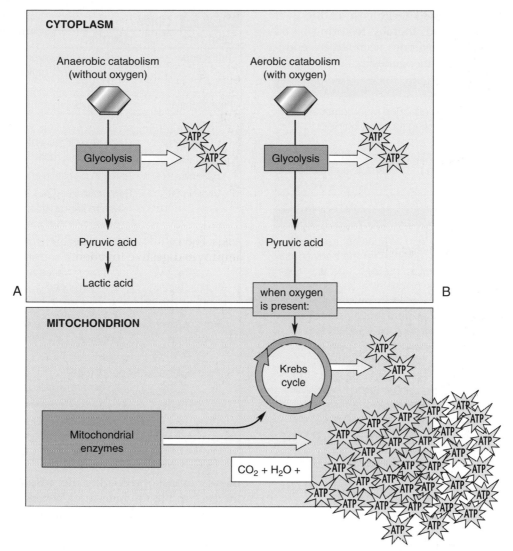

FIG. 4.3 Breakdown of glucose. (A) Anaerobic catabolism, to lactic acid and a little ATP. (B) Aerobic catabolism, to carbon dioxide, water, and lots of ATP.

fragments are completely broken down to carbon dioxide and water. This process is accompanied by the release of a large amount of energy (ATP). Two sets of enzymes exist in the mitochondria: the enzymes of the Krebs cycle and the enzymes of the electron transport chain. Both sets of enzymes work together to produce ATP aerobically.

Three important points about aerobic catabolism should be considered. First, the chemical reactions occurring in the mitochondria require oxygen. If the cells are deprived of oxygen, they soon become low in energy and cannot carry out their functions. This need for oxygen is why we breathe continuously—to ensure a continuous supply of oxygen to the cells. Second, when glucose is broken down completely to carbon dioxide and water, all the stored energy is released. Some of the energy is transferred to ATP, and the rest is released as heat. Thus, the aerobic breakdown of glucose produces much more ATP than the anaerobic breakdown of glucose. Third, if oxygen is not available to the cell, the

pyruvic acid cannot enter the mitochondria. Instead, the pyruvic acid is converted to lactic acid in the cytoplasm. The buildup of lactic acid is the reason that a lack of oxygen in a critically ill patient causes lactic acidosis.

THE MAKING OF GLUCOSE

As we have seen, glucose can be broken down in the cells as a source of energy. The body requires a constant supply of glucose for fuel. Dietary carbohydrates provide glucose, as does the conversion of glycogen into glucose. In addition, the body is capable of making glucose from noncarbohydrate substances. Protein, for example, can be broken down and the breakdown products used to make glucose. The making of glucose from nonglucose sources, especially protein, is called *gluconeogenesis*. **Gluconeogenesis** (gloo-koh-nee-oh-JEN-eh-sis) is an important mechanism in the regulation of blood sugar. For example, if blood sugar declines, protein is converted to glucose in the liver and released into the blood, thereby restoring blood sugar to normal. Many hormones secreted by endocrine glands stimulate gluconeogenesis.

? Re-Think

1. Define glycolysis, noting its effect on blood glucose.
2. Define gluconeogenesis, noting its effect on blood glucose.
3. What purpose is served by gluconeogenesis?
4. Compare ATP production in the anaerobic and aerobic catabolism of glucose.

◎ Sum It Up!

The body, like a factory, requires raw material for growth, repair, and operation. The raw materials for the body come in the form of food: carbohydrates, proteins, and fats. Metabolism refers to the millions of chemical reactions that make the body run. Anabolic reactions are involved in the synthesis of complex substances from simpler substances. Catabolic reactions break down complex substances into simpler substances, generally in an effort to liberate energy stored within the food substances. Carbohydrates and fats are the body's primary fuel. Glucose can be broken down and used as fuel in two ways: anaerobically (glycolysis), yielding little ATP, and aerobically, within the mitochondria (Krebs cycle and electron transport chain enzymes), yielding large amounts of ATP. In addition to the consumption of dietary carbohydrates, glucose can also be made by glycolysis and from the breakdown products of protein by a process called *gluconeogenesis*.

LIPIDS (FATS)

Lipids are organic compounds that are commonly called *fats* and *oils*. Fats are solid at room temperature, whereas oils are liquid. Most of the lipids are eaten as fatty meats, egg yolks, dairy products, and oils. The lipids found most commonly in the body include triglycerides, phospholipids, and steroids. Other relatives of lipids, called *lipoid substances*, are listed in Table 4.2.

The building blocks of lipids are **fatty acids** and **glycerol**. The lipid illustrated in Fig. 4.4A is a triglyceride (try-GLI-ser-ride). It has three (tri) long chains of fatty acids attached to one small glycerol molecule. A phospholipid is formed when a phosphorus-containing group attaches to one of the glycerol sites (see Fig. 4.4B). Phospholipids are important components of the cell membrane. (Do not confuse glycerol with glycogen.)

The steroid is a third type of lipid. The most important steroid in the body is **cholesterol** (see Fig. 4.4C).

Although cholesterol is consumed in the diet, the body can also synthesize cholesterol in the liver. In fact, most of our cholesterol is made by the liver from saturated fat. This observation raises an interesting point regarding the dietary control of cholesterol. The

Table 4.2   Lipids

LIPID TYPE	FUNCTION
Triglyceride	In adipose tissue: protect and insulate body organs; major source of stored energy
Phospholipid	Found in cell membranes
Steroid	
Cholesterol	Used in synthesis of steroids; component of cell membranes
Bile salt	Assist in digestion and absorption of fats
Vitamin D	Synthesized in skin on exposure to ultraviolet radiation; contributes to calcium and phosphate homeostasis
Hormones from adrenal cortex, ovaries, testes	Adrenal cortical hormones are necessary for life and affect every body system; ovaries and testes secrete sex hormones
Lipoid substances	
Fat-soluble vitamins (A, D, E, K)	Variety of functions (identified in later chapters)
Prostaglandins	Found in cell membranes; affect smooth muscle contraction
Lipoproteins	Help transport fatty acids; high-density lipoprotein (HDL) is "good cholesterol" and low-density lipoprotein (LDL) is "bad cholesterol"

dietary intake of a healthy diet results in only a slight increase in blood cholesterol, whereas the dietary intake of saturated fats (meat, eggs, cheeses) accounts for a significant increase of blood cholesterol as it is used by the liver to synthesize cholesterol. Thus, the focus of dietary control of blood cholesterol is the restriction of saturated fats. Despite all the bad press about it, cholesterol performs several important functions. For example, cholesterol is found in all cell membranes and is necessary for the synthesis of vitamin D in the skin. It is also used in the ovaries and testes in the synthesis of the sex hormones.

USES OF LIPIDS

What about the bacon you ate for breakfast? There is good news and bad news. The good news is that lipids are needed by the body (1) as a source of energy, (2) as a component of cell membranes and myelin sheath (coverings of nerve cells), and (3) in the synthesis of steroids. The bad news is that fat can be put into long-term storage. Fat can make you fat! It can also be deposited in areas where it is not wanted, such as inside your blood vessels. Cholesterol-related fatty plaques develop in the walls of the blood vessels (coronary arteries) that supply the heart. Over time, the plaques harden the arteries and block the flow of blood to the heart, resulting in the death of heart muscle (commonly called a *heart attack*).

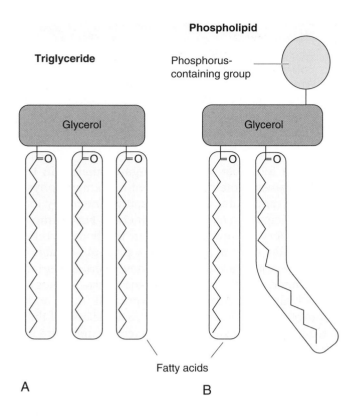

Triglyceride

Phospholipid

Phosphorus-containing group

Glycerol

Glycerol

Fatty acids

A

B

Steroid (cholesterol)

H_3C

CH_3

CH_3

CH_3

CH_3

CH_3

HO

C

FIG. 4.4 **Lipids: A. triglyceride, B. phospholipid, C. steroid**

🔼 Ramp It Up!

Cholesterol, Triglycerides, and Lipoproteins

Cholesterol and triglycerides are lipids that we love to hate, often for very good reason. Both have been implicated in coronary artery heart disease. Cholesterol and triglycerides are lipids and therefore are not soluble in water. Both, however, must be transported by the blood, a water (or aqueous) solution. How is the solubility problem solved? Enter the lipoproteins! They make the cholesterol and triglycerides soluble in water. Read on.

LIPOPROTEINS

A lipoprotein has a basic lipid-soluble core composed of cholesterol and triglycerides, surrounded by a single layer of phospholipid. It is the phospholipid coat that makes the lipid water-soluble. In addition to increasing the solubility of the lipid core, the phospholipid layer contains receptors.

These receptors play a role in the delivery and excretion of cholesterol and triglycerides.

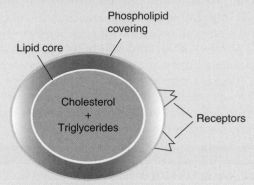

There are six major classes of lipoproteins, but we will describe only three: very low-density lipoprotein (VLDL), low-density lipoprotein (LDL), and high-density lipoprotein (HDL). This classification is based on the density, which is determined by the percentage composition of lipid and protein. Protein is more dense than lipid. Thus, lipoproteins that have a greater proportion of protein than lipid have a relatively high density. Conversely, lipoproteins with a lower percentage of protein have a lower density.

VERY LOW-DENSITY LIPOPROTEIN (VLDL)

VLDLs contain mostly triglycerides and little cholesterol as the core lipid; the triglycerides in VLDL account for almost all the triglycerides in the blood. The role of VLDLs is to transport triglycerides to adipose tissue and muscle. It is unclear about the role of VLDLs in heart disease, but marked elevations cause pancreatitis. The degradation of VLDLs produces LDLs.

LOW-DENSITY LIPOPROTEIN (LDL)

LDLs contain cholesterol as the core lipid and account for most (60% to 70%) of the cholesterol in the blood. The role of LDLs is to deliver cholesterol to nonhepatic (non-liver) tissue. Cells of the target tissues have membrane receptors that recognize and bind to LDLs; on binding, the cholesterol is ingested by the cells by endocytosis. Of all lipoproteins, LDLs make the greatest contribution to atherosclerotic heart disease and are therefore called "bad" cholesterol.

There are a number of drugs that reduce LDLs. The most effective drugs are the "statins," such as lovastatin and pravastatin. The statins reduce LDLs by decreasing the hepatic synthesis of cholesterol and increasing the number of receptors on the liver cells (hepatocytes). The increased number of hepatic receptor sites increases the elimination of cholesterol into the bile.

HIGH-DENSITY LIPOPROTEIN (HDL)

HDLs contain cholesterol as the primary core lipid and account for 20% to 30% of all cholesterol in the blood. HDLs carry cholesterol from the peripheral tissues to the liver for excretion into the bile. Thus, HDLs promote the removal of cholesterol from the blood. Unlike LDLs, which increase the risk of coronary heart disease, elevation of HDLs reduces the risk. Because HDLs are thought to be cardioprotective, they are called "good" cholesterol. Adherence to dietary guidelines, weight reduction, and exercise elevate HDLs.

Like glucose, fatty acids and glycerol can be broken down to release the stored energy. Because the fatty acids are long structures, however, they must be chopped into tiny units before entering the mitochondria and being catabolized within the Krebs cycle. The aerobic burning of the fatty acid units in the mitochondria releases a huge amount of energy that is captured as ATP. Because the fatty acids are much longer than the glucose molecules, the amount of energy released in the burning of fatty acids is much greater than the amount released in the burning of glucose.

Do You Know...

That Griz Does Not Urinate During His Hibernating Months?

Nature encourages the grizzly bear ("Griz") to overeat and gain weight. By doing so, Griz is able to hibernate during the winter months because he can live off the fat stored during the summer feeding frenzy. While hibernating, the bear's fat is gradually broken down, and the energy that is released is sufficient to keep him alive.

What, then, about the waste produced by his metabolizing body? The bear has apparently developed the metabolic ability to convert his waste (urea) into a substance that can be used by the body. He literally recycles the "waste" that is normally excreted in urine. An understanding of this recycling process would certainly benefit the many persons who require dialysis because of kidney failure.

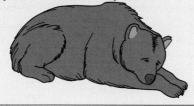

MAKING FAT

Like Griz, we too can go on a feeding frenzy and gain pound after pound! However, we do not hibernate and fast and therefore do not easily shed those excess pounds. The extra doughnut eaten today is worn on your hips tomorrow. When excess calories are consumed, the hormones and enzymes that promote fat synthesis are stimulated. The fat is deposited in adipose tissue throughout the body.

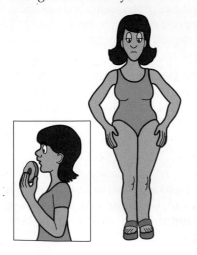

 Re-Think

1. What is a triglyceride?
2. Why is it unwise to feed an infant only "fat-free" milk?
3. Why does the catabolism of a fatty acid yield so much more ATP than does the catabolism of glucose?

PROTEINS

Protein is the most abundant organic matter in the body. Because proteins are present in so many physiologically important compounds, it is safe to say that they participate in every body function. For example, almost every chemical reaction in the body is regulated by an enzyme, which is a protein substance. Most hormones are proteins; they exert important widespread effects throughout the body. Hemoglobin, which delivers oxygen to every cell in the body, is a protein. Finally, muscles contract because of their contractile proteins. As you can see, proteins are essential to life.

AMINO ACIDS

The building blocks of protein are **amino acids**. About 20 amino acids are used to build body protein. Most amino acids come from protein foods, especially lean meat, milk, and eggs. More than half of the amino acids can be synthesized by the body. If the diet lacks the amino acid alanine, for example, alanine can be synthesized in the liver.

Some amino acids, however, cannot be synthesized by the body and must be obtained from dietary sources. Because dietary intake of these amino acids is essential, these amino acids are called *essential amino acids*. The amino acids that can be synthesized by the liver are called *nonessential amino acids*, meaning that these amino acids are not absolutely necessary in the diet. See Box 4.1 for a list of common amino acids.

NOTE: The word *nonessential* does not mean that these amino acids are not essential to the body. The term refers to the ability of the body to synthesize these amino acids when they are not included in the diet.

Like carbohydrates and lipids, amino acids are composed of carbon, hydrogen, and oxygen. In addition to these three elements, amino acids also contain nitrogen. The nitrogen appears as an amine group (NH_2). At the other end of the amino acid is the acid group (—COOH); hence, the name *amino acid*. Note the amine group and the acid group in Fig. 4.5A; the amino acid alanine is used as an example.

Amino acids are joined together by peptide bonds. A **peptide bond** is formed when the amine group (NH_2) of one amino acid joins with the acid group (—COOH) of a second amino acid. A peptide is formed when several amino acids are joined together by peptide bonds (see Fig. 4.5B). A polypeptide is formed when many amino acids are joined together. Proteins are very large polypeptides. Most proteins are composed of more than one polypeptide chain. The polypeptide chains are curly and coil around each other, creating a large and uniquely shaped protein. The amino acid sequence and the size and shape of the protein are important to its function. If the amino acids are not assembled in the correct order, the shape of the protein changes and its function is impaired. For example, in sickle cell anemia, only one of the amino acids is "out of order" in the hemoglobin protein, the major component of a red blood cell. The improperly constructed hemoglobin causes the red blood cells to sickle and break apart.

Proteins can bond with other organic compounds. For example, the combination of a sugar and a protein forms a glycoprotein, whereas the combination of a lipid and protein creates a lipoprotein.

USES OF PROTEINS

Proteins are used in three ways. The most important use is in the synthesis of hormones, enzymes, antibodies, plasma, muscle proteins, hemoglobin, and most cell membranes. In one way or another, proteins play a key role in every physiological function. The various types of proteins and their functions are listed in Table 4.3. With such a large demand for protein, most of the amino acids are carefully conserved by the body and used in the synthesis of protein.

Proteins have two less common uses. First, protein can be broken down and used as fuel, as a source of energy for ATP production. This process, however, is not desirable. The preferred energy sources are glucose and fat. Second, protein can be broken down and converted to glucose (gluconeogenesis). This mechanism is used by the body to ensure that the blood glucose level does not become too low to sustain life. In severe starvation, the body catabolizes its own protein, including the heart muscle, in order to survive.

❓ Re-Think

1. What is the most important use of amino acids?
2. What is the difference between an essential and nonessential amino acid?
3. Why do peptide bonds form between amino acids and not between glycogen molecules?

BREAKDOWN OF PROTEIN AND THE PROBLEM WITH AMMONIA

Because amino acids contain nitrogen, as well as carbon, hydrogen, and oxygen, the breakdown of protein poses a special problem. Carbon, hydrogen, and oxygen can be broken down into carbon dioxide and water and eliminated from the body. The nitrogen part of the amino acid, however, must be handled in a special way, primarily by the liver. Nitrogen is either recycled and used to synthesize different amino acids or converted to urea and excreted.

Formation of Urea

Some of the nitrogen released by the breakdown of amino acids is converted to **urea** by the liver (Fig. 4.6). Note the nitrogen in the structural formula of urea. Blood then carries the urea, a nitrogenous waste, from the liver to the kidneys, where it is eliminated in the urine. This is important clinical information and forms the basis for several diagnostic tests.

A diagnostic test called the *blood urea nitrogen* (BUN) test measures the amount of urea in the blood. A change in BUN can be caused by either poor liver function (cannot make urea) or poor kidney function (cannot excrete it).

Box 4.1 Common Amino Acids

Alanine	Leucine*
Arginine	Lysine*
Asparagine	Methionine*
Aspartic acid	Phenylalanine*
Cysteine	Proline
Glutamic acid	Serine
Glutamine	Threonine*
Glycine	Tryptophan*
Histidine*	Tyrosine
Isoleucine*	Valine*

*Essential amino acids.

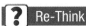

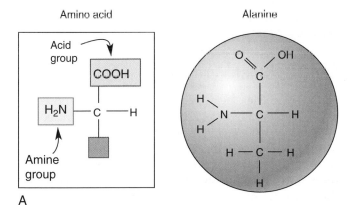

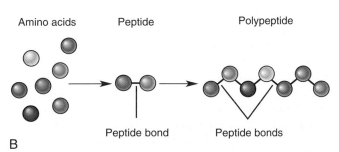

FIG. 4.5 Amino acids and proteins. (A) The structure of an amino acid (alanine). (B) The assembly of amino acids to form a polypeptide. Note the peptide bonds.

Table **4.3** Proteins

TYPE	FUNCTION
Structural proteins	
Components of cell membranes	Perform many functions: determine pore size; allow hormones to "recognize" cell
Collagen	Structural component of muscle and tendons
Keratin	Part of skin and hair
Peptide hormones	Many hormones are proteins; have widespread effects on many organ systems (e.g., insulin, growth hormone)
Hemoglobin	Transports oxygen
Antibodies	Protect body from disease-causing microorganisms
Plasma proteins	Used in blood clotting, fluid balance, and defense against disease
Muscle proteins	Enable muscles to contract
Enzymes	Regulate the rates of chemical reactions

Worrying about ammonia. Why does the liver "worry" about **ammonia**? Under normal conditions, the liver extracts ammonia (NH_3) from the blood and converts it to urea. Why? Ammonia is toxic to brain cells and causes disorientation and a diminished level of consciousness. In liver failure, the extraction of ammonia from the blood is diminished, so blood levels of ammonia rise. The toxic effect of ammonia on the brain is called *hepatic encephalopathy* (heh-PAT-ik en-sef-al-OP-eh-thee).

 Re-Think

1. Why is urea production so important?
2. What happens if a damaged liver is unable to make urea?
3. Why may an elevated BUN indicate poor kidney function?

 Sum It Up!

There are three types of lipids: triglycerides, phospholipids, and steroids. Cholesterol is the most important steroid. Lipids are used in the synthesis of cell membranes and steroids and in the storage of energy; they are catabolized as fuels. Amino acids are used primarily in the synthesis of body proteins: hormones, enzymes, antibodies, plasma proteins, and structural components of cells. Amino acids join together by peptide bonds, whereby the amine group ($-NH_2$) of one amino acid joins with the acid group ($-COOH$) of a second amino acid. In addition to carbon, hydrogen, and oxygen, the catabolism of proteins produces nitrogen that is toxic to the brain. The hepatic (liver) production and renal (kidney) excretion of the nitrogenous waste, urea, is the biochemical solution to ammonia (NH_3) toxicity.

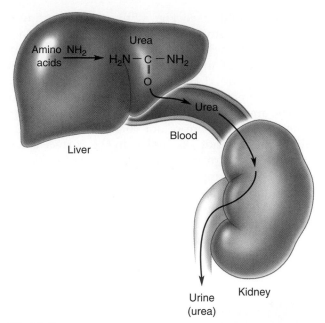

FIG. **4.6** Urea: formation in the liver and excretion by the kidney.

PROTEIN SYNTHESIS AND DNA

Proteins play a crucial role in every body function. Protein synthesis involves the arrangement of amino acids in a specific sequence. Because the sequencing of amino acids is so precise, there is an elaborate protein-synthesizing mechanism in each cell. How does the cell know the exact pattern of amino acid assembly? The pattern of amino acid assembly is coded and stored in the **deoxyribonucleic** (de-OX-see-rye-boh-noo-KLAY-ik) **acid (DNA)** in the nucleus. In fact, the essential role of DNA is to serve as a code for the structure of protein.

DNA STRUCTURE

DNA is a nucleic acid. Nucleic acids are composed of smaller units called *nucleotides* (Fig. 4.7A). A nucleotide has three parts: a sugar, a phosphate group, and a base. Nucleotides are joined together to form long strands. Two strands of nucleotides are arranged in a twisted ladder formation (the double helix) to form DNA (see Fig. 4.7B). The two sides of the DNA ladder are composed of sugar and phosphate molecules. The rungs, or steps, of the ladder are composed of bases, one base from each side. The names of the bases in DNA are adenine (A), cytosine (C), guanine (G), and thymine (T). Note the different shapes of the bases in the rungs of the ladder. Note also that the bases have a particular arrangement. Adenine can pair only with thymine, and cytosine can pair only with guanine. Adenine and thymine are base pairs, as are cytosine and guanine. This system is called **base pairing**.

THE GENETIC CODE

The protein-synthesizing code is stored within the DNA. More specifically, the information is stored, or encoded, within the sequence of bases along one strand (one side of the ladder) of DNA (Fig. 4.8). Because the DNA is arranged in hereditary units called *genes*, the code is called the **genetic code**. (Genes and heredity are discussed further in Chapter 27.)

Reading the Code

A single strand of DNA (see Fig. 4.8) reads vertically (according to the bases in the rungs), such as GAC-GCCCAA. GAC (a sequence of three bases) codes for a particular amino acid, GCC codes for another amino acid, and CAA codes for a third amino acid. The list of bases in triplicate is called **base sequencing**. In this way, DNA codes for the proper sequence of amino acids and therefore the synthesis of protein.

NOTE: Do not confuse base pairing with base sequencing. *Base pairing* describes the way in which two strands of DNA are linked together by the bases. *Base sequencing* describes the sequence, or order, of the bases along a single strand of DNA. The code is stored within the sequence of bases.

Copying the Code: mRNA

The code for protein synthesis is stored in the nucleus in the DNA. DNA does not leave the nucleus because it is too large to fit through the pores of the nuclear membrane. Protein synthesis, however, occurs along the ribosomes in the cytoplasm. The big question? How does the code get out of the nucleus and into the cytoplasm? The copying and delivery of the code is done by a second nucleic acid called **ribonucleic** (rye-boh-noo-KLAY-ik) **acid (RNA)**.

RNA is a nucleic acid composed of nucleotides and resembles the structure of DNA. RNA differs from DNA in three ways:

1. The sugars are different. The sugar in DNA is deoxyribose, whereas the sugar in RNA is ribose.
2. DNA has two strands, whereas RNA has only one strand.
3. There is a difference in one of the bases. Both DNA and RNA contain cytosine (C), guanine (G), and adenine (A). The fourth base differs. DNA contains thymine (T), whereas RNA contains uracil (U). The uracil in RNA forms a base pair with adenine. The differences between DNA and RNA are summarized in Table 4.4.

There are three types of RNA, but we are concerned only with messenger RNA (mRNA) and transfer RNA (tRNA). Messenger RNA copies the code from DNA in the nucleus and then carries the code, or message, to the ribosomes in the cytoplasm. Because this type of RNA acts as a messenger, it is called *mRNA*.

Transfer RNA (tRNA) is found attached to individual amino acids within the cytoplasm and, through its own base sequencing, can "read" the code on the mRNA sitting on the ribosome. Each individual amino acid is carried by tRNA to its proper site on the mRNA. The amino acids are assembled in the proper sequence as the polypeptide (protein) is formed.

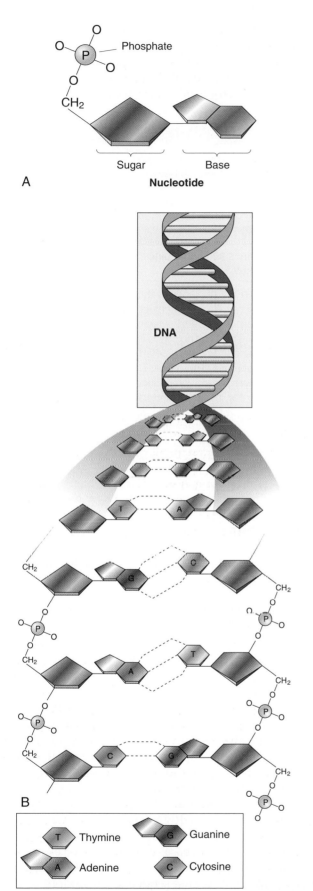

FIG. 4.7 (A) Nucleotide. (B) The ladder structure of DNA. Note the base pairing of the DNA strands.

mRNA as Copycat

Refer to Fig. 4.8 as we see how mRNA copies the code. DNA separates and exposes the base sequences, GACGCCCAA. A strand of mRNA reads the base sequence by forming base pairs. The strand of mRNA has this code: CUGCGGGUU. (The mRNA is not shown.) The copying of the code by mRNA is called **transcription**.

NOTE: Transcription is a base-pairing event. Following transcription, the mRNA takes the code to the ribosomes in the cytoplasm, where the amino acids will be assembled.

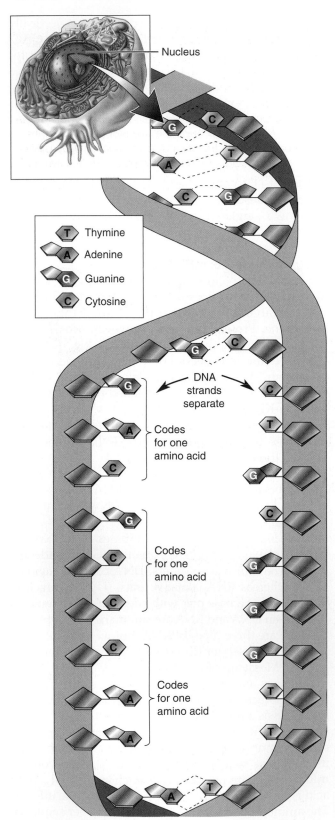

FIG. 4.8 DNA: genetic code and base sequencing.

Thymine

Adenine

Guanine

Cytosine

Nucleus

DNA strands separate

Codes for one amino acid

Codes for one amino acid

Codes for one amino acid

? Re-Think

1. List three differences between DNA and RNA.
2. What is the difference between base pairing and base sequencing?
3. Explain how the base sequence codes for a protein.

Do You Know...

What Are Purines and Pyrimidines, and Why Are Cancer Drugs Aimed at Them?

The bases in the nucleotides that make up DNA and RNA are classified as either purines or pyrimidines. Adenine and guanine are purines, and cytosine, thymine, and uracil are pyrimidines. This terminology is important to know because some anticancer drugs are called *purine analogs* and others *pyrimidine analogs*. This means that the drugs resemble purines and pyrimidines. When incorporated into the DNA or RNA molecules, the drugs introduce errors into the genetic code, impair protein synthesis, and kill the cancer cell. Unfortunately, the drugs are also incorporated into many normal cells, thereby causing their death and producing many of the toxic effects of cancer therapy. No wonder these anticancer drugs are classified as cytotoxic agents; they are toxic to both cancer and normal cells.

STEPS IN PROTEIN SYNTHESIS

How do DNA and RNA control protein synthesis? See Fig. 4.9 and identify the following five steps in protein synthesis:

1. When a particular protein is to be synthesized, the strands of DNA in the nucleus separate. The exposed sequence of bases on the separated DNA strand is copied onto a strand of mRNA (transcription).
2. The mRNA leaves the nucleus and travels to the ribosomes in the cytoplasm.
3. The code on the mRNA (now sitting on a ribosome) determines which amino acids can attach to it. For example, the code may specify that only the amino acid alanine can bind to site 1 and only the amino acid cysteine can bind to site 2. How does alanine (located in the cytoplasm) know that it should move to the ribosome for protein assembly? Alanine is attached to tRNA. The tRNA contains bases, a sequence called its *anticodon*, that can recognize and pair with the bases on mRNA. For example, if mRNA contains the base sequence GCA, then only a tRNA with the base sequence (anticodon) of CGU can attach to that site. The reading of the mRNA code by tRNA is called **translation**. Like transcription (nucleus), translation (cytoplasm–ribosomes) is a base-pairing event.

4. The amino acids are lined up in proper sequence along the ribosome. A peptide bond forms between each amino acid, creating a growing peptide chain.

5. When all the amino acids have been assembled in the exact sequence dictated by the code, the protein chain is terminated. A complete protein has been created. The protein is now ready for use in the cell or for export to another site outside the cell.

Table 4.4   Comparison of DNA and RNA Structures

	DNA	RNA
Sugar	Deoxyribose	Ribose
Base	Adenine	Adenine
	Guanine	Guanine
	Cytosine	Cytosine
	Thymine	Uracil
Strands	Double (two)	Single (one)

 Re-Think

1. Differentiate between the roles of mRNA and tRNA. Use the word *anticodon* in your response.
2. What is the difference between transcription and translation?

Sum It Up!

Body structure and function are largely determined by the specific proteins synthesized by the cells. Because of the crucial roles played by proteins, an elaborate cellular mechanism guides the assembly of the amino acids into proteins. Your protein blueprint, or genetic code, is stored in the DNA in the nucleus. When there is a need for protein synthesis, the code must be transferred to the ribosome by mRNA, where amino acid assembly takes place. Protein synthesis occurs in five steps (see Fig. 4.9).

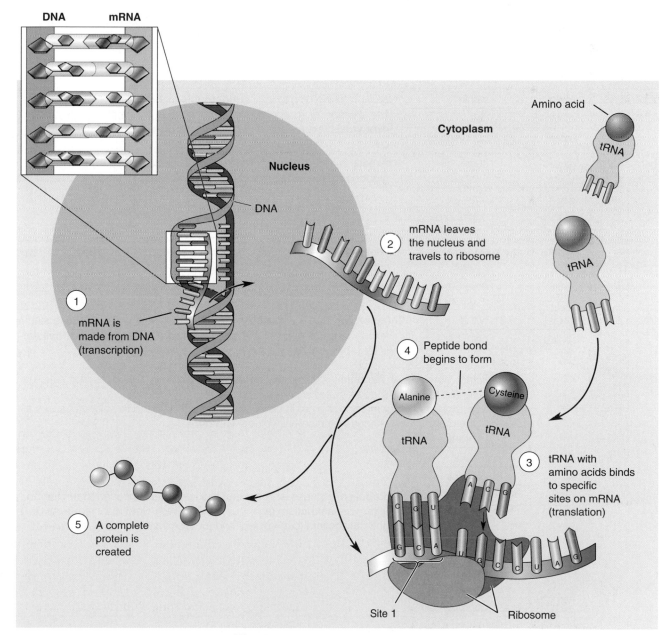

FIG. 4.9 Steps (1 to 5) in protein synthesis.

As You Age

1. Age brings a decrease in the number and function of organelles such as mitochondria. Because mitochondria play a key role in metabolism, a decrease in mitochondrial function affects metabolism.
2. In general, metabolism slows with aging. This effect is a result of a decrease in hormonal secretion, particularly the thyroid hormones. A decreased metabolism has

several effects: less tolerance to cold, a tendency to gain weight, and metabolic effects, such as a decreased efficiency in using glucose.
3. The rate of protein synthesis decreases. Tissue growth and repair slow down, as does the synthesis of other proteins, such as digestive enzymes.

Medical Terminology and Disorders   Cell Function and Disorders of the Cell

MEDICAL TERM	WORD PARTS	WORD PART MEANING OR DERIVATION	DESCRIPTION
Words			
anaerobic	an-	without	An **anaerobic** reaction occurs in the absence of oxygen. For example, lactic acid is produced by the anaerobic metabolism of glucose. **Aerobic** (with oxygen) catabolism of glucose is more efficient with regard to energy (ATP) production.
	-aer/o-	air or gas	
	-ic	pertaining to	
cytology	cyt/o-	cell	Broadly, **cytology** is *a branch of biology concerned with the study of cell structure and function.* From the medical perspective, cytology is a branch of pathology that is concerned with the diagnosis of disease and disorders through examination of tissue samples. The Pap smear is a **cytological** examination used to detect cancer.
	-logy	study of	
endocytosis	endo-	within	"Cellular drinking" is a type of **endocytosis** that moves water into the cell. *The ejection of a digestive enzyme from a pancreatic cell* is called **exocytosis** (ex/o = outside), or the movement of the enzyme out of the cell.
	-cyt/o-	cell	
	-osis	condition of	
gluconeogen-esis	gluc/o-	sugar, glucose	A diabetic is hyperglycemic (elevated blood glucose), in part, because of **gluconeogenesis,** the making of new glucose from a nonglucose source.
	-neo-	new	
	-gen/o-	origin, production	
glycolysis	glyc/o-	sugar, glucose	**Glycolysis** is *the anaerobic breakdown (catabolism) of glucose to lactic acid.*
	-lysis	breakdown, dissolution	
intracellular	intra-	within	**Intracellular** (intra = within) refers to *the space inside a cell*. **Extracellular** (extra = outside) refers to *the space outside the cell*. The **intercellular** (inter = between) space is *the space between the cells.*
	-cell/u-	cell	
	-ar	pertaining to	
isotonic	iso-	*same* with regard to stretch of the membrane	An **isotonic** (same stretch) **solution** is *a solution that does not cause a change in cell volume or pressure.* Submersion of a cell in either a hypotonic or hypertonic solution causes a change in intracellular volume and pressure.
	-ton/o-	tension	
	-ic	pertaining to	
metabolism	meta-	beyond	**Metabolism** includes all of the enzymatic reactions needed to run the body. It includes **anabolism** (ana = up, and a Greek word meaning "to throw") and **catabolism** (cat = down, and a Greek word meaning "to throw").
	-bol-	From a Greek word, *ballein,* meaning "to throw"	
	-ism	condition of	

Medical Terminology and Disorders | Cell Function and Disorders of the Cell—cont'd

MEDICAL TERM	WORD PARTS	WORD PART MEANING OR DERIVATION	DESCRIPTION
monosaccha-ride	mono-	one	Glucose is a **monosaccharide,** or *a simple sugar*. Sucrose is table sugar, or a **disaccharide** (di = two). Glycogen is a **polysaccharide** (poly = many).
	-saccharide	From a Greek word meaning "sugar"	
synthesis	syn-	together, with	**Synthesis** means *the putting together of simpler substances to make a larger, more complex substance.*
	-thesis	From a Greek word meaning "to put"	
transport	trans-	across	**Transport** means *to carry from one place to another*. Most water and dissolved solute is transported by diffusion.
	-port	From a Latin word meaning "to carry"	

Disorders

Adaptive Cellular Changes

atrophy	a-	without	*A cellular adaptive process that results in a decrease in the size of a tissue or organ caused by a decrease in the number of cells or a reduction in cell size.* Numerous causes: resulting from a disease such as muscular dystrophy; diminished blood supply, muscle inactivity, nutritional deficiency, and the natural aging process.
	-troph-	develop-ment; nourish-ment	
	-y	condition of	
hypertrophy	hyper-	excessive	*An increase in the size (not number) of cells.* **Hypertrophy** is *a response to increased workload*. Lifting weights hypertrophies arm and shoulder muscles.
	-troph-	development	
	-y	condition of, process	
hyperplasia	hyper-	excessive	*An increase in the number of cells caused by an increase in cell division.* There is compensatory and hormonal hyperplasia. An increase in the number of liver cells subsequent to the removal of part of the liver is an example of **compensatory hyperplasia.** The uterine response to estrogen is an example of **hormonal hyperplasia.**
	-plasia	formation	
metaplasia	meta-	beyond, after, change	*A reversible cellular transformation (from one cell type to another).* Cigarette smoking can cause the transformation of columnar epithelium into squamous epithelium; cessation of smoking can reverse the cellular change.
	-plasia	formation	

Maladaptive Cellular Changes

dysplasia	dys-	faulty	*A maladaptive cellular disorder in which the cells show evidence of abnormal differentiation, resulting in changes in cell size, shape, and appearance.* Dysplasias, such as cervical dysplasia, are considered malignant precursors.
	-plasia	formation	
anaplasia	ana-	up; apart	*A serious maladaptive* (mal = bad) *cellular change.* Cells are poorly differentiated (immature and embryonic). Anaplastic cell growth is characteristic of malignant (cancerous) cells.
	-plasia	formation	

Get Ready for Exams!

Summary Outline

To carry on its functions, the cell must metabolize carbohydrates, proteins, and fats.

I. Metabolism
  A. Anabolism: chemical reactions that build more complex substances from simpler substances
  B. Catabolism: chemical reactions that break down complex substances into simpler substances

II. Carbohydrates: Structure and Function
  A. Carbohydrates: composed of carbon, hydrogen, and oxygen; classified as monosaccharides, disaccharides, and polysaccharides
  B. Glucose: the primary source of energy
  C. Glucose: can be stored as glycogen or converted to and stored as fat
  D. Glucose: can be catabolized anaerobically and aerobically. Anaerobically, glucose is incompletely broken down (glycolysis) into lactic acid and small amounts of ATP. Aerobically, glucose is broken down completely (Krebs cycle) into carbon dioxide (CO_2) and water (H_2O) and large amounts of energy (ATP).
  E. Glucose: can be synthesized from nonglucose substances such as protein; called gluconeogenesis

III. Lipids
  A. Most common lipids are triglycerides, phospholipids, and steroids
  B. Cholesterol: the most important steroid; made soluble by lipoprotein; called "good" and "bad"
  C. Lipids: used primarily in the synthesis of membranes and fuel
  D. Long fatty acid chains: broken down into two-carbon units and metabolized by the enzymes of Krebs cycle and electron transport chain enzymes to CO_2 and H_2O, releasing large amounts of energy (ATP)

IV. Proteins
  A. Proteins: composed of amino acids linked together by peptide bonds in a specific sequence
  B. Proteins: used primarily in the synthesis of hormones, enzymes, antibodies, plasma proteins, muscle proteins, hemoglobin, and cell membranes; also used as fuel and for gluconeogenesis
  C. Urea synthesis: special handling of protein nitrogen by enzymes in the liver

V. Protein Synthesis and DNA
  A. DNA (deoxyribonucleic acid)
    1. DNA: stores the code for protein synthesis
    2. DNA: double-stranded series of nucleotides, arranged in a twisted ladder formation
    3. Nucleotide: composed of a sugar, a phosphate group, and a base. For DNA, the sugar is deoxyribose; the bases are adenine, thymine, cytosine, and guanine.
    4. Genetic code: stored in a sequence of three bases
    5. Base pairs with DNA and RNA

  B. RNA
    1. Ribonucleic acid (RNA): similar structure to DNA, with the following differences. In RNA, the sugar is ribose, RNA is single-stranded, and the RNA bases are adenine, uracil, cytosine, and guanine.
    2. Two types of RNA: messenger RNA (mRNA) and transfer RNA (tRNA)
    3. Transcription: DNA and mRNA (occurs within nucleus)
    4. Translation: mRNA and tRNA (occurs within cytoplasm/ribosomes)
  C. Protein synthesis: five steps, summarized in Fig. 4.9

Review Your Knowledge

Matching: Carbohydrates, Proteins, and Fats
Directions: Match the following words with their descriptions. Some words may be used more than once.

a. glycogen
b. amino acids
c. lipids
d. urea
e. monosaccharides
f. glucose
g. disaccharides
h. fatty acids and glycerol

1. ___ Nitrogen-containing waste product
2. ___ Building blocks of proteins
3. ___ Classification of steroids and triglycerides
4. ___ Sucrose, maltose, and lactose
5. ___ Monosaccharide that is chief fuel for the body
6. ___ Building blocks held together by peptide bonds
7. ___ Building blocks of lipids
8. ___ Storage form of glucose
9. ___ Glucose, fructose, and galactose
10. ___ Animal starch stored in the liver and skeletal muscles

Matching: Biochemistry Terms
Directions: Match the following words with their descriptions. Some words may be used more than once.

a. glycolysis
b. Krebs cycle and electron transport chain enzymes
c. gluconeogenesis
d. enzyme
e. ketone bodies

1. ___ Series of aerobic reactions that occur within the mitochondria
2. ___ Series of anaerobic reactions that occur within the cytoplasm
3. ___ Process of converting protein to glucose
4. ___ Catalyst
5. ___ Series of reactions that convert glucose to lactic acid
6. ___ Metabolic consequence of rapid and incomplete breakdown of fatty acids

Matching: Genetic Code and Protein Synthesis
Directions: Match the following words with their descriptions.

a. mRNA
b. ribose
c. base pairing
d. DNA
e. base sequencing

1. ___ Double-stranded nucleotide that stores the genetic code
2. ___ The manner in which the genetic code is stored
3. ___ The manner whereby one strand of a nucleotide interacts with another
4. ___ Single-stranded nucleotide that brings the code from the nucleus to the ribosomes
5. ___ A sugar used in the formation of a nucleotide

Multiple Choice

1. Which of the following is true of the Krebs cycle and electron transport chain enzymes?
   a. Are located within the mitochondria
   b. Function anaerobically
   c. Result in lactic acid production
   d. Are responsible for glycolysis

2. Which of the following is *not* characteristic of glycolysis?
   a. Occurs within the cytoplasm
   b. Operates anaerobically
   c. Forms lactic acid
   d. Completely metabolizes glucose to CO_2, H_2O, and energy

3. Characteristics of urea include which of the following?
   a. Formed in the liver
   b. Contains nitrogen
   c. Excreted by the kidneys
   d. All of the above

4. Which of the following is true of amino acids?
   a. Joined together by peptide bonds
   b. Are the building blocks of polysaccharides
   c. Classified as monosaccharides, disaccharides, and polysaccharides
   d. Classified as saturated and unsaturated

5. Monosaccharides
   a. include glucose, fructose, and galactose.
   b. include sucrose, lactose, and maltose.
   c. are classified as saturated and unsaturated.
   d. are the building blocks of protein.

6. Which of the following is descriptive of glycogen?
   a. Can be converted to glucose, thereby elevating the blood glucose level
   b. Combines with three fatty acids to form a lipid
   c. Contains nitrogen
   d. Is a disaccharide

7. Gluconeogenesis is a series of
   a. reactions that catabolize glycogen to glucose.
   b. reactions that use protein to make glucose.
   c. anaerobic reactions that catabolize glucose to lactic acid.
   d. reactions that convert lactic acid to ketoacids.

8. Peptide bonds are formed between
   a. glycerol and fatty acids.
   b. glucose, fructose, and galactose.
   c. alanine, phenylalanine, and arginine.
   d. urea and ammonia.

9. When blood sugar declines, hepatic glycogen is converted into
   a. ammonia.
   b. urea.
   c. glucose.
   d. glycerol.

10. Translation
    a. is a base-pairing event between DNA and mRNA.
    b. is a base-sequencing event confined to the nucleus.
    c. is a base-pairing event between mRNA and tRNA along the ribosome.
    d. refers to the copying of DNA by mRNA.

11. What is determined by the sequence of bases in DNA and RNA?
    a. The order of amino acids in the formation of a protein
    b. The directions for the formation of glycogen from glucose
    c. The directions for the assembly of fats from fatty acids and glycerol
    d. The directions for the release of energy from ATP

12. Adenine, thymine, cytosine, and guanine are
    a. monosaccharides that provide the energy for protein synthesis.
    b. bases that form the rungs or steps of DNA.
    c. essential amino acids.
    d. Krebs cycle enzymes.

13. The double helix refers to
    a. the growing peptide sitting along the ribosome.
    b. the transcribed strand of mRNA.
    c. transcription and translation.
    d. the double-stranded DNA arrangement into a twisted ladder structure.

14. DNA is arranged in hereditary units called
    a. genes.
    b. ribosomes.
    c. lysosomes.
    d. peptides.

15. Which of the following represents base pairing?
    a. ATT, CCG, CCC
    b. AT, CG, GC, AU
    c. Alanine, phenylalanine, glycine, arginine
    d. Sugar–phosphate, sugar–phosphate

Go Figure

1. Which of the following is true according to Fig. 4.1?
   a. The assembly of amino acids into protein is called protein catabolism.
   b. Anabolic reactions are represented by the destruction of the brick wall.
   c. Catabolic reactions generally release energy.
   d. Anabolic reactions are generally accompanied by the release of energy. .

2. Which of the following is true according to Fig. 4.2 and Table 4.1?
   a. A disaccharide contains two polysaccharides.
   b. When enzymatically split, sucrose yields glucose and lactose.
   c. When enzymatically split, maltose yields two glycogens.
   d. Excess glucose is stored as glycogen in the liver and skeletal muscle.

3. Which of the following is true according to Fig. 4.3?
   a. Most ATP is generated by glycolysis.
   b. Glycolysis is an aerobic catabolic pathway.
   c. Under aerobic conditions, the end-products of glycolysis enter the mitochondria, where they are completely metabolized to CO_2, water, and ATP.
   d. Fig. 4.3A illustrates glycolysis, whereas Fig. 4.3B, illustrates gluconeogenesis.

4. Which of the following is true according to Fig. 4.3A?
   a. Pyruvic acid is aerobically metabolized to lactic acid.
   b. Lactic acid is generated under anaerobic conditions.
   c. Lactic acid is produced within the mitochondrion under aerobic conditions.
   d. Mitochondrial ATP production is dependent on the production of lactic acid.

5. Which of the following is true according to Table 4.2 and Fig. 4.4?
   a. Cholesterol and adrenal cortical hormones are steroids.
   b. All lipoid substances are steroids.
   c. All cholesterol is "bad."
   d. Glycerol, an alcohol, can only combine with long-chain fatty acids.

6. Which of the following is true according to Box 4.1 and Fig. 4.5?
   a. All amino acids in Box 4.1 contain an $-NH_2$ and $-COOH$ group.
   b. All amino acids in Box 4.1 are essential.
   c. The only amino acids that form peptide bonds are alanine and phenylalanine.
   d. Peptide bonds form when the $-COOH$ group of one amino acid combines with the $-COOH$ group of a second amino acid.

7. Which of the following is true according to Fig. 4.6?
   a. Urea is a nitrogen-containing waste product produced in the kidney.
   b. Urea is transported from the kidneys to the liver, where it is excreted into the bile and eliminated from the body.
   c. Urea is produced in the liver and excreted by the kidneys in the urine.
   d. Urea is produced in the blood and excreted by both the liver and the kidneys.

8. Which of the following is true according to Fig. 4.7?
   a. DNA is single stranded.
   b. The bases are called ribose and deoxyribose.
   c. The rung of the DNA ladder is formed by sugar–phosphate bonds.
   d. A nucleotide is composed of three parts: a sugar, phosphate, and base.

9. Which of the following is true according to Fig. 4.8?
   a. Cytosine can base pair with thymine.
   b. Adenine can base pair with thymine.
   c. Structurally, adenine resembles thymine more than it resembles guanine.
   d. Thymine can base pair with both adenine and guanine.

10. Which of the following is true according to Fig. 4.9?
    a. mRNA is transcribed from DNA in the nucleus.
    b. DNA is transcribed from mRNA in the nucleus.
    c. mRNA cannot leave the nucleus.
    d. The assembly of amino acids into peptide strands occurs in the nucleus.

11. Which of the following is true according to Fig. 4.9?
    a. The assembly of amino acids occurs along the ribosomes in the cytoplasm.
    b. mRNA carries the genetic code from the nucleus to the ribosomes in the cytoplasm.
    c. Translation involves base pairing between mRNA and tRNA in the cytoplasm.
    d. All of the above are true.

Microbiology Basics

Objectives

1. Define *disease* and *infection*.
2. List the characteristics of the different types of pathogens, including the types of bacteria by shape.
3. Describe the types of bacteria by staining characteristics.
4. Define portals of exit and portals of entry.
5. List common ways in which infections are spread.
6. Identify the microbiological principles described in Five Germ-Laden Stories.

Key Terms

bacteria (p. 66)
carrier (p. 67)
colonization (p. 65)
contacts (p. 67)
disease (p. 65)
fungus (p. 68)
helminths (p. 69)
infection (p. 65)

local infection (p. 65)
microbiota (p. 66)
mycotic infection (p. 68)
normal flora (p. 66)
nosocomial infection (p. 74)
parasites (p. 68)
pathogens (p. 65)
protozoa (p. 68)

rickettsia (p. 68)
spores (p. 68)
sporozoa (p. 68)
systemic infection (p. 65)
vector (p. 69)
viruses (p. 68)
zoonosis (p. 75)

For as long as humans have roamed the earth, we have been plagued by disease, especially infectious disease. A long and colorful history of medicine relates many tales of how we learned to dose, purge, lance, and in-cant. Sometimes we managed to arrest and cure the disease, but many times we killed the patient long before we killed the germs. The battle against disease is far from over. The microbial warriors are tough; they mount a great offensive and are very persistent! Although we may not tremble at the thought of the Black Death that terrorized Europe in the 1300s, we tremble at the thought of other plagues around today, as well as those that can erupt tomorrow. We are liv-ing through the terror of infection by the Ebola virus, and we dread an outbreak of avian or swine flu, the contamination of a minor abrasion with flesh-eating streptococcus, and the possibility of contracting mad cow disease, of all things! What about the new genera-tion of life-threatening "superbugs" that are resistant to all antibiotics? And lately? The growing threat of mosquito-borne illnesses. In the past we confronted the challenges of yellow fever and malaria. Today, the mosquitoes have made their threatening presence known through recent outbreaks of infections by the Zika virus.

This chapter provides background information about microbiology—the world of microorganisms, those tiny critters that keep scientists glued to their microscopes. Chapter 21 describes the body's response to this microbial challenge.

WHAT IS DISEASE?

Disease is a failure of the body to function norma-lly. There are many types of diseases, not all caused by germs. These include inherited diseases, diseases caused by birth defects, age-related degenerative dis-eases, diseases caused by nutritional deficiencies, tu-mors, and diseases related to trauma and environmen-tal toxins. This chapter focuses on infectious disease. Although most microorganisms are harmless or even beneficial to the body, some are harmful, causing dis-ease and sometimes death. A leading cause of disease in humans is the invasion of the body by **pathogens**, or disease-producing microorganisms. The invasion of the body by a pathogen and the symptoms that devel-op in response to this invasion are called an **infection**. A **local infection** is restricted to a small area, whereas a **systemic infection** is more widespread throughout the body. A systemic infection is spread by the blood; it af-fects the entire body and generally makes you feel sick. With regard to a wound, there is often an attempt to differentiate between colonization and infection. **Colo-nization** means that the microorganism is present and growing but is not causing illness. Infection means that the microorganism is present and is causing illness.

Table 5.1   Key Microbiological Terms

TERM	DEFINITION
Antibiotic	Chemical used to treat bacterial infections. A broad-spectrum antibiotic destroys many different types of bacteria, whereas a narrow-spectrum antibiotic destroys only a few types.
Commensal	Organisms living in a harmonious and beneficial relationship with each other. The organisms derive nutritional or other environmental benefits from the other. Commensal bacteria are part of the normal flora.
Communicable disease	Any disease that can be spread from one host to another. A noncommunicable disease is an infectious disease that cannot be transmitted directly or indirectly from host to host. For example, a bladder infection caused by *Escherichia coli* cannot be spread from the infected person to another person. A contagious disease is a communicable disease that is easily spread from one person to another. Measles and chickenpox are contagious diseases because they are easily spread.
Epidemic disease	A disease acquired by many people in a given area over a short period. An endemic disease is always present in a population. A pandemic is a worldwide epidemic.
Epidemiology	The study of the occurrence and distribution of a disease in a population.
Incubation period	The lapsed period of time from the exposure of a person to a pathogen to the development of the symptoms of the disease.
Normal flora	A group of microorganisms that colonize a host without causing disease. Normal flora colonize the mouth, intestinal tract, vagina, nasal cavities, and other areas of the body. Microorganisms that are not pathogenic in one area may become pathogenic when transferred to another area. For example, when the *E. coli* bacterium that is part of the normal flora of the large intestine is unintentionally transferred to the urinary bladder, it causes a bladder infection. Some body fluids such as blood, urine, and cerebrospinal fluid are sterile and do not have a normal flora.
Nosocomial infection	A hospital-acquired infection.
Reservoir of infection	A continual source of infection. A reservoir of infection can be living organisms such as humans and other animals; nonliving objects are substances that are contaminated with the pathogen. A contaminated nonliving object is called a *fomite,* such as a dirty glass and used needles. Contaminated soil and water also serve as inanimate reservoirs of infection.
Resistance	The ability to ward off diseases. A lack of resistance is called *susceptibility*.
Sterilization	A process that destroys all living organisms.
Vector	A carrier of pathogens from host to host. The mosquito is the animal vector carrying the plasmodium (malaria) to humans. A contaminated syringe is a nonliving vector (fomite).

Obviously, a wound that is colonized may eventually become infected. Table 5.1 describes several key terms used in discussing microbiology.

 Re-Think

1. What is a pathogen?
2. Differentiate between a local and systemic infection.
3. Differentiate between colonization and infection.

TYPES OF PATHOGENS

The groups of microorganisms (some of which are pathogens) are bacteria, viruses, fungi, and protozoa. Other larger, disease-causing organisms include worms and arthropods (Fig. 5.1).

MICROORGANISMS (MICROBES)

Bacteria (sing., bacterium) are single-celled organisms found everywhere. They were first observed under the microscope by van Leeuwenhoek, who called them "little beasties." Most bacteria consider living conditions within the human body to be ideal, so they move right in. The good news is that many bacteria perform useful roles. For example, **microbiota** or **normal flora** (microorganisms that normally and harmoniously live in or on the human body without causing disease) prevents the overgrowth of other organisms, keeping them under control. Some bacteria synthesize needed substances such as vitamin K. The bad news is that bacteria can also cause disease; in fact, bacteria make up the largest group of pathogens. When bacteria successfully invade the human body, they cause damage in two ways: (1) by entering and growing in the human cell and (2) by secreting toxins that damage the cells.

Bacteria are classified into three groups based on shape: (1) coccus (round), (2) bacillus (rod-shaped), and (3) curved rod. Rickettsiae and chlamydiae are also classified as bacteria, although they differ in several important ways from cocci, bacilli, and curved rods.

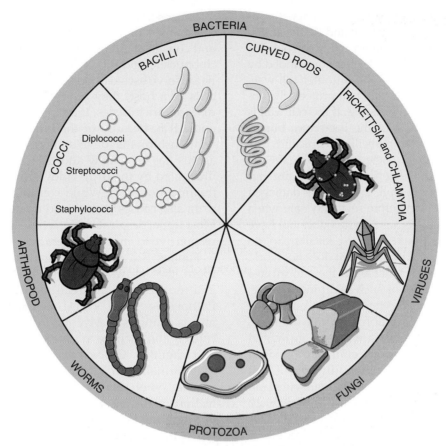

FIG. 5.1 Pathogens: microorganisms and larger disease-causing organisms.

The cocci are round cells and are arranged in patterns. Cocci that are arranged in pairs are called diplococci (dip-loh-KOHK-eye). Streptococci (strep-toh-KOHK-eye) are arranged in chains, like a chain of beads. Staphylococci (staf-il-oh-KOHK-eye) look like bunches of grapes and are arranged in clusters. The cocci cause many diseases, including gonorrhea, meningitis, and pneumonia. The bacilli (bah-SIL-ee) are long and slender and are shaped like a cigar. Diseases caused by bacilli include tetanus, diphtheria, and tuberculosis. The curved rods include the vibrio, the spirillum (spy-RIL-um), and the spirochete (SPY-ro-keet). The vibrios have a slight curve and resemble a comma. Cholera is caused by a vibrio (*Vibrio cholerae*). The spirillum is a long cell that coils like a corkscrew. Tightly coiled spirilla that are capable of waving and twisting motions are called spirochetes. The most famous spirochete, *Treponema pallidum,* causes syphilis. Syphilis has been around for centuries. Its origin, if nothing else, is colorful. The French called syphilis the Italian disease, and, of course, the Italians reciprocated, calling it the French disease. The Polish referred to it as the German disease and—you guessed it—the Germans called it the Polish disease! Regardless of its origin, syphilis is well traveled.

 Do You Know...

What Maria, Sophia, and Leah Have in Common?

"Hey! Maria, Sophia, and Leah ... y'all got gonorrhea," shouts their main squeeze. Mr. Busy has just been informed that he has gonorrhea, a sexually transmitted infection caused by *Neisseria gonorrhoeae*. As the girls now know, gonorrhea is highly contagious. Today has been hectic for our **carrier**, Mr. B. He began treatment with the antibiotic ciprofloxacin and is currently burning up the phone lines informing his sexual partners (called **contacts** in public health jargon) of probable and almost certain infection. It is crucial that all four be treated for gonorrhea to prevent the "ping-pong effect": treatment and cure, followed by reexposure and reinfection. By this time next week, Maria, Sophia, and Leah should also be taking ciprofloxacin and sitting at home in front of the flat-screen contemplating the definition of "safe sex."

 Do You Know...

That "Lues, Lues" Is Not a Hit Tune?

"Lues, Lues" sounds like an oldie-but-goody hit tune. In fact, it is an oldie, but definitely not a goody. *Lues* refers to syphilis. Lesions associated with syphilis are referred to as *luetic* lesions. Got lues? "Singin' nothing but the blues ..."

There are two clinically important characteristics of bacteria: (1) the presence of a cell wall and (2) the ability to form **spores**. Although the human cell is surrounded by the cell membrane, the bacterial cell is surrounded by two structures: a cell membrane and an outer cell wall. The bacterial cell wall is a rigid wall that protects the underlying cell membrane from bursting. If the cell wall is damaged, the cell membrane of the bacterium bursts, killing the bacterium. Enter penicillin! Penicillin prevents cell wall synthesis in the bacterium, causing the cell membrane to burst and the bacterium to die. Because human cells do not have a cell wall, they are not damaged by penicillin; penicillin is therefore relatively safe when administered to humans. Because a virus does not have an outer cell wall, it is not affected by penicillin. So, do not take penicillin for a viral infection—it does not work.

Many bacteria form spores that allow them to survive harsh environmental conditions such as drying, heating, and exposure to certain disinfectants. Spores enable the bacteria to exist in a "sleepy," or dormant, state until conditions improve. Then the bacteria wake up, grow, and resume their usual activities. For example, *Clostridium botulinum,* the organism that causes a deadly form of food poisoning (botulism), is a spore former and can withstand several hours of exposure to boiling water. Obviously, spore-forming microorganisms have great survival skills and present a challenge in infection control procedures.

Rickettsia (ri-KET-see-ah) and chlamydia (cla-MID-ee-uh) are classified as bacteria. However, they are smaller than most bacteria and must reproduce within the living cells of a host. Because they require a living host, they are called **parasites**. The rickettsiae are often carried by fleas, ticks, and body lice. For example, the rickettsia that causes Rocky Mountain spotted fever is carried by the tick. Body lice carry the rickettsia responsible for epidemic typhus. The chlamydiae are smaller than rickettsiae and cause several major human diseases. One of the most prevalent sexually transmitted diseases in the United States today is caused by *Chlamydia trachomatis*. Chlamydial infection is also responsible for trachoma, a serious eye infection that is a leading cause of blindness in the world. Like other bacterial infections, rickettsial and chlamydial infections are treated with antibiotics.

 Do You Know...

Who Russ T. Nale Is?

By stepping on his namesake, Russ T. Nale accomplished two things. First, he allowed a potentially lethal pathogen, *Clostridium tetani*, to enter his body. Second, he had a deep puncture wound that encouraged the growth of the pathogen. Because little bleeding is associated with a puncture wound, the pathogen was not washed out of the wound. More important, however, a deep puncture wound prevents air (oxygen) from entering the wound. Because this pathogen grows anaerobically (without oxygen), the conditions associated with a puncture wound are ideal. Sure hope Russ is up to date on his tetanus shots!

Viruses (from the Latin *virus,* meaning "poison") are the smallest of the infectious agents. They are not cells and consist of either ribonucleic acid (RNA) or deoxyribonucleic acid (DNA) surrounded by a protein shell. Because viruses can only reproduce within the living cells of a host, they are parasites. Examples of viral diseases are measles, mumps, influenza, poliomyelitis, and AIDS. Because of the intimacy of the virus–host relationship, the development of nontoxic antiviral agents has been slow and difficult. This point is well illustrated by the drug zidovudine (AZT), used in the treatment of AIDS. While exerting antiviral effects, the drug also causes widespread damage to the host cells. Most upper respiratory infections are viral and are not responsive to antibiotic therapy.

Fungus is a plantlike organism, such as a mushroom, that grows best in dark, damp places. Yeasts and molds (such as bread mold) are types of fungi. Pathogenic fungi cause **mycotic infections** (*myco* means "fungus"). Mycotic infections are usually localized and include athlete's foot, ringworm, thrush, and vaginitis. *Candida albicans* is a yeastlike fungus that normally inhabits the mouth, digestive tract, and vagina. When *Candida* overgrows, it can cause an infection in the mouth (thrush), intestinal symptoms, or vaginitis. Systemic fungal infections are rare, but when they occur, they are life-threatening and difficult to cure.

 Do You Know...

About the Ring of Ringworm?

Ringworm is an infection of the skin caused not by worms, but a fungus. Why the circular or ring shape? The fungus grows outward from the center. The fungi in the center of the lesion die before the outer circle of fungi die. This type of fungal growth pattern leaves a clear or healed center surrounded by living fungi.

NOTE: There is a ringworm bush *(Cassia alata)* whose leaves produce a juice that is used as a cure for ringworm and poisonous bites. The two explanations for the name *ringworm* are as follows: (1) an ancient and mistaken belief existed that worms caused the infection; and (2) it was named after the ringlike or circular appearance of the lesion. Both theories have a "ring" of truth.

Protozoa (pro-toe-ZO-ah) are single-celled, animal-like microbes. The four main types of protozoa are amebas (ah-MEE-bah-z), ciliates (SIL-ee-atz), flagellates (FLAH-jel-atz), and **sporozoa** (spor-uh-ZOH-uh). Protozoa are found in the soil and in most bodies of water. Amebic dysentery and giardiasis are caused by protozoan parasites. The parasites are ingested in contaminated water and food and cause severe diarrhea. Malaria is caused by a sporozoan called a plasmodium. *Plasmodium malariae* is carried by a mosquito, which is capable of spreading malaria over a wide region. Indeed, malaria still causes more than 3 million deaths per year in the more tropical regions of the world. Two other members of the sporozoa group pose a serious health threat to those persons with impaired immune systems. *Pneumocystis jiroveci* and *Cryptosporidium* cause infections in persons with AIDS and other immunocompromised persons.

? Re-Think

1. List the types of microorganisms.
2. List the three groups of bacteria.
3. What is a parasite?
4. What is a normal flora? What is the consequence of disturbing the intestinal normal flora?

OTHER (MULTICELLULAR) DISEASE-CAUSING ORGANISMS

Other disease-causing organisms that are larger than microorganisms include multicellular organisms such as parasitic worms and arthropods.

Parasitic worms, called **helminths**, are multicellular animals that are parasitic and pathogenic to humans. In other words, worms can be germs. The identification of most worm infestations requires microscopic examination of body samples (usually stool) and reveals the presence of the adult worms or the larval forms. The worms are classified as roundworms or flatworms. Roundworms include ascarides, pinworms, hookworms, trichinae, and the tiny worms that cause filariasis (fi-LAR-eye-ah-sys) or elephantiasis. Infestation by pinworms is common in children and is very hard to control. The pinworms live in the intestinal tract but lay their eggs on the outer perianal area. The deposition of the eggs causes itching (pruritus). A child may then scratch the anal area and transfer the eggs to his or her mouth and onto others. The eggs are swallowed, and the newly hatched pinworms grow into adulthood in the intestine. Most worm infestations are transmitted by the fecal–oral route (in which hands contaminated by feces introduce the worms, eggs, or larvae into the mouth). Trichinosis is transmitted by ingestion of undercooked, contaminated pork; and filariasis is transmitted by biting insects.

The flatworms include the tapeworms and the flukes. Tapeworms that live in the intestines may grow from 5 to 50 feet in length. Imagine hosting a 50-foot tapeworm! Flukes are flat, leaf-shaped worms that invade the blood and organs such as the liver, lungs, and intestines. Because these large flatworms feed on the human host, infestation causes weight loss, anemia, and generalized debilitation. Infestation by worms is treated with drugs called *anthelmintics* (which means "against worms").

Arthropods are animals with jointed legs and include insects. They are of concern for two reasons. Arthropods such as mites and lice are ectoparasites,

meaning that they live on the surface of the body, skin, and mucous membranes. Ectoparasites cause itching and discomfort but are not life-threatening. More seriously, arthropods such as mosquitoes, biting flies, fleas, and ticks act as vectors of disease. (A **vector** is an object, living or nonliving, that transfers a pathogen from one organism to another.) The bite of the arthropod vector introduces pathogens into the host (the person or organism that is infected by a pathogen), causing infection. For example, the mosquito (arthropod vector) can carry the pathogens for malaria and encephalitis. The tick can carry the pathogens that cause Lyme disease and Rocky Mountain spotted fever.

? Re-Think

1. What is a helminth?
2. What is the arthropod vector of the Zika virus?
3. What is meant by the fecal–oral route? How would you prevent the spread of an organism that is spread by this route of transmission?

LABORATORY IDENTIFICATION OF PATHOGENS

Many laboratory procedures and techniques are used to identify pathogens. One of these techniques is called *staining* and involves the use of dyes. A second technique is a culture.

Many bacteria are classified according to staining characteristics using the Gram stain (a dye). A gram-positive bacterium is one that stains purple or blue. *Streptococcus* is an example of a gram-positive bacterium. A gram-negative bacterium such as *Escherichia coli* does not absorb the purple Gram stain. Instead, a gram-negative bacterium picks up a pink or red stain. Because most bacteria are gram-positive or gram-negative, Gram staining is an important first step in the identification of the causative organism of an infection.

Another stain is called the *acid-fast stain*. The bacterium is first stained with a red dye and then washed with an acid. Most bacteria lose the red stain when washed with acid. However, several bacteria retain the red stain and are therefore called *acid-fast*. The most famous of the acid-fast bacteria is the *Mycobacterium tuberculosis*, the causative organism of tuberculosis (TB). This organism is commonly called the *acid-fast bacillus*. Some bacteria do not stain with any of the commonly used dyes. Thus, spirochetes and rickettsiae must be stained with special dyes and techniques.

Sometimes the physician wants to identify the specific pathogen growing in an infected wound and orders a wound culture to be done. A sample of the wound exudate (pus) is placed on culture medium (food that supports the growth of the pathogens). The pathogens are incubated and allowed to grow and multiply. The pathogens can then be stained and identified. The growth of pathogens in a culture medium is called a *culture*. The cultured pathogens can also be tested for their susceptibility to various antibiotics (culture and sensitivity test). For example, if an antibiotic is placed in the same culture and stops the growth of the pathogen, the pathogen is assumed to be responsive or sensitive to the effects of the antibiotic. The antibiotic is given to the patient to treat the infection. Other antibiotics may have no effect on the growth of the pathogens in the culture and therefore would not be used in the treatment of the infection.

You will often be asked to collect samples for laboratory analysis. Specific rules must be followed for each specimen. For example, in collecting a urine specimen that will be analyzed for the presence of pathogens, you must be careful not to contaminate the urine with microorganisms from your hands or unsterile containers. The proper identification of the pathogen depends on correct technique.

 Re-Think

1. What does it mean to say that a bacterium is gram-positive or gram-negative?
2. Why is the tubercle bacillus called the "acid-fast" bacillus?
3. Why may a specimen be cultured before an antibiotic is prescribed?

THE SPREAD OF INFECTION

To understand how infection is spread, we must know how germs move—in, out, and about (Fig. 5.2).

PORTALS OF ENTRY AND EXIT

How do pathogens enter the body? Pathogens enter the body by portals of entry, which include the respiratory, gastrointestinal, and genitourinary tracts; and eye, skin, and parenteral route. The parenteral route includes those injuries that penetrate the skin or mucous membranes, such as bites, cuts, and surgery. A break in the skin is an excellent way for pathogens to enter the body. This is the reason why health care workers wear gloves when handling blood or other body fluids. In the event that the body fluids are contaminated (with, say, the AIDS or hepatitis viruses), the gloves prevent the entrance of the virus through tiny cuts or abrasions. Most pathogens enter the body through the respiratory tract (inhaled droplets of water and dust) and the gastrointestinal tract (by eating spoiled food or placing contaminated hands in the mouth).

How do pathogens leave the body of an infected person? Pathogens leave an infected body by portals of exit, which include the respiratory, gastrointestinal, or genitourinary tracts; the skin (intact and broken); eyes

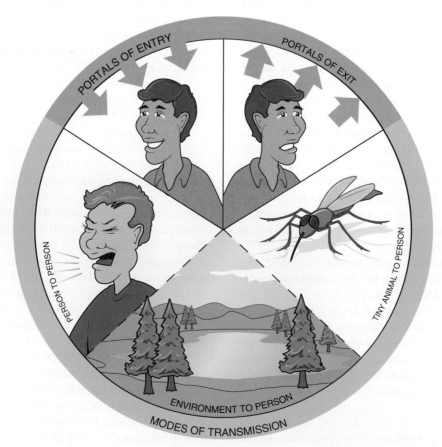

FIG. 5.2 Spread of infection: portals of entry, portals of exit, and modes of transmission.

(tears), and breasts (milk). The most common portals of exit are the respiratory and gastrointestinal tracts. For example, the common cold virus is often sneezed or coughed into room air from the respiratory passages of the infected person, whereas the *Salmonella* organism in a person with typhoid fever exits the body in the stool. Discharge from the urogenital tract is also an important means of spreading infection (sexually transmitted diseases). By knowing the portal of exit of each pathogen, one can set up procedures for preventing the spread of the infection. For example, by knowing that *Salmonella typhi* is excreted in the stool, we know that the patient's underwear and bed linens are contaminated with the pathogens. We can then take measures to clean the soiled clothing and linens, thereby preventing the spread of the disease. By far, the most important procedure in preventing the spread of infection is handwashing!

 Re-Think

Give an example of a portal of entrance and portal of exit. Explain in terms of the fecal–oral route. Work the term *handwashing* into your answer!

HOW PATHOGENS SPREAD

We know how pathogens enter and leave the body—but how do they move about, or "spread"? Pathogens are spread from person to person, environment to person, and from "tiny animals" (insects) to persons (see Fig. 5.2).

PERSON-TO-PERSON CONTACT

Suppose you have a cold and go to work. Within a week, everyone in the office has your cold. What happened? First, whenever you sneezed, the cold virus was sprayed into the room air in little droplets of nasal discharge. These droplets were then inhaled by your coworkers. The virus was spread by droplet contact. Second, your hands were contaminated with the virus, and you touched many objects in the office (e.g., doorknobs, desktops, other people's hands after handshaking), thereby contaminating these objects. Others touched the contaminated objects and eventually introduced the virus into their own bodies. The spread of infection from person to person is effective. One of the best ways to prevent respiratory infections is to avoid crowds during cold and flu season. Another way is to avoid contact with a fomite or vector. The doorknob is considered to be both a vector and a fomite. Remember that a vector is an object, living or nonliving, that transfers a pathogen from one organism to another. A *fomite* is a nonliving vector. Other fomites include soiled handkerchiefs and eating utensils.

ENVIRONMENT-TO-PERSON CONTACT

The environment-to-person mode of transmission includes contact with contaminated water, air, food, or soil. For example, you can develop typhoid fever if you drink a glass of water contaminated by *S. typhi*. Similarly, you can develop food poisoning if you eat food contaminated with *E. coli*.

"TINY ANIMAL"-TO-PERSON CONTACT

The "tiny animal"-to-person mode of transmission includes the use of insects (and other "crawling critters") in the spread of disease; these tiny animals are living vectors. For example, a mosquito bites a person with malaria. The malaria-causing plasmodium matures in the stomach of the mosquito. The plasmodium-loaded mosquito then bites another person and voilà!—malaria. You can understand why the eradication of mosquitoes is key in malaria control. A final stomach-churning example is flies hopping from dog feces to food on a picnic table. The pathogens from the dog feces are transferred by the fly feet to the food, which is then eaten by you.

Note that the mosquito and fly both spread disease. The mosquito, however, plays a more complicated and biological role. The plasmodium (causative organism of malaria) requires the mosquito as part of its life cycle; it matures in the stomach of the mosquito. Because of this role, the mosquito is called a *biological vector*. The lowly fly does not participate in the life cycle of the pathogen; it merely walks on the dog feces, and the germs stick to the feet of the fly. The fly then flies onto your food and deposits the germs on your food. The fly is only a *mechanical vector* but a very effective germ spreader.

 Re-Think

1. Explain how a doorknob can act both as a vector and fomite during flu season.
2. Describe why the malaria-causing mosquito acts as a biological vector, whereas the common housefly usually acts as a mechanical vector.

FIVE GERM-LADEN STORIES

The following five stories illustrate important microbiological principles and introduce you to the language of microbiology. "Dr. Semmelweis Screams, 'Wash Those Mitts!'" is a tragic story of handwashing, nosocomial infection, and the arrogance of the scientific community. "Flora and Her Vaginal Itch" addresses the normal flora and superinfection. "Rick, Nick, and the Sick Tick" describes disease transmission by an arthropod vector and differentiates between a communicable and contagious disease. "Why Typhoid Mary Needed to Lose Her Gallbladder" describes the carrier state and the efficiency of the fecal–oral route in disease transmission. Finally, "A Pox News Alert!" focuses on the pox throughout history and some of the current concerns. As you read the stories, refer to Table 5.1 for the definitions of unfamiliar terms; the table defines and expands the microbiological principles illustrated in the stories Table 5.2 identifies other pathogenic microorganisms.

DR. SEMMELWEIS SCREAMS, "WASH THOSE MITTS!"

Dr. Ignaz Semmelweis was an assistant at the First Obstetrical Clinic in Vienna (circa 1850). At that time, an alarmingly high mortality rate was associated with puerperal fever or childbirth fever. Puerperal fever begins as an infection of the uterus after childbirth and is commonly caused by a strain of beta-hemolytic streptococcus. Puerperal fever progresses from an infection of the uterus to peritonitis and to generalized septicemia, ending in an agonizing death.

Semmelweis made the following two keen observations while caring for his patients:

1. A woman became ill immediately after being examined by a medical student who had previously examined a woman dying of puerperal fever.
2. If a medical student cut himself while attending a woman with puerperal fever, his wound became infected, and he subsequently died of puerperal sepsis.

Dr. Semmelweis concluded that puerperal fever is caused by conveyance to the pregnant woman

Table 5.2	Disorders Caused by Pathogens
PATHOGEN	**DISORDER**
Cocci	
Neisseria	*N. gonorrhoeae* causes gonorrhea and inflammation of the mucous membranes of the reproductive and urinary tracts. May cause sterility and pelvic inflammatory disease (PID). Infants of infected mothers may develop ophthalmia neonatorum. *N. meningitidis* causes meningitis, or inflammation of the membranes covering the brain and the spinal cord.
Staphylococcus	*S. aureus* causes skin infections such as boils and impetigo, pneumonia, kidney and bladder infections, osteomyelitis, septicemia, and food poisoning. *S. aureus* is a leading cause of nosocomial (hospital-acquired) infections.
Streptococcus	*S. pneumoniae* causes pneumonia, middle ear infection, and meningitis. *S. pyogenes* causes septicemia, strep throat, middle ear infection, scarlet fever, pneumonia, and endocarditis. An immunological response can cause rheumatic fever with permanent damage to the heart valves, and glomerulonephritis (kidney damage).
Bacilli	
Bordetella pertussis	*Bordetella* causes pertussis (whooping cough), a severe infection of the trachea and bronchi characterized by episodes of violent coughing. The "whoop" is an effort to inhale after the coughing bouts.
Clostridium	*C. botulinum* causes botulism, a potentially fatal form of food poisoning caused by improper processing of foods. *C. perfringens* causes gas gangrene, in which death of the tissue is accompanied by the production of a gas. *C. tetani* causes tetanus, or lockjaw.
Escherichia coli	*E. coli* is part of the normal flora of the intestines. *E. coli* causes local and systemic infections, food poisoning, diarrhea, septicemia, and septic shock; it is a leading cause of nosocomial infection.
Haemophilus	*H. aegyptius* causes conjunctivitis, a highly contagious infection that occurs in areas where there are many young children. *H. influenzae* causes meningitis in children and upper respiratory infection in older adults.
Helicobacter pylori	*H. pylori* causes gastritis and ulceration of the stomach and duodenum.
Legionella pneumophila	*L. pneumophila* is responsible for Legionnaires' disease, a type of pneumonia. The organism contaminates water supplies, as in air-conditioning units.
Mycobacterium tuberculosis	*M. tuberculosis* causes tuberculosis (TB). The organism, also called the tubercle bacillus, causes primary lesions called tubercles. The bacillus most commonly affects the lungs. The incidence of TB is high in the homeless population, persons with AIDS, and closed populations such as in prisons. Formerly called the "white plague," TB is making a comeback in a more virulent and drug-resistant strain.
Pseudomonas aeruginosa	*P. aeruginosa* is the common cause of wound and urinary tract infections in debilitated patients, such as patients with severe burns, cancer, and other chronic conditions.

Table 5.2	Disorders Caused by Pathogens—cont'd
PATHOGEN	**DISORDER**
Salmonella	*S. enteritidis* causes salmonellosis, food poisoning characterized by severe diarrhea. *S. typhi* causes typhoid fever, an intestinal infection. Typhoid fever is rare in the United States because of the chlorination of the water supply, but the incidence increases during periods of flooding when the water supply is contaminated with sewage.
Shigella dysenteriae	*S. dysenteriae* causes dysentery.
Curved Rods	
Borrelia burgdorferi	*B. burgdorferi* causes Lyme disease and is characterized by a rash, palsy, and joint inflammation. It is transmitted by a small deer tick.
Treponema pallidum	*T. pallidum* causes syphilis.
Vibrio cholerae	*V. cholerae* causes cholera.
Rickettsia and Chlamydia	
Rickettsia	*R. prowazekii* causes epidemic typhus, which is transmitted to humans by lice. *R. rickettsii* causes Rocky Mountain spotted fever, which is transmitted to humans by ticks. *R. typhi* causes endemic or murine typhus, which is transmitted to humans by fleas.
Chlamydia	*C. trachomatis* causes trachoma, the leading cause of blindness in the world. Another form causes nongonococcal urethritis, the most common sexually transmitted disease in the United States.
Viruses	
Chikungunya fever	The word literally means "that which bends up," a reference to the extreme musculoskeletal pain associated with the viral infection. Caused by a mosquito-borne (*Aedes*) virus.
Dengue fever	Also called "breakback fever" because of the pain associated with the disease. Caused by mosquito-borne (*Aedes*) dengue viruses
Ebola	A lethal viral infection also called hemorrhagic fever; spread most often by contact with infected body secretions.
Encephalitis viruses	Encephalitis is the inflammation of the brain.
Hepatitis viruses	Several forms of hepatitis exist, causing inflammation of the liver, as follows: Hepatitis A is spread by the fecal–oral route. Hepatitis B is spread by sexual activity or contact with contaminated blood and body fluids. Hepatitis C is caused by contaminated blood transmitted via transfusions, through needles in drug abuse, and to health care workers on the job. Hepatitis can become chronic, develop into a carrier state, or deteriorate to hepatic failure.
Herpes simplex viruses	*Type 1:* Cold sores or fever blisters appear on the lip, in the oral cavity, or in the nose. The virus lies dormant in the nerves between attacks. *Type 2:* Genital herpes is a common sexually transmitted disease characterized by painful lesions in the genitalia.
Herpes varicella-zoster	Chickenpox (varicella) is a mild infection characterized by generalized skin lesions. On remission of the infection, the virus becomes dormant and may reactivate in later years as shingles (herpes zoster).
Human papillomavirus (HPV)	HPV causes genital warts, which are transmitted sexually.
Influenza viruses	Influenza ("flu") is caused by different strains of the influenza viruses. The word *influenza* has its origin in astrology. The ancients believed that illness (later diagnosed as viral infection) was under the *influence* of the planets.
Measles virus	Measles (rubeola) is an acute respiratory inflammation characterized by fever, sore throat, skin rash, and Koplik's spots (white spots in the mouth).
Mumps virus	Mumps is epidemic parotitis (inflammation of a salivary gland).
Polio virus	Poliomyelitis (infantile paralysis) is an acute infection that may destroy nerve cells in the spinal cord, causing paralysis.
Rhabdovirus	Rabies is a fatal disease characterized by headache, fever, seizures, and spasm of the throat muscles while swallowing (hydrophobia). It is spread by the saliva of infected animals such as dogs and other wild animals (e.g., bats, raccoons).
Rhinoviruses	Rhinoviruses are responsible for the common cold (coryza).
Rubella virus	Causes German measles. The virus causes severe teratogenic birth defects that occur during the first trimester, such as blindness, deafness, brain damage, and heart defects.

Continued

Table 5.2	Disorders Caused by Pathogens—cont'd
PATHOGEN	**DISORDER**
Zika virus	Named after the Zika forest in Uganda where it was first identified. It is spread by the bite of an *Aedes* mosquito. The infection is usually mild; however, the virus crosses the placenta of the pregnant woman and can cause microcephaly in the fetus. Another complication of Zika virus infection is Guillain-Barré syndrome.
Fungi	
Tinea	Tinea causes ringworm, a highly contagious fungal infection of the skin. One form of ringworm (tinea pedis) is found on the foot and is called *athlete's foot*. Other forms of ringworm are found on the scalp (tinea capitis) and on the bearded areas of the face and neck (tinea barbae). (Ringworm is not caused by a worm, nor is the lesion always ring-shaped.)
Protozoa	
Entamoeba histolytica	*E. histolytica* causes amebic dysentery.
Giardia lamblia	Giardiasis is characterized by gastrointestinal discomfort and diarrhea.
Trichomonas vaginalis	Trichomoniasis is a sexually transmitted disease.
Worms	
Ascaris	These are long worms that live in the small intestine.
Hookworm (*Necator*)	Larval worms burrow their way through the skin of a bare foot, migrate to the intestine, and hook on to the intestinal wall. The worms feed on the blood of the host, causing anemia, fatigue, and wasting.
Pinworm (*Enterobius*)	Pinworm is the most common worm infestation in the United States.
Tapeworms (*Taenia*, others)	Tapeworms are acquired by eating poorly cooked contaminated food, such as beef, fish, and pork.

of "putrid particles derived from living organisms through the agency of the examining fingers." This conclusion was impressive because he linked the disease to the putrid particles—tiny disease-producing critters that would not be discovered and linked to disease officially for another 25 years.

As a result of his observations, Semmelweis demanded that his medical students wash their hands with a disinfectant before examining each patient. "Wash those mitts!" he screamed, and wash they did. Mortality rates in his clinic decreased from 18% to 1%. You might conclude that Semmelweis eliminated puerperal fever and was honored by his colleagues. Not so! They ridiculed him for his insistence on handwashing. He eventually became so distraught that he deliberately cut his finger and contaminated his injury with the vaginal discharge of a woman with puerperal fever. Ranting and raving, he was committed to the Budapest Insane Asylum, where he quickly died of the disease that he had worked so hard to eradicate.

With the passing of Semmelweis, the practice of handwashing was discontinued, and the mortality rate from puerperal fever again soared. Puerperal fever, although rarely seen today, is a great example of a nosocomial infection. A **nosocomial** (noh-soh-CO-mee-al) **infection** is a hospital-acquired infection that is most often transmitted from patient to patient by direct contact (through the agency of the examining finger, according to Semmelweis). Today, a nosocomial infection is transmitted by health professionals who *do not wash their hands*. We go from patient to patient, carrying germs from one to another. Historically, nosocomial infections have been a tremendous problem. Today, 15% of hospitalized patients develop a nosocomial infection. "Wash those mitts!" echoes through the centuries but generally falls on deaf ears.

 Re-Think

Explain why the same problem dealt with by Semmelweis is the same as today's issue with nosocomial infection.

FLORA AND HER VAGINAL ITCH

Stuffed up and miserable, Flora went to her physician. She was given an antibiotic for a sinus infection. Within a week, the sinus infection was cured; the misery, however, had headed south. Flora now had an antibiotic-induced vaginal discharge.

The vagina is normally inhabited by a population of diverse microbes. These microbes are permanent residents and, when present in normal amounts, do not produce disease. This population of microbes within the vagina is called the *normal flora*. Other body cavities or areas such as the skin, large intestine, mouth, and respiratory tract contain their own diverse populations of microbes and therefore have their own normal flora.

The presence of a normal flora within the vagina prevents the overgrowth of yeast called *Candida albicans* that is present in small numbers within the vagina. If the normal flora is destroyed by an antibiotic, the yeast grows uncontrollably and causes candidiasis, a vaginal yeast infection, characterized by discharge, odor, and itching. Candidiasis is an example of a superinfection. Organisms that do not cause disease in their normal habitat become pathogenic when allowed to overpopulate the area. What was the cause of Flora's itch? Flora's normal flora had become abnormal. Watch those antibiotics!

 Re-Think

Why may antibiotic therapy cure one infection but cause a superinfection in the same patient?

RICK, NICK, AND THE SICK TICK

One week after returning from a camping trip with his friend Nick, Rick went to his physician feeling awful. He had chills, a high fever, headache, muscle pain, and a red measles-like spotted rash that was prominent on the palms of his hands and the soles of his feet. On examination, the physician removed a tick from Rick's back. He was diagnosed with Rocky Mountain spotted fever (RMSF) and treated with the antibiotic tetracycline. Microbiologically speaking, Rick had become the perfect host (an organism who had become infected with a pathogen).

Enough about Rick! What's with the tick? The tick that bit Rick was sick; it was infected with the pathogen called *Rickettsia rickettsii*, the causative organism of RMSF. When the tick bit Rick, the infected saliva was injected into the bite site. The rickettsia then feasted on Rick's blood by growing, multiplying, and eventually causing the signs and symptoms that sent Rick to the doctor.

The tick acts as an arthropod vector for RMSF. An animal vector is an organism that transmits a pathogen such as rickettsia. An arthropod is a class of tiny animals that have jointed legs. In this case, the arthropod is the sick tick. The rickettsia is transmitted by saliva (the bite of the tick) or the feces of the tick that are rubbed into the bite. The tick also serves as a reservoir of infection, which harbors pathogens; in this case, the tick is the reservoir.

The tick is not killed by the rickettsia. Mama tick coexists with the rickettsia and passes the rickettsia through her eggs to her baby ticks, thereby perpetuating and expanding generations of sick ticks.

Why didn't Nick catch Rick's infection? RMSF is considered a communicable disease inasmuch as the infection can be spread (through the bite of a tick). RMSF, however, is not considered a contagious disease—that is, one easily spread from host to host like a common cold or impetigo. Thus, Nick remained well, despite his close association with Rick.

One last thing about RMSF: it is an example of **zoonosis**, an animal disease that is transmissible to humans. Other zoonotic diseases include malaria and endemic typhus.

 Re-Think

Explain the role of the arthropod vector in Rocky Mountain spotted fever.

WHY TYPHOID MARY NEEDED TO LOSE HER GALLBLADDER

Mary Mallon (Typhoid Mary) lived in New York in the early 1900s. While employed as a cook, she unintentionally infected many persons with typhoid fever. Hearing several rumors of Mary's unfortunate associations with this disease, her wealthy employer hired a sanitary engineer, George Soper, to investigate the sudden outbreak of typhoid fever within the former's home. Soper soon informed Mary that she was a carrier of the germ that caused typhoid fever. Mary vehemently denied that she was the infecting culprit because she herself did not feel ill. Understandably, she chased Soper from her kitchen with a carving fork. But Soper was correct—Mary was indeed a carrier of typhoid fever.

The *S. typhi* bacterium, the causative organism of typhoid fever, is transmitted by the fecal–oral route through contaminated food or water. Mary's vocation as a cook was a perfect way to spread the salmonella organism via her contaminated hands touching food. Carriers of typhoid fever never rid their systems of *Salmonella;* instead, they harbor the organisms in the bile stored within the gallbladder. Salmonella-laden bile then enters the intestine and contaminates the feces. Removal of the gallbladder rids the body of the salmonella, thereby eliminating the carrier state. Surgical removal of the gallbladder would have made an enormous difference in Mary's life. Unfortunately, surgery was not an option, and Mary was forced into isolation on a coastal island, where she lived unhappily for 26 years.

 Re-Think

How may a cholecystectomy (gallbladder removal) and antibiotics have rendered Mary "safe"?

A POX NEWS ALERT!

Pox News, responding to an ancient medieval curse "A pox be upon you," has issued an update on the pox. Here it is, fair and balanced!

- There has been much confusion about the pox throughout history. The ancients referred to any infectious disease as a "dose of the pox." (Because pox infection was so ugly and visible, the ancients commonly invoked pox curses on their enemies.) Later, the term *pox* was restricted to any disease characterized by a vesicular skin lesion. The term *pox* focuses only on the skin lesion and does not address its cause or treatment. Today, the medical focus is placed on the type of virus that causes a pox.

- Pox diseases are not limited geographically, nor are they restricted to humans. There are "flocks of pox": monkey pox, parrot pox, camel pox, squirrel pox, goat pox, fox pox, ox pox—even plants have pox (plum pox).

- What about chickenpox? Chickenpox is caused by the varicella-zoster virus, a member of the herpesvirus group. It is characterized by a vesicular pox, accompanied by severe pruritus, and is capable of causing pockmarks. Why the name *chickenpox*? Explanations abound. In England, children were often called "chickens." Because chickenpox is primarily a disease of children, the pox was dubbed "childrenpox." Others suggest that the name is derived from the appearance of the pockmarks it looks like the skin has been pecked by a chicken. Others observe the pox as resembling chick peas. There's no telling what it means.

- Think that's strange? Pox News has learned that some parents are throwing "pox parties" in which they are deliberately exposing their unvaccinated children to those who currently have chickenpox! Some parents are convinced that the chickenpox vaccine is unsafe and that the only safe way to build up immunity is to "get" a real case of chickenpox. When a child contracts chickenpox, the child's friends are invited to a party. The infected child is told to blow a whistle and to then pass the whistle to the friends. The whistle, acting as a vector, then spreads the virus from child to child. The practice is effective but dangerous; whereas most children recover uneventfully from chickenpox, some develop serious complications. In particular, children who are immunocompromised may develop a lethal multiple organ infection by the virus; this carries a 17% mortality. Pox parties are probably not the best approach to infectious disease control.

- Poxes come in different sizes. There is the dreaded lethal smallpox and the infamous Great Pox. Pox News, however, has just learned that the Great Pox is no pox at all; its pocky lesion is a chancre and is caused by a spirochete called *Treponema pallidum*. Yikes! The Great Pox is syphilis, the source of untold misery. Just ask Beethoven, Hitler and his lovely bunker mate Eva B, and Henry VIII and his tower ladies, to mention a few. As for the "Chief of Grief" (syphilis), its cause was accurately described by the ancients: "It is taken when one pocky person doth synne (sin) in lechery with one another." Prevention is obvious: "Sin thou not with a pocky person."

 Do You Know...

That Dr. Herbie Zoster Hung Out His Shingle?

Meet Dr. Herbie Zoster, a herpes specialist, according to his newly hung shingle. Today, he is seeing his first patient, Ms. Vera Cella. Ms. Cella is miserable; she has a string of painful skin lesions around her waist. Dr. Zoster makes an immediate diagnosis: It is shingles, medically known as *herpes zoster*. Shingles is an acute infection of the peripheral nervous system caused by the varicella-zoster virus, the same virus that causes chickenpox. After a person recovers from chickenpox, the virus hides in a posterior root ganglion. Later in life, often in response to stress or immunosuppressive therapies, the virus leaves the ganglion and travels along the sensory neurons to the skin. This results in a line of skin blisters along the infected nerve and severe pain. As a complication, some persons develop a postherpetic neuralgia (pain that lingers long after the skin lesions have cleared). Yes, shingles can be triggered by exposure to a child with chickenpox.

 Re-Think

What is the relationship between chickenpox and shingles?

 Sum It Up!

Infectious disease has plagued us forever. Today the battle continues against the tiny but tough disease-producing organisms called pathogens. Pathogens include bacteria, viruses, fungi, protozoa, parasitic worms, and arthropods. To understand the transmission of an infection, one should know the portals of entry (how the pathogen enters the body), the portals of exit (how the pathogen leaves the body), and how the pathogen is spread (person-to-person, environment-to-person, or "tiny animal"-to-person). Important microbiological principles are illustrated in Five Germ-Laden Stories.

Get Ready for Exams!

Summary Outline

The human body is often invaded by disease-producing organisms; these pathogens disrupt normal structure and function and are a common cause of disability and death.

I. Disease and Pathogens
  A. Disease is a failure of the body to function normally.
  B. Infections are diseases caused by pathogens.

II. Types of Pathogens
  A. Microorganisms
    1. Bacteria (cocci, bacilli, curved rods, chlamydia, rickettsia)
    2. Viruses
    3. Fungi
    4. Protozoa (amebas, ciliates, flagellates, sporozoa)
  B. Other larger pathogens
    1. Worms
    2. Arthropods

III. Laboratory Identification
  A. Staining (Gram stain, acid-fast stain)
  B. Cultures

IV. Spread of Infection
  A. Portals of entry: most pathogens enter the body through the respiratory tract and the gastrointestinal tract.
  B. Portals of exit: the most common portals of exit are the respiratory and gastrointestinal tracts.
  C. Modes of transmission
    1. Person-to-person transmission
    2. Environment-to-person transmission
    3. "Tiny animals"-to-person transmission

V. Five Germ-Laden Stories
  A. "Dr. Semmelweis Screams, 'Wash Those Mitts!'"
  B. "Flora and Her Vaginal Itch"
  C. "Rick, Nick, and the Sick Tick"
  D. "Why Typhoid Mary Needed to Lose Her Gallbladder"
  E. "Pox News Alert!"

Review Your Knowledge

Matching: Microorganisms and Other Pathogens
Directions: Match the following words with their descriptions. Some words are used more than once.

a. virus
b. bacteria
c. arthropods
d. worms
e. fungi
f. protozoa

1. ___ Coccus, bacillus, curved rods
2. ___ RNA or DNA surrounded by a protein shell; parasitic
3. ___ Yeasts and molds
4. ___ Ascarides, trichinae, flukes
5. ___ Helminths
6. ___ Ectoparasites
7. ___ Mycotic infections
8. ___ Chlamydia and rickettsia
9. ___ Animals with jointed legs
10. ___ Arranged in pairs, chains, and bunches of grapes
11. ___ Amebas, ciliates, flagellates, and sporozoa

Multiple Choice

1. A vaginal yeast infection *(Candida albicans)* is most apt to develop
   a. as a consequence of antibiotic therapy.
   b. in response to eating contaminated food.
   c. as an allergic response to penicillin.
   d. in response to being bitten by a "sick tick."

2. The plasmodium
   a. is pathogenic to mosquitoes.
   b. causes malaria.
   c. is an arthropod.
   d. is a biological vector.

3. Cocci, bacilli, and curved rods
   a. are eradicated by anthelmintics.
   b. cause mycotic infections.
   c. are types of bacteria.
   d. always act as pathogens.

4. Which of the following is most descriptive of *Staphylococcus?*
   a. Viral
   b. Parasitic
   c. Gram-positive
   d. Chainlike arrangement

5. Spores
   a. allow the bacterium to stain blue (gram-positive).
   b. only develop in parasites.
   c. are characteristic of arthropods.
   d. make a bacterium heat-resistant and hard to kill.

Go Figure

1. Which of the following is correct according to Figs. 5.1 and 5.2?
   a. Cocci are classified as viruses.
   b. Strep and staph are classified as bacilli.
   c. Worms can be pathogenic.
   d. A virus is classified as an arthropod vector.

2. Which of the following is correct according to Figs. 5.1 and 5.2 and Table 5.1?
   a. The normal flora in the large intestine differs from the normal flora in the nose.
   b. A nosocomial infection is hospital-acquired.
   c. Fungi can be pathogenic.
   d. All of the above are true.

Tissues and Membranes

http://evolve.elsevier.com/Herlihy

Objectives

1. List the four major types of tissues.
2. Do the following regarding epithelial tissue:
   - Describe the characteristics and functions of epithelial tissue.
   - Explain how epithelial tissue is classified.
   - List the types of epithelial tissue membranes.
   - Differentiate between endocrine and exocrine glands.
3. Describe the characteristics and functions of connective tissue, and list the types of connective tissue membranes.
4. Describe the characteristics and functions of nervous and muscle tissues.
5. Explain the process of tissue repair after an injury.
6. Differentiate between mucous and serous membranes.

Key Terms

adipose tissue (p. 83)
areolar tissue (p. 83)
chondrocytes (p. 85)
columnar epithelium (p. 79)
connective tissue (p. 82)
cuboidal epithelium (p. 79)
endocrine glands (p. 82)

epithelial tissue (p. 78)
exocrine glands (p. 82)
fascia (p. 83)
intercellular matrix (p. 82)
ligaments (p. 83)
mucous membranes (p. 88)
muscle tissue (p. 86)

nervous tissue (p. 86)
osseous tissue (p. 86)
parietal layer (p. 89)
serous membranes (p. 89)
squamous epithelium (p. 79)
tendons (p. 83)
visceral layer (p. 89)

In Chapter 3, we studied a typical cell. We explained how it divides into millions of identical cells and how they differentiate into cells with unique shapes, sizes, and functions. In this chapter, we see how these cells are arranged to perform specific functions.

Tissues are groups of cells that are similar to each other in structure and function. Four major types of tissues are epithelial, connective, nervous, and muscular. The study of tissues is called *histology*.

EPITHELIAL TISSUE

WHERE IS IT FOUND?

Epithelial (ep-i-THEE-lee-al) tissue, also called *epithelium*, forms large continuous sheets. Epithelial tissue helps form the skin and covers the entire outer surface of the body. Sheets of epithelium also line most of the inner cavities such as the mouth, respiratory tract, and reproductive tract. Types of epithelial tissue are listed in Table 6.1.

WHAT DOES IT DO?

Epithelial tissue is primarily concerned with protection and transport (see Table 6.1). The skin, for example, protects the body from sunlight and from invasion by disease-producing bacteria. The epithelial tissue lining the respiratory passages helps clean inhaled air. The epithelium of the respiratory tract secretes mucus and is lined with cilia. The mucus traps the dust inhaled in the air, and the constantly waving cilia move the dust and mucus toward the throat. The dust and mucus are then either coughed up or swallowed and eliminated in the stools.

Epithelial tissue also functions in the transport of substances across membranes. Epithelium is abundant in organs like those in the digestive tract, which must absorb large amounts of water and digested food. Finally, epithelial tissue forms glands that secrete a variety of hormones and enzymes.

WHAT IS IT LIKE?

Epithelial tissue has the following characteristics:
- Epithelial tissue forms continuous sheets (Fig. 6.1). The cells fit together snugly like tiles.
- Epithelial tissue has two surfaces. One surface is always unattached, like the surface of the outer skin or the inner lining of the mouth. The undersurface of the epithelium is attached to a basement membrane,

Table 6.1   Types of Epithelial Tissue

TYPE	LOCATION	FUNCTION
Simple		
Simple squamous	Walls of blood vessels (capillaries) Alveoli (air sacs in lungs) Kidneys	Permits the exchange of nutrients and wastes Allows diffusion of oxygen and carbon dioxide Filtration of water and electrolytes
Simple cuboidal	Lining of kidney tubules Various glands (thyroid, pancreas, salivary glands)	Absorption of water and electrolytes Secretion of enzymes and hormones
Simple columnar	Digestive tract	Protection, absorption, and secretion of digestive juice; often contains goblet cells (mucus)
Pseudostratified columnar	Lining of respiratory tract Lining of reproductive tubes (fallopian tubes)	Protection and secretion; cleans respiratory passages; sweeps egg toward uterus
Stratified		
Stratified squamous	Outer layer of skin Lining of mouth, esophagus, anus, and vagina	Protects body from invading microorganisms; withstands friction
Transitional	Urinary bladder	Permits expansion of an organ

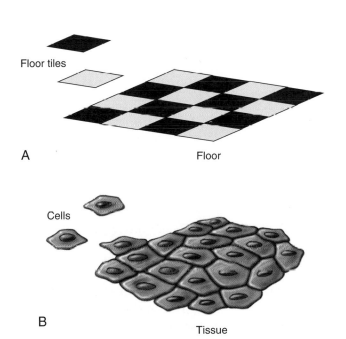

FIG. 6.1 (A) A tile floor. **(B)** Tight-fitting cells of epithelial tissue.

which is a very thin material that anchors the epithelium to the underlying structure.

- Epithelial tissue has no blood supply of its own; it is avascular. For its nourishment, it depends on the blood supply of underlying connective tissue.
- Because epithelial tissue is so well nourished from the underlying connective tissue, it is able to regenerate, or repair itself, quickly if injured.

? Re-Think

1. List four types of tissue.
2. List three words that describe epithelial tissue.
3. Define the word *avascular*. If epithelial tissue is avascular, how does it receive its blood supply?

CLASSIFICATION

Epithelial tissue is classified according to its shape and the numbers of layers. It has three shapes: squamous, cuboidal, and columnar (Fig. 6.2 and Table 6.1). The **squamous** (SKWAY-muss) **epithelium** cells are thin and flat, like fish scales. (The word *squamous* comes from *squam*, meaning "scale.") The **cuboidal epithelium** cells are cubelike and look like dice. The **columnar epithelium** cells are tall and narrow and look like columns.

Epithelial cells are arranged in a single layer or multiple layers (see Fig. 6.2). One layer of cells is a simple epithelium. Two or more layers of cells are a stratified (STRAT-i-fyed) epithelium.

Both the shape and the number of layers describe the various types of epithelium. For example, simple squamous epithelium refers to a single layer of squamous cells. Stratified squamous epithelium contains multiple layers of squamous cells. Note that Fig. 6.2 shows stratified squamous epithelium but not stratified cuboidal or columnar tissue because they are found in very few organs.

SIMPLE EPITHELIA

Because simple epithelia are so thin, they are concerned primarily with the movement, or transport, of various substances across the membranes from one body compartment to another (Fig. 6.3).

Simple squamous epithelium is a single layer of squamous cells with an underlying basement membrane. Because this tissue is so thin, simple squamous epithelium is found where substances move by rapid diffusion or filtration. For example, the walls of the capillaries (the smallest blood vessels) are composed of simple squamous epithelium. The walls of the

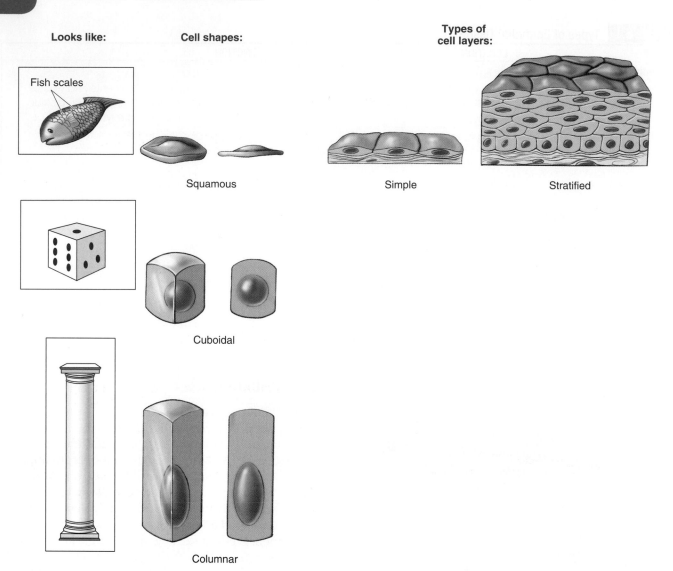

FIG. 6.2 Classification of epithelial tissue: shapes and layers of cells.

alveoli (air sacs of the lungs) are also composed of simple squamous epithelium. This tissue allows the rapid diffusion of oxygen from the alveoli into the blood.

Simple cuboidal epithelium is a single layer of cuboidal cells resting on a basement membrane. This epithelial layer is most often found in glands and in the kidney tubules, where it functions in the transport and secretion of various substances.

Simple columnar epithelium refers to a single layer of columnar cells resting on its basement membrane. These tall, tightly packed cells line the entire length of the digestive tract and play a major role in the absorption of the products of digestion. Lubricating mucus is produced by goblet cells, which are modified columnar cells.

Pseudostratified (SOOD-oh-STRAT-i-fyed) columnar epithelium is a single layer of columnar cells. Because the cells are so irregularly shaped, they appear multilayered—hence the term *pseudostratified*, meaning

"falsely stratified." Their function is similar to that of simple columnar cells: They facilitate absorption and secretion.

STRATIFIED EPITHELIA

Stratified epithelia are multilayered (from 2 to 20 layers) and are therefore stronger than simple epithelia. They perform a protective function and are found in tissue exposed to everyday wear and tear, such as the mouth, esophagus, and skin. Stratified squamous epithelium is the most widespread of the epithelial tissue.

Transitional epithelium is found primarily in organs that need to stretch, such as the urinary bladder. This epithelium is called *transitional* because the cells slide past one another when the tissue is stretched. The cells appear stratified when the urinary bladder is empty (unstretched) and simple when the bladder is full (stretched).

Epithelial Tissue

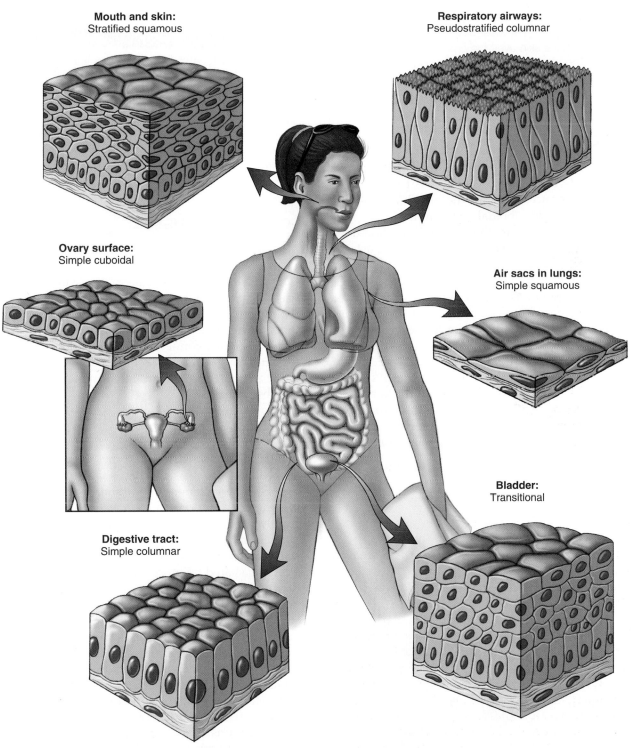

Mouth and skin:
Stratified squamous

Respiratory airways:
Pseudostratified columnar

Ovary surface:
Simple cuboidal

Air sacs in lungs:
Simple squamous

Bladder:
Transitional

Digestive tract:
Simple columnar

FIG. 6.3 Types and location of epithelial tissue.

Do You Know...

What Causes a Pressure, or Decubitus ("Lying Down"), Ulcer?

A decubitus ulcer is another name for a bedsore or a pressure ulcer. The ulcer is caused by an interruption of the blood supply to a tissue. Decubitus ulcers often develop in patients who have been bedridden or confined to a wheelchair for long periods. Decubitus comes from a Latin word meaning to lie down. The ulcers are caused by the weight of the body on the skin overlying a bony area (e.g., elbow, heel, hip). The weight of the body compresses the blood vessels, cutting off the supply of blood to the tissues. Deprived of its blood supply, the tissue dies, forming an ulcer.

GLANDULAR EPITHELIA

The function of glandular epithelium is secretion. A gland is made up of one or more cells that secrete a particular substance. Much of the glandular tissue is composed of simple cuboidal epithelium.

Two types of glands are the exocrine glands and the endocrine glands. The **exocrine glands** have ducts, or tiny tubes, into which the exocrine secretions are released before reaching body surfaces or body cavities. The exocrine secretions include mucus, sweat, saliva, and digestive enzymes. The ducts carry the exocrine secretions outside the body. For example, sweat flows from the sweat glands through ducts onto the surface of the skin for evaporation (Fig. 6.4).

The **endocrine glands** secrete hormones, such as insulin. Endocrine glands do not have ducts and are therefore called *ductless glands*. Because endocrine glands are ductless, the hormones are secreted directly into the blood. The blood then carries the hormones to their sites of action.

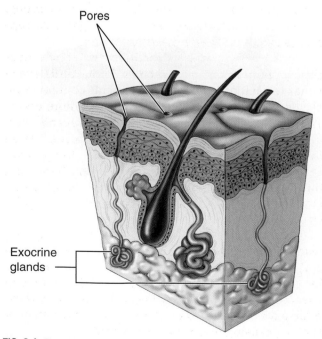

Pores

Exocrine glands

FIG. 6.4 **Exocrine gland, a sweat gland.**

 Re-Think

1. With regard to classification, what are two differences between simple columnar epithelial tissue and stratified squamous epithelial tissue?
2. What is the primary function of simple squamous epithelium?

 Sum It Up!

Tissues are groups of cells that are similar to each other in structure and function. The four types of tissues are epithelial, connective, nervous, and muscle. Epithelial tissue covers the body (as the skin) and lines cavities that open to the outside; it is primarily concerned with protection, secretion, filtration, and absorption. The shape of epithelial tissue is described as squamous, cuboidal, and columnar. Depending on the number of layers, epithelial tissue is described as simple or stratified.

CONNECTIVE TISSUE

WHERE IS IT FOUND?

Connective tissue is the most abundant of the four tissue types and is widely distributed throughout the body. Connective tissue is found in blood, under the skin, in bone, and around many organs. As the name suggests, connective tissue connects, or binds together, the parts of the body. Other functions include support, protection, fat storage, and transport of substances.

WHAT DOES IT LOOK LIKE?

Although connective tissue types may not resemble each other very closely, they share two characteristics. First, most connective tissue, with the exception of ligaments, tendons, and cartilage, has a good blood supply. Ligaments, tendons, and cartilage have a poor blood supply. As any athlete knows, an injury to these structures usually heals very slowly. The second characteristic shared by most connective tissue is an abundance of **intercellular matrix**.

CONNECTIVE TISSUE CELLS

Each major type of connective tissue contains immature or "blast" cells. Fibroblasts are cells found in loose and dense fibrous tissue. Chondroblasts (KON-drohblasts) are found in cartilage and osteoblasts are found in bone. Blast cells secrete matrix that is characteristic of the tissue. In addition to fibroblasts, connective tissue contains other types of cells, such as macrophages, adipocytes, and cells that fight infection and inflammation.

The intercellular matrix is what makes the various types of connective tissue so different. Matrix is composed of fibrous protein and ground substance. The hardness of the matrix varies from one cell type to the next. The intercellular matrix may be liquid as in blood, gel-like as in fat tissue, rubbery as in cartilage, or hard as in bone. The amount of matrix also varies from one cell type to the next. In fat tissue, the cells are close together, with little intercellular matrix. Bone and cartilage, however, have few cells and large amounts of intercellular matrix.

Also found in the matrix of most connective tissue are protein fibers. These fibers are secreted by fibroblasts, and the fiber types include collagen, elastin, and reticular fibers (fine collagen). Collagen fibers are strong and flexible but are not easily stretched. Elastin fibers are not very strong, but they are stretchy, like a rubber band.

 Re-Think

Compare the amount of intercellular material of epithelial tissue with the amount of intercellular matrix of connective tissue.

TYPES OF CONNECTIVE TISSUE

The many types of connective tissue are loose connective tissue, dense fibrous connective tissue, cartilage, bone, and the "liquid" connective tissue (blood and lymph; Fig. 6.5). Table 6.2 describes these types.

LOOSE CONNECTIVE TISSUE

Loose connective tissue contains fibers that are loosely arranged around cells. There are three types of loose connective tissue: areolar tissue, adipose tissue, and reticular connective tissue (see Fig. 6.5).

Areolar (ah-REE-oh-lar) **tissue** is made up of collagen and elastin fibers in a gel-like intercellular matrix. Areolar tissue is soft and surrounds, protects, and cushions many of the organs, acting as "tissue glue." It is the most widely distributed type of connective tissue.

Adipose (AD-i-pohs) **tissue** or fat is composed primarily of adipocytes, or cells that store fat (see Fig. 6.5). The more fat that is stored, the larger the adipocyte. Fat performs several important functions:

- Fat serves as the body's reservoir of energy. When the body needs energy, the fat is broken down, and the energy is released. Unfortunately, fat storage often exceeds energy requirements.
- Fat assists in body temperature regulation. Adipose tissue forms the tissue layer underlying the skin (the subcutaneous layer). Because of its location, adipose tissue can insulate the body from extremes of outside temperature. For example, in a cold environment, adipose tissue prevents the loss of heat from the body. This protection is best appreciated in observing the fat content of animals living in arctic conditions. The walrus, for example, has huge layers of fat tissue (blubber).

Because of the insulating qualities of the blubber, the walrus can swim in deep cold waters without freezing to death. Think of how long you could sit on an iceberg, even if you had a few extra pounds.

- Fat acts as a cushion. For example, a pad of fat behind the eyeball protects the eye from the hard bones of the eye socket.
- Fat protects some organs by anchoring them in place. The kidney, for example, has a layer of fat tissue that helps hold it in place. In extremely thin individuals, this fat tissue may be absent, allowing the kidney to move around (a "floating kidney").

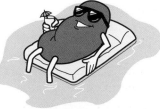

Reticular tissue is characterized by a network of delicately interwoven cells and reticular (fine collagen) fibers. It forms the internal framework for lymphatic tissue such as the spleen, lymph nodes, and bone marrow.

 Re-Think

1. List the three types of loose connective tissue.
2. Describe four functions of adipose tissue.

DENSE FIBROUS CONNECTIVE TISSUE

Dense fibrous connective tissue is composed of fibroblasts and an intercellular matrix that contains many collagen and elastic fibers. Collagen is the main type of fiber in dense fibrous tissue. The fibers form strong, supporting structures such as tendons, ligaments, capsules, fascia, and the dermal layer of skin.

Tendons are cordlike structures that attach muscles to bones. **Ligaments** cross joints and attach bones to each other. Because ligaments contain more elastic fibers than tendons, they stretch more easily. The ability to stretch is important; it prevents tearing of the ligaments when the joints bend. Dense fibrous connective tissue also forms tough capsules around certain organs (kidney and liver) and forms sheets of tissue called **fascia** (FASH-uh) that covers, supports, and anchors organs to nearby structures.

If stretching is excessive, as with athletic injuries, tendons and ligaments can tear, causing severe pain and impaired mobility. A ruptured Achilles tendon, for example, is a serious injury. The Achilles tendon attaches the leg muscles to the heel of the foot. If excessive force is exerted on the tendon, it may snap or rupture, causing loss of foot movement.

Connective Tissue

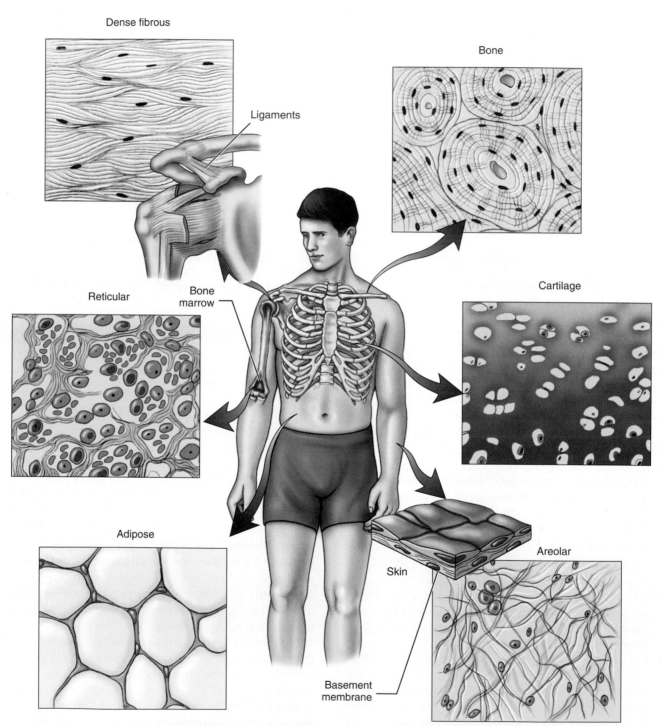

Dense fibrous

Ligaments

Bone

Reticular

Bone marrow

Cartilage

Adipose

Skin

Areolar

Basement membrane

FIG. 6.5 **Types and location of connective tissue. (Blood and lymph are not shown.)**

Table 6.2 Types of Connective Tissue

TYPE	LOCATION	FUNCTION
Loose Connective		
Areolar	Beneath skin and most epithelial layers; between muscles	Binds together, protects, cushions; "tissue glue"
Adipose	Beneath skin (subcutaneous) Around kidneys and heart Behind eyeballs	Cushions, insulates, stores fat
Reticular	Lymphoid tissue such as lymph nodes, spleen, and bone marrow	Forms internal framework of lymphoid organs
Dense Fibrous Connective		
	Tendons, ligaments, capsules, and fascia Skin (dermis)	Binds structures together
Cartilage		
Hyaline	Ends of long bone at joints Connects ribs to sternum Rings in trachea of respiratory tract Nose Fetal skeleton	Supports, protects, provides framework
Fibrocartilage	Intervertebral discs (in backbone) Pads in knee joint Pad between pubic bones (symphysis pubis)	Cushions, protects
Elastic cartilage	External ear and part of larynx	Supports, provides framework
Bone		
	Bones of the skeleton	Supports, protects, provides framework
Blood		
	Blood vessels throughout the body	Transports nutrients, hormones, respiratory gases (oxygen and carbon dioxide), waste
Lymph		
	Lymphatic vessels throughout the body	Drains interstitial fluid; involved in immune response

 ### Do You Know...

Why Overweight Men and Women "Round Out" into Different Shapes?

Overeating results in the storage of fat in adipose tissue. Because fat metabolism is affected by the sex hormones estrogen and testosterone, storage sites differ for males and females. In the male, excess fat is stored primarily in the abdominal region, whereas in the female, excess fat is stored around the breasts and hips. Excess adipose tissue, especially that which deposits in the abdominal region, becomes metabolically active and secretes hormones that adversely affect metabolism. The "spare tire" hormones increase blood glucose, increase resistance to insulin, and increase blood pressure, none of which is healthy.

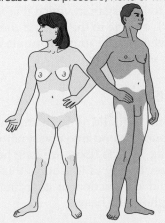

 ### Do You Know...

About Cooper's Droop?

As we age, the effects of gravity take over and some parts of the anatomy "head south." Breast tissue is anchored to the underlying structures by strands of connective tissue called *suspensory ligaments* (Cooper's ligaments). As we age, the tissue weakens and, sadly, sagging happens. The sorry saga of the sagging breasts is called *Cooper's droop*.

 ### Re-Think

What is the difference between a tendon and a ligament? Between fascia and a capsule?

CARTILAGE

Cartilage is formed by chondroblasts that eventually mature into **chondrocytes**, or cartilage cells. The chondroblasts secrete a protein-containing intercellular matrix that becomes firm, smooth, and rubbery. Although the matrix of cartilage is solid, it is not as hard as that of bone. Except for fibrocartilage, most cartilage is covered by perichondrium (pair-i-KON-dree-um), a layer of connective tissue that carries blood vessels to the cartilage. The blood vessels supply oxygen and nutrients to the cartilage. Located between the perichondrium and the cartilage is a storage supply of chondroblasts. The stored chondroblasts provide for cartilage growth throughout life.

Types of Cartilage

Three types of cartilage are hyaline cartilage, elastic cartilage, and fibrocartilage. Hyaline cartilage is found in (1) the larynx, or voicebox, (2) the ends of long bones at joints, (3) the nose, and (4) the area between the breastbone and the ribs. Fig. 6.5 illustrates the attachment of the ribs to the breastbone by hyaline cartilage. Hyaline cartilage is found in larger quantities in the fetal skeleton. As the fetus matures, however, most of the cartilage is converted to bone.

BONE

Bone tissue is also called **osseous** (OS-ee-us) **tissue.** Immature bone cells are called *osteoblasts.* Osteoblasts secrete an intercellular matrix that includes collagen, calcium salts, and other minerals. The collagen provides flexibility and strength; the mineral-containing matrix as a whole makes the bone tissue hard. The hardness of the bone enables it to protect organs such as the brain and to support the weight of the body for standing and moving. Bone also acts as a storage site for mineral salts, especially calcium (see Chapter 8). Osteoblasts mature into osteocytes.

When mineralization of bone tissue is diminished, as in osteoporosis, the bone is weakened and tends to break easily. Adequate dietary intake of calcium is essential for strong bones. Calcium is needed throughout the life cycle but is especially important during childhood and pregnancy, when bones are growing, and after menopause, when estrogen levels in women decline. Estrogen normally encourages the deposition of calcium in bone tissue, as does exercise and weight-bearing activity.

BLOOD AND LYMPH

Blood and lymph are two types of connective tissue that have a liquid intercellular matrix. Blood consists of blood cells surrounded by a fluid intercellular matrix called *plasma.* Unlike other connective tissues, which contain collagen and elastin fibers in the intercellular matrix, plasma contains nonfibrous plasma proteins (see Chapter 15). Lymph is the fluid that is found in lymphatic vessels (see Chapter 20).

? Re-Think

1. Differentiate between a chondroblast, chondrocyte, and perichondrium.
2. Differentiate between osseous tissue, osteoblasts, and osteocytes.
3. What is the difference in the intercellular matrix of cartilage, bone, and blood?

NERVOUS TISSUE

Nervous tissue makes up the brain, spinal cord, and nerves. Nervous tissue consists of two types of cells: neurons and neuroglia (Fig. 6.6).

NEURONS

Neurons are nerve cells that transmit electrical signals to and from the brain and spinal cord. The neuron has three parts: (1) the dendrites, which receive information from other neurons; (2) the cell body, which contains the nucleus and is essential to the life of the cell; and (3) the axon, which transmits information away from the cell body.

Neuroglia (noo-ROG-lee-ah), or glia, are cells that support and take care of the neurons. The word *glial* means "gluelike" and refers to the ability of these cells to support, or bind together, the vast network of neurons. (Nervous tissue is described more fully in Chapters 10 to 13.)

MUSCLE TISSUE

Muscle tissue is composed of cells that shorten, or contract. In doing so, they cause movement of a body part. Because the cells are long and slender, they are called *fibers* rather than *cells.* The three types of muscle are skeletal, smooth, and cardiac (Fig. 6.7).

SKELETAL MUSCLE

Skeletal muscle is generally attached to bone (the skeletal system). Because of the appearance of striations (STRYE-ay-shuns) or stripes, *skeletal muscle* is also called *striated muscle.* Skeletal muscles move the skeleton, maintain posture, and stabilize joints.

SMOOTH MUSCLE

Smooth muscle, also called *visceral muscle,* is generally found in the walls of the viscera, or organs, such as the stomach, intestines, and urinary bladder. It is also found in tubes such as the bronchioles (breathing passages) and blood vessels. The function of smooth muscle is related to the organ in which it is found. For example, smooth muscle in the stomach helps mash and churn food, whereas the smooth muscle in the urinary bladder helps expel urine.

CARDIAC MUSCLE

Cardiac muscle is found only in the heart, where it functions to pump blood into a vast network of blood vessels. Cardiac muscle fibers are long branching cells that fit together tightly at junctions; this arrangement promotes rapid conduction of coordinated electrical signals throughout the heart.

Nervous Tissue

Neuron

Neuroglia (glia)

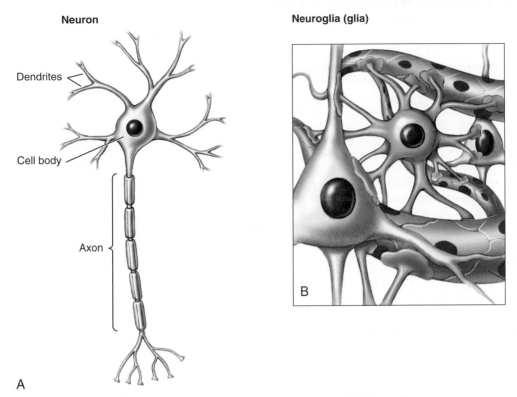

Dendrites

Cell body

Axon

A

B

FIG. 6.6 Two types of nervous tissue. (A) Neuron. (B) Neuroglia.

Muscle Tissue

Skeletal

Cardiac

Smooth

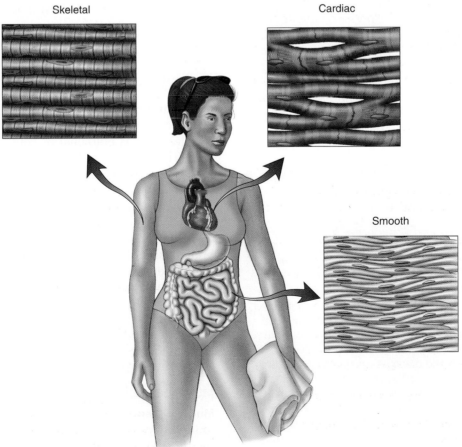

FIG. 6.7 Types of muscle tissue: skeletal, cardiac, and smooth.

? Re-Think

List the four types of tissue, and state the general function of each type.

 Sum It Up!

Connective tissue is the most widespread and diverse of the tissue types; its abundant intercellular matrix can be solid, rubbery, gel-like, or liquid. Connective tissue generally connects and binds together parts of the body. Nervous tissue is found in the brain, spinal cord, and nerves and is concerned with the transmission of information throughout the entire body. Muscle tissue is composed of cells that can contract and thus produce movement of body parts. The three types of muscle are skeletal, smooth, and cardiac.

TISSUE REPAIR

How does tissue repair itself after an injury? Two types of tissue repair are regeneration and fibrosis. Regeneration refers to the replacement of tissue by cells that are identical to the original cells. Regeneration occurs only in tissues whose cells undergo mitosis, such as the skin.

Fibrosis is the replacement of injured tissue by the formation of fibrous connective tissue, or scar tissue. The fibers of scar tissue pull the edges of the wound together and strengthen the area. Damaged skeletal muscle, cardiac muscle, and nervous tissue do not undergo mitosis and must be replaced by scar tissue. The steps involved in tissue repair are illustrated and described in Fig. 6.8. The injured skin of some persons exhibits excessive fibrosis, leading to the formation of keloids. Keloid (KEE-loyd) scars develop most often on the upper trunk and earlobes and are of concern cosmetically. Unfortunately, they tend to recur when surgically removed. Some tribespeople practice scarification during which the skin is sliced in hopes of inducing keloid scar formation. The keloid scar pattern reflects a significant event or rite of passage in the person's life.

 Do You Know...

What a Confederate Medical Officer Observed about a Maggot-Infested Battle Wound?

He observed that the wound was "cleaner" than wounds not infested with maggots. The incidence of septicemia (blood poisoning) was also lower in patients with maggot-infested wounds. Maggots are fly larvae; in the battlefield, the infected wound attracted flies that promptly laid their eggs, producing the larvae. Hungry maggots feasted on dead and infected tissue, thereby débriding the wound. (Débridement (day-BREED-ment) is the process of removing necrotic tissue from a wound to promote the growth of healthy tissue.) Despite our disgust at such dining practices, maggots have recently been re-employed in the hospital setting to clean up infected wounds. Maggots, hatched and dispatched under sterile conditions, perform their duties under a new fancy name: bio-débridement. Maggots are placed in the infected wound and allowed to "do their thing." New name, same old maggot.

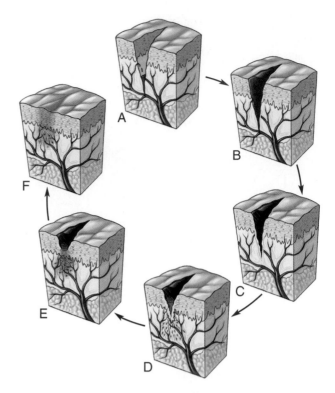

FIG. 6.8 Steps in tissue repair. (A) A deep wound to the skin severs blood vessels, causing blood to fill the wound. (B) A blood clot forms and, as it dries, it forms a scab. (C and D) The process of tissue repair begins. Scar tissue forms in the deep layers. (E) At the same time, surface epithelial cells multiply and fill the area between the scar tissue and the scab. (F) When the epithelium is complete, the scab detaches. The result is a fully regenerated layer of epithelium over an underlying area of scar tissue.

MEMBRANES

CLASSIFICATION OF MEMBRANES

Membranes are thin sheets of tissue that cover surfaces, line body cavities, and surround organs. Membranes are classified as epithelial or connective tissue (Table 6.3). (The connective tissue membranes are described in Chapters 8 and 10.)

EPITHELIAL MEMBRANES

The epithelial membranes include the cutaneous membrane (skin), the mucous membranes, and the serous membranes (Fig. 6.9). Although called *epithelial*, these membranes contain both an epithelial sheet and an underlying layer of connective tissue.

CUTANEOUS MEMBRANE

The cutaneous membrane is the skin and will be described in Chapter 7.

MUCOUS MEMBRANES

Mucous membranes line all body cavities that open to the exterior of the body (see Fig. 6.9). They include the digestive, urinary, reproductive, and respiratory

Table **6.3**   Types of Membranes

TYPE	LOCATION
Epithelial Membranes	
Cutaneous membrane	Skin (outer layer)
Mucous membrane	Digestive tract lining Urinary tract lining Reproductive tract lining Respiratory tract lining

Serous membrane
  Pleurae
  Pericardium
  Peritoneum
	
	Thoracic cavity; pleural cavity
	Thoracic cavity around the heart; pericardial cavity
	Abdominopelvic cavity

Connective Tissue Membranes	
Synovial	Lines joint cavities; secretes synovial fluid
Periosteum	Covers bone; contains the blood vessels that supply the bone
Perichondrium	Covers cartilage; contains capillaries that nourish the cartilage
Meninges	Covers brain and spinal cord
Fascia (various kinds)	Appears throughout body

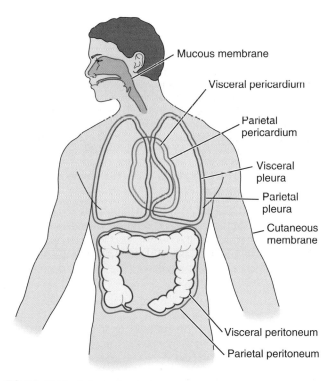

FIG. 6.9 **Epithelial membranes.**

tracts. For example, the digestive tract opens to the exterior of the body at the mouth and anus, whereas the respiratory tract opens to the exterior at the nose and mouth. Mucous membranes usually contain stratified squamous epithelium or simple columnar epithelium. Most mucous membranes are adapted for absorption and secretion. Mucous membranes secrete mucus, which keeps the membrane moist and also lubricates it. For example, in the digestive tract, the mucus allows food to move through the tract with little friction.

SEROUS MEMBRANES

Serous membranes line the ventral body cavities that are not open to the exterior of the body. If you were to enter the abdominal or thoracic cavity surgically, you would be looking at serous membranes. Serous membranes secrete a thin, watery, serous fluid. The fluid allows the membranes to slide past one another with little friction.

A serous membrane is composed of simple squamous epithelium resting on a thin layer of loose connective tissue. Serous membranes line a cavity and then fold back onto the surface of the organs within that cavity. Thus, part of the membrane lines the wall of the cavity, and the other part covers the organ or organs within that cavity. The part of the membrane that lines the walls of the cavity (like wallpaper) is the **parietal layer**, and the part of the membrane that covers the outside of an organ is the **visceral layer**.

The three serous membranes are the pleura, pericardium, and peritoneum (see Fig. 6.9):

1. Pleurae are found in the thoracic cavity. The parietal pleurae line the wall of the thoracic cavity, and the visceral pleurae cover each lung. The space between the pleural layers is called the *pleural cavity*; the membranes are lubricated by pleural fluid. Why is pleurisy so painful? Pleurisy refers to an inflammation of the pleurae and a decrease in serous fluid. As the inflamed and "dry" pleural membranes slide past one another during breathing movements, the person experiences pain.
2. The pericardium is found in the thoracic cavity and partially surrounds the heart. There is a parietal and visceral pericardium that offers slinglike support to the heart. The space between the pericardial membranes is called the *pericardial cavity*; the membranes are lubricated by pericardial fluid. Pericardial structure is described further in Chapter 16.

3. The peritoneum is found within the abdominal cavity. The parietal peritoneum lines its walls, and the visceral peritoneum covers some of the abdominal organs (see Chapter 23).

Infection in the abdominal cavity often involves the peritoneum. For example, a ruptured appendix allows the escape of intestinal contents, loaded with bacteria, into the peritoneal cavity. This leakage causes a life-threatening infectious condition called *peritonitis*.

 Re-Think

1. List the two classifications of membranes.
2. List and locate three epithelial membranes.

 Sum It Up!

Membranes are sheets of tissue. Membranes cover surfaces, line body cavities, and surround organs. Membranes are classified as epithelial membranes or connective tissue membranes. The epithelial membranes include cutaneous (skin), mucous, and serous membranes. The location and functions of the epithelial and connective tissue membranes are summarized in Table 6.3.

 As You Age

1. Because tissues consist of cells, cellular aging alters the tissues formed by the cells. Alterations in tissues, in turn, affect organ function. For example, by age 85, lung capacity has decreased by 50%, muscle strength has decreased by about 45%, and kidney function has decreased by 30%.
2. Collagen and elastin decrease in connective tissue. Consequently, tissues become stiffer, less elastic, and less efficient in their functioning.
3. Lipid and fat content of tissues change. In men, a gradual increase in tissue lipids and fat occurs until age 60, and then a gradual decrease follows. In women, lipids and fats accumulate in the tissues continuously; no decline occurs as in men.
4. The total amount of water in the body gradually decreases. The change in body fat and the decrease in water are major reasons why older adults respond differently to drugs than the younger population does.
5. Tissue atrophy causes a decrease in the mass of most organs.

Medical Terminology and Disorders   Disorders of Tissues and Membranes

MEDICAL TERM	WORD PARTS	WORD PART MEANING OR DERIVATION	DESCRIPTION
Words			
biopsy	bi/o-	life	A **biopsy** is *the removal and examination of tissue from a living body for diagnostic purposes.*
	-opsy	view of	
diagnosis	dia	apart	**Diagnosis** is *the process of identifying a disease or disorder by examination of the patient and all relevant data.* A correct diagnosis allows the physician to give the patient his **prognosis** (pro = before; gnos/o = knowing), *a forecast of the probable course of the disease.*
	-gnos/o-	distinguishing, learning, knowing	
endocrine	endo-	within	An endocrine gland secretes hormones that circulate through the blood and function within the body. For example, insulin is secreted by a gland called the *pancreas* and is carried throughout the body in the blood. An exocrine (exo = outside) gland secretes substances into ducts that carry the secretion to the outside of the body, as in sweat and sebum.
	-crin/o-	secrete	
histology	hist/o-	tissue	**Histology** is *the study of tissues.*
	-logy	study of	
necrosis	necr/o-	death	**Necrosis** refers to *the process of death of the cells or tissues, especially in a localized area.* Tissue that is deprived of its blood supply necroses, or dies.
	-osis	condition of	
Disorders			
adhesions	ad-	to, toward, or near	**Adhesions** are *bands of "internal scar tissue" that bind or constrict organs.* Surgery and infection are common causes. As part of the healing process, fibrin and other tissue repair cells penetrate the fibrous bands, contributing to the formation of the adhesion. Adhesions are particularly common in the abdominopelvic cavity. An example of an adhesion-related consequence is intestinal obstruction.
	-hension	From a Latin word meaning "sticking to"	
connective tissue diseases			*A group of diseases that attack the connective tissues of the body.* The connective tissues are composed of two major structural proteins: collagen and elastin. *Diseases that affect collagen specifically* are also referred to as *collagen diseases.* Many connective tissue diseases are associated with abnormal immune system activity. A wide variety of symptoms can occur depending on the location of the connective tissue. Systemic autoimmune connective tissue diseases include systemic lupus erythematosus (SLE) and scleroderma.

Medical Terminology and Disorders   Disorders of Tissues and Membranes—cont'd

MEDICAL TERM	WORD PARTS	WORD PART MEANING OR DERIVATION	DESCRIPTION
gangrene		From a Greek word meaning "to gnaw"	**Gangrene** is *a condition in which an insufficient blood supply causes tissue necrosis.* Two types of gangrene are dry and wet gangrene. Dry gangrene is caused by ischemia (poor blood supply). Wet gangrene involves infection of a wound that impairs both arterial and venous blood flow and cell function.
neoplasm	neo- -plasm	newly formed material	A **neoplasm** is *an abnormal proliferation of cells, the growth being excessive and uncoordinated with surrounding cells.* The excessive growth most often forms a lump or a solid tumor. Neoplasms may be benign, premalignant, or malignant. Examples of benign (meaning "well," as opposed to malignant) neoplasms include fibromas, adenomas, lipomas, and skin moles. They are localized, do not become malignant, and do not metastasize. An example of a premalignant neoplasm is carcinoma-in-situ; it remains localized for a while but becomes cancerous given enough time. Hence, the urgency for early diagnosis and treatment. Malignant (from a Latin word meaning "acting from malice") neoplasms are called *cancers.* Because they are invasive and metastatic (spreading), they eventually kill the host. The primary neoplasm is *the original or first tumor;* untreated, it spreads or metastasizes throughout the body. A **secondary neoplasm** refers to *a cancerous tumor that is the result of metastasis (metastatic lesion). Carcinomas and sarcomas are malignant tumors. A* **carcinoma** *is a malignant tumor that arises from epithelial tissue. A* **sarcoma** *is a malignant tumor that arises from connective tissue.*

Get Ready for Exams!

Summary Outline

Tissues are groups of cells similar to each other in structure and function. Membranes are thin sheets of tissue that cover surfaces, line body cavities, and surround organs.

I. **Types of Tissue**
   A. Epithelial tissue
      1. Covers surfaces, lines cavities, and engages in secretion/absorption and protective functions
      2. Classified according to cell shape (squamous, cuboidal, and columnar) and layers (simple and stratified)
      3. Types and functions are summarized in Table 6.1.
   B. Connective tissue
      1. Primary function of connective tissue is to bind together the parts of the body. Other functions include support, protection, storage of fat, and transport of substances. See Table 6.2.
      2. Has an abundant intercellular matrix that may be liquid, gel-like, or hard; often contains protein fibers that are secreted by the cells
      3. Types of loose connective tissue: areolar, adipose, and reticular
      4. Dense fibrous connective tissue forms tendons, ligaments, capsules, fascia, and the dermal layer of skin.
      5. Types of cartilage: hyaline, elastic, and fibrocartilage
      6. Bone (osseous tissue) has a hard intercellular matrix that includes collagen, calcium salts, and other minerals.
      7. Blood and lymph have a watery intercellular matrix.
   C. Nervous tissue
      1. Nervous tissue: found in the nerves, brain, and spinal cord
      2. Two types of nervous tissue: neurons (transmit electrical signals) and neuroglia (support and take care of the neurons)
   D. Muscle tissue
      1. Muscle cells contract, thereby causing movement.
      2. Three types of muscle: skeletal, smooth, and cardiac

II. **Tissue Repair**
   A. Tissue repair by regeneration: replacement of tissue by cells that undergo mitosis
   B. Tissue repair by fibrosis: formation of scar tissue

III. **Membranes**
   A. Epithelial membranes (see Table 6.3)
      1. Cutaneous membrane: the skin
      2. Mucous membrane: lines all body cavities that open to the exterior of the body
      3. Serous membranes: line the ventral body cavities, which are not open to the exterior of the body
      4. Layers of serous membranes: a parietal layer that lines the wall of the cavity and a visceral layer that covers the outside of an organ
      5. Three serous membranes: pleurae, pericardium, and peritoneum
   B. Connective tissue membranes (see Table 6.3): includes synovial, periosteum, pericardium, meninges, and fascia

Review Your Knowledge

Matching: Tissues

Directions: Match the following words with their descriptions. Some words may be used more than once.

a. epithelial

b. connective

c. muscle

d. nervous

1. ___ Important functions: secretion, absorption, excretion, and protection

2. ___ Blood, bone, cartilage, and adipose tissue

3. ___ Classified as squamous, cuboidal, or columnar

4. ___ Endocrine and exocrine glands arise from this type of tissue

5. ___ Binds together parts of the body; examples include tendons, ligaments, and fascia

6. ___ Skeletal, cardiac, and smooth

7. ___ Has the greatest amount of intercellular matrix

8. ___ Chondrocytes and osteocytes are included in this tissue

9. ___ Intercellular matrix may be liquid, gel, or rigid

10. ___ Dendrites, axons, and glia

Matching: Membranes

Directions: Match the following words with their descriptions.

a. visceral pleura

b. parietal peritoneum

c. connective tissue membranes

d. mucous membranes

e. parietal pleura

1. ___ Membranes lining all body cavities that open to the outside of the body

2. ___ Serous membrane that lines the walls of the thoracic cavity

3. ___ Serous membrane that lines the walls of the abdominopelvic cavity

4. ___ Serous membrane that covers each lung

5. ___ Synovial membranes: periosteum, perichondrium, and meninges

Multiple Choice

1. Which of the following is *not* characteristic of epithelial tissue?
   a. Arranged like floor tiles
   b. Simple, cuboidal, and columnar
   c. Large amount of mineral-containing intercellular matrix
   d. Gives rise to endocrine and exocrine glands

2. Adipose tissue is
   a. a type of connective tissue that stores fat.
   b. described as striated and voluntary.
   c. classified as endocrine and exocrine.
   d. classified as skeletal, cardiac, and smooth.

3. Characteristics of osseous tissue include which of the following?
   a. Contains hard mineral-containing intercellular matrix
   b. Contains osteocytes
   c. Is a type of connective tissue
   d. All of the above

4. With regard to the pleural membranes,
   a. there is a visceral and parietal pleural membrane.
   b. they are connective tissue membranes.
   c. they are mucous membranes.
   d. they are located in the dorsal cavity.

5. The pleurae and peritoneum
   a. are serous membranes.
   b. are located within the thoracic cavity.
   c. are located within the abdominal cavity.
   d. surround the lungs and the heart.

6. Epithelial tissue is avascular, meaning that it
   a. is shaped like a fish scale.
   b. contains no blood vessels.
   c. has no intercellular matrix.
   d. cannot repair itself.

7. The intercellular matrix of connective tissue
   a. is less apparent than the intercellular matrix of epithelial tissue.
   b. is absent in blood and lymph.
   c. is classified as squamous, cuboidal, or columnar.
   d. can be hard, liquid, or gel-like in consistency.

Go Figure

1. Which of the following is correct according to Figs. 6.1 and 6.2 and Table 6.1?
   a. Cuboidal epithelium is flatter than squamous epithelium.
   b. Simple squamous epithelium is ideally suited for the movement of nutrients, waste, and gases.
   c. Simple squamous epithelium is thick and easily withstands stretch and abrasion.
   d. Epithelial tissue is characterized by an abundance of intercellular matrix.

2. Which of the following is correct according to Fig. 6.3 and Table 6.1?
   a. The air sacs in the lungs are composed of stratified columnar epithelium, thereby facilitating the exchange of oxygen and carbon dioxide.
   b. The linings of the mouth and digestive tract are composed of transitional epithelium, thereby allowing for expansion.
   c. Transitional epithelium is found primarily in the urinary bladder.
   d. Pseudostratified epithelium has three layers (strata) of columnar cells.

3. Which of the following is correct according to Fig. 6.4 and Table 6.1?
   a. Exocrine glands pour their secretions into ducts.
   b. The ducts carrying exocrine secretions empty into the blood.
   c. Exocrine glands secrete only sweat.
   d. Glandular tissue is composed primarily of adipose tissue.

4. Which of the following is correct according to Fig. 6.5 and Table 6.2?
   a. All connective tissue has a hard intercellular matrix.
   b. Bone is classified as dense fibrous connective tissue.
   c. The skeleton consists only of bone.
   d. Adipose tissue stores fat.

5. Which of the following is correct according to Fig. 6.5 and Table 6.2?
   a. Tendons, ligaments, capsules, and fascia are composed primarily of dense fibrous connective tissue.
   b. Fibro-, hyaline, and elastic refer to types of loose connective tissue.
   c. Glandular tissue, both endocrine and exocrine, is composed primarily of dense fibrous connective tissue.
   d. Connective tissue is classified as squamous, cuboidal, columnar, and simple/stratified.

6. Which of the following is correct according to Fig. 6.6?
   a. Dendrites and axons are parts of the glial cells.
   b. There are two types of nervous tissue: axons and dendrites.
   c. Dendrites are the blue structures that wrap around the axon.
   d. The neuron has a cell body, axon, and dendrites.

7. Which of the following is correct according to Fig. 6.6?
   a. Smooth muscle is confined to the heart.
   b. *Skeletal, cardiac,* and *smooth* are terms that describe visceral muscle.
   c. Both skeletal and cardiac muscle are striped or striated.
   d. Smooth muscle is striped or striated, like skeletal muscle.

8. Which of the following is correct according to Fig. 6.9?
   a. The terms *parietal* and *visceral* only refer to serous membranes located within the thoracic cavity.
   b. Pleural membranes surround the lungs and heart.
   c. The visceral and parietal peritoneal membranes are located in the abdominopelvic cavity.
   d. The cutaneous membrane lines the mouth and digestive tract.

Integumentary System and Body Temperature

Objectives

1. List seven functions of the skin.
2. Discuss the structure of the skin, including the following:
   - Describe the two layers of skin: the epidermis and the dermis.
   - Define *stratum germinativum* and *stratum corneum*.
   - List the two major functions of the subcutaneous layer.
3. List the factors that influence the color of the skin.
4. Describe the accessory structures of the skin: hair, nails, and glands.
5. Define *thermoregulation*, and describe the way that the body conserves and loses heat.
6. Differentiate between insensible and sensible perspiration.

Key Terms

apocrine glands (p. 101)
ceruminous glands (p. 101)
conduction (p. 102)
convection (p. 102)
cutaneous membrane (p. 95)
dermis (p. 95)
eccrine glands (p. 101)
epidermis (p. 95)
evaporation (p. 102)

fingerprints (p. 96)
hyperthermia (p. 102)
hypothermia (p. 102)
insensible perspiration (p. 101)
integument (p. 95)
keratin (p. 95)
melanin (p. 97)
nonshivering thermogenesis (p. 103)
pyrexia (p. 104)

radiation (p. 102)
sebaceous glands (p. 100)
sensible perspiration (p. 101)
stratum corneum (p. 96)
stratum germinativum (p. 95)
subcutaneous layer (p. 97)
sudoriferous glands (p. 101)
thermoregulation (p. 102)
vernix caseosa (p. 100)

Oh no, a zit! How many times have you looked in the mirror only to see a pimple, rash, wrinkle, or unwanted hair? No other organ in the body is so scrutinized, scrubbed, lifted, and painted over as the skin. Yet, year after year, the skin withstands the effects of harsh weather, the burning rays of the sun, constant bathing, friction, injury, and microorganisms that are constantly trying to penetrate its surface.

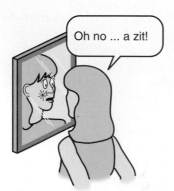

The skin, its accessory structures (sweat glands, oil glands, hair, and nails), and the subcutaneous tissue below the skin form the integumentary system.

FUNCTIONS OF THE INTEGUMENTARY SYSTEM

The integumentary (in-teg-yoo-MEN-tar-ee) system is a complex organ that performs many different functions:

- Acts as a mechanical barrier. It keeps harmful substances out of the body and helps retain water and electrolytes. The acid pH of the skin surface serves as a protective chemical barrier.
- Protects the internal structures and organs from injuries caused by blows, cuts, harsh chemicals, sunlight, burns, and pathogenic microorganisms.
- Participates in the immune response against invading microbes by housing specialized cells, called *dendritic* or *Langerhans'* cells. When the skin is broken, the dendritic cells alert the immune system so that it can ward off infection.
- Performs an excretory function. Although excretion is a minor role, the skin is able to excrete water, salt, and small amounts of waste, such as urea.
- Acts as a gland by synthesizing vitamin D when exposed to sunlight. Vitamin D is necessary for the absorption of calcium from the digestive tract.
- Performs a sensory role by housing the sensory receptors for touch, pressure, pain, and temperature.

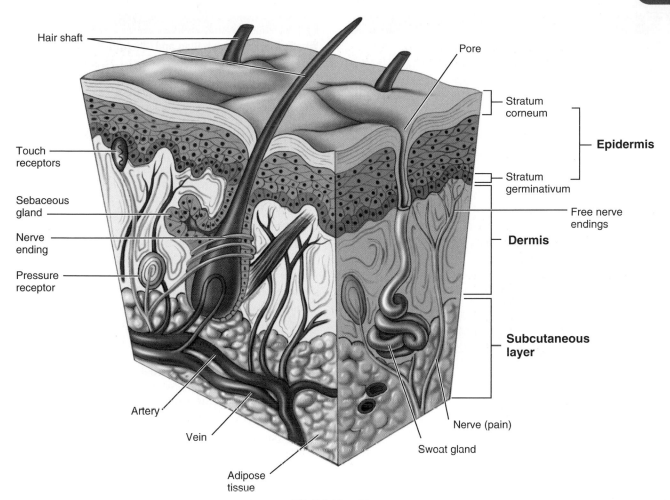

FIG. 7.1 **The skin.**

In this way, the skin helps detect information about the environment.

- Plays an important role in the regulation of body temperature.

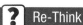 Re-Think

1. What are the functions of the integumentary system?
2. Explain how the skin acts as a mechanical barrier.

STRUCTURE OF THE SKIN

The skin is called the **integument** or **cutaneous membrane** and is considered an organ; it is the largest organ in the body. The skin has two distinct layers—the outer, or surface, layer is the **epidermis** and the inner layer is the **dermis**. The dermis is anchored to a subcutaneous layer (Fig. 7.1). The study of skin and skin disorders is referred to as *dermatology*.

LAYERS OF THE SKIN

EPIDERMIS

The epidermis (ep-i-DER-mis) is the thin outer layer of the skin and is composed of stratified squamous epithelium. Like all epithelial tissue, the epidermis is avascular; it has no blood supply of its own. Oxygen and nutrients, however, diffuse into the lower epidermis from the rich supply of blood in the underlying dermis. The epidermis can be divided into five layers. Two of the layers are the deeper stratum germinativum and the more superficial stratum corneum.

The **stratum germinativum** (jer-mi-nah-TIV-um) lies on top of the dermis and thus has access to a rich supply of blood. The cells of this layer are continuously dividing, producing millions of cells per day. As the cells divide, they push the older cells up toward the surface of the epithelium. As the cells move away from the dermis, two changes take place. First, as they move away from their source of nourishment, the cells begin to die. Second, the cells undergo a process of keratinization, whereby a tough protein, **keratin** (KER-ah-tin), is deposited within the cell. The keratin hardens and flattens the cells as they move toward the surface of the skin. In addition to hardening the cells, the keratin makes the skin water-resistant. Have you ever noticed that your hand does not dissolve when you place it in water?

Do You Know...

If Toad Did It?

Did Toad have anything to do with the wart on Helga's nose? No. A wart is an epidermal growth on the skin and is caused by a virus. Although Toad is innocent of this charge, there are several other health concerns. Toad skin can harbor and therefore transmit *Salmonella*, and some toad skins secrete toxins that are harmful to pets and humans. However, from Toad's perspective, handling can damage his skin.

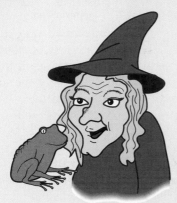

The **stratum corneum** is the surface layer of the epidermis and is composed of about 30 layers of dead, flattened, keratinized cells. The dead cells are continuously sloughed off, exfoliated (eks-FOH-lee-a-tid), or desquamated (des-kwah-MAY-tid) through wear and tear. The dead sloughed cells are called *dander*; when dander is clumped together by the oil on the skull, it is called *dandruff*. The sloughed cells are replaced by other cells that are constantly moving up from the deeper layers. You shed about 40,000 skin cells each minute; each month you have a new layer of epithelium. Interesting fact: the ink used in creating a tattoo must be deposited into the dermis because of the sloughing characteristic of the epidermis. Ouch!

DERMIS

The dermis is located beneath the epidermis and is the largest portion of the skin; it is composed of dense fibrous connective tissue. It contains numerous collagen and elastin fibers surrounded by a gel-like substance. The fibers make the dermis strong and stretchable; note how well the skin stretches during pregnancy and weight gain. Sometimes, however, excessive stretching of the skin causes small tears in the skin, producing white lines. These lines are called *stretch marks*, or striae (STRYE-ay). The thickness of the epidermis and dermis varies according to the location on the body. Look at the skin on the palms of your hands and the soles of your feet; it is much thicker here than it is over your inner arm or eyelids.

 Do You Know...

What's in That Bathtub Ring and What Are You Dusting?

The bathtub ring: What's in it? Dirt, grime...and, yes, a piece of yourself—dead skin (stratum corneum). How much dead skin? A person sheds about 1.5 lb per year, or about 105 lb over a lifetime. This means that you will scrape the equivalent of your entire body from the sides of your tub and watch it go down the drain. Also, about 75% of household dust is human skin flakes. What doesn't wash down the drain gets sucked up by a vacuum cleaner.

Dead skin on your furniture? Dust not only looks nasty but also feeds critters such as the house dust mite *(Dermatophagoides)*. Those who have been diagnosed as having house dust allergy will be relieved to know that they are really allergic to the inhaled feces of the dust mite.

The wavy boundary between the epidermis and dermis resembles the ridges of corrugated cardboard. The interlocking ridges prevent the slippage of the skin layers. More importantly, for you forensic sleuths, the ridges form the **fingerprints**. Also! Here is a problem that had baffled investigators in child abduction cases. Why do a child's fingerprints vanish so quickly at the crime scene? Finally, the answer! An adult's fingerprints are oil-based. On the other hand, a child's fingerprints, before puberty when the oil-secreting glands kick in, are water-based. When the water evaporates, the fingerprints evaporate. Not good for evidence collecting.

Although derived from the epidermis, the accessory structures such as the hair, nails, and certain glands are embedded within the dermis. Also located within the dermis are blood vessels, nervous tissue, and some muscle tissue. Many of the nerves have specialized endings called *sensory receptors* that detect pain, temperature, pressure, and touch.

 Re-Think

1. What are the two layers of the skin?
2. What "happens" in the stratum germinativum?
3. Describe two changes that the cells undergo as they "ascend" to the stratum corneum.

THE SKIN TELLS A STORY

- The skin reflects disease processes in the body. For example, a person with herpes zoster (shingles)—an inflammation of nerves caused by the chickenpox virus—develops painful skin lesions along the path of the nerve. A person with a severe generalized staphylococcal infection may develop scalded skin syndrome, a condition in which the skin appears scalded and peels off in layers. Many clinical disorders present initially with skin rashes; the rashes offer clues to the underlying problems.
- Drug reactions are often revealed by skin changes. For example, a person allergic to penicillin may develop hives, or urticaria (er-ti-KAIR-ee-ah). Similarly, a person allergic to sulfa drugs may develop a generalized rash that can progress to a lethal syndrome called *Stevens–Johnson syndrome*.

- The skin responds to chronic irritation. Epidermal cell growth increases in response to certain stimuli. For example, constant irritation or rubbing of an area causes the rate of epidermal cell division to increase, producing a thickened area called a *callus*. Constant rubbing of a toe by a poorly fitting shoe can also produce an overgrowth of epidermal cells arranged in a conical shape. This overgrowth is called a *corn*.
- The skin mirrors your stress level. How many times have you become stressed out and then broke out? The skin truly reveals on the outside what is going on inside!

 Do You Know...

About Margarita Dermatitis?

Exposure to the ultraviolet radiation of sunshine while mixing up tangy margaritas can cause a severe skin reaction called margarita dermatitis. Margarita dermatitis is a *phytophotodermatitis* (from the words parts meaning "plant," "light," "skin," and "inflammation") that resembles a second-degree burn: blistering, pain, and related misery. The skin reaction is apparently caused by the exposure of skin to the lime juice used in the preparation of a margarita. Although lime is the usual toxic culprit, the dermatitis can also develop in response to other citrus fruits and celery. If left untreated, severe dermatitis may cause an irreversible hyperpigmentation of the affected skin. So, party on….in the shade.

SUBCUTANEOUS LAYER

The dermis lies on the subcutaneous layer. This layer is not considered part of the skin; it lies under the skin and is therefore called the **subcutaneous layer**, or the hypodermis. The subcutaneous layer is composed primarily of loose connective and adipose tissue. The subcutaneous tissue performs two main roles: it helps insulate the body from extreme temperature changes in the external environment, and it anchors the skin to the underlying structures. A few areas of the body have no subcutaneous layer and the skin anchors directly to the bone. Look at the skin over your knuckles. It is wrinkled and creased because it attaches directly to bone. Imagine what you would look like if all your skin were anchored directly to underlying bone.

 Do You Know...

How You Inject a Medication into the Subcutaneous Layer?

When injecting medication subcutaneously, you need to use a correctly sized needle and insert the needle at the proper angle. The needle penetrates the epidermis and dermis so that the tip of the needle is located in the subcutaneous layer, where the medication is deposited.

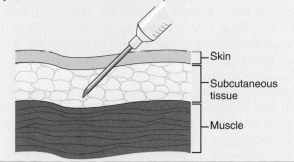

THE SKIN, DRUGS, AND CHEMICALS

The skin can absorb many chemicals; this is good news and bad news. The good news is concerned with drug absorption. Drugs can be placed on the surface of the skin and absorbed transdermally (across the skin) to achieve a systemic effect (throughout the body). For example, nitroglycerin can be applied using an adhesive patch on the skin. The drug penetrates the skin, is absorbed by the dermal blood vessels, and is transported by the blood throughout the body where it exerts its effects. The skin can also be used to detect allergies by injecting antigens (possible allergic substances) intradermally. An allergic response will appear as a skin reaction (redness, swelling, and itching). Drugs can also be applied topically; the drug is meant to exert its effect on the surface of the skin. Lastly, the subcutaneous route is a common way to inject drugs.

The bad news? Skin can absorb toxins; these include pesticides, cleaning fluids, the acetone in nail polish remover, mercury, and many other toxic chemicals that we encounter daily. Farm workers exposed to chemical sprays are commonly treated for pesticide poisoning. Interesting! Green, a favorite color in Victorian England, sometimes proved to be a lethal fashion statement. Seems that green was made from an arsenic-based dye that was readily absorbed across the skin. Not so today…green is good. Do not underestimate the ability of the skin to absorb toxins!

 Re-Think

Describe the role of the skin in drug administration (i.e., four routes of administration).

SKIN COLOR

Why are there different colors of skin? Skin color is determined by many factors: some genetic, some physiological, and some caused by disease. When we think of skin color, we generally think of black, brown, yellow, and white, as well as the many shades in between! These skin colors are genetically determined.

Deep within the epidermal layer of the skin are cells called *melanocytes*. Melanocytes (meh-LAN-oh-sytes) secrete a skin-darkening pigment called **melanin**; the melanin stains the surrounding cells, causing them to darken. The more melanin secreted, the darker the skin color. Interestingly, we all have the same numbers of melanocytes. What determines our skin color is not the numbers of melanocytes but the amount of melanin secreted. The following factors play a role in changes in skin color:

- *Melanin.* Can melanocytes increase their secretion of melanin? Yes! When exposed to the ultraviolet radiation of sunlight, the melanocytes secrete more melanin. The skin darkens in an attempt to protect the deeper layers from the harmful effects of radiation. This effort creates the famous summer tan. A number of conditions involve malfunctioning melanocytes. If the melanocytes completely fail to secrete melanin, the skin, hair, and the colored part of the eye (iris) are white. This condition is referred to as *albinism*. Other persons develop a condition called *vitiligo* (vit-i-LYE-go). This condition involves a loss of pigment (melanin) in certain areas of the skin, creating patches of white skin. Melanin can also stain unevenly. Freckles and moles are examples of melanin that becomes concentrated in local areas.

- *Carotene.* The yellowish tint of carotene in most persons is hidden by the effects of melanin. Because people of Asian descent have little melanin in their skin, the carotene gives their skin a yellow tint.
- *Blood.* What accounts for the pinkish color of fair-skinned people? So little melanin is produced that the blood in the dermal blood vessels is visible, thereby providing a pinkish tinge to the skin. Poorly oxygenated blood causes the skin to look blue. This condition is called *cyanosis* (sye-ah-NO-sis). Embarrassment causes the blood vessels in the skin to dilate. This condition increases blood flow to the skin, causing the person to blush or flush. What about the saying, "He was white as a sheet"? A person who is scared experiences a constriction of the blood vessels in the skin and a decrease in the amount of oxygenated blood. The resulting pale or ashen color is called *pallor.* A black and blue discoloration (bruise) indicates that blood has escaped from the blood vessels into the injured tissue. A black and blue area is called an *ecchymosis* (ek-ih-MOH-sis).
- *Bilirubin.* Skin color may also change in response to disease processes. A person with liver disease is unable to excrete a pigment called *bilirubin* (bil-ih-ROO-bin). This pigment is instead deposited in the skin, causing it to turn yellow—a condition known as *jaundice.*
- *Diet.* Finally, skin color may also change in response to diet. For example, it is possible to impart a yellow tint to the skin by overeating carotene-rich vegetables such as carrots.

Sum It Up!

The integumentary system is composed of the skin and accessory organs (hair, nails, and glands). It is a complex organ that performs many functions. It affords protection for the entire body, acts as a barrier, regulates temperature, detects sensations (e.g., touch, pressure, temperature, and pain), synthesizes vitamin D, participates in the immune response, and acts as an excretory organ. The skin is composed of two layers: the epidermis and dermis. The dermis sits on a subcutaneous layer called the *hypodermis*. There are different colors of skin. Our natural skin color is genetically determined; we are light-skinned, dark-skinned, and many shades in between. Our skin color changes in response to certain stimuli or underlying conditions; these changes include tanning, blushing, cyanosis, and jaundice. The skin can also reveal certain disease states, such as allergic responses, infections, liver disease, and stress. The skin often announces on the outside what is happening on the inside.

 Re-Think

Describe the underlying causes of the following color changes: cyanosis, flushing, pallor, jaundice, tanning, and vitiligo.

ACCESSORY STRUCTURES OF THE SKIN

The skin is the home of several accessory structures, including the hair, nails, and glands.

HAIR

Thousands and thousands of years ago, we humans were a hairy lot. Like our furry friends, our pets, we depended on a thick crop of hair to keep us warm. Today, most of the hair covering our bodies is sparse and very fine, with the exception of the hair on our heads (and for some, that too is sparse). The main function of our sparse body hair is to sense insects on the skin before they can sting us. Some body parts are hairless. These include the palms of the hands, soles of the feet, lips, nipples, and parts of the external reproductive organs.

Some areas of hair perform other functions. For example, the eyelashes and eyebrows protect the eyes from dust and perspiration. The nasal hairs trap dust and prevent it from being inhaled into the lungs. The hair of the scalp helps keep us warm and, of course, plays an important cosmetic role.

Hair growth and distribution are influenced by the sex hormones estrogen and testosterone. The onset of puberty is heralded by the growth of hair in the axillary and pubic areas in males and females. In the man, the surge of testosterone also produces a beard and hairy chest. Estrogen, of course, does not have this effect. When a woman has too much testosterone, excessive hair growth occurs, including facial hair. The excessive growth of hair is called *hirsutism* (HER-soo-tiz-em), from a Greek word meaning "shaggy." One more thing: apparently, hair growth responds rather well to mind–body signals. The beards of men who have been at sea for an extended period experience a growth spurt of hair when told that they are going ashore.

The chief parts of a hair are the shaft (the part above the surface of the skin) and the root (the part that extends from the dermis to the surface) (Fig. 7.2). Each hair arises from a group of epidermal cells that penetrate the dermis. This downward extension of epidermal cells forms the hair follicle. The epidermal cells of the hair follicle receive a rich supply of blood from the dermal blood vessels. As these cells divide and grow, the older cells are pushed toward the surface of the skin. As they move away from their source of nourishment, the cells die. Like other cells that compose the skin, the hair cells also become keratinized. The hair that we brush, blow-dry, and curl every day is a collection of dead, keratinized cells.

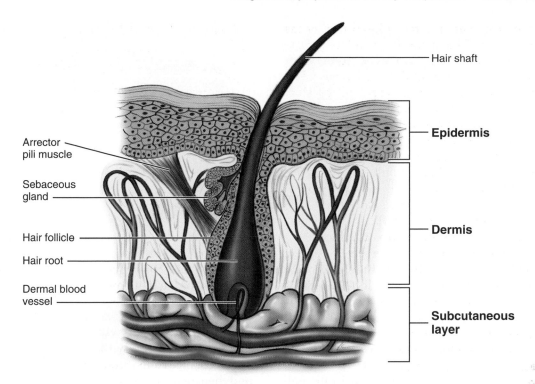

- Hair shaft
- **Epidermis**
- **Dermis**
- **Subcutaneous layer**
- Arrector pili muscle
- Sebaceous gland
- Hair follicle
- Hair root
- Dermal blood vessel

FIG. 7.2 **Hair follicle and parts of the hair.**

Hair color is determined by the type and amount of melanin secretion. An abundance of melanin produces dark hair, whereas less melanin produces blond hair. With age, the melanocytes become less active; the absence of melanin produces white hair. Gray hair is caused by a mixture of pigmented and nonpigmented hairs. Interestingly, red hair is caused by a modified type of melanin that contains iron. And… redheads require more anesthesia before surgery than people with other colored hair.

Curly, wavy, or straight—this is determined by the shape of the hair shaft. A round shaft produces straight hair, whereas an oval shaft produces wavy hair. Curly and kinky strands of hair are the result of flat hair shafts. Hair can be curled by chemically flattening the hair shafts.

How does Frightened Kitty get her hair to stand on end? Attached to the hair follicle is a group of smooth muscle cells called the *arrector pili* (ah-REK-tor PYE-lye) muscles (see Fig. 7.2). Contraction of these muscles causes the hair to stand on end. When frightened, the cat's brain sends its panic message along the nerves to these muscles. The muscles then contract and pull the hair into an upright position. Kitty looks more ferocious with her fur standing on end, and the spiked look helps frighten off her attackers. Her fur also stands on end when she is cold; the raised fur traps heat and helps keep her warm.

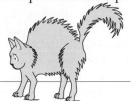

Although humans may not benefit as much from hair as do our furry friends, we respond to fear and cold in the same way. Contraction of the arrector pili muscles also causes our hair to stand on end. As the hair stands, it pulls the skin up into little bumps. This reaction is the basis of goose flesh, or goose bumps. Unlike Kitty, the erect human hair does not do much to trap heat.

Cosmetically, hair is important. Hair loss to the point of baldness is distressing—enter the comb-over. Loss of hair is called *alopecia* (al-o-PEE-sha), which comes from a word meaning "fox mange." The most common type of baldness is male pattern baldness, which is a hereditary condition characterized by a gradual loss of hair with aging—hair today, gone tomorrow! A second common cause of hair loss is related to drug toxicity, as with chemotherapy or radiation therapy. Anticancer drugs are so cytotoxic that they often destroy hair-producing epithelial cells. When drug therapy is terminated, the cells regenerate and start to grow hair again. Interestingly, the new hair may be a different color or texture from the original (pre-drug) hair.

Forensically, hair is a gold mine. For example, arsenic is called *inheritance powder* because it is a long-time favorite for dispatching wealthy family members. Chronic arsenic poisoning is difficult to detect medically, but analysis of the hair not only detects the presence of arsenic; it can also detect the time course of the poisoning.

? Re-Think

1. What is the function of the hair follicle?
2. What effect do the sex hormones, such as estrogen and testosterone, have on hair growth and distribution?
3. Differentiate between hirsutism and alopecia.

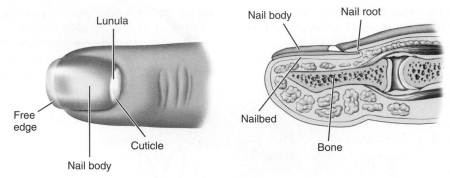

FIG. 7.3 Nail.

NAILS

Nails are thin plates of stratified squamous epithelial cells that contain a very hard form of keratin (Fig. 7.3). The nails are found on the distal ends of the fingers and toes and protect these structures from injury.

Each nail has the following structures: a free edge, a nail body (fingernail), and a nail root. The cells of the nail body develop and are keratinized in the nail root. The extent of nail growth is represented by the half-moon–shaped lunula (LOO-nyoo-lah), located at the base of the nail. As the nail body grows, it slides over a layer called the *nail bed,* a part of the epidermis. The pink color of nails is caused by the blood vessels in the underlying dermal layer beneath the nail. The cuticle is a fold of stratum corneum that grows onto the proximal portion of the nail body.

Like the skin, the nails also tell stories. The condition of the nails provides important diagnostic information regarding systemic disease. Nails should be examined for shape, dorsal curvature, adhesion to the nail bed, color, and thickness. Some clinical observations include the following:

- *Clubbing.* Chronic lung and heart disease cause clubbing, a condition that indicates that the fingertips have received an insufficient supply of oxygenated blood over a period of time. Clubbing involves changes in the fingertips and nails; the fingertips enlarge, and the nails become thick, hard, shiny, and curved at the free end. With severe clubbing, the nail may detach from its base.
- *In the pink…or not.* Nail color should be pink. Poor oxygenation makes the blood appear bluish-red (cyanosis), which in turn makes the nails appear bluish. Other color changes include pigment bands; these dark bands are normally seen in dark-skinned individuals. When present in light-skinned persons, the bands may indicate melanoma.
- *Brittle.* Nails may also be described as brittle; this is generally caused by poor oxygenation, thyroid gland dysfunction, and nutritional anemia.

? Re-Think

1. What is clubbing, and why is it indicative of heart and/or lung disease?

GLANDS

Two major exocrine glands are associated with the skin: the sebaceous glands and the sweat glands (Fig. 7.4).

Most **sebaceous** (seh-BAY-shus) **glands**, or oil glands, are associated with hair follicles and are found in all areas of the body that have hair. They secrete an oily substance called *sebum* that flows into the hair root and then out onto the surface of the skin. A small number of sebaceous glands open directly onto the surface of the skin. The sebum lubricates and helps waterproof the hair and skin, as well as inhibits the growth of bacteria on the surface of the skin. With aging, sebum production gradually decreases. This change accounts, in part, for the dry skin and brittle hair seen in older persons. The sebaceous glands play a unique role in the fetus. Babies are born with a covering that resembles cream cheese. The covering is called the **vernix caseosa** (VERN-iks kay-see-OH-sah) and is secreted by the sebaceous glands. The vernix caseosa protects the skin of the fetus from the macerating effects of amniotic fluid.

Sometimes, the sebaceous glands become blocked by accumulated sebum and other debris. When the sebum

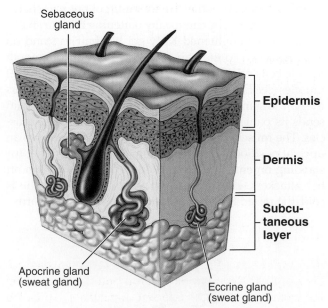

FIG. 7.4 Skin glands: sebaceous glands and sweat glands (apocrine and eccrine glands).

is exposed to the air and dries out, it turns black, forming a blackhead. When the blocked sebum becomes infected with staphylococci, it is a pimple (pustule). You have seen the contents of a pimple. Blackhead and pimple formation is common among adolescents because sebaceous gland activity responds to the hormonal changes associated with puberty. Babies may also have a problem with their sebaceous glands. The sebaceous glands on the scalp can oversecrete sebum, producing oily scales. Because this condition occurs during infancy, the cradle period, it is called *cradle cap*.

Do You Know...

About Blackheads, Pimples, and Worms?

There is a long history of persons squeezing (not a good idea!) or expressing the contents (sebum) of a blackhead or comedo. The expressed sebum resembles a long worm. The ancients concluded that the skin was being eaten into by a worm—hence, the word *comedo* (from a Latin word meaning "to eat into").

The sweat glands, or **sudoriferous** (soo-dor-IF-er-us) **glands**, are located in the dermis (see Fig. 7.4). As the name implies, these glands secrete sweat; the sweat is secreted into a duct that opens onto the skin as a pore. An individual has approximately 3 million sweat glands.

Two types of sweat glands are the apocrine and eccrine sweat glands. The **apocrine** (AP-oh-krin) **glands** are usually associated with hair follicles and are found in the axillary and genital areas. The apocrine glands respond to emotional stress and become active when the person is frightened, upset, in pain, or sexually excited. Because the development of these glands is stimulated by the sex hormones, they become more active during puberty. The sweat produced by these glands does not have a strong odor. If allowed to accumulate on the skin, however, the substances in sweat are degraded by bacteria into chemicals with a strong unpleasant odor. This is called *body odor* and is the reason we use deodorant.

Do You Know...

'Bout Them "Apples"?

In some species of animals, the olfactory area of the brain, the "smell brain," is the largest part of the brain. The survival of these animals depends heavily on the sense of smell. Humans also have a smell brain that, although very small, plays a powerful role in our emotional responses and is responsible for some very strange responses. For example, in Elizabethan times, lovers exchanged "love apples." And where did they get them? They made them. A woman peeled a common apple and placed it in her armpit until it was saturated with her perspiration (thanks to the apocrine glands). The sweat-soaked apple was then given to her lover to smell—for his pleasure, at his leisure.

Some of these secretions act as sex attractants. Watch how eagerly Rover sniffs when a potential mate is in the immediate area. These sex attractants are called *pheromones* (FAIR-o-mohns). The vaginal secretions of an ovulating female contain pheromones called *copulines*. The copulines can cause a testosterone surge (and an urge to merge) in the male.

The **eccrine** (EK-rin) **glands** are the more numerous and widely distributed of the sweat glands. They are located throughout the body and are especially numerous on the forehead, neck, back, upper lip, palms, and soles. Unlike apocrine glands, the eccrine glands are not associated with hair follicles.

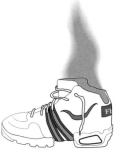

The sweat secreted by the eccrine glands plays an important role in body temperature regulation. As sweat evaporates from the skin surface, heat is lost. These are the glands that sweat profusely on hot days or during periods of strenuous exercise. Unlike the apocrine glands, which become active during puberty, the eccrine glands function throughout an entire lifetime. Eccrine secretion is composed primarily of water and a few salts.

Modified sweat glands include the mammary glands and ceruminous (ser-ROO-mi-nus) glands. The mammary glands are located in the breasts and secrete milk. (The secretion of milk is discussed further in Chapter 26.) The **ceruminous glands** are found in the external auditory canal of the ear. They secrete cerumen (seh-ROO-men), or ear wax. This yellow, sticky, waxlike secretion repels insects and traps foreign material. Silkworms and spiders use modified sweat glands to secrete silk and weave intricate webs.

Think all sweat looks the same? Not so! Some dyes, foods, and drugs are excreted in the sweat and may color the sweat in a variety of bright hues. This condition is called *chromhidrosis*.

Re-Think

1. What are the two major exocrine glands of the skin?
2. List the two types of sweat glands.
3. What are sudoriferous glands?
4. What is the function of vernix caseosa?

Do You Know...

Why Perspiration Is Sensible...or Insensible?

About 500 mL/day of water is normally lost through the skin and is called **insensible perspiration**. If the epidermis is damaged, as in severe burns, the rate of insensible perspiration increases enormously; the fluid loss is so great that the untreated patient may die from shock because of low blood volume. The eccrine glands are largely responsible for **sensible perspiration**. As body temperature rises, as in exercise, the eccrine glands increase the secretion of sweat, thereby cooling the body. When operating maximally, the eccrine glands can secrete 1 gallon of sweat per hour in an attempt to cool the body.

Sum It Up!

The skin is the home of several accessory structures, including the hair, nails, and glands. There are two major exocrine glands: the sebaceous glands and the sweat glands (also called *sudoriferous glands*). There are two types of sweat glands: the eccrine glands and the apocrine glands. Modified sweat glands include the ceruminous glands, which secrete ear wax, and the mammary glands, which secrete milk.

BODY TEMPERATURE

Normal body temperature is said to be 98.6°F, although it can range from 97° to 100°F. The temperature, however, fluctuates about 1.8°F in a 24-hour period, being lowest in the early morning and highest in the late afternoon. Body temperature also differs from one part of the body to another. The inner parts of the body (cranial, thoracic, and abdominal cavities) reflect the higher core temperature. The more surface areas (skin and mouth) reflect the cooler shell temperature. For example, the rectal temperature measures core temperature and ranges between 99° to 99.7°F, whereas the oral temperature is about 1°F lower.

Body temperature is maintained by balancing heat production and heat loss. The mechanism whereby the body balances heat production and heat loss is called **thermoregulation**. Failure to thermoregulate causes body temperature to fluctuate; an excessive decrease in body temperature is called **hypothermia**, and an excessive increase is called **hyperthermia**. Extreme changes in body temperature are often fatal.

 Do You Know...

Why You Shouldn't Offer a Hypothermic Individual a Rum Punch?

Although this is a thoughtful gesture, the alcohol in the rum causes dilation of the blood vessels in the skin, thereby increasing blood flow and the loss of heat. Mr. Hypothermia needs his heat. He may prefer the rum punch, but he is better served with a cup of hot tea.

HEAT PRODUCTION

Heat is thermal energy and is produced by the millions of chemical reactions occurring in the cells of the body. The heat is distributed throughout the body by the blood. The heat produced by metabolizing cells is the basis of body temperature. In the resting state, the greatest amount of heat is produced by the muscles, liver, and endocrine glands. The resting brain produces only about 15% of the heat. Interestingly, the studying brain does not produce much more heat.

The amount of heat produced can be affected by many factors, such as food consumption, the amounts and types of hormones secreted, and physical activity. With exercise, the amount of heat produced by the muscles may increase enormously. The hormonal effects on heat production are dramatically illustrated by

persons with thyroid gland disease. The hypothyroid person generally has a lower-than-normal body temperature, but the hyperthyroid person has an elevated temperature. In fact, an extreme hyperthyroid state (thyroid storm) can elevate body temperature into a range that is potentially lethal.

HEAT LOSS

Most heat loss (80%) occurs through the skin. The remaining 20% is lost through the respiratory system (lungs) and in the excretory products (urine and feces). Heat loss occurs by four means: radiation, conduction, convection, and evaporation.

The amount of blood in the dermal blood vessels influences the amount of heat that can be lost or dissipated by radiation, conduction, and convection. **Radiation** means that heat is lost from a warm object (the body) to the cooler air surrounding the warm object. Thus, a person loses heat in a cold room. **Conduction** is the loss of heat from a warm body to a cooler object in contact with the warm body. For example, a person (warm object) becomes cold when sitting on a block of ice (cooler object). Clinically, a cooling blanket may reduce a dangerously high fever. **Convection** is the loss of heat by air currents moving over the surface of the skin. For example, a fan moves air across the surface of the skin, thereby constantly removing the layer of heated air next to the body.

Finally, heat may be lost through evaporation. **Evaporation** occurs when a liquid becomes a gas. For example, during strenuous exercise, sweat on the surface of the skin evaporates and cools the body. Note that the evaporation of water is associated with a loss of heat. On a hot, humid day, water cannot evaporate from the surface of the skin. Hence, heat loss is diminished. This is why we feel the heat so intensely on a hot, humid day.

Check out some of the thermoregulatory mechanisms of some of our animal friends. Squirrels cool off by waving their bushy tails, and elephants flap their wonderful ears. And we all know that Rover pants. On a less appealing note, the vulture cannot sweat and cools itself by excreting waste along its own legs. The vulture? Not a house-friendly pet.

 Re-Think

1. Differentiate between core and shell temperature.
2. What is the origin of body temperature?
3. Define *thermoregulation*.

REGULATION

Normal body temperature is regulated by several mechanisms. The thermostat of the body is located in a part of the brain called the *hypothalamus*. The hypothalamus (hye-poh-THAHL-ah-mus) senses changes in body temperature and sends information to the skin (blood vessels and sweat glands) and skeletal muscle.

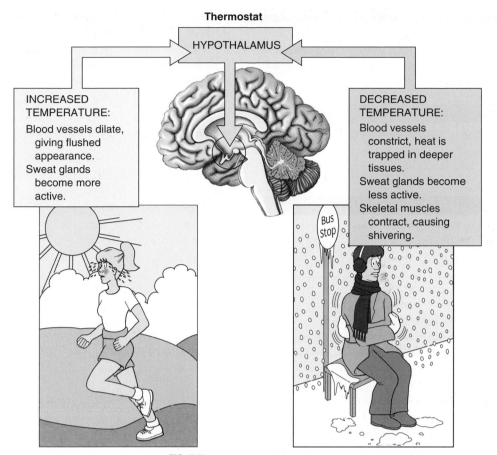

FIG. 7.5 **Temperature regulation.**

With exercise and temperature elevation, the blood vessels dilate, thereby allowing more blood to flow to the skin. This activity transfers heat from the deeper tissues to the surface of the body. Note how flushed our jogger is because of the blood coming to the surface (Fig. 7.5). Temperature elevation also stimulates the activity of the sweat glands. As the sweat evaporates from the surface of the body, heat is lost. Under extreme conditions of heat, 12 L of sweat can be secreted in a 24-hour period. These two activities lower body temperature.

What about Mr. Ear Muffs in Fig. 7.5? How does his body respond as his temperature decreases? First, the blood vessels constrict, reducing blood flow to the skin. This response traps the blood and heat in the deeper tissues, preventing heat loss. Second, the sweat glands become less active, also preventing heat loss. Third, skeletal muscles contract vigorously and involuntarily, causing shivering and an increase in the production of heat. These three activities raise body temperature. Contraction of the arrector pili muscles causes goose bumps, indicating a decline in body temperature, but contributes minimally to heat production. In furry animals the story is a little different; contraction of the arrector pili muscles pulls the fur upright, thereby trapping warm air. So, it's not good to shave Rover in the winter.

NEWBORNS AND BODY TEMPERATURE

In the delivery room, everyone is relieved when Baby (neonate) takes her first breath and delivers her first wail. Next to establishing respiratory activity, however, is the infant's need to regulate body temperature. In short, the neonate produces only about two-thirds of the heat produced by an adult, but loses twice as much. Several factors contribute to the excess heat loss:

- The neonate generally has a large surface area that increases heat loss. (The curled-up position of the infant decreases surface area and conserves heat.) Interestingly, considerable heat is lost from the head area; hence, the use of caps in the newborn nursery.
- The neonate generally has only a thin layer of subcutaneous fat. (Fat acts as an insulator, thus preventing heat loss.)
- The neonate cannot shiver. (Shivering produces heat.)

The neonate, like a squirrel, produces heat by a process called **nonshivering thermogenesis.** A neonate has brown adipose tissue (BAT), or brown fat, scattered throughout its body, especially around the neck and shoulder area. Metabolism of BAT generates more heat than the metabolism of ordinary adipose tissue (white fat). The heat produced by BAT is picked up by the blood and dispersed throughout the body.

Although we are generally concerned about excessive heat loss in the neonate, we must also be concerned about excess heat. An infant has a very limited capacity to dissipate heat and is therefore at risk for hyperthermia. Do not leave Baby in a hot car!

Re-Think

1. Explain why shivering and vasoconstriction increase body temperature.
2. Explain how the body cools itself.

Ramp It Up!

Temperature Terms and the Body Thermostat

Unlike your cold-blooded pet boa, you are warm-blooded and therefore maintain your body temperature within a narrow range. Body temperature, however, changes under many clinical conditions and gives rise to several confusing terms. Refer to the diagram of the thermometer as we define these terms. The temperatures on the thermometer were recorded orally; temperatures recorded by other techniques (rectal or axillary) are higher or lower.

- *Normothermia.* This refers to the normal range of body temperature from 97° to 99.6°F (36.1° to 37.6°C).
- *Fever (pyrexia).* The right side of the thermometer illustrates an increase in temperature that is called a *fever,* or **pyrexia**. Pyrogenic cytokines, often secreted by pathogens, increase the hypothalamic set point (thermostat). Then, vasoconstriction (to conserve heat) and shivering (to produce heat) cause the body temperature to reach the elevated set point. The set point can be lowered, usually by resolving its cause (often infection) or by the use of a fever-lowering drug (e.g., aspirin), called an *antipyretic.* Then the body loses heat through vasodilation and sweating. Laypersons often describe this late phase as the "fever has broken." A very high, life-threatening fever is called *hyperpyrexia* (105.8°F [41°C]).
- *Hyperthermia.* The left side of the thermometer illustrates hyperthermia and hypothermia. Hyperthermia refers to an elevation of body temperature caused by the inability of the body to get rid of excess heat; the body simply cannot cool itself. The cause of hyperthermia is most often environmental; the person is subjected to prolonged exposure to high temperatures, as in an infant being left in a car during the hot weather. Unlike fever, hyperthermia is not caused by resetting the thermostat; the set point is normal. Treatment measures focus on cooling the body; antipyretics are not effective because the set point is normal. In the advanced state (104°F [40°C]), hyperthermia is called *heat stroke* or *sunstroke* and represents thermoregulatory failure. Death ensues without immediate treatment.
- *Hypothermia.* This refers to a decrease in body temperature and is usually caused by prolonged exposure to cold, as in falling through ice into cold water. Body temperature becomes too low for the body to sustain body metabolism. Death usually ensues when the body temperature drops below 95°F (35°C).

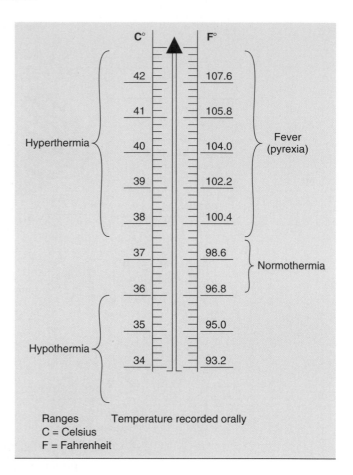

WHEN SKIN IS BURNED

Large areas of skin are often lost because of burns. Burns are classified according to the depth of the burn and the extent of the surface area burned (Fig. 7.6A). On the basis of depth, burns are classified as partial-thickness burns or full-thickness burns. Partial-thickness burns are further divided into first-degree and second-degree burns. A first-degree burn is red, painful, and slightly edematous (swollen). Only the epidermis is involved. Sunburn is an example of a first-degree burn. A second-degree burn involves damage to both the epidermis and dermis. With little damage to the dermis, the symptoms of a second-degree burn include redness, pain, edema, and blister formation. With greater damage to the dermis, the skin may appear red, tan, or white.

Full-thickness burns are also called *third-degree burns.* With a burn this severe, both the epidermis and dermis are destroyed, often with destruction of the deeper underlying layers. Although first- and second-degree burns are painful, third-degree burns are painless because the sensory receptors have been destroyed. Third-degree burns may appear white, tan, brown, black, or deep cherry red.

The extent of the burn injury is initially evaluated according to the rule of nines (see Fig. 7.6B). In this system, the total body surface area is divided into regions.

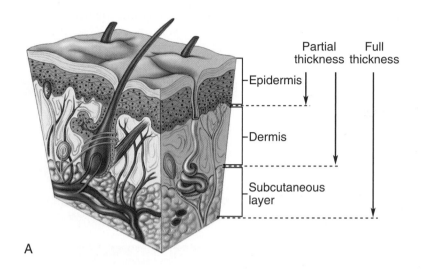

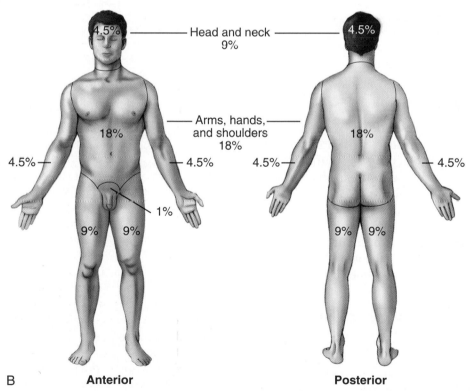

FIG. 7.6 (A) Parts of the skin damaged by burns. Partial-thickness (first- and second-degree burns) and full-thickness burns (third-degree burns). (B) The rule of nines.

The assigned percentages are related to the number 9. For example, the head and neck are considered to be 9% of the total body surface area. Each upper limb is 9%, whereas each lower limb is 18% (9 × 2). Note the percentages assigned to each specific body region. To determine proper treatment, the clinician needs to evaluate the depth and extent of the burn injury.

ESCHAR

Severe burns are associated with eschar (ESS-kahr) formation. Eschar is dead, burned tissue that forms a thick, inflexible, scablike layer over the burned surface. Eschar is a problem for two reasons. First, it may surround an area, such as a leg, and act like a tourniquet, thereby cutting off the flow of blood to the extremity. More seriously, if the eschar surrounds the chest, it prevents chest expansion and breathing. Second, eschar, which is initially sterile, becomes a breeding ground for bacteria and secretes potentially lethal toxins into the blood. These toxins adversely affect various organs in the body, such as the lungs and kidneys. Because eschar can have such serious consequences, it is often slit (escharotomy) to allow expansion of the burned area or removed to rid the body of a source of toxin.

 Re-Think

Explain why an extensive body burn causes fluid and electrolyte imbalance.

A NOTE ABOUT SKIN CARE

The skin is constantly exposed to all sorts of insults, such as the drying effects of soap and water, the damaging effects of the ultraviolet radiation of the sun, friction, numerous bumps, and exposure to sharp objects. Although we cannot avoid normal wear and tear, we can protect the skin in several ways. For example, we can lessen exposure of the skin to ultraviolet radiation. Sunbathing is deadly to the skin. Sun exposure both dries and irreversibly damages the skin. It also makes the skin leather-like and increases the risk of skin cancer and malignant melanoma.

 Do You Know...

What "Vagabond Syndrome" Is and Why It Makes You "Feel Lousy"?

The skin of people who continuously harbor body lice becomes hardened and darkly pigmented; this condition is known as *vagabond syndrome*. Chronic infestation of lice also causes the person to feel tired and irritable—hence the term *feeling lousy*.

Skin care is particularly important in older adults. The skin of an older person is normally drier, more easily injured, and slower to heal. Because the skin is so dry, excessive use of soap should be

discouraged. Limiting the use of soaps and excessive bathing can help prevent additional drying of the skin. Moreover, maintaining the acid surface of the skin discourages the growth of bacteria. In addition to becoming drier with aging, the skin changes in another important way. Both the dermis and underlying subcutaneous layer become thinner. As a result, older people bruise more easily because the blood vessels are not as well protected. In addition, heat is lost from the blood vessels, so older people often feel cold.

 Sum It Up!

Body temperature is caused by metabolizing cells. Metabolism, in turn, is affected by several factors: food consumption, hormones, exercise, and disease states. Thermoregulatory mechanisms balance heat production and heat loss. These mechanisms include the coordinated activities of the hypothalamus, blood vessels, and sweat glands. Because the skin performs so many vital functions, burns severely compromise many organ systems, often causing death.

As You Age

1. Aging causes a generalized thinning of the epidermis; the epidermal cells reproduce more slowly and are larger and more irregular. These changes result in thinner, more translucent skin.
2. Melanocyte activity decreases, resulting in decreased protection from ultraviolet light and greater susceptibility to sunburn and skin cancer. Selected melanocytes increase melanin production, resulting in brown spots, or age spots, especially in areas exposed to the sun.
3. The dermis becomes thinner, with a decreased amount of collagen and decreased number of elastin fibers. The result is increased fragility of the skin, as well as increased wrinkles. The skin also heals more slowly.
4. There is a decreased number of dermal blood vessels with a slower rate of repair. This change causes the skin to become more susceptible to small hemorrhages and pressure ulcers.
5. Blood vessels in the subcutaneous tissue decrease, so drugs administered subcutaneously are absorbed more slowly.
6. The amount of adipose tissue in the subcutaneous layer decreases, resulting in increased and wrinkled skin that has a decreased ability to maintain body temperature. The person tends to feel cold.
7. Sebaceous gland activity decreases, resulting in dry, coarse, itchy skin.
8. Sweat gland activity decreases, resulting in decreased ability to regulate body temperature and intolerance to cold.
9. The rate of melanin production by the hair follicle decreases. As a result, hair may become lighter in color, turning gray or white. Hair does not replace itself as often and becomes thinner.
10. Blood supply to the nail bed decreases. Consequently, the nails can become dull, brittle, hard, and thick; their growth rate also slows.

MEDICAL TERM	WORD PARTS	WORD PART MEANING OR DERIVATION	DESCRIPTION
Words			
cutaneous	cutane/o-	skin	**Cutaneous** means "relating to the skin," which is comprised of two layers: the epidermis and the dermis.
	-ous	pertaining to	
dermis	derm/o-	skin	The **dermis** is *the thick layer of skin under the epidermis.* Drugs may be administered using the skin.
epidermis	epi-	upon	The **epidermis** is *the layer that lies upon the dermis and forms the outer layer of skin.*
	derm/o-	skin	
melanocyte	melan/o-	black	A **melanocyte** is *an epidermal cell that secretes melanin, a pigment that darkens the skin.*
	-cyte	cell	
thermogenesis	therm/o-	heat	**Thermogenesis** refers to *the production of heat by physiological processes, as in shivering.*
	-genesis	production	
xeroderma	xer/o-	dry	**Xeroderma** refers to *dry skin.*
	-derm/a	skin	
Disorders			
Cancers of the Skin			
nonmelanomas	non-	not	**Nonmelanomas** are *neoplasms that arise from epithelial tissue and most commonly occur on sun-exposed areas of the body.* **Actinic keratosis** (kerat/o- = hard), or **solar keratosis,** is *a premalignant form of squamous cell carcinoma.* **Basal cell carcinoma (BCC)** is *the most common skin cancer and arises from epidermal basal cells that fail to mature and keratinize.* **Squamous cell carcinoma (SCC)** *arises from squamous epithelial cells.*
	-melan/o-	black	
	-oma	tumor	
malignant melanoma	melan/o-	From the Greek *melas-,* for "dark"	**Malignant melanoma** is *a malignant neoplasm of the melanocytes.* Because of its tendency to metastasize extensively, it is the most deadly form of skin cancer. All moles should be monitored. Remember the **ABCD**s of "mole watch": **A**symmetry, **B**order irregularity, **C**olor, **D**iameter.
	-oma	tumor	
Cutaneous Lesions			
macule	-ule	-ule means "little one"	A **macule** is a flat lesion, also called a blemish. Macules include **freckles, flat mole (nevus), vitiligo, port-wine stains,** the rash of **measles** and **smallpox,** some **drug-induced reactions,** and **petechiae** (pinpoint hemorrhages under the skin). A congenital nevus is a **birthmark.** There are many types of nevi, including **hemangiomas (strawberry mark),** a vascular nevus.
papule		From a Latin word meaning "pustule"	*An elevated lesion that looks like a solid blister.* Examples of a papule include elevated moles **(nevi), lichen planus, insect bites,** some **skin cancers,** and **verrucae** (wart). A **wart** is a contagious viral infection caused by one of the many human papillomaviruses (HPVs). A **nodule** is *a firm papule that extends into the dermis or subcutaneous tissue. Nodules include cysts, lipomas, and fibromas.*
pustule		From a Latin word meaning to "swell up" or "blow up"	*A small pus-containing elevation of the skin that is seen in conditions such as acne and impetigo.* A **pimple** is *a small pustule.*
wheal		From an Old English word meaning "to go round," as a wheel	Also called a **hive.** Multiple hives are called **urticaria,** a pruritic or itchy skin eruption. Urticaria is usually an allergic response to medication, food, and insect venom.
vesicle	vesic/o-	From a Latin word meaning "little bladder"; vesic/o- refers to *bladder,* -icle refers to *small*	Also called a **blister.** *A vesicle is a round lesion filled with serous fluid.* Vesicular lesions characterize herpes zoster (shingles), herpes simplex infection, and contact dermatitis. A larger vesicle is called a **bulla.**
	-icle		
ulcer		From a Latin word meaning "wound"	*A crater-like lesion formed by the loss of the epidermis and dermis.* Examples include a decubitus ulcer and a chancre. A **decubitus ulcer** is *a pressure-induced ulcer.* A **chancre,** meaning "little ulcer," is *the lesion that develops in response to infection by* Treponema pallidum *(syphilis).*

Continued

Medical Terminology and Disorders   Disorders of the Integumentary System—cont'd

MEDICAL TERM	WORD PARTS	WORD PART MEANING OR DERIVATION	DESCRIPTION
Disorders of Pigmentation			
hypopigmenta-tion	hypo-	insufficient	**Vitiligo** and **albinism** are conditions of **hypopigmentation,** in which *the melanocytes fail to secrete melanin.*
	-pigment-	pigment	
	-a/tion	state or condition	
hyperpigmen-tation	hyper-	more than normal	**Hyperpigmentation** is *a condition wherein there is an abnormally high amount of pigment in the skin.* **Dermal melanocytosis (mongolian spots)** is congenital; the spots appear as a blue-gray pigmentation in the sacral area. **Melasma,** related to hormone sensitivity, occurs during pregnancy **("mask of pregnancy")** and with the use of oral contraceptives. **Lentigo** refers to brown to black flat lesions, called **"liver spots,"** often seen in older persons **(senile lentigo).** The spots may occur in sun-exposed areas **(solar lentigo).** Infections, allergic reactions, and trauma can also induce a **post-inflammatory hyperpigmentation.**
	-pigment-	coloring matter	
	-a/tion	state or condition	
Infections of the Skin			
bacterial	bacteri-	Derived from New Latin, from Greek *baktērion,* for "staff"	**Impetigo** (from a word meaning "to attack") is *a bacterial infection that appears most often on the face and is caused by beta-hemolytic streptococci or staphylococci.* It is characterized by vesiculopustular lesions that are itchy and have a thick, honey-colored crust. A **furuncle** is *a deep staphylococcal infection around a hair follicle.* A **carbuncle** is *a group of interconnecting furuncles.* **Cellulitis** is *an inflammation of the subcutaneous tissue and is most commonly caused by* S. aureus *or streptococci.*
	-al	pertaining to	
viral		From a Latin word meaning "poison"	The most common viral infections of the skin are herpes simplex, herpes zoster, and warts. Herpes comes from a word meaning "to creep along," a reference to the progression of the vesicular development. The *herpes varicella* virus causes **chickenpox** (see Chapter 5), a highly contagious infection characterized by pruritic crusty vesicles. **Warts (verrucae)** are hyperkeratotic papular growths caused by the human papillomavirus (HPV).
fungal infec-tions		From a Latin word meaning "mushroom," in reference to the appearance of fungi	**Dermatophytosis,** or "ringworm," refers to *infection by a group of fungi called dermatophytes and occurs primarily in the skin, nails, and hair.* Ringworm conditions are named according to location: **tinea pedis (athlete's foot), tinea cruris ("jock itch"), tinea capitis (scalp), tinea corporis (body), tinea faciei (face), tinea manuum (hands). Candidiasis,** also called **moniliasis,** is a yeast infection caused by *Candida albicans.* **Cutaneous candidiasis** appears primarily in moist areas such as the thigh and beneath the breasts. Other common sights of infection are the mouth and vagina.
infestations and insect bites			There are numerous possibilities with regard to insect bites and infestations. The physiological response is due to a reaction to the venom, or to a reaction to the ova, body parts, or feces of the invading organism. *Infestation with lice* is called **pediculosis** (head, body, and pubic). **Scabies** develops in response to a parasitic mite that seeks out skin creases or folds in which to deposit eggs.
Disorders of the Hair and Nails			
onychocryp-tosis	onych/o-	nail	An **onychocryptosis** is *an ingrown nail, usually on the big toe.* It is most often caused by improper cutting of the toenails or the wearing of tight shoes.
	-crypt/o-	hidden, secret	
	-osis	condition of	
onychomycosis	onych/o-	nail	**Onychomycosis** is called *"ringworm of the nail,"* a fungal infection.
	-myc/o-	fungus	
	-osis	condition of	

Medical Terminology and Disorders   Disorders of the Integumentary System—cont'd

MEDICAL TERM	WORD PARTS	WORD PART MEANING OR DERIVATION	DESCRIPTION
paronychia	para-	alongside of	A **paronychia** is *a skin infection around the nail usually at the site of a hangnail or cuticle.*
	-onych/o-	nail	
	-ia	condition of	
trichotillomania	trich/o-	hair	**Trichotillomania** is *an impulse-control disorder in which the person compulsively twists strands of hair until they break off.*
	-tilo-	From a Latin word meaning "I pull out"	
	-mania	abnormal impulse	
Skin Diseases			
acne		From a Latin word meaning "point," as in the point of a pimple	**Acne vulgaris**—*common acne*—is characterized by scaly red skin, comedones (whiteheads and blackheads), papules, nodules, and pustules. These changes are due to sebaceous ducts that are plugged by sebum and dead skin cells.
dermatitis	dermat/o-	skin	**Dermatitis** is *a general term referring to inflammation of the skin.* There are different forms of dermatitis, including contact, seborrheic, and atopic dermatitis. Contact dermatitis may be allergic or irritant dermatitis. Allergic contact dermatitis is a skin allergy to something that touches the skin, as in poison ivy. Irritant contact dermatitis is dermatitis that develops in response to repeated exposure to an irritating substance. Atopic dermatitis, also called *eczema,* from a Greek word meaning "to erupt," is often associated with allergies and asthma. Atopic refers to the genetic predisposition to the allergen. Seborrheic dermatitis is a greasy (skin oil, or sebum), white to yellow scaling on the face (forehead, side of nose), scalp, or genitals.
	-itis	inflammation	
psoriasis	psor-	From a Greek word meaning "to have the itch"	An autoimmune disease often confused with eczema. Psoriasis affects the life cycle of skin cells, causing them to build up on the surface of the skin. The accumulation of skin cells forms thick silvery scales and itchy and painful red patches.

Get Ready for Exams!

Summary Outline

The integumentary system includes the skin, accessory structures, and subcutaneous tissue that covers the body, protects the internal organs, and plays an important role in the regulation of body temperature.

I. Structures: Organs of the Integumentary System
  A. Skin
   1. Called the cutaneous membrane or integument
   2. Functions: acts as mechanical barrier, protects internal organs, performs immune function, excretes waste, synthesizes vitamin D, houses sensory receptors, contributes to temperature regulation
   3. Has two layers: an outer layer called the epidermis and an inner layer called the dermis
   4. The epidermis has five layers. The stratum germinativum is the layer in which cell division takes place. The outer layer is the stratum corneum and consists of flattened, dead, keratinized cells.
   5. The dermis is the largest part of the skin and contains blood vessels, nerves, and sensory receptors.
   6. The dermis lies on the subcutaneous tissue.

   7. Skin color is determined by many factors, some genetic, some physiological, and some caused by disease. Melanin causes skin to darken. Carotene causes skin to appear yellow. The amount of blood in the skin affects skin color (e.g., flushing), as does the appearance of abnormal substances such as bilirubin (jaundice) and a low blood oxygen content (cyanosis).
  B. Accessory structures of the skin
   1. The location of the hair determines its function. Eyebrows and eyelashes protect the eyes from dust and perspiration.
   2. Main parts of a hair: shaft, root, and follicle
   3. Hair color: determined by the amount and type of melanin
   4. Nails are thin plates of stratified squamous epithelial cells that contain a hard form of keratin.
   5. Two major exocrine glands: sebaceous glands and sweat glands
   6. Sebaceous glands secrete sebum (lubricates hair and skin). In the fetus, these glands secrete vernix

caseosa, a cheeselike substance that coats the skin of a newborn.

7. Two types of sweat glands (sudoriferous glands): apocrine glands and eccrine glands (especially important in temperature regulation)
8. Modified sweat glands: Mammary glands secrete milk, and the ceruminous glands secrete ear wax.

C. Subcutaneous tissue (hypodermis)
   1. Anchors the dermis to underlying structures
   2. Acts as an insulator; it prevents heat loss.

II. Regulation of Body Temperature (Thermoregulation)

A. Heat production
   1. Heat produced by metabolizing cells constitutes the body temperature.
   2. Shivering and nonshivering thermogenesis

B. Heat loss
   1. Most of the heat (80%) is lost through the skin.
   2. Heat loss occurs through radiation, conduction, convection, and evaporation.
   3. Normal body temperature: set by the body's thermostat in the hypothalamus
   4. Heat: lost through sweating and vasodilation. Heat is conserved by vasoconstriction and produced by shivering.

III. When Skin Is Burned

A. Physiological effects
   1. Short-term effects (e.g., fluid and electrolyte losses, shock, inability to regulate body temperature, infection)
   2. Long-term effects (e.g., scarring, loss of function, and cosmetic and emotional problems)

B. Classification of burns
   1. Classified according to the thickness of the burn (partial, full); also first-, second-, and third-degree burns
   2. The rule of nines is a way to evaluate burns.

Review Your Knowledge

Matching: Skin
Directions: Match the following words with their descriptions. Some words may be used more than once.

a. keratin
b. dermis
c. subcutaneous layer
d. epidermis

1. ___ Thin outer layer of skin
2. ___ Layer that sits on the hypodermis and supports the epidermis
3. ___ A protein that flattens, hardens, and makes the skin water-resistant
4. ___ A layer of insulation
5. ___ Contains the stratum germinativum and stratum corneum
6. ___ Contains blood vessels that nourish the stratum germinativum

Matching: Glands
Directions: Match the following words with their descriptions. Some words may be used more than once.

a. eccrine
b. sebaceous
c. ceruminous
d. mammary

1. ___ Oil glands
2. ___ Glands that secrete vernix caseosa
3. ___ Glands that play a crucial role in body temperature regulation
4. ___ Modified sweat glands that secrete ear wax
5. ___ Modified sweat glands that secrete milk
6. ___ Classified as sudoriferous
7. ___ Most related to blackhead, pimple, and cradle cap
8. ___ Secretes sweat during intense exercise

Matching: Colors
Directions: Match the following words with their descriptions. Some words may be used more than once.

a. jaundice
b. cyanosis
c. melanin
d. vitiligo
e. ecchymosis
f. pallor

1. ___ Tanning pigment
2. ___ Condition in which the skin has a bluish tint because of poor oxygenation
3. ___ Yellowing of the skin because of bilirubin
4. ___ Patches of white skin caused by loss of pigmentation
5. ___ Black-and-blue mark; bruising
6. ___ Ashen color due to decreased amount of oxygenated blood

Multiple Choice

1. Which of the following is most apt to increase body temperature?
   a. Dilation of the blood vessels in the skin
   b. Shivering
   c. Secretion of the eccrine glands
   d. Secretion of sebum

2. The stratum germinativum
   a. is a dermal layer.
   b. gives rise to epidermal cells.
   c. contains the blood vessels that nourish the epidermis.
   d. is part of the hypodermis.

3. The epidermis is nourished by the
   a. air in the environment that diffuses into the pores.
   b. blood vessels in the hair shafts.
   c. blood vessels in the underlying dermis.
   d. oxygen and glucose in the sebum.

4. Which of the following is true of the stratum corneum?
   a. Continuously produces epidermal cells
   b. Secretes keratin for making the skin water-resistant
   c. Is the dead layer that is sloughed off
   d. Continuously secretes bilirubin

5. Which of the following best describes the function of the stratum germinativum?
   a. Desquamation
   b. Mitosis
   c. Keratinization
   d. Shivering thermogenesis

6. Secretion of the eccrine glands
   a. "oils" the hair shafts.
   b. produces vernix caseosa that protects the skin of the fetus.
   c. lowers body temperature.
   d. tans the skin.

7. Cyanosis occurs when
   a. the blood in the cutaneous blood vessels is unoxygenated.
   b. bilirubin deposits in the skin and mucous membrane.
   c. cutaneous blood vessels dilate.
   d. sebum is exposed to air and changes color.

8. Which of the following pertains to the terms *apocrine, sudoriferous, eccrine,* and *sebaceous*?
   a. Sweat glands
   b. Vernix caseosa
   c. Sebum
   d. Exocrine glands

9. Shivering thermogenesis
   a. is due to metabolism of brown fat.
   b. increases body temperature.
   c. is primarily due to the contraction of the arrector pili muscles.
   d. is triggered by hypoxemia and cyanosis.

10. Blushing, flushing, and pallor are due to
    a. deposition of melanin in the dermal cells.
    b. changes in blood flow through the dermal blood vessels.
    c. the rate of keratinization of the epidermal cells.
    d. staining of tissues by bilirubin.

11. Which of the following is true of the group of smooth muscle cells attached to a hair follicle?
    a. Called the arrector pili muscles
    b. Cause "goose bumps" when contracted
    c. Contract in response to fear and exposure to cold temperatures
    d. All of the above

12. Which of the following is least descriptive of the sebaceous glands?
    a. Sebum
    b. Vernix caseosa
    c. Oily
    d. Sweat

13. With which skin function are the words core and shell most concerned?
    a. Bilirubin metabolism
    b. Vitamin D synthesis
    c. Thermoregulation
    d. Skin color determination

14. Which of the following word roots refers to nail?
    a. Trich/o-, as in trichotillomania
    b. Onych/o, as in paronychia
    c. Melan/o, as in melanoma
    d. Dermat/o, as in dermatologist

15. Pyrexia, antipyretic, and pyrogenic all refer to
    a. pathogens.
    b. fever.
    c. infection.
    d. antibiotics.

Go Figure

1. Which of the following is correct according to Fig. 7.1?
   a. There is a rich supply of blood vessels within the epidermis.
   b. The dermis sits on the epidermis.
   c. Blood vessels, touch receptors, and free nerve endings are located within the dermis.
   d. The stratum corneum and the stratum germinativum are dermal layers.

2. Which of the following is correct according to Fig. 7.2?
   a. The hair root arises from the adipose tissue in the subcutaneous layer.
   b. The hair arises from epidermal cells embedded within the dermis.
   c. The arrector pili muscles attach the epidermis to the hypodermis.
   d. Dermal cells arise within the stratum germinativum.

3. Which of the following is correct according to Figs. 7.1 and 7.2?
   a. All glands arise from cells at the base of the hair shaft.
   b. All touch and pressure receptors are located within the stratum corneum.
   c. Some epidermal cells are embedded within the dermis.
   d. All sensory receptors are located in the hypodermis.

4. Which of the following is correct according to Fig. 7.4?
   a. Sebaceous, eccrine, and apocrine glands are ductless glands.
   b. Eccrine glands are generally located at the base of the hair root.
   c. Sweat glands are located within the dermis.
   d. All ductless glands are sweat glands.

5. Which of the following is correct according to Fig. 7.5?
   a. Blood vessel constriction and shivering increase body temperature.
   b. The body's "thermostat" is located in the brain.
   c. Blood vessel dilation and sweating lower body temperature.
   d. All of the above are true.

6. Which of the following is correct according to Fig. 7.6B?
   a. The rule of nines evaluates the depth of a burn.
   b. A partial-thickness burn refers to a burn injury involving the skin and underlying muscle and bone.
   c. Burns described as partial thickness and full thickness are determined by the rule of nines.
   d. A person with burns over the anterior and posterior aspects of the lower extremities has burns over 36% of the body.

Skeletal System

Objectives

1. List the functions of the skeletal system and the classification of bones by size and shape.
2. Differentiate between the composition and location of compact and spongy bone.
3. Describe the structure of a long bone.
4. Describe the roles of osteoblasts and osteoclasts, and explain how bones grow in length and width.
5. List the bones of the axial skeleton, and label important landmarks on selected bones.
6. List the bones of the appendicular skeleton, and label important landmarks on selected bones.
7. List the main types and functions of joints, and describe the types of joint movement.

Key Terms

abduction (p. 137)
adduction (p. 139)
appendicular skeleton (p. 118)
articulation (p. 116)
axial skeleton (p. 118)
circumduction (p. 139)
compact bone (p. 114)
diaphysis (p. 116)
epiphyseal disc (p. 116)

epiphysis (p. 116)
extension (p. 137)
flexion (p. 137)
fontanels (p. 122)
haversian system (p. 115)
ossification (p. 116)
osteoblasts (p. 114)
osteoclasts (p. 117)
osteon (p. 115)

pectoral girdle (p. 128)
pelvic girdle (p. 118)
periosteum (p. 116)
pronation (p. 128)
spongy bone (p. 114)
supination (p. 128)
suture (p. 122)
synovial joint (p. 134)
vertebral column (p. 118)

The skeletal system consists of the bones, joints, and cartilage and ligaments associated with the joints. Bone tissue is living and metabolically active, but because it contains so much nonliving material, such as calcium and phosphorus, it appears dead or dried up. In fact, the word *skeleton* comes from a Greek word meaning "dried-up body."

The skeletal system, however, is anything but dead. It contains 206 bones that are very much alive and perform a number of important functions. This is how busy bone is...the average 70-year-old person has replaced seven complete skeletons during his or her lifetime!

 Do You Know...

About Growing Down with Osteoporosis?

Osteoporosis is a common bone disorder, especially in postmenopausal women. Osteoporosis is characterized by a decline in bone-making activity and the loss of bone tissue. As tissue is lost, the bones weaken and break. Common sites of fracture caused by osteoporosis are the hip, wrist, and vertebrae. Osteoporosis may also affect the vertebral column. As the vertebrae collapse, nerves may be pinched, causing severe pain. The collapsed vertebrae also cause a shortening of the vertebral column (growing down) and a change in its curvature. This change in shape, in turn, often impairs the functioning of organs such as the lungs.

ARRANGEMENT AND FUNCTIONS OF BONES

The bones of the skeletal system are arranged to provide a framework for our bodies (Fig. 8.1). The skeletal system gives us our basic shape. Imagine what you would look like without bones!

THE SKELETAL SYSTEM: WHAT IT DOES

In addition to shaping us up, the skeletal system performs other functions:
- The bones of the lower extremities support the weight of the body.
- The bones support and protect the soft body organs.
- With the assistance of muscles, the skeletal system enables the body to move about.
- Bones store a number of minerals, the most important being calcium and phosphorus.
- Red bone marrow produces blood cells.

MANY SIZES AND SHAPES OF BONES

Bones come in many sizes and shapes, from the pea-sized bones in the wrist to the 24-inch femur in the

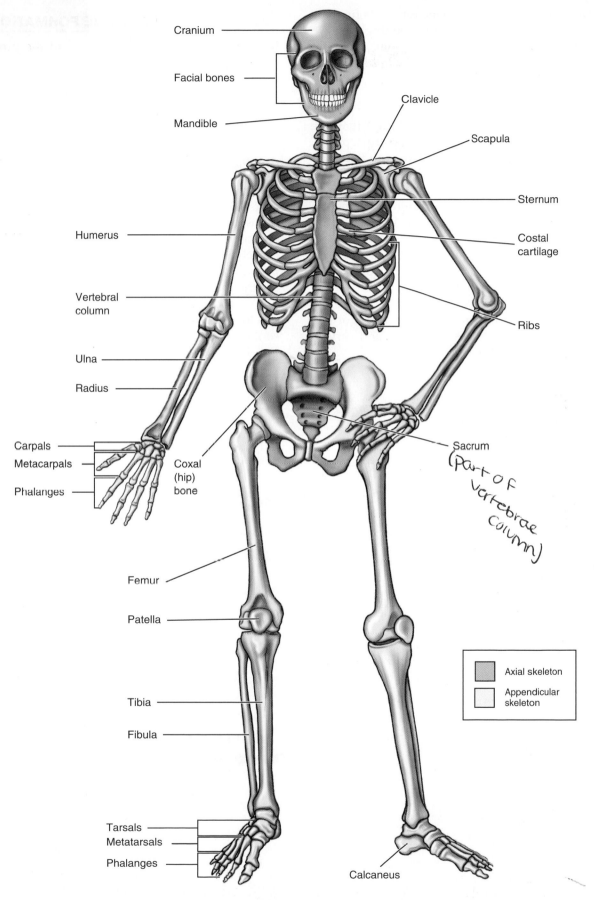

Cranium

Facial bones

Mandible

Clavicle

Scapula

Sternum

Costal cartilage

Humerus

Vertebral column

Ribs

Ulna

Radius

Carpals

Metacarpals

Phalanges

Coxal (hip) bone

Sacrum

(Part of Vertebrae Column)

Femur

Patella

Tibia

Fibula

Tarsals

Metatarsals

Phalanges

Calcaneus

Axial skeleton

Appendicular skeleton

FIG. 8.1 Skeleton. Axial skeleton *(pink)* and appendicular skeleton *(tan)*.

thigh. The size and shape of a bone reflect its function (Fig. 8.2). The long, strong femur in the thigh, for example, supports a great deal of weight and can withstand considerable force. Some of the skull bones, on the other hand, are thin, flat, and curved. Their function is to encase and protect the brain.

Bones are classified as follows:

- *Long bones.* Long bones are longer than they are wide. They are found in the arms, forearms, palms, fingers, thighs, legs, and instep. Although it is obvious that the femur (thigh) and the humerus (arm) are long bones, even small bones such as the metacarpals and finger bones are considered long bones.
- *Short bones.* Short bones are shaped like cubes and are found primarily in the wrists and ankles.
- *Flat bones.* Flat bones are thin, flat, and curved. They form the ribs, breastbone, cranium, and bones of the shoulder girdle.
- *Irregular bones.* Irregular bones are differently shaped and are not classified as long, short, or flat. They include the hip bones, vertebrae, and various bones in the skull.

BONE TISSUE AND BONE FORMATION

Bone is also called *osseous tissue,* and the process of bone formation is called *ossification.* Bone cells, called **osteoblasts**, secrete an intercellular matrix, containing calcium, other minerals, and protein fibers. The osteoblasts mature into osteocytes that sit within the hard bone matrix and maintain the bone.

COMPACT AND SPONGY BONE

There are two types of bone: compact and spongy (Fig. 8.3). **Compact bone** refers to dense, hard bone tissue found primarily in the shafts of long bones and on the outer surfaces of other bones. Spongy, or cancellous, bone is less dense. **Spongy bone** is located primarily at the ends of long bones and in the center of other bones.

Compact and spongy bone tissues look different under the microscope. Compact bone is tightly packed, so its density can provide a great deal of strength (see Fig. 8.3B). The microscopic unit of compact bone is the

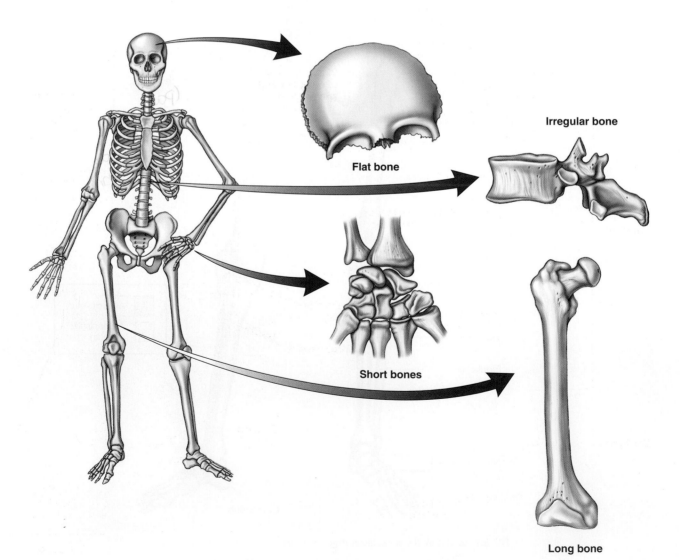

Flat bone

Irregular bone

Short bones

Long bone

FIG. 8.2 Types of bones: long, short, flat, and irregular.

osteon, or haversian (hah-VER-shun) system. Each haversian system consists of mature osteocytes arranged in concentric circles around large blood vessels. The area surrounding the osteocytes is filled with protein fibers, calcium, and other minerals. The protein fibers provide elasticity, and the minerals make bone tissue hard and strong. Each haversian system looks like a long cylinder.

Compact bone consists of many haversian systems running parallel to each other. Communicating blood vessels run laterally and connect the haversian systems with each other and with the periosteal lining that surrounds the bone. The network of blood vessels ensures that the bone tissue receives an adequate supply of blood. Blood supplies tissues with oxygen and nutrients.

Spongy, or cancellous, bone has a much different structure than compact bone (see Fig. 8.3B). Unlike compact bone, spongy bone does not contain haversian systems. In spongy bone, the bone tissue is arranged in plates called *trabeculae* (trah-BEK-yoo-lay). These bony plates are separated by holes that give spongy bone a punched-out Swiss cheese appearance. The holes are important for two reasons: (1) they decrease the weight of the bone, and (2) they contain red bone marrow. The red bone marrow richly supplies the spongy bone with blood and also produces blood cells for use throughout the body. Spongy bone is located in the short, flat, and irregular bones. It is also found in the ends of long bones.

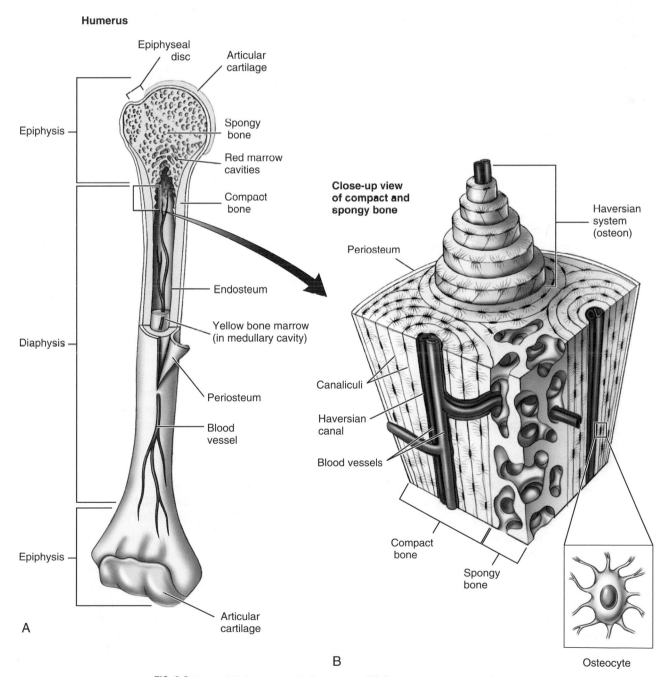

FIG. 8.3 Bone. (A) Anatomy of a long bone. (B) Compact and spongy bone.

? **Re-Think**

1. What are the four shapes/sizes of bone?
2. What are two types of bone tissue?
3. What is the structure of an osteon, or haversian system?

LONG BONES

The arrangement of the compact and spongy tissue in a long bone accounts for its strength. Long bones also contain sites of growth and reshaping and structures associated with joints. Locate the parts of a long bone in Fig. 8.3A:

- *Diaphysis.* The **diaphysis** (dye-AF-i-sis) is the long shaft of the bone. It is composed primarily of compact bone and therefore provides considerable strength.
- *Epiphysis.* The enlarged ends of the long bone are the epiphyses. The **epiphysis** (eh-PIF-i-sis) of a bone articulates, or meets, with a second bone at a joint. Each epiphysis consists of a thin layer of compact bone overlying spongy bone. The epiphyses are covered by cartilage.
- *Epiphyseal disc.* A growing long bone contains a band of hyaline cartilage located near the proximal and distal ends of long bones. This band of cartilage is the **epiphyseal disc,** or growth plate. It is here that longitudinal bone growth occurs.
- *Medullary cavity.* The medullary cavity is the hollow center of the diaphysis. In infancy, the cavity is filled with red bone marrow for blood cell production. In the adult, the medullary cavity is filled with yellow bone marrow and functions as a storage site for fat. The inside of the medullary cavity is lined with connective tissue called the *endosteum* (en-DOS-tee-um).
- *Periosteum.* The **periosteum** is a tough, fibrous, connective tissue membrane that covers the outside of the diaphysis. It is anchored firmly to the outside of the bone on all surfaces except the articular cartilage. The periosteum protects the bone, serves as a point of attachment for muscle, and contains the blood vessels that nourish the underlying bone. Because the periosteum carries the blood supply to the underlying bone, injury to this structure has serious consequences to the health of the bone. Like any other organ, the loss of blood supply can cause its death.
- *Articular cartilage.* The articular cartilage is found on the outer surface of the epiphysis. It forms a smooth, shiny surface that decreases friction within a joint. Because a joint is also called an **articulation**, this cartilage is called *articular cartilage.*

OSSIFICATION

The process of bone formation is called *ossification.* **Ossification** begins in the late embryonic period with

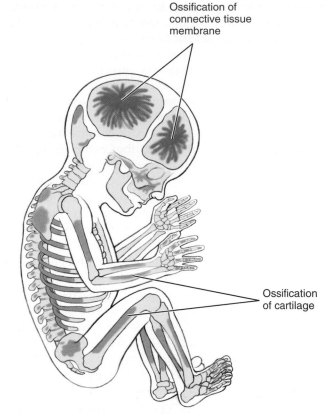

FIG. 8.4 Ossification.

the formation of fibrous connective tissue and hyaline cartilage that is shaped like a miniskeleton (Fig. 8.4). As the fetus matures, the cartilage and connective tissue change into bone. Ossification occurs in two ways: intramembranous ossification and endochondral ossification.

OSSIFICATION OF FLAT BONES: INTRAMEMBRANOUS OSSIFICATION

In the fetus, the flat bones (those in the skull) consist of thin connective tissue membranes. Ossification begins when osteoblasts, or bone-forming cells, migrate to the region of the flat bones. The osteoblasts secrete calcium and other minerals into the spaces between the membranes, thereby forming bone. This type of ossification involves the replacement of thin membrane with bone.

OSSIFICATION OF LONG BONES: ENDOCHONDRAL OSSIFICATION

Most bones are formed by endochondral ossification as bone tissue replaces cartilage. The fetal skeleton is composed largely of cartilage, and the layout of the cartilage in the fetus provides a model for bone formation (see Fig. 8.4). As the fetus matures, osteoblasts invade the cartilage and gradually replace the cartilage with bone. This process continues in each long bone until all but the articular cartilage and epiphyseal disc have been replaced by bone. By the time the fetus has fully matured, most cartilage of the body has been replaced by bone. Only isolated pieces of cartilage remain, such as the bridge of the nose, parts of the ribs, and the epiphyses of long bones.

GROWING BONES

Maturation from infancy to adulthood is characterized by two types of bone growth: (1) bones grow longitudinally and determine the height of an individual, and (2) bones grow thicker and become wider to support the weight of the adult body.

GROWING TALLER

Longitudinal bone growth occurs at the epiphyseal disc (also called the *growth plate;* see Fig. 8.3A). The cartilage adjacent to the epiphysis continues to multiply and grow toward the diaphysis. The cartilage next to the diaphysis, however, is invaded by osteoblasts and becomes ossified. As long as the cartilage continues to form within the epiphyseal disc, the bone continues to lengthen. Longitudinal bone growth ceases when the epiphyseal disc becomes ossified and fused.

The epiphyseal disc is sensitive to the effects of certain hormones, especially growth hormone and the sex hormones. Growth hormone stimulates growth at the epiphyseal disc, making the child taller. The sex hormones estrogen and testosterone, however, cause the epiphyseal disc to fuse, thereby inhibiting further longitudinal growth. Because the epiphyseal disc is especially sensitive to the effects of the female hormone estrogen, girls tend to be shorter than boys. After puberty, which is associated with increasing plasma levels of sex hormones, longitudinal growth eventually ceases.

The "What-Ifs" of the Epiphyseal Disc

- What if there is an oversecretion or undersecretion of growth hormone? Gigantism occurs with hypersecretion, whereas a type of dwarfism develops with hyposecretion.
- What if the epiphyseal disc is injured? Longitudinal bone growth is impaired in the injured bone. A child who injures the epiphyseal disc in a leg bone, for example, may end up with that leg considerably shorter than the noninjured leg.
- What if a young athlete uses anabolic steroids to enhance performance? Steroids induce premature fusion of the epiphyseal plate, thereby permanently stunting growth.

GROWING THICKER AND WIDER

During and long after longitudinal bone growth has ceased, bones continue to increase in thickness and width. The bones are continuously being reshaped. Bone remodeling is accomplished by the combined actions of osteoblasts, which are bone-forming cells, and **osteoclasts**, which are bone-destroying cells. Osteoblasts on the undersurface of the periosteum

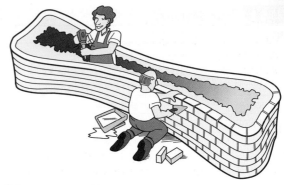

FIG. 8.5 **Bone remodeling.**

continuously deposit bone on the external bone surface.

Fig. 8.5 shows how osteoblastic activity works like a bricklayer. Whereas osteoblasts build new bone, osteoclasts, found on the inner bone surface surrounding the medullary cavity, break down bone tissue, thereby hollowing out the interior of the bone. Osteoclastic activity is like sculpting. The bricklayer and the sculptor gradually create a large, wide, hollow bone that is strong but not too heavy.

The process whereby osteoclasts break down bone matrix is called *bone resorption* (not to be confused with *reabsorption*). Bone resorption not only widens bone but also moves calcium from the bone to the blood. In this way, bone resorption also plays a crucial role in the regulation of blood calcium levels. The influence of parathyroid hormone on bone resorption is described in Chapter 14.

Factors that stimulate bone growth are weight-bearing and exercise; both activities keep calcium in the bone and increase bone mass. The bones of bedridden or sedentary people tend to lose bone mass and are more easily broken when stressed. The weightlessness experienced by astronauts similarly causes a loss of bone mass and easily broken bones. The beneficial effects of exercise on bone strength cannot be overemphasized.

 Re-Think

1. Referencing the long bone, describe the function of the diaphysis, epiphysis, epiphyseal disc and the red bone marrow.
2. Differentiate between the functions of osteoblasts and osteoclasts.
3. Describe how a bone grows in length and in width.
4. Describe how bone resorption is involved in bone growth.

BUMPS AND GROOVES

The surface of bone appears irregular and bumpy as a result of numerous ridges, projections, depressions,

Table 8.1   Bone Markings

BONE MARKINGS	DEFINITION
Projections or Processes	
Condyle	A large rounded knob that usually articulates with another bone
Epicondyle	An enlargement near or above a condyle
Head	An enlarged and rounded end of a bone
Facet	A small flattened surface
Crest	A ridge on a bone
Process	A prominent projection on a bone
Spine	A sharp projection
Tubercle (tuberosity)	A knoblike projection
Trochanter	A large tubercle (tuberosity) found only on the femur
Depressions or Openings	
Foramen	An opening through a bone; usually serves as a passageway for nerves, blood vessels, and ligaments
Fossa	A depression or groove
Meatus	A tunnel or tubelike passageway
Sinus	A cavity or hollow space

and grooves called *bone surface markings*. The projecting bone markings (the markings that stick out) serve as points of attachment for muscles, tendons, and ligaments. The grooves and depressions form the routes traveled by blood vessels and nerves as they pass over and through the bones and joints. The projections and depressions also help form joints. The rounded head of the proximal arm bone, for example, fits into a round depression in a shoulder bone, forming the shoulder joint. The specific bone markings are summarized in Table 8.1. Note the various markings on individual bones as they are described.

BROKEN BONES

Occasionally, a bone breaks, or fractures (Fig. 8.6). A simple fracture is a break in which the overlying skin remains intact; local tissue damage is minimal. A compound fracture is a broken bone that has also pierced the skin. The ends of the broken bone usually cause extensive tissue damage. The risk of infection is a concern with a compound fracture.

A greenstick fracture is an incomplete break in the bone and usually occurs in children. Why is it called a greenstick fracture? If you were to bend a branch of a young tree, the branch would not snap and break apart completely. It would, instead, bend and perhaps break incompletely. The branch responds this way because it is young and pliable, much like a child's bone.

There are many other types of bone fractures. For example, there is a spiral fracture in which the line of

the fracture extends in a spiral direction along the diaphysis. It is caused when the bone is subjected to a twisting type of force. There is a comminuted fracture in which there are more than two bone fragments; the small fragments seem to be floating. An impacted fracture is a comminuted fracture in which the two parts of the broken bone have been jammed into each other. The list of fractures goes on!

Sum It Up!

The skeletal system consists of bones, joints, cartilage, and ligaments found in and around the joints. Bones are composed of two types of osseous tissue: compact (dense bone) and spongy (cancellous bone). Bones come in a variety of sizes and shapes and are classified as long, short, flat, or irregular. We begin life in the womb as a skeleton-like frame made of cartilage and thin connective tissue membrane. With maturation, the process of ossification changes most of the cartilage and certain connective tissue membranes into bone. As a person matures, the skeleton enlarges as the bones grow longer, wider, and thicker.

DIVISIONS OF THE SKELETAL SYSTEM

The skeleton is divided into the axial skeleton and appendicular skeletons (see Fig. 8.1). The **axial** (AK-see-all) **skeleton** includes the bones of the cranium, face, middle ear bones, hyoid bone, **vertebral column**, and bony thorax. The **appendicular skeleton** includes the bones of the **pelvic girdle**, the upper extremities (arms, forearms, wrist, palms, and fingers), and lower extremities (thighs, legs, ankles, instep, and toes). The names of the 206 bones of the skeleton are listed in Table 8.2.

AXIAL SKELETON

SKULL

The skull sits on top of the vertebral column and is formed by two groups of bones: the cranium and the facial bones (Fig. 8.7).

Cranium

The cranium is a bony structure that encases and protects the brain. The cranium is composed of eight bones, most of which are curved and flat.

- *Frontal bone.* The frontal bone forms the forehead and the upper part of the bony structure surrounding the eyes.
- *Parietal bones.* The two parietal (pah-RYE-i-tal) bones form the upper sides of the head and the roof of the cranial cavity (top of the head).
- *Temporal bones.* The two temporal bones are on the sides of the head, close to the ears (commonly called the *temples*). Several important bone markings are found on the temporal bones. They include the external auditory meatus (mee-AY-tus), an opening for the ear; the zygomatic (zye-goh-MAT-ik)

Closed (simple)   **Open (compound)**

Incomplete (greenstick)

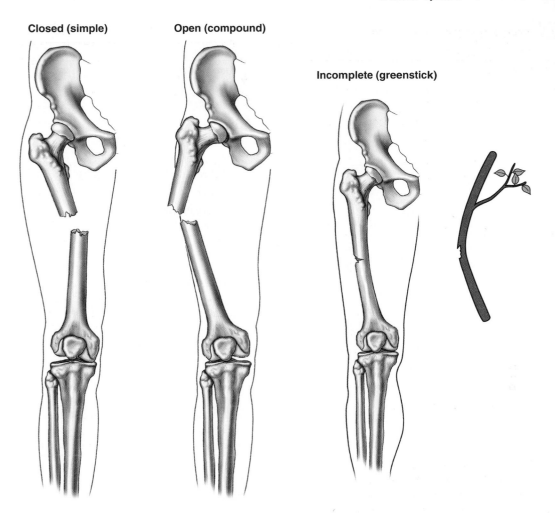

FIG. 8.6 Common types of fractures: simple, compound, incomplete (greenstick).

process, which articulates with the cheekbone (not to be confused with the zygomatic bones); the sty-loid process, a sharp projection used as a point of attachment for several muscles associated with the tongue and larynx; and the mastoid process, which forms a point of attachment for some of the muscles of the neck. Here's an interesting note about the temporal bone. *Tempor* is a Latin word meaning "time." As men age, over time, they usually develop their first gray hairs over the temple area. So, the name of the temporal bone is a reference to aging.

- *Occipital bone* (see Fig. 8.7C). The occipital (ok-SIP-it-al) bone is located at the back and base of the cranium. The large hole in the occipital bone is called the *foramen magnum.* The foramen allows the brain stem to extend downward and become the spinal cord. On either side of the foramen magnum are bony projections, called *occipital condyles* (KON-dylz), that sit on the first vertebra of the vertebral column. Unfortunately, the foramen magnum can act as a deathtrap, because it provides the only escape hatch in the cranium in the event that the brain

swells. The increased intracranial pressure created by the swollen brain pushes the brain through the foramen magnum into the spinal region. The downward displacement or herniation of the brain exerts pressure on the brain stem, causing respiratory arrest and death.

- *Sphenoid bone.* The sphenoid (SFEE-noyd) bone is a butterfly-shaped bone that forms part of the floor and sides of the cranium (see Fig. 8.7C). The sphenoid bone also helps form the orbits surrounding the eyes. In the midline of the sphenoid bone is a depression called the *sella turcica* (Turk's saddle); it forms the seat for the pituitary gland (not shown).

- *Ethmoid bone.* The ethmoid (ETH-moyd) bone is an irregularly shaped bone located between the eye orbits; it is the major supporting bony structure of the nasal cavity. A projection of the ethmoid bone forms a point of attachment for the meninges, the membranes that surround the brain and contain cerebrospinal fluid. The location and shape of the ethmoid bone have important clinical implications. A sharp blow to the ethmoid bone can drive the pointed bone into the brain, causing

Table 8.2   Bones of the Adult Skeleton

BONES	NUMBER	BONES	NUMBER
Axial Skeleton (80)		**Thoracic Cage (25)**	
Skull (28)		True ribs	14
Cranium (8)		False ribs	10
Frontal	1	Sternum	1
Parietal	2	**Appendicular Skeleton (126)**	
Temporal	2	**Pectoral Girdle (4)**	
Occipital	1	Scapula	2
Sphenoid	1	Clavicle	2
Ethmoid	1	**Upper Limbs (60)**	
Facial (14)		Humerus	2
Maxilla	2	Radius	2
Zygomatic	2	Ulna	2
Palatine	2	Carpals	16
Mandible	1	Metacarpals	10
Lacrimal	2	Phalanges	28
Nasal	2	**Pelvic Girdle (2)**	
Inferior concha	2	Coxal	2
Vomer	1	**Lower Limbs (60)**	
Middle Ear Bones (6)		Femur	2
Malleus	2	Tibia	2
Incus	2	Fibula	2
Stapes	2	Patella	2
Hyoid Bone (1)		Tarsals	14
Vertebral Column (26)		Metatarsals	10
Cervical vertebrae	7	Phalanges	28
Thoracic vertebrae	12	**Total Number of Bones**	206
Lumbar vertebrae	5		
Sacrum	1		
Coccyx	1		

*Know

severe brain injury and death. Because the shattered bone tears the meninges, cerebrospinal fluid leaks into the nasal passages. This type of injury also creates a direct opening into the brain for pathogens and subsequent infections of brain tissue, so watch that karate chop to the face. The impact of the face with the steering wheel during a car wreck can also drive the shattered ethmoid bone into the brain.

Facial Bones

The face has 14 facial bones, most of which are paired (see Fig. 8.7B). Only the mandible and the vomer are single bones.

- *Mandible.* The mandible (MAN-di-bal), the lower jaw bone, carries the lower teeth. The anterior portion of the mandible forms the chin. The mandible forms the only freely movable joint in the skull. Two posterior upright projections on the

mandible have bony processes that articulate with the temporal bones at the temporomandibular joint (TMJ). The TMJ can be felt as the depression immediately in front of the ear. Tension or stress often causes pain in the TMJ. This condition is often associated with tooth grinding (bruxism) during sleep. Bony processes on the mandible serve as points of attachment for chewing muscles.

- *Maxilla.* Two maxillary bones fuse to form the upper jaw. The maxilla (mak-SIH-lah) carries the upper teeth. An extension of the maxilla, the palatine process, forms the anterior portion of the hard palate (roof) of the mouth (see Fig. 8.7C). These bones also form parts of the nasal cavity and the eye orbits.

- *Palatine bones.* Two palatine (PAL-ah-tine) bones form the posterior part of the hard palate and the floor of the nasal cavity. Failure of the palatine

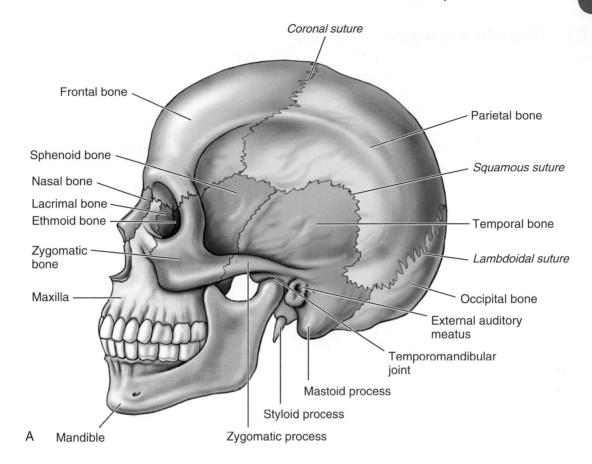

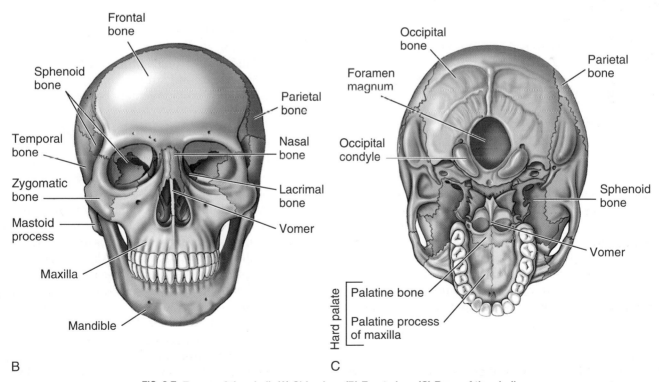

FIG. 8.7 Bones of the skull. (A) Side view. (B) Front view. (C) Base of the skull.

and/or maxillary bones to fuse causes a cleft palate (an opening in the roof of the mouth), making suckling very difficult for an infant and contributing to a host of other developmental issues. Fortunately, a cleft palate can be surgically repaired.

- *Zygomatic bones.* The zygomatic bones are the cheekbones. They also form a part of the orbits of the eyes.
- *Other facial bones.* Several other bones complete the facial structure, including the lacrimal bones, nasal bones, vomer, and inferior nasal conchae.

Do You Know...

About Two Drug-Induced Jaw-Breaking Events?

The mandible often takes it on the chin! A rather common mandibular event is the alcohol-fueled Saturday night brawl that often culminates in a broken jaw. Unlike a broken leg bone, which can be immobilized by a cast, the mandible (lower jaw) can be immobilized only by wiring it to the maxilla (upper jaw). Can't talk, can't eat, can't expel vomit. In fact, people with wired jaws must have access to wire cutters in case they vomit. What about nutrition? Puréed food is delivered through a straw.

A second mandibular malady is a drug-induced "Fossy jaw." Alendronate (Fosamax), which belongs to a group of drugs called *bisphosphonates*, is used in the prevention and treatment of osteoporosis in postmenopausal women. It works by inhibiting bone resorption by osteoclasts. A rare but distressing side effect of Fosamax is osteonecrosis of the jaw, characterized by loose teeth and a crumbling jaw bone—hence the term *dead jaw*, or *Fossy jaw*. In addition to osteonecrosis, a small group of patients treated with bisphosphonates also experienced a distinctive type of low-energy fracture of the femur. One theory has suggested that by suppressing bone turnover (diminished osteoclastic activity), normal wear-and-tear microscopic bone cracks are not repaired daily and ultimately progress to bone weakening and fracture.

 Re-Think

1. What are the two groups of bones that form the skull?
2. List the cranial bones that articulate with the parietal bone.
3. What are the functions of the foramen magnum and occipital condyles?
4. With regard to head injury, why is the foramen magnum called a "deathtrap"?

Sinuses

Sinuses are air-filled cavities located in several of the bones of the skull. They perform two important functions: (1) they lessen the weight of the skull, and (2) they modulate the sound of the voice.

The four sinuses are called the *paranasal sinuses* because they surround and connect with the nasal structures (Fig. 8.8). The names of the four sinuses reflect their location within the various skull bones: frontal sinus, ethmoidal sinuses, sphenoidal sinus, and maxillary sinuses.

Because the sinuses connect with the nasal passages and the throat, infections may spread from the nose and throat into the sinuses. An inflammation of the sinus is called *sinusitis*. Why do allergies sometimes make your face hurt? Allergies often cause the mucous membranes that line the facial sinuses to oversecrete mucus. The mucus forms an excellent medium for bacterial growth. As the mucus accumulates and the membranes swell, pressure and discomfort are often experienced in the facial

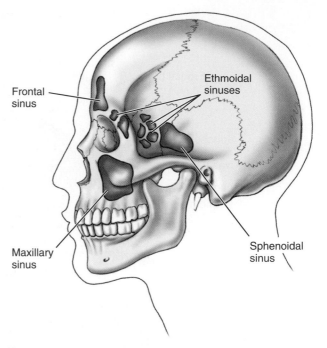

FIG. 8.8 Sinuses.

region, which overlies the sinuses (around the eyes and nose).

How the Skull Bones Are Held Together

The bones of the adult skull form a unique type of joint called a **suture** (see Fig. 8.7A). The sutures join together the bones of the skull, much like a zipper. The major sutures include the coronal suture, the lambdoidal suture, and the squamosal suture. Unlike other joints in the body, no significant movement occurs between cranial bones.

The Infant Skull

The two major differences between the infant and adult skulls are the fontanels and unfused sutures in the infant skull.

The infant skull has areas that have not yet been converted to bone. Instead, they are covered by a fibrous membrane. Because these areas are soft to touch, they are called a baby's *soft spots*. Also, the rhythm of the baby's pulse can be felt in these soft spots, and so they are called **fontanels** (FON-tah-nels), meaning "little fountains."

The two major fontanels are the larger, diamond-shaped anterior fontanel and the smaller, posterior occipital fontanel. Two smaller fontanels are located more laterally—the anterolateral and posterolateral fontanels (Fig. 8.9). By the time a child reaches 2 years of age, these fontanels have been gradually converted to bone and can no longer be felt.

The fontanels are one reason why infant skull bones are more movable than those of the adult skull. Another reason is that the sutures of the infant skulls are not fused. Unfused sutures allow the skull to be compressed

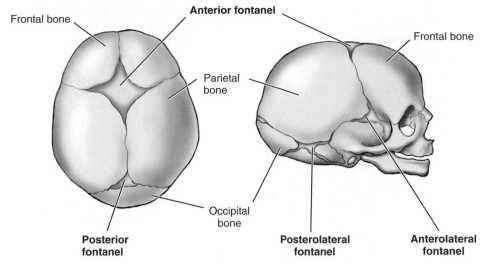

Frontal bone

Anterior fontanel

Parietal bone

Posterior fontanel

Occipital bone

Frontal bone

Posterolateral fontanel

Anterolateral fontanel

FIG. 8.9 Fontanels in the infant skull.

during birth. They also allow for the continued growth of the brain and skull after birth and throughout infancy. It also explains why your adorable newborn may look like a "conehead." The fetal skull is too large to fit through the birth canal, so the movable bones overlap, thereby decreasing the diameter of the head. Fortunately, the pointy skull reshapes shortly after birth.

Occasionally, the sutures of the infant skull fuse too early, preventing the growth of the brain. This condition is called *microcephalia* and is characterized by a small cranium, restricted brain growth, and impaired intellectual functioning. Sometimes the skull expands too much. For example, if excessive fluid accumulates within the brain of an infant, the bones are forced apart, and the skull enlarges. This condition is called *hydrocephalus* (or "water on the brain").

Observation of the fontanels can provide valuable information regarding brain swelling. What does a bulging or sunken fontanel indicate? If an infant suffers a head injury or infection, the brain may swell. Because the fontanel is soft tissue, it will bulge outward in response to increasing pressure within the skull. Conversely, the fontanels may become sunken in the presence of dehydration.

 Re-Think

1. Why does your face "hurt" in response to sinusitis?
2. What are fontanels?
3. Why is it important that the infant sutures are unfused?

Hyoid Bone

The hyoid (HYE-oyd) bone is a U-shaped bone located in the upper neck. It anchors the tongue and is associated with swallowing. The hyoid bone is often fractured during strangulation. Watch for this during an autopsy, you forensic sleuths!

Bones of the Middle Ear

Each ear contains three small bones called *ossicles* (see Chapter 13 for the role of the ossicles in hearing).

VERTEBRAL COLUMN

The Back and Its Stack of Bones

The vertebral column, also called the backbone or spine, extends from the skull to the pelvis (Fig. 8.10). The vertebral column consists of 26 bones, called *vertebrae* (VER-teh-bray), aligned and stacked in a column. Sitting between each vertebra is a cartilaginous disc. The vertebral column performs four major functions:

- Forms a supporting structure for the head and thorax
- Forms an attachment for the pelvic girdle
- Encases and protects the spinal cord
- Provides flexibility for the body

The vertebrae are named according to their location. Seven cervical vertebrae (C1 to C7) are located in the neck region. If you bend your head forward and run your hand down the cervical vertebrae, you will feel a large bump; this large vertebra is C7, which is called the *vertebra prominens* (VER-teh-bra PRAH-meh-nenz) and is used as a landmark in assessing surface anatomy. Twelve thoracic vertebrae (T1 to T12) are located in the chest region, and the five lumbar vertebrae (L1 to L5) are located in the lower back region. If you place your hands on your hips, you are at the level of L4. In addition, five sacral vertebrae fuse into one sacrum. The sacrum forms the posterior wall of the pelvis. How did the sacrum get its name? The ancients thought that the seat of the soul was located at the base of the spine and therefore called the sacred area the "sacrum." The tailbone is called the *coccyx* (KOHK-iks) because it resembles the beak of a cuckoo bird.

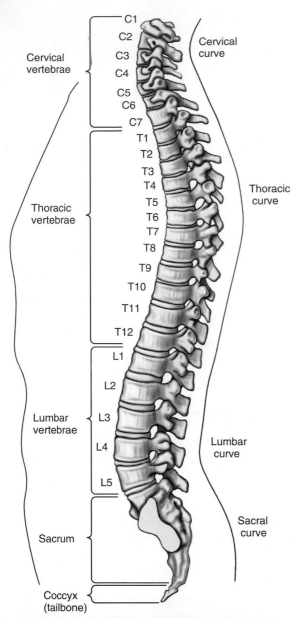

FIG. 8.10 Vertebral column: cervical vertebrae (7), thoracic vertebrae (12), lumbar vertebrae (5), sacrum, and coccyx. Vertebral curves: cervical, thoracic, lumbar, and sacral.

 Do You Know...

Why Your Spine Hates Texting?

Poor spine! All hunched over from heavy backpacks and various other totes. Not only do we get to carry all our stuff everywhere, but something new is bothering the spine. The latest in spine aggravation is "texting," the nonstop bending of our heads to check and dispatch our messages. The texting craze has us permanently hunched, even while sitting. A new report from the New York Spine Surgery and Rehabilitation Center names the disorder "text neck" and has implicated it as a major source of chronic back pain. The rehab center provides this explanation. Your "squash" weighs about 10 to 12 lb, a weight that is easily supported by your spine and muscles. When your head tips forward, as in texting, the spine and muscles experience a much heavier weight, maybe as much as 60 lbs. Over time, the increased weight causes wear and tear on the spine and chronic back pain.

Two Special Vertebrae: Atlas (C1) and Axis (C2)

The first and second cervical vertebrae have several special features and names (Fig. 8.11). The first cervical vertebra (C1) is called the *atlas*. The atlas has no body but does have depressions into which fit the bony projections of the occipital bone of the skull. The atlas supports the skull and allows you to nod "yes." The atlas is named after a figure in Greek mythology, Atlas, who carried the earth on his shoulders.

The second cervical vertebra (C2) is called the *axis*. The axis has a projection, called the *dens* (nicknamed for the toothlike odontoid process), which fits into the atlas and acts as a pivot or swivel for the atlas. The axis allows your head to rotate from side to side as you say "no." A strong blow to the top of the head can force the dens through the foramen magnum and into the base of the brain, causing sudden death. Not good! In children, the fusion between the dens and the axis is incomplete. Shaking a child can easily dislocate the dens, causing injury to the spinal cord and brain.

Characteristics of Vertebrae

The vertebra is an irregular bone that contains several distinct structures (see Fig. 8.11). The body of the vertebra is padded by a cartilaginous disc and supports the weight of the vertebra sitting on top of it. Some processes provide sites of attachment for ligaments, tendons, and muscles; other processes articulate with bones such as the ribs. The vertebral foramen is the opening for the spinal cord; the vertebral foramen of the stacked vertebrae form the vertebral canal. The vertebrae are aligned so that if you run your hand down your back, you will feel the spinous processes. For this reason, the vertebral column is also called the *spine*. Note that the vertebrae become larger as the vertebral column descends. The larger lower vertebrae support a heavier load.

The bodies of the vertebrae are padded and separated by cartilaginous discs. The intervertebral discs act as shock absorbers. They also act as "spacers" between vertebrae, allowing peripheral nerves to connect to the spinal cord without being squashed. (Ouch!)

SOME VERTEBRAL COLUMN CONCERNS

- The vertebra has a barlike lamina. Spina bifida refers to the failure of the lamina to fuse during fetal development. The vertebral defect allows the spinal cord to protrude onto the surface of the back. Depending on the level of the defect, compression of the spinal cord then causes paralysis and loss of bladder and bowel control.
- A surgical procedure called a *laminectomy* may be performed to access the intervertebral disc; the opening allows the surgeon to remove a damaged, or "slipped," disc. Occasionally, several vertebrae are fused together to stabilize a part of the vertebral column. This procedure is called *spinal fusion*.

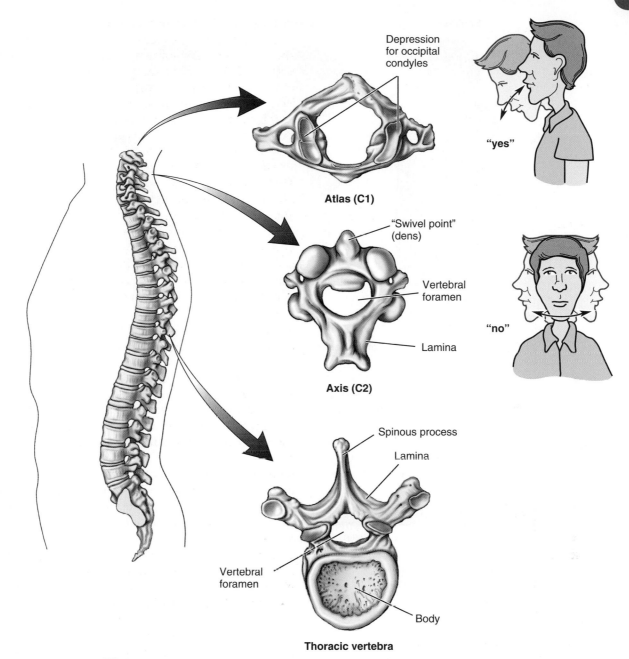

FIG. 8.11 Anatomy of a vertebra: the atlas (C1) and axis (C2), and a thoracic vertebra.

- Note that the spinal cord descends from the base of the brain through the vertebral foramen of the stack of vertebrae. Injury to the vertebral column at any point can compress or sever the spinal cord, causing paralysis. You must use extreme caution while treating or moving a person with a spinal cord injury. Immobility is a key term in the first-aid treatment of suspected spinal cord injury.

Curvatures

When viewed from the side, the vertebral column has four normal curvatures (see Fig. 8.10): the cervical, thoracic, lumbar, and sacral curves. The directions of the curvatures are important. The cervical and the lumbar curvatures bend toward the front of the body. The thoracic and sacral curvatures bend away from the front of the body. These curves center the head over the body, thereby providing the balance needed to walk in an upright position.

The curvature of the fetal spine is different. Its single C-shaped curvature bends away from the front of the body. Its shape reflects the curled-up position of the fetus during the 9 months in the cozy, but cramped, uterine living quarters. The cervical curvature develops about 3 to 4 months after birth as infants start to hold up their heads. The lumbar curvature develops at about 1 year of age, when children begin standing and walking.

Fig. 8.12 illustrates several abnormal curvatures of the spine. Scoliosis (skoh-lee-OH-sis) refers to a lateral curvature, usually involving the thoracic vertebrae. If severe, a lateral curvature can compress abdominal organs. It can also diminish expansion of the rib cage and

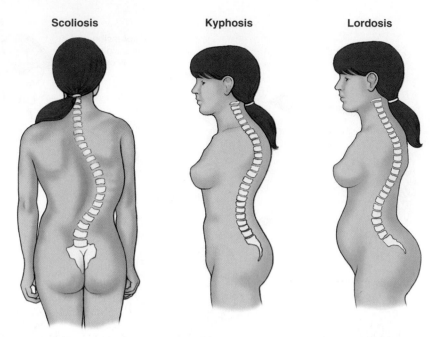

FIG. 8.12 Abnormal curvatures of the vertebral column: scoliosis, kyphosis, and lordosis.

therefore impair breathing. Kyphosis (kye-FOH-sis) is an exaggerated thoracic curvature; it, too, can impair breathing and is sometimes called *hunchback*. Lordosis is an exaggerated lumbar curvature and is sometimes called *swayback*. These abnormalities may be caused by a genetic defect or may develop in response to disease or poor posture.

 Re-Think

1. How does the structure and function of C1 and C2 differ from that of other vertebrae?
2. What is the function of the vertebral foramen?
3. Why are the lumbar vertebrae larger than the cervical vertebrae?
4. List the four curvatures of the vertebral column.

THORACIC CAGE

The *thorax* (THOH-raks) is a term that refers to the chest region. The thoracic cage is the skeletal part of the chest; it is a bony, cone-shaped cage that surrounds and protects the lungs, heart, large blood vessels, and some of the abdominal organs, such as the liver, spleen, and kidneys (Fig. 8.13). The thoracic cage plays a crucial role in breathing. If you put your hand on your chest and take a deep breath, you will feel your thoracic cage move up and out. It also helps support the bones of the shoulder. The thoracic cage is composed of the sternum, ribs, and thoracic vertebrae.

Sternum

The sternum, or breastbone, is a dagger-shaped bone located along the midline of the anterior chest. The three parts are the manubrium (man-OO-bree-ahm), body, and xiphoid (ZYE-foyd) process. The xiphoid process is the tip of the sternum and serves as a point of attachment

for some abdominal muscles. Note the suprasternal notch (also called the *jugular* notch), a depression on the upper part of the manubrium between the two clavicles; it is used as a landmark to locate other structures.

Ribs

Twelve pairs of ribs attach posteriorly to the thoracic vertebrae. Anteriorly, the top seven pairs of ribs attach directly to the sternum by costal cartilage and are called *true ribs*. The next five pairs attach indirectly to the sternum by cartilage or do not attach at all and are called *false ribs*. The bottom two pairs of false ribs lack sternal attachment and are therefore called *floating ribs*. Because of their location and lack of sternal support, the floating ribs are easily broken. Note that the ribs are numbered, which allows us to describe the location of thoracic structures. The spaces between the ribs (intercostal spaces) are also numbered. For example, the heart is located between the second rib and fifth intercostal space (the space between the fifth and sixth ribs). You will spend a lot of time counting ribs and intercostal spaces as part of your clinical practice.

Lines and Angles

Note the red lines on Fig. 8.13.
- Midsternal line—an imaginary line drawn vertically from the suprasternal notch through the middle of the sternum.
- Midclavicular lines (right and left)—imaginary lines drawn vertically from the midpoints of the clavicles (collarbones) and parallel to the midsternal line.
- Costal margins—the edges of the cartilage that form an angle as they converge near the xiphoid process.
- Costal angle—the angle formed by the intersection of the costal margins; it should be less than

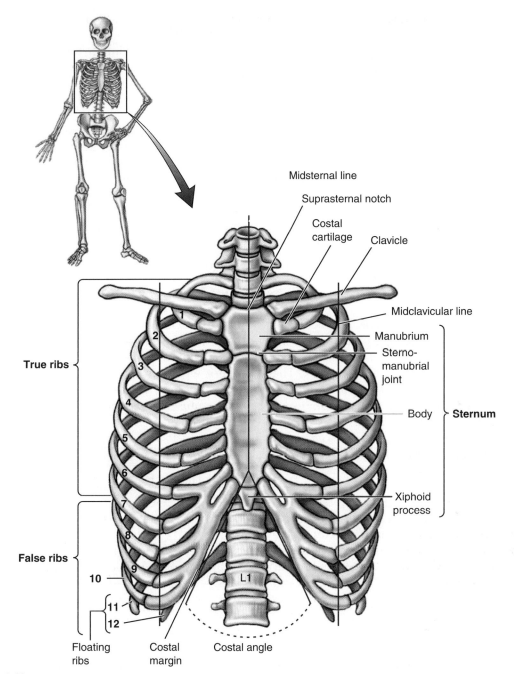

FIG. 8.13 Thoracic cage: the sternum, ribs, and thoracic vertebrae. Note in red: costal margin, costal angle, midsternal line, and midclavicular lines.

90 degrees. The costal angle can change size; for example, during pregnancy, the angle increases. It also increases when the chest diameter expands with certain lung diseases, such as emphysema.
- Angle of Louis (sternomanubrial joint)—a joint that is referenced in counting ribs. The joint is located at the level of the second rib.

? Re-Think

1. What bones form the thoracic cage?
2. With what bony structures do the ribs articulate?
3. Differentiate between the true, false, and floating ribs.
4. Why is the sternomanubrial joint an important landmark?

◎ Sum It Up!

The skeleton is divided into the axial and appendicular skeletons. The axial skeleton includes the bones of the skull (facial and cranial), hyoid bone, bones of the middle ear, bones of the vertebral column, and bones of the thoracic cage (ribs and sternum). The skull contains the facial bones, cranial bones, and air-filled cavities called *sinuses*. The skull of a newborn contains fontanels, which are membranous areas that allow brain growth. The vertebral column is formed from 24 vertebrae, one sacrum, and one coccyx. The vertebrae are separated by cartilaginous discs. The vertebral column of the adult has four curvatures: cervical, thoracic, lumbar, and sacral. The thoracic cage is a bony cone-shaped cage formed by the sternum, 12 pairs of ribs, and thoracic vertebrae.

APPENDICULAR SKELETON

The appendicular skeleton is composed of the bones of the shoulder girdle, upper limbs, pelvic girdle, and lower limbs (see Fig. 8.1).

SHOULDER GIRDLE

The shoulder girdle is also called the **pectoral girdle**. Each shoulder girdle contains two bones: one clavicle (KLAV-i-kul) and one scapula (SKAP-yoo-lah) (Fig. 8.14). The shoulder girdle supports the upper limbs and serves as a place of attachment for muscles. The shoulder girdle is designed for great flexibility; move your shoulder and arm around and note how many different movements you can make. Compare this with the limited movement you have at the elbow and the knee.

Clavicle

The clavicle is also called the *collarbone*. It looks like a long, slender, S-shaped rod and articulates with both the sternum and scapula. The clavicle helps stabilize the shoulder; the attachment, however, is weak. The clavicle is easily dislocated and is the most frequently broken bone in the body.

Scapula

The scapula, also called the *shoulder blade* or *wing bone*, is a large flat bone shaped like a triangle. The two scapulae are located on the posterior thorax. Two large processes on the scapula allow it to articulate with the clavicle and serve as points of attachment for arm and chest muscles. The glenoid cavity on the scapula is the site where the head of the humerus (arm bone) fits, thereby allowing you to rotate your arm at the shoulder. Note the acromion process and coracoid process on the scapula near the glenoid cavity. Both processes serve as points of attachment for ligaments and muscles. The acromion process forms the "pointy" part of the shoulder and articulates with the clavicle.

 Do You Know...

About Xtreme Modeling and Toe Cleavage?

The saying, "You can never be too thin" (or off-balance) has taken on a new meaning. In addition to a starvation diet, Xtreme Modeling has taken surgical aim at the skeletal system. It's called "remodeling the model." How so? Surgeons have successfully shortened or removed toes, thereby allowing the foot to fit into stylish "pointy" shoes. More importantly, toe removal also creates revealing toe cleavage. The toe is not the only osseous victim of this skeletal redesign. Removal of the lower floating ribs further slims the slim. When accompanied by high colonic irrigations (enemas), our remodeled model easily slips into the elusive size 0. Of obvious concern: the risk of general anesthesia, the loss of ribs that normally protect the kidneys, and the loss of toes that assist in walking, balance, and overall comfort! Go figure!

UPPER LIMBS

The upper limbs contain the bones of the arm (humerus), forearm (ulna and radius), and hand (carpals, metacarpals, and phalanges).

Humerus

The humerus is the arm bone. The proximal humerus contains a head, which fits into the glenoid cavity of the scapula, allowing the arm to rotate at the shoulder joint. At the distal end of the humerus are several processes that allow it to articulate with the bones of the forearm. The olecranon (oh-LEK-rah-non) fossa is a depression of the humerus that holds the olecranon process of the ulna when the elbow is extended (not bent).

Radius

The radius is one of two bones of the forearm. It is located on the lateral or thumb side when the palm of the hand is facing forward. The head of the radius articulates with the humerus and proximal ulna, whereas the distal end articulates with the distal ulna and the carpal or wrist bones. The radial tuberosity at the proximal end of the radius is the site of attachment for one of the muscles responsible for bending the forearm at the elbow.

 Do You Know...

Why Hitting Your Funny Bone Doesn't Feel Funny?

When you hit your elbow and get that sharp pain that is associated with the "funny bone," you are actually hitting the ulnar nerve. The unprotected ulnar nerve lies over the distal end of the humerus and is therefore vulnerable to being bumped. Why do we call it funny? Maybe because of its location near the humerus, a "humorous" name for a bone.

Ulna

The ulna is the second bone of the forearm. The longer of the two bones, the ulna, is located on the medial or little finger side of the forearm. It has processes and depressions that allow it to articulate with the humerus and radius proximally and with the radius distally. The olecranon process of the ulna is what you feel as the bony point of the elbow. Note that the distal ends of both the ulna and radius have a pointed styloid process; the styloid processes can be felt at the wrist.

Also note the relationship of the radius to the ulna when the hand moves from a palm-up (**supination**) to a palm-down (**pronation**) position. When the palm is up, the two bones are parallel. When the palm is down, the two bones cross to achieve this movement.

Hand

The hand is composed of a wrist, palm, and fingers. The wrist contains eight bones called *carpal bones*, which are tightly bound by ligaments. Five metacarpal bones form the palm of the hand; each metacarpal bone is in line with a finger. Feel your metacarpal

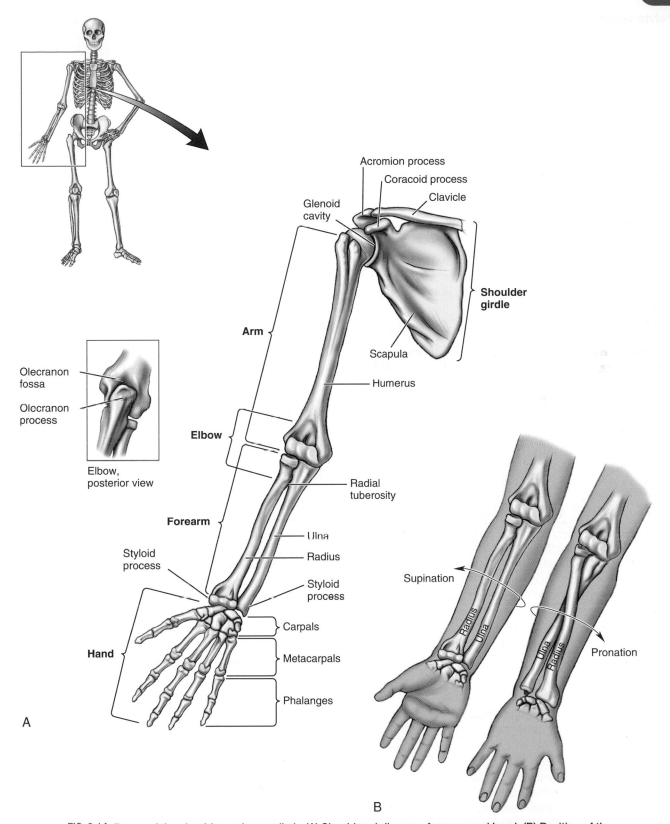

FIG. 8.14 **Bones of the shoulder and upper limb. (A) Shoulder girdle, arm, forearm, and hand. (B) Position of the radius and ulna during supination and pronation.**

bones on the back of your hand; note how each aligns with your fingers. The 14 finger bones are called *pha-langes* (fah-LAN-jeez), or digits. Note that each digit has three bones except the thumb (called the *pollex*), which has only two bones. The heads of the phalanges are prominent as the knuckles when a fist is made.

? Re-Think

1. List the bones of the pectoral girdle.
2. List the bones of the upper extremities
3. What "happens" at the glenoid cavity?
4. What bones form the elbow? What is the olecranon process?

Pelvic Girdle

The pelvic girdle is composed of two coxal bones that articulate with each other anteriorly and with the sacrum posteriorly (Fig. 8.15A). The pelvic girdle performs three functions: (1) it bears the weight of the body; (2) it serves as a place of attachment for the thighs; and (3) it protects the organs located in the pelvic cavity, including the urinary bladder and reproductive organs.

Pelvis

The pelvis is formed by the pelvic girdle, sacrum, and coccyx.

Male and Female Differences. The differences between the female and male pelvis are related to the childbearing role of the female. In general, the female pelvis is broader and shallower than the male pelvis. The male pelvis is narrow and funnel-shaped (see Figs. 8.15C and D).

Do You Know...

About Dr. Pollex and Mr. Blackberry's Thumb?

Mr. Blackberry went to his family physician, Dr. Pollex, with a chief complaint of extreme pain in his left thumb. He writhed in pain and sobbed uncontrollably as he punched numbers into his cell and frantically sent text messages to everyone he had ever met. Dr. Pollex, however, was all over it. "Thumb abuse!" he roared. He explained to Mr. Blackberry. "Your thumb [pollex] was not designed to click away 24/7; it's aching for relief. The sheath around your thumb is inflamed and swollen." The digit doc assured Mr. Blackberry that with rest and retraining, he would soon be clicking away again. Other digits could be trained to share the clicking load. Thumb pain resulting from repetitive thumb-clicking marathons is a trendy new malady called *Blackberry thumb,* a reference to the once popular handheld device.

Coxal Bone

The coxal bone is the hip bone (see Fig. 8.15B). Each coxal bone is composed of three parts: the ilium, ischium, and pubis. The three bones join together to form a depression called the *acetabulum* (ass-it-TAH-buhl-um). The acetabulum is important because it receives the head of the femur and therefore enables the thigh to rotate at the hip joint.

Ilium. The ilium (IL-ee-um) is the largest part of the coxal bone. The ilium is the flared upper part of the bone and can be felt at the hip. The outer edge of the ilium is called the *iliac crest.* The ilium connects in the back with the sacrum, forming the sacroiliac joint. The greater sciatic notch is the site where blood vessels and the sciatic nerve pass from the pelvic cavity into the posterior thigh region. Like the sternum, the ilium produces blood cells and is a site for bone marrow biopsy.

Ischium. The ischium (ISH-ee-um) is the most inferior part of the coxal bone. The ischium contains three im-

portant structures: the ischial tuberosity, ischial spine, and lesser sciatic notch. The ischial tuberosity is the part of the coxal bone on which you sit. The ischial spine projects into the pelvic cavity and narrows the outlet of the pelvis. If the spines of a woman's two ischial bones are too close together, the pelvic outlet becomes too small to allow for the birth of a baby. The measurement of the distance between the two spines therefore provides valuable information about the adequacy of the pelvis for childbearing.

Pubis. The pubis is the most anterior part of the coxal bone. The two pubic bones meet in front as the symphysis (SIM-fi-sis) pubis. A disc of cartilage separates the pubic bones at the symphysis pubis. In women, the disc expands in response to the hormones of pregnancy, thereby enlarging the pelvic cavity to provide a bigger space for the growing fetus. The symphysis pubis is a forensic gold mine. It is an accurate indicator of age, gender, and evidence of past pregnancies.

A large hole called the *obturator foramen* is formed as the pubic bone fuses with a part of the ischium. The obturator is the largest foramen in the body.

What is meant by the true pelvis and false pelvis? The false pelvis is the area surrounded by the flaring parts of the two iliac bones (see Fig. 8.15C). The true pelvis lies lower and is smaller than the false pelvis. The true pelvis is a ring formed by the fusion of the pelvic bones. The pelvic brim is the border between the false and true pelvises. The true pelvis has an inlet and outlet area. In women, the size of these areas is important because they must be large enough to allow for childbirth.

Re-Think

1. Name the three bones that form the coxal bone.
2. What is the function of the acetabulum?
3. Locate the symphysis pubis. Explain how it affects the size of the pelvis during pregnancy.

LOWER LIMBS

The lower limb includes the bones of the thigh, kneecap, leg, and foot (Fig. 8.16).

Femur

The femur is the thigh bone; it is the longest and strongest bone in the body. The femur articulates proximally with the coxal bone to form the hip joint and distally with the bones of the leg to form the knee joint. The head of the femur sits in the acetabulum of the coxal bone and allows the thigh to rotate at the hip joint. The head of the femur attaches to the rest of the femur by the neck. A number of bony processes are on the femur. The most important are the greater and lesser trochanters (tro-KAN-ters). These trochanters provide sites of attachment for many muscles.

In older persons, the neck of the femur is easily broken during a fall and is known as a *broken hip.* Forced

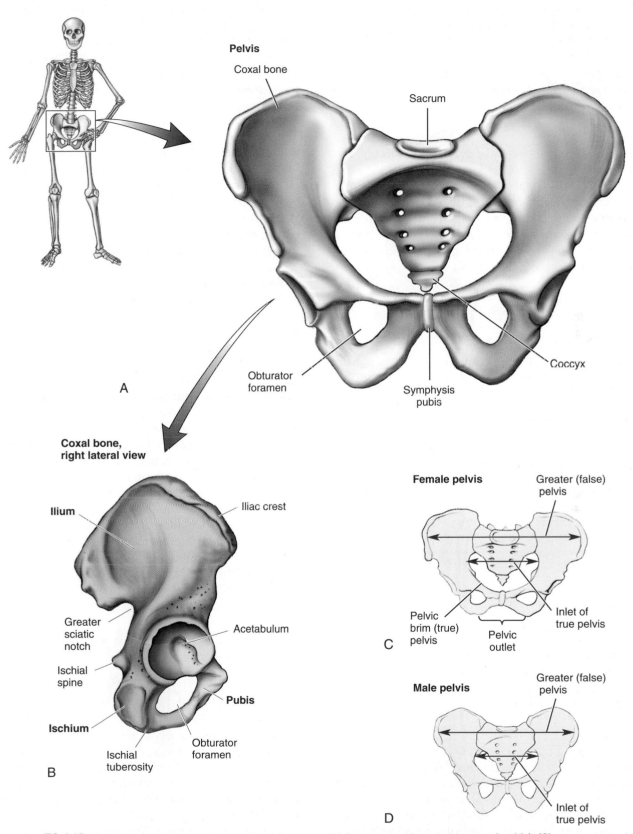

FIG. 8.15 Pelvic cavity. (A) Bones that make up the pelvis. (B) Coxal bone (ilium, ischium, and pubis). (C) Female pelvis. (D) Male pelvis.

immobility (bed rest) often results in serious complications. For example, because of the weight of the injured leg, an immobile bedridden person may experience an outward rotation of the hip. If allowed to develop, this outward rotation makes walking very difficult and therefore delays rehabilitation. Other hazards of immobility, such as blood clots and pneumonia, contribute to the seriousness of a fractured hip.

Patella

The patella is the kneecap. It is a triangular bone located within a tendon that passes over the knee. It articulates with both the distal femur and protects the anterior surface of the knee joint. Interestingly, an infant is born without kneecaps; somewhere between the ages of 2 and 6 years, in response to weight bearing, a small sesamoid bone (one that looks like a sesame seed) in the patellar region enlarges, thereby forming the kneecap.

Tibia and Fibula

The tibia and the fibula form the leg. The tibia is the shinbone and articulates with the distal femur at the knee. The tibia is the larger weight-bearing bone of the leg. A protuberance called the *tibial tuberosity* is the site of attachment for the muscles and ligaments from the thigh. At the distal end of the tibia, a protuberance called the *medial malleolus* (mah-LEE-oh-lis) articulates with the talus, a tarsal bone.

The fibula (FIB-yoo-lah) is a long, thin bone positioned laterally alongside the tibia in the leg. The proximal end of the fibula articulates with the tibia. It does not articulate with the femur, is not part of the knee, and bears much less weight than does the tibia. The distal end forms the lateral malleolus, which articulates with the talus. The articulation of the distal tibia (medial malleolus) and fibula (lateral malleolus) with the talus forms the ankle joint or talocrural joint. Skiers often twist their ankles and break the fibula at the lateral malleolus. You don't need snow, however, to hobble. Just roll the ankle, and you too can be on crutches!

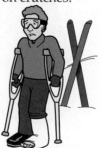

How do we remember the positions of the leg bones? The **tib**ia is the **T**hick **I**nner **B**one; the fibu**la** is **LA**teral to the tibia.

Foot

Each foot (Fig. 8.17) has an ankle, instep, and five toes. Seven tarsal bones form the ankle. The most proximal of the tarsal bones, the talus, articulates with the tibia

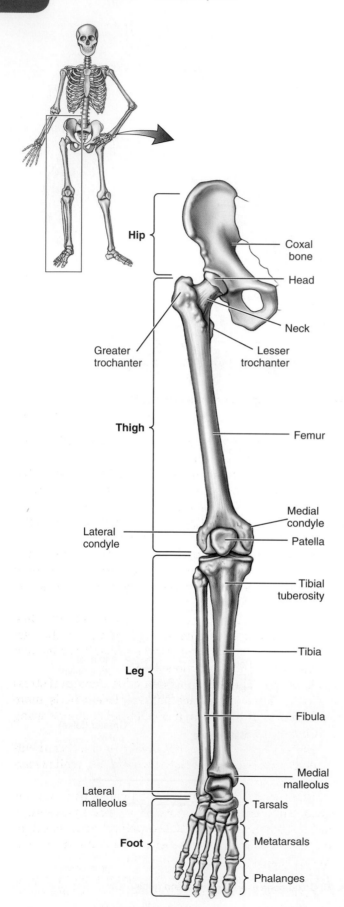

FIG. 8.16 **Bones of the hip and lower limb: thigh, leg, and foot.**

Hip
- Coxal bone
- Head
- Neck
- Lesser trochanter

Greater trochanter

Thigh
- Femur

Lateral condyle

Medial condyle

Patella

Tibial tuberosity

Leg
- Tibia
- Fibula
- Medial malleolus

Lateral malleolus

Foot
- Tarsals
- Metatarsals
- Phalanges

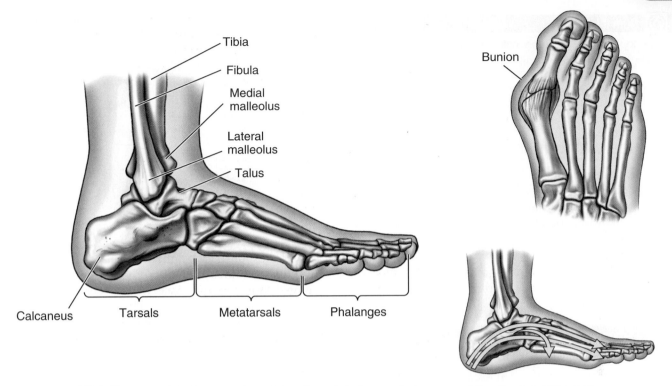

FIG. 8.17 Bones of the foot: tarsals, metatarsals, and phalanges. Arches support the structure of the foot.

and fibula. Most of the weight of the body is supported by two of the tarsal bones, the talus and the calcaneus (kal-KAY-nee-us), or heel bone. The instep of the foot is formed by five metatarsal bones. The ball of the foot is formed by the distal ends of the metatarsals. The tarsals, metatarsals, and associated tendons and ligaments form the arch of the foot. If the ligaments and tendons weaken, the arches can fall, and the person is said to have flat feet. The toes contain 14 phalanges. The great toe is called the *hallux*.

Foot Notes and Toe Woes: We all know about the thrill of victory (looking great in heels and flaunting the latest in toe cleavage). What about the "agony of de-feet"? Think about it. Sometimes we jam our square feet into pointy shoes, creating an unnatural, uncomfortable, and crippling tiptoe gait. The entire weight of the body is pushed forward to the balls of the feet. What do we get for this stylish effort?

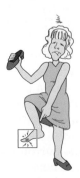

- *Bunions.* Bunions develop in response to excessive force, whereby the big toe is compressed and forced toward the second toe. The joint becomes distorted, inflamed, and painful.
- *Neuromas.* The shift of body weight to the balls of the feet causes painful and debilitating nerve growths (neuromas) between the toes.
- *Metatarsalgia.* The shift of body weight causes metatarsalgia, or pain in the ball of the foot.
- *Shortening of the Achilles tendon.* The tiptoe position causes contraction of the Achilles tendon; the shortened tendon makes the use of flat shoes uncomfortable.
- *Pump bump.* Excess pressure of the heel of the shoe on bone causes an enlargement (bump) on the heel bone. Pump bump is so common that it has its own medical name: Haglund's deformity.
- *Knee pain.* The shift in weight adds unnatural stress to the knee joint; knee joint replacement is more common in women and is often related to wearing abusive footwear.
- *Last but not least.* There have been several documented cases of death associated with falling while wearing platform shoes.

What to do? Although it can be performed, the surgical removal of toes is not the answer. Instituting a fashion change is certainly less painful than redesigning the foot. In any event, heels are definitely an anatomical step in the wrong direction!

? Re-Think

1. List the bones that articulate with the femur.
2. What bones articulate at the knee?
3. What bones form the ankle? foot?

Sum It Up!

The appendicular skeleton includes bones of the pectoral girdle (clavicle, scapula), upper extremities (humerus, radius, ulna, carpals, metacarpals, phalanges), pelvic girdle (coxal bones), and lower extremities (femur, patella, tibia, fibula, tarsals, metatarsals, phalanges).

JOINTS (ARTICULATIONS)

A joint, or articulation, is the site where two bones meet. Joints perform two functions: they hold the bones together, and they provide flexibility to a rigid skeleton. Without joints, we would move around stiffly like robots. Think of how awkward a basketball player would look if the entire skeleton were rigid. There is a branch of science that studies joints, called *arthrology;* the branch of medicine that studies disease of the joints is called *rheumatology.*

Do You Know...

What Dripping "Humours" Have to Do with Gout?

The typical cartoon of a person experiencing gout is that of an older, red-faced, obese, well-off man. His elevated, throbbing big toe fits the picture perfectly. Gout is caused by an increase of uric acid in the blood. The uric acid deposits in joints, where it forms tiny sharp crystals (called *tophi*) that inflame the joint and cause intense pain. Foods high in uric acid can bring on an attack of gout. A diet of meat and alcohol (the rich man's diet) can cause it; hence, the caricature of a glutton—wealthy, obese, and red-faced—comes to mind. The term *gout* comes from *gutta*, a Latin word meaning "to drop." It was originally believed that gout was caused by unhealthy humours (fluids) or poisons that dropped or dripped into the joints, particularly the joint of the great toe. This disease was so common that the pubs often had gout stools for their portly porkers. Remember this:

G	**g**reat toe
O	**o**ne joint, usually the great toe
U	**u**ric acid
T	**t**ophi
Y	**Y**ikes, that hurts!

Joints can be classified into three groups according to the amount of movement: immovable, slightly movable, and freely movable (Table 8.3). Joints can also be classified according to the types of tissues—fibrous, cartilaginous, or synovial—that bind the bones at the joint.

JOINT CLASSIFICATION

IMMOVABLE JOINTS

 Immovable joints permit no movement. The sutures in the skull are immovable joints. The sutures are formed as the irregular edges of the skull bones interlock and are bound by fibrous connective tissue. When fused, they look like zippers.

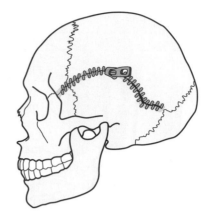

SLIGHTLY MOVABLE JOINTS

Slightly movable joints permit limited movement. Limited movement is usually achieved by bones connected by a cartilaginous disc. For example, movement of the spinal column occurs at the intervertebral discs. Also, during pregnancy, the symphysis pubis allows the pelvis to widen.

FREELY MOVABLE JOINTS

Freely movable joints provide much more flexibility and movement than the other two types of joints. Most of the joints of the skeletal system are freely movable. All freely movable joints are known as **synovial** (si-NO-vee-all) **joints** (Fig. 8.18).

- A typical synovial joint like the knee includes the following structures:
- *Articular cartilage.* The articulating surface of each of the two bones is lined with articular cartilage, forming a smooth surface within the joint.
- *Joint capsule.* The joint capsule is made of fibrous connective tissue. It encloses the joint in a strong sleevelike covering.
- *Synovial membrane.* Lining the joint capsule is the synovial membrane. This membrane secretes synovial fluid into the joint cavity.
- *Synovial fluid.* Synovial fluid lubricates the bones in the joint, thereby decreasing the friction within the joint. Synovial fluid gets its name from an ovum or egg because the thick consistency of the synovial fluid resembles the consistency of an egg white.
- *Bursae.* Many synovial joints contain bursae (sing., bursa). Bursae are small sacs of synovial fluid between the joint and the tendons that cross over the joint. Bursae permit the tendons to slide as the bones move. Excessive use of a joint may cause a painful inflammation of the bursae, called *bursitis.* Tennis elbow is bursitis caused by excessive and improper use of the elbow joint.
- *Supporting ligaments.* Surrounding the joint are supporting ligaments. There are collateral ligaments found on the sides of the knee and cruciate ligaments (anterior and posterior) found inside the knee. These ligaments join the articulating bones together and

Table 8.3   Types of Joints

TYPE	DESCRIPTION	EXAMPLES
Immovable	Suture, or "zipper"	Cranial bones
Slightly movable	Disc of cartilage between two bones	Intervertebral discs; symphysis pubis
Freely movable	Ball-and-socket	Shoulder (scapula and humerus): hip (coxal bone and femur)
	Hinge	Elbow (humerus and ulna): knee (femur and tibia); fingers
	Pivot	Atlas and axis; allows for rotation (side-to-side movement) of the head, indicating "no"
	Saddle	Thumb (carpometacarpal joint); sternoclavicular joint
	Gliding	Carpals
	Condyloid	Temporal bone and mandible (jaw); knuckles

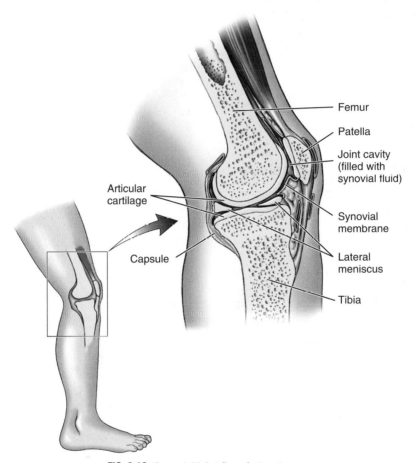

FIG. 8.18 Synovial joint (knee) structures.

stabilize the joint. Sometimes a ligament is stretched or torn, causing pain and loss of mobility.

NAMING JOINTS

The joints of the body are named so as to provide information about the articulating bones. The joints are named according to the bones they connect. Refer to Fig. 8.19 as we identify several joints. The temporomandibular joint connects the temporal bone in the skull with the mandible (lower jaw). The tibiofemoral joint is the articulation between the tibia and the femur—the knee. The knuckles refer to the metacarpophalangeal joints. The name indicates that the metacarpal bone articulates with a phalange (finger). Some names specify the bony process rather than the bone. For example, the glenohumeral joint names the glenoid cavity of the scapula and humerus, the arm bone that fits into the glenoid cavity. The acromioclavicular joint is the articulation between the acromion process of the scapula and the clavicle. Finally, locate the sternomanubrial joint (breastbone); it is a landmark used to count ribs.

MOVING SYNOVIAL JOINTS

The body contains many types of freely movable synovial joints. The type of motion and the degree of flexibility vary with each type of joint. For example, if you

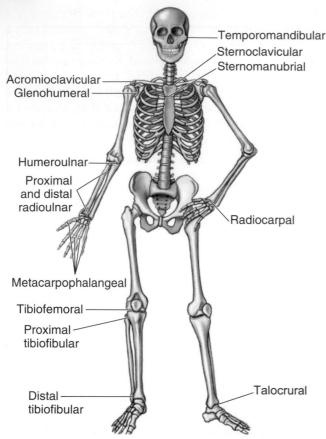

FIG. 8.19　Naming joints.

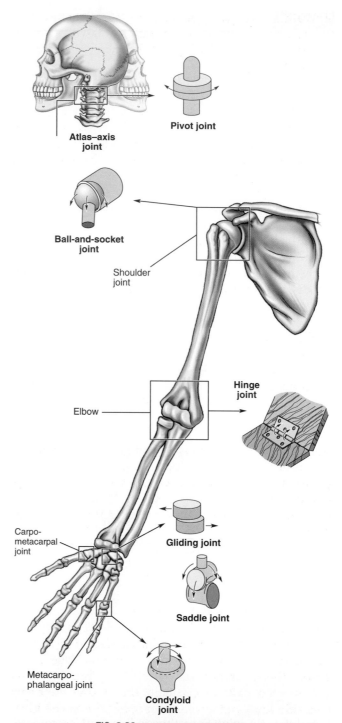

FIG. 8.20　Freely movable joints.

move your elbow, your forearm will move like two boards joined by a hinge. This motion is very different from the arm-swinging motion at the shoulder joint. Both the elbow and shoulder joints are freely movable, but the types of movement differ.

Six types of freely movable joints are classified according to the type of movement allowed by the joint (Fig. 8.20; see Table 8.3).

HINGE JOINT

The hinge joint allows movement similar to the movement of two boards joined together by a hinge. The hinge allows movement in one direction, where the angle at the hinge increases or decreases. Hinge joints include elbows, knees, and fingers. Move each of these joints to clarify the movement described here.

BALL-AND-SOCKET JOINT

A ball-and-socket joint is formed when the ball-shaped end of one bone fits into the cup-shaped socket of another bone, allowing the bones to move in many directions around a central point. The shoulder and hip joints are ball-and-socket joints. The head of the humerus fits into the glenoid cavity of the scapula in the shoulder joint. The head of the femur fits into the acetabulum of the coxal bone in the hip joint.

Move your shoulder all around (as in pitching a softball) and note the freedom of movement. Compare

this movement with the limited movement at the elbow or knee hinge joints. Although the ball-and-socket joint allows for a wide range of movement, it also predisposes the joint to easy displacement. When a strong force (as in falling) is applied to the shoulder, for example, a dislocation may occur.

PIVOT JOINT

A pivot joint allows for rotation around the length of a bone. The pivot joint allows only for rotation. An example is the side-to-side movement of the head indicating "no." This rotation occurs as the atlas (first cervical vertebra) swivels around, or pivots, on the axis (second cervical vertebra). This joint is called the *atlantoaxial joint.*

SADDLE JOINT

A saddle joint is formed when the surfaces of both articulating bones are saddle-shaped; the saddle shape of one bone is concave whereas the saddle shape of the second bone is convex. The position of the articulating bones is like a rider in a saddle. The clearest example of a saddle joint is the carpometacarpal joint at the base of the thumb, which allows the thumb a wide range of motion. Move your thumb all around to check out its versatility. Now, touch the tip of each finger with your thumb, a movement referred to as *opposition.* Interestingly, having an opposable thumb is one of the bragging points for being classified as human!

GLIDING JOINT

A gliding joint is formed by the interaction of the flat surfaces of the articulating bones. A gliding joint allows for a limited but complex gliding movement. Gliding joints are found in the wrist (intercarpal joints), ankle (intertarsal joints), and vertebral column.

CONDYLOID JOINT

A condyloid (KON-di-loyd) joint is formed when the oval articular surface of one bone fits into the oval depression of the second articulating bone. The radiocarpal joint (wrist) and the metacarpophalangeal joints (knuckles) at the bases of the fingers are examples of condyloid joints.

CLINICALLY "BIG" SYNOVIAL JOINTS

KNEE

The knee joint, called the *tibiofemoral joint,* is a hinge joint. In addition to all the structures contained in a synovial joint, the knee joint contains extra cushioning in the form of pads of cartilage. These pads absorb the shock of walking and jumping. Two crescent-shaped pads of cartilage, the medial meniscus (min-ISS-kiss) and lateral meniscus, rest on the tibia. Like other synovial joints, the knee joint is reinforced and aligned by supporting ligaments, the cruciate (KROO-she-ate) ligaments in particular. There is an anterior cruciate ligament (ACL) and a posterior cruciate ligament (PCL). All athletes are very aware of these joint-stabilizing structures. Football penalties, in particular, acknowledge the seriousness of the hinged nature of the knee by assessing a 15-yard penalty for clipping—an attempt to convert a hinge joint to a ball-and-socket arrangement.

SHOULDER

The shoulder joint is called the *glenohumeral joint,* indicating that the head of the humerus fits into the glenoid cavity of the scapula. The shoulder joint is a ball-and-socket joint that permits the greatest range of motion. The joint is stabilized by surrounding skeletal muscles, tendons, and ligaments. The rotator cuff muscles and tendons, in particular, hold the head of the humerus in the glenoid cavity. The wide range of motion of the shoulder joint comes at a price. The shoulder joint is the most frequently dislocated joint.

ELBOW

The elbow is called the *humeroulnar joint.* A lesser component of the elbow is the humeroradial joint. The olecranon process of the ulna forms the pointy part of the elbow when it is flexed. The elbow is a hinge joint that is very stable; nonetheless, it can be injured. For example, "nursemaid's elbow" is caused by an impatient parent dragging a toddler by the arm. The upward twisting pull causes a partial dislocation of the child's elbow and possible damage to the growth plate (epiphyseal disc).

HIP

The hip, called the *coxal joint,* is a ball-and-socket joint formed where the head of the femur articulates with the acetabulum, the depression formed by the three coxal bones. The hip is strengthened by surrounding muscles, tendons, and ligaments. A fractured hip refers to a break in the neck of the femur.

 Re-Think

1. Give one example of each type of joint: immovable, slightly movable, and freely movable.
2. Classify each of the following freely movable joints: tibiofemoral, humeroulnar, glenohumeral, atlas–axis, talocrural, and hip.

Types of Joint Movements

Movements at freely movable joints occur when the muscles that lie across the joints contract and exert pressure on the attached bone. These movements are illustrated in Fig. 8.21 and defined as follows:

- **Flexion.** This is the bending of a joint that decreases the angle between the bones (bending the leg at the knee or the fingers).
- **Extension.** This is the straightening of a joint so that the angle between the bones increases (e.g., straightening the leg at the knee or the fingers to open the hand).
- *Plantar flexion.* This is bending the foot down, as in toe dancing.
- *Dorsiflexion.* This is bending the foot up toward the leg.
- *Hyperextension.* This is overextending the joint beyond its normally straightened position, as in moving the hand toward the upper surface of the wrist.
- **Abduction.** This is movement away from the midline of the body (move your leg sideways, away from your body).

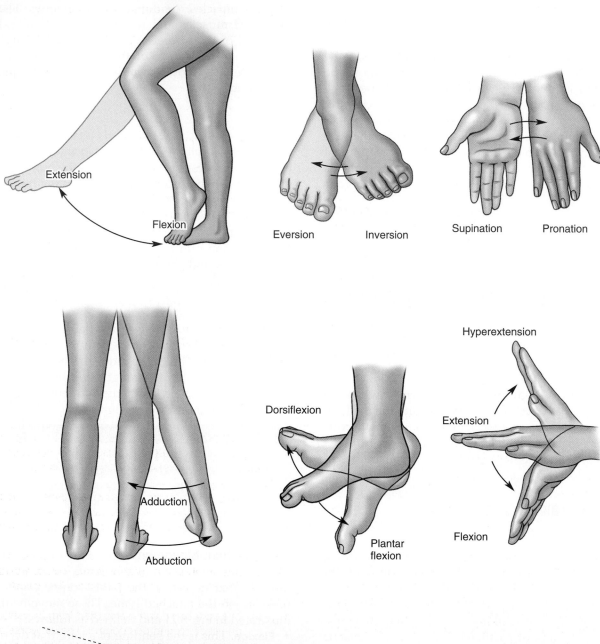

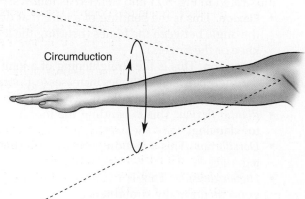

FIG. 8.21 Types of movements at joints.

- **Adduction.** This is movement toward the midline of the body (return your leg toward your body).
- *Inversion.* This is turning the sole of the foot inward so that it faces the opposite foot.
- *Eversion.* This is turning the sole of the foot outward.
- *Supination.* This is turning the hand so that the palm faces upward.
- *Pronation.* This is turning the hand so that the palm faces downward.
- **Circumduction.** This is a combination of movements, as in the circular arm movement that a softball pitcher makes while pitching the ball.

Re-Think

Refer to Fig. 8.19 and describe the type of joint movements of the following parts: left hand at the wrist, right leg at the knee, right forearm at the elbow, left forearm at the elbow, and right hand at the wrist.

Sum It Up!

A joint, or articulation, is the place where two or more bones meet. The three types of joints are immovable joints, slightly movable joints, and freely movable joints.

Freely movable joints are synovial joints. Types of freely movable joints include hinge, ball-and-socket, pivot, gliding, saddle, and condyloid joints. Because of the diverse types of joints, the skeleton is capable of a variety of movements.

As You Age

1. Because of loss of calcium and organic material, bones are less strong and more brittle. Many older women develop osteoporosis. As a result, bones fracture more easily. Moreover, fractured bones heal incompletely and more slowly.
2. As sex hormones in the blood decrease, there is a decrease in new bone growth and in bone mass, thus increasing the susceptibility to osteoporosis.
3. Tendons and ligaments are less flexible. As a result, joints have a decreased range of motion. A thinning of the articular cartilage and bony overgrowths in the joints contributes to joint stiffness.
4. The intervertebral discs shrink. Because of the compressed discs and the loss of bone mass, body height decreases and the thoracic spine curves (causing kyphosis).

Note: The Medical Terminology and Disorders table appears in Chapter 9.

Get Ready for Exams!

Summary Outline

The skeletal system supports the weight of the body, supports and protects body organs, enables the body to move, acts as a storage site for minerals, and produces blood cells.

I. **Bones: An Overview**
   A. Sizes, shapes, and markings
      1. Bones are classified as long, short, flat, and irregular.
      2. Bone markings: projections and depressions; function as sites of muscle attachments and passages for nerves and blood vessels
      3. Composed of compact (dense) bone and spongy (cancellous) bone
   B. Parts of a long bone
      1. Diaphysis (shaft)
      2. Epiphyses (ends), covered by articular cartilage
      3. Other components: medullary cavity, periosteum, bone marrow, epiphyseal disc, endosteum, and articular cartilage
   C. Ossification
      1. Intramembranous
      2. Endochondral
   D. Bone growth
      1. Bones grow longitudinally at the epiphyseal disc to determine height.
      2. Bones grow thicker and wider to support the weight of the body.

II. **Divisions of the Skeletal System**—The names of the 206 bones of the skeleton are listed in Table 8.2.
   A. Axial skeleton
      1. The axial skeleton includes the bones of the skull (cranium and face), hyoid bone, bones of the middle ear, bones of the vertebral column, and thoracic cage.
      2. The skull of a newborn contains fontanels, which are membranous areas that allow brain growth.
      3. The skull contains air-filled cavities called *sinuses.*
      4. The vertebral column is formed from 24 vertebrae, one sacrum, and one coccyx. The vertebrae are separated by cartilaginous discs. The vertebral column of the adult has four curvatures: cervical, thoracic, lumbar, and sacral.
      5. The thoracic cage is a bony cone-shaped cage formed by the sternum, 12 pairs of ribs, and thoracic vertebrae.
   B. Appendicular skeleton
      1. The appendicular skeleton includes the bones of the extremities (arms and legs) and the bones of the hip and pectoral (shoulder) girdles.
      2. The pectoral (shoulder) girdle consists of the scapula and the clavicle.
      3. The pelvic girdle is formed by the two coxal bones and is secured to the axial skeleton at the sacrum.

III. Joints—A joint or articulation is the site where two bones meet.
   A. Types of joints (based on the degree of movement)
   1. Immovable joints
   2. Slightly movable joints
   3. Freely movable joints or synovial joints—structures within a synovial joint (knee) are the articular cartilage, joint capsule, synovial membrane, synovial fluid, bursae, and supporting ligaments.
   4. The types of freely movable joints include hinge, ball-and-socket, pivot, gliding, saddle, and condyloid joints.
   B. Joint movement
   1. Flexion, extension, and hyperextension
   2. Abduction and adduction
   3. Inversion and eversion
   4. Supination and pronation
   5. Circumduction
   6. Plantar flexion and dorsiflexion

Review Your Knowledge

Matching: Long Bone
Directions: Match the following words with their descriptions.

a. epiphysis
b. spongy bone
c. epiphyseal disc
d. diaphysis
e. medullary cavity
f. haversian system
g. osteoblast
h. osteoclast
i. red bone marrow
j. periosteum

1. ___ Shaft of a long bone
2. ___ Site of longitudinal bone growth
3. ___ Bone-building cell
4. ___ Site of blood cell production
5. ___ Tough outer covering of the bone
6. ___ Enlarged end of a long bone
7. ___ Cancellous bone
8. ___ Osteon
9. ___ Bone-eroding cell that helps in bone remodeling
10. ___ Hollow center of a long bone

Matching: Names of Bones
Directions: Match the following words with their descriptions.

a. femur
b. scapula
c. mandible
d. ulna
e. sternum
f. coxal bone
g. tibia
h. calcaneus
i. frontal
j. phalanges

1. ___ Manubrium, body, xiphoid process
2. ___ Acetabulum formed by parts of this bone
3. ___ Contains the glenoid cavity that holds the head of the humerus
4. ___ Contains the "pointy" olecranon process
5. ___ The thick inner bone of the leg
6. ___ Heel bone
7. ___ Fingers and toes
8. ___ The head of this bone that articulates with the acetabulum
9. ___ Lower jaw bone
10. ___ Forms the forehead

Matching: Joints and Joint Movement
Directions: Match the following words with their descriptions. Some words may be used more than once.

a. ball-and-socket
b. adduction
c. flexion
d. pronation
e. dorsiflexion
f. circumduction
g. extension
h. plantar flexion
i. abduction
j. supination

1. ___ Type of joint movement at the elbow (angle decreases)
2. ___ Turning the forearm so that the palm of the hand "looks" at the sky
3. ___ Movement away from the midline of the body
4. ___ Toe dancing
5. ___ Movement of the ulna toward the humerus
6. ___ Type of joint at the shoulder and hip
7. ___ Shoulder movement, as in pitching a softball
8. ___ Movement toward the midline of the body
9. ___ Turning the forearm so that the hand "looks" at the floor
10. ___ Straightening the bended knee

Multiple Choice

1. Which of the following bones form the upper extremity?
   a. Femur, tibia, fibula
   b. Carpals, tarsals, phalanges
   c. Humerus, ulna, radius
   d. Manubrium, body, xiphoid process

2. Osteoclastic activity
   a. is responsible for longitudinal bone growth.
   b. lowers blood calcium levels.
   c. stimulates bone breakdown.
   d. regulates the production of blood cells.

3. The medial and lateral malleoli are closest to the
   a. hip.
   b. ankle.
   c. hallux.
   d. tibiofemoral joint.

4. Which of the following is most descriptive of the radiocarpal, humeroulnar, metacarpophalangeal, and distal radioulnar joints?
   a. Classified as sutures
   b. Permit hinge movement only
   c. Permit ball-and-socket movement
   d. Located in the upper extremities

5. Which of the following is *not* true of the acetabulum?
   a. Formed by the ilium, ischium, and pubis
   b. Receives the head of the femur
   c. Articulates with the greater trochanter
   d. Forms a ball-and-socket joint

6. Which of the following is a correct combination?
   a. Occipital bone; pectoral girdle
   b. Foramen magnum; suture
   c. Maxilla; cranium
   d. Mandible; facial bone

7. The atlas and axis
   a. are pelvic bones.
   b. are processes located on the posterior scapula.
   c. form the glenoid cavity.
   d. are vertebrae that allow the head to move.

8. To determine the approximate length of the humerus, you would measure from the
   a. olecranon process to the styloid process of the radius.
   b. acromion to the olecranon process.
   c. suprasternal notch to the xiphoid process.
   d. greater trochanter to the medial malleolus.

9. Depression of the red bone marrow
   a. causes a life-threatening decline in blood cells.
   b. stunts longitudinal bone growth.
   c. causes arthritis.
   d. causes loss of bone mineralization and osteoporosis.

10. Identify the movement at the elbow that decreases the angle at the humeroulnar joint.
    a. Extension
    b. Adduction
    c. Pronation
    d. Flexion

11. Which of the following is *not* true of the skull?
    a. The joint between the frontal and parietal bones is called the *coronal suture.*
    b. The lambdoidal suture is an immovable joint.
    c. Cranial bones include the zygomatic, frontal, occipital, and temporal bones.
    d. Facial bones include the maxilla, mandible, and zygomatic bones.

12. Which of the following is true of the foramen magnum?
    a. It is a large hole through which the brain exits the cranium.
    b. It is located within the frontal bone.
    c. It is part of C1, the atlas.
    d. It is a suture between the frontal and parietal bones.

13. The manubriosternal joint identifies the location of the
    a. foramen magnum.
    b. glenohumeral joint.
    c. second rib.
    d. vertebra prominens.

14. C1 to C7, T1 to T12, and L1 to L5 are
    a. responsible for the lumbar curve.
    b. vertebrae.
    c. cranial sutures.
    d. part of the appendicular skeleton.

15. The epiphyseal disc is
    a. located in the medullary cavity.
    b. composed of cartilage and is involved in the growth of long bones.
    c. composed exclusively of osteoclasts.
    d. the site of blood cell formation.

Go Figure

1. Which of the following is correct according to Figs. 8.1 and 8.2?
   a. The appendicular skeleton is composed of only long bones.
   b. The axial skeleton is composed of only flat bones.
   c. The cranial bones, facial bones, bony thorax, and vertebral column are parts of the axial skeleton.
   d. Flat bones are confined to the appendicular skeleton.

2. Which of the following is correct according to Fig. 8.3?
   a. The osteon is called the *haversian system.*
   b. The osteon has a punched-out, Swiss cheese appearance.
   c. Only spongy bone contains osteocytes.
   d. Neither compact nor spongy bone has a blood supply.

3. Which of the following is correct according to Fig. 8.3?
   a. The periosteum is a tough outer layer of the diaphysis.
   b. Yellow bone marrow occupies the spaces found within spongy bone.
   c. The articular cartilage lines the medullary cavity.
   d. Red bone marrow fills the medullary cavity in the adult long bones.

4. Which of the following is correct according to Fig. 8.7?
   a. The temporomandibular joint is a suture.
   b. The coronal suture is the immovable joint between the parietal and occipital bones.
   c. The squamous and the lambdoidal sutures are immovable joints involving the maxilla and mandible.
   d. The temporomandibular joint is the articulation between a facial bone and a cranial bone.

5. Which of the following is correct according to Fig. 8.7?
   a. The external auditory meatus, styloid process, mastoid process, and zygomatic process are parts of the zygomatic bone.
   b. The zygomatic process of the temporal bone articulates with the cheekbone.
   c. The chin is a maxillary structure.
   d. The occipital bone forms the forehead.

6. Which of the following is correct according to Fig. 8.7?
   a. The sphenoid bone is a butterfly-shaped bone that forms the base of the cranium.
   b. The foramen magnum is a large hole in the occipital bone.
   c. The palatine bones and part of the maxilla form the roof of the mouth.
   d. All of the above are true.

7. Which of the following is correct according to Fig. 8.9?
   a. The posterior fontanel is the largest of the fontanels.
   b. The infant skull has only two fontanels, the anterior and posterior fontanels.
   c. Fontanels are patches of spongy bone in the infant skull.
   d. The sutures in the infant skull are unfused.

8. Which of the following is correct according to Fig. 8.10 and Fig. 8.12?
   a. The adult vertebral column is perfectly straight, with no curvatures.
   b. Kyphosis refers to a lateral curvature of the spine.
   c. Both the cervical and lumbar curvatures are concave.
   d. Scoliosis is the official name for the humpback curvature.

9. Which of the following is correct according to Fig. 8.11?
   a. The most prominent part of the atlas and the axis is the body of the vertebrae.
   b. The spinal cord descends through the vertebral foramen.
   c. All vertebrae have a structure called the "dens."
   d. All vertebrae structurally resemble the atlas and axis.

10. Which of the following is correct according to Fig. 8.13?
   a. The manubrium, body, and clavicle are the parts of the sternum.
   b. The second rib is at the level of the sternomanubrial joint.
   c. The floating ribs are classified as true ribs.
   d. The clavicle articulates with the body of the sternum.

11. Which of the following is correct according to Fig. 8.13?
   a. The floating ribs articulate with the xiphoid process.
   b. The midclavicular line runs parallel to the midsternal line.
   c. The costal margin is part of the sternum.
   d. The costal angle is formed by the cartilaginous attachment of the true ribs to the sternum.

12. Which of the following is correct according to Fig. 8.14?
   a. The radial tuberosity slides into the olecranon fossa when the forearm is extended at the elbow.
   b. The carpals, metacarpals, and phalanges form the hand.
   c. The olecranon process is a depression on the distal humerus.
   d. The glenoid cavity is a socket located on the proximal humerus.

13. Which of the following is correct according to Fig. 8.14?
   a. The radius and ulna are parallel when the forearm is supinated.
   b. The acromion and coracoid processes are projections on the clavicle.
   c. Pronation and supination are dependent upon the ball-and-socket motion at the glenoid cavity.
   d. The metacarpals and phalanges are "twisted" when the forearm supinates.

14. Which of the following is correct according to Fig. 8.15?
   a. The femur articulates at the acetabulum.
   b. The acetabulum is formed by the pubis, ischium, and ilium.
   c. The coxal bone is formed by the ilium, pubis, and ischium.
   d. All of the above are true.

15. Which of the following is correct according to Fig. 8.16?
   a. The medial malleolus and lateral malleoli are located on the distal tibia.
   b. The femur articulates distally with the fibula to form the knee.
   c. The patella articulates with both the fibula and tibia.
   d. The femur articulates with the acetabulum of the coxal bone.

16. Which of the following is correct according to Fig. 8.16?
   a. The medial and lateral condyles of the femur are closer to the hip than to the knee.
   b. The medial and lateral malleoli are closer to the knee than to the ankle.
   c. The lesser and greater trochanters are closer to the hip than to the knee.
   d. The tibial tuberosity is closer to the ankle than to the knee.

17. Which of the following is correct according to Fig. 8.17?
   a. The calcaneus is the heel bone.
   b. The calcaneus, talus, and lateral malleolus are tarsal bones.
   c. The phalanges form the arch of the foot.
   d. The lateral and medial malleoli articulate with all the metatarsal bones.

18. Which of the following is correct according to Fig. 8.19 and Table 8.3?
   a. The radiocarpal joint is an immovable joint.
   b. The humeroulnar joint at the elbow is both a freely movable and ball-and-socket joint.
   c. The tibiofemoral joint is both a freely movable and hinge joint.
   d. The temporomandibular joint is an immovable joint.

19. Which of the following is correct according to Fig. 8.19 and Table 8.3?
   a. The proximal tibiofibular joint is closer to the ankle than is the distal tibiofibular joint.
   b. The humeroulnar joint is a slightly movable joint.
   c. The metacarpophalangeal joints are in the hand.
   d. The sternomanubrial joint is a hinge joint.

20. Which of the following is correct according to Fig. 8.19 and Fig. 8.21?
   a. Flexion of the forearm occurs at the humeroulnar joint.
   b. Plantar flexion occurs at the tibiofemoral joint.
   c. Circumduction of the arm is achieved by the humeroulnar joint.
   d. Extension of the forearm occurs at the radiocarpal joint.

21. Which of the following is correct according to Fig. 8.19 and Fig. 8.21?
   a. Flexion of the leg at the knee is a hinge movement.
   b. Flexion of the leg at the knee occurs at the tibiofemoral joint.
   c. Abduction and adduction of the thigh are hip movements.
   d. All of the above are true.

Muscular System

Objectives

1. Identify three types of muscle tissue.
2. Compare the structure of the whole muscle and the structure of a single muscle fiber.
3. Describe the sliding filament mechanism of muscle contraction.
4. Explain the role of calcium and adenosine triphosphate (ATP) in muscle contraction.
5. Describe the relationship between skeletal muscles and nerves, including the motor unit and its relationship to recruitment and the events that occur at the neuromuscular junction.
6. Discuss single-fiber and whole-muscle responses, including the following:
   - Define *twitch* and *tetanus.*
   - Identify the sources of energy for muscle contraction.
   - Trace the sequence of events from nerve stimulation to muscle contraction.
7. Define muscle terms, and state the basis for naming muscles.
8. Identify and list the actions of the major muscles.

Key Terms

acetylcholine (ACh) (p. 148)
actin (p. 146)
antagonist (p. 153)
aponeurosis (p. 146)
cardiac muscle (p. 144)
contraction (p. 144)
cross-bridges (p. 146)
fascia (p. 145)
insertion (p. 153)
motor unit (p. 148)
muscle fiber (cell) (p. 145)

myosin (p. 146)
neuromuscular junction (NMJ) (p. 148)
origin (p. 153)
prime mover (p. 153)
recruitment (p. 148)
relaxation (p. 146)
sarcomere (p. 146)
sarcoplasmic reticulum (SR) (p. 146)
skeletal muscle (p. 143)
sliding filament mechanism (p. 146)

smooth muscle (p. 143)
striated muscle (p. 143)
synergist (p. 153)
tendon (p. 146)
tetanus (p. 149)
thick filament (p. 146)
thin filament (p. 146)
tonus (p. 151)
troponin–tropomyosin complex (p. 147)
twitch (p. 151)

The word *muscle* comes from the Latin word *mus,* meaning "little mouse." As muscles contract, the muscle movements under the skin resemble the movement of mice scurrying around—thus the name *mus,* or *muscle.* Muscle tissue makes up 40% to 50% of body weight.

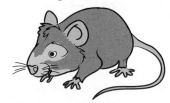

TYPES AND FUNCTIONS OF MUSCLES

The three types of muscles are skeletal, smooth, and cardiac (Fig. 9.1). Smooth muscle is discussed throughout the book, and cardiac muscle is discussed in Chapters 16 and 17. In this chapter, the focus is on skeletal muscle.

SKELETAL MUSCLE

Skeletal muscle is generally attached to bone. Because skeletal muscle can be controlled by choice (I choose to move my arm), it is also called *voluntary muscle.* The skeletal muscle cells are long, shaped like cylinders or tubes, and composed of proteins arranged to make the muscle appear striped, or **striated** (STRYE-ay-ted). Skeletal muscles produce movement, maintain body posture, and stabilize joints. They also produce considerable heat and therefore help maintain body temperature. If damaged, skeletal muscle has a limited capacity for regeneration.

SMOOTH MUSCLE

Smooth muscle is generally found in the walls of the viscera, such as the stomach, and is called *visceral*

Cellular appearance:

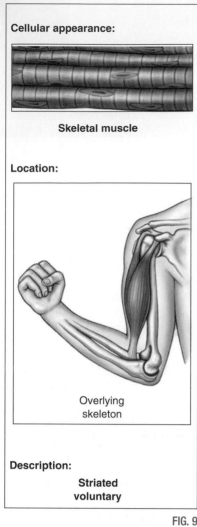

Skeletal muscle

Smooth muscle

Cardiac muscle

Intercalated discs

Location:

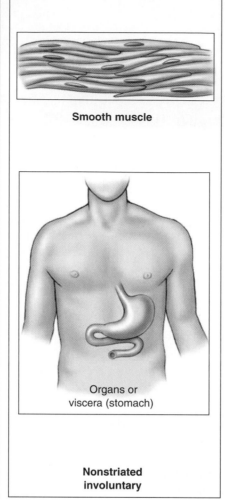

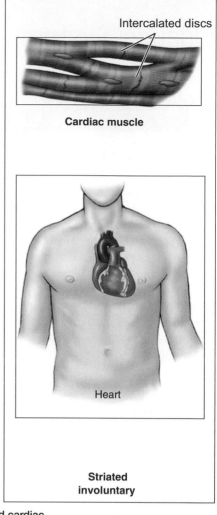

Overlying
skeleton

Organs or
viscera (stomach)

Heart

Description:

**Striated
voluntary**

**Nonstriated
involuntary**

**Striated
involuntary**

FIG. 9.1 Three types of muscle: skeletal, smooth, and cardiac.

muscle. It is also found in tubes and passageways such as the bronchioles (breathing passages) and blood vessels. Because smooth muscle functions automatically, it is called *involuntary muscle.* Unlike skeletal muscles, smooth muscle does not appear striped, or striated, and is therefore called *nonstriated muscle.*

Smooth muscle **contraction** has two unique characteristics in comparison with skeletal muscle contraction. First, smooth muscle contraction is slower and continues for a longer period. This characteristic allows for a continuous partial contraction of the smooth muscle, called *smooth muscle tone.* Smooth muscle tone plays an important role physiologically. For example, the muscle tone of the smooth muscle in blood vessels helps maintain blood pressure. If the muscle tone were to decrease, the person might experience a life-threatening decline in blood pressure. In addition to its contractile ability, smooth muscle has a greater degree of stretchiness as compared with skeletal muscle. This allows the walls of organs such as the uterus, urinary bladder, and stomach to expand

to store their contents temporarily. Contraction of the smooth muscle of the organ then expels its content. For example, the urinary bladder expands to store urine. When the bladder fills, the smooth muscle of the urinary bladder contracts, thereby expelling the urine. Similarly, contraction of the smooth muscles of the stomach mixes solid food into a paste and then pushes it forward into the intestine. If injured, smooth muscle has a better capacity for regeneration than does skeletal muscle.

CARDIAC MUSCLE

Cardiac muscle is found only in the heart, where it functions to pump blood throughout the body. Cardiac muscle cells are long branching cells that fit together tightly at junctions called *intercalated discs.* These tight-fitting junctions promote rapid conduction of electrical signals throughout the heart. Cardiac muscle is classified as striated and involuntary muscle. If damaged, as in a heart attack, cardiac muscle has no capacity for regeneration.

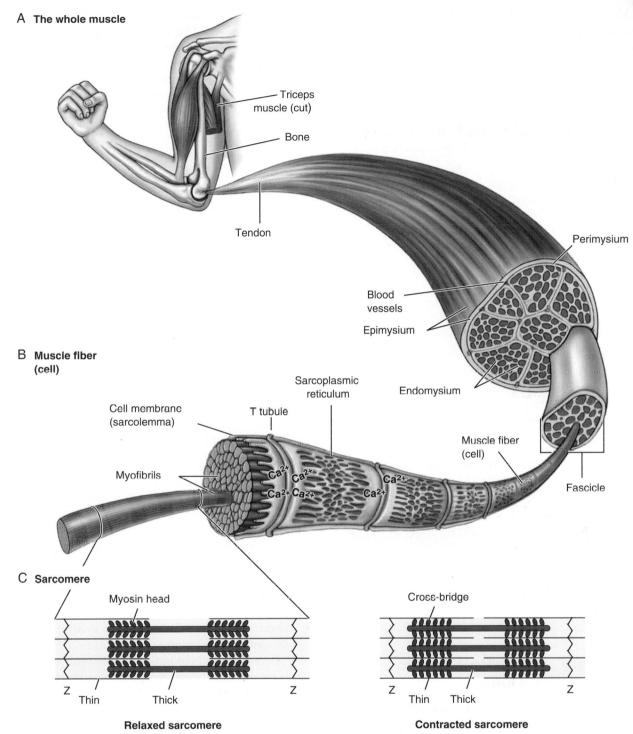

FIG. 9.2 Muscle structure. (A) Structure of a whole muscle attached to the bone by a tendon. (B) Structure of a muscle fiber (muscle cell). (C) Sarcomeres, relaxed and contracted.

STRUCTURE OF THE WHOLE MUSCLE

MUSCLE

If you touch your anterior thigh, you will feel a large muscle. What you are actually feeling are thousands of elongated **muscle fibers (cells)**, blood vessels, nerves, that are packaged together by various layers of connective tissue.

LAYERS OF CONNECTIVE TISSUE

A large skeletal muscle is surrounded by layers of tough connective tissue called **fascia** (FASH-uh) (Fig. 9.2A). This outer layer of fascia is called the *epimysium*. Another layer of connective tissue, called the *perimysium,* surrounds smaller bundles of muscle fibers. The bundles of muscle fibers are called *fascicles* (FAS-i-kuls). Individual muscle fibers are found within the fascicles and are surrounded by a third layer of connective tissue called the *endomysium*. The epimysium, perimysium, and endomysium extend toward and attach to the bone as a **tendon**, a long cordlike structure. In the limbs, the extensive amount of fascia separates the muscles into isolated sections or compartments.

 Do You Know...

What Muscle Compartments Have to Do with Crush Injuries?

In the limbs, the extensive amount of fascia separates the muscles into isolated compartments. Each muscle compartment also receives blood vessels and nerves necessary for muscle function. With a severe crush injury, the muscle is damaged; it becomes inflamed and leaks fluid into the compartment. Pressure within the compartment increases and compresses the nerves and blood vessels. Deprived of its oxygen and nourishment, the muscle and nerves begin to die—a condition called *compartment* or *crush syndrome*. Immediate treatment involves reduction of the compartment pressure by surgically slicing the fascia lengthwise. Failure to restore blood flow to the muscle results in permanent muscle and nerve damage.

MUSCLE ATTACHMENTS

Muscles form attachments to other structures in three ways: (1) the tendon attaches the muscle to the bone, (2) muscles attach directly (without a tendon) to a bone or to soft tissue, and (3) a flat sheetlike fascia called **aponeurosis** (ap-oh-nyoo-ROH-sis) connects muscle to muscle or muscle to bone.

 Re-Think

1. List the three types of muscles.
2. With regard to muscle types, what is meant by striated/ nonstriated and voluntary/involuntary?
3. How does the connective tissue of muscle relate to the development of compartment syndrome?

STRUCTURE AND FUNCTION OF A SINGLE MUSCLE FIBER

The muscle cell is an elongated muscle fiber (see Fig. 9.2B). The muscle fiber has more than one nucleus and is surrounded by a cell membrane called a *sarcolemma*. At several points, the cell membrane penetrates deep into the interior of the muscle fiber, forming transverse tubules (T tubules). Within the muscle fiber is a specialized endoplasmic reticulum called the **sarcoplasmic reticulum (SR)**.

Each muscle fiber is composed of long cylindrical structures called *myofibrils* (my-oh-FYE-brils). Each myofibril is made up of a series of contractile units called **sarcomeres** (SAR-koh-meers) (see Fig. 9.2C). Each sarcomere extends from Z line to Z line and is formed by a unique arrangement of contractile proteins, referred to as **thin** and **thick filaments**. The thin

filaments extend toward the center of the sarcomere from the Z lines. The thin filament is composed of two proteins called **actin** and the *troponin–tropomyosin* (troh-POH-nin–troh-poh-MY-oh-sin) *complex*. The actin contains binding sites for the **myosin**. The thicker myosin filaments sit between the thin filaments. Extending from the thick myosin filaments are structures called *myosin heads*. The arrangement of the thin and thick filaments in each sarcomere gives skeletal and cardiac muscle their striated appearances. Be sure you understand sarcomere structure; otherwise, you will not understand how the sliding filaments cause muscle contraction. Read on.

 Do You Know...

Why Beef Is Red and Chicken Meat Is White?

Certain muscle fibers contain a reddish-brown protein called *myoglobin*. The myoglobin stores oxygen in the muscle and gradually releases it when the muscle starts to work. Fibers that contain myoglobin are red because of the iron pigment. This is the red meat of a steak. Fibers that do not contain myoglobin are white, as in the meat of chicken.

HOW MUSCLES CONTRACT

SLIDING FILAMENT MECHANISM

The **sliding filament mechanism** describes how muscle contracts. Muscles can only pull, not push! To pull, muscles contract. When muscles contract, they shorten. Muscles shorten because the sarcomere length shortens, and the sarcomere length shortens because the thin and thick filaments slide past each other. Note how much shorter the contracted sarcomere appears compared with the relaxed sarcomere (see Fig. 9.2C). The following statements explain how the sarcomere shortens.

- When the contractile apparatus is stimulated, the sarcomere is flooded with calcium. This enables the myosin heads to make contact with special sites on the actin, forming temporary connections called **cross-bridges**.
- Once the cross-bridges are formed, the myosin heads rotate, pulling the actin toward the center of the sarcomere. The rotation of the myosin heads causes the thin filaments to slide past the thick filaments. (Sarcomere length shortens.)
- Muscle **relaxation** occurs when the cross-bridges are broken, and the thin and thick filaments return to their original positions. (The sarcomere lengthens.)

Because of this sliding activity of the thin and thick filaments, muscle contraction is called the sliding filament mechanism of muscle contraction. *Repeat:* Sarcomere length shortens not because the thin and thick filaments shrink or shrivel up, but because they slide past one another. The sliding is like a trombone. The trombone shortens because the parts slide past one another, not because the metal shrinks. The thin and thick filaments do the same thing—they slide.

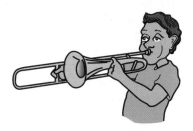

THE ROLE OF CALCIUM AND ADENOSINE TRIPHOSPHATE

Calcium and adenosine triphosphate (ATP) play important roles in the contraction and relaxation of muscle. Calcium is necessary for the formation of the actin-myosin connections called *cross-bridges*. Calcium is stored in the sarcoplasmic reticulum (SR), away from the thin and thick filaments. When the muscle membrane is stimulated, calcium is released from the SR and floods the sarcomere. The calcium exposes a site on the actin that is necessary for the binding of the myosin heads, the formation of cross-bridges, and sarcomere shortening (muscle contraction). When calcium is pumped back into the SR, the cross-bridges are broken, and the muscle relaxes. The energy released by ATP is necessary for cross-bridges to both form and disengage. (See the Ramp It Up!: The Troponin–Tropomyosin Complex and Calcium box for further details of calcium and the thin filament.)

 Ramp It Up!

The Troponin–Tropomyosin Complex and Calcium

Muscle contraction occurs when the myosin heads bind to actin, thereby causing the thin and thick filaments to slide past one another. The sliding occurs only in the presence of calcium. What role does calcium play in muscle contraction and relaxation?

Panel A illustrates the components of the thin filament in the relaxed state. The thin filament is composed of two proteins: actin and the **troponin–tropomyosin complex.** (The cup-shaped troponin sits on the tropomyosin.) The actin protein contains sites to which myosin heads bind. In the relaxed state the myosin-binding sites on actin are blocked by the troponin–tropomyosin complex. Thus, cross-bridge formation and muscle contraction cannot occur.

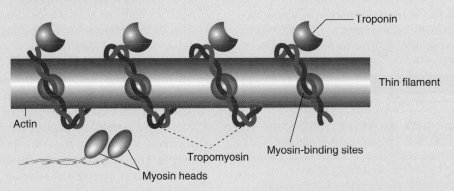

Panel A: Thin Filament

Panel B illustrates the effects of calcium. When the calcium is released from the sarcoplasmic reticulum, it floods the troponin sites. The activation of the troponin with calcium causes the tropomyosin to move, thereby exposing the myosin-binding sites on actin. The myosin heads can now bind to the actin, forming cross-bridges. The swiveling of the cross-bridges causes the sliding movements of the thin and thick filaments and muscle contraction. What causes the muscle to relax? Calcium is pumped back into the SR away from the troponin. The troponin–tropomyosin complex then moves back to its original position (panel A) where it blocks the myosin-binding sites on actin. Thus, the removal of calcium causes muscle relaxation.

An interesting clinical point! When muscle tissue (skeletal and cardiac) is injured, the contents of the muscle cell leak into the blood. Thus, following a heart attack, enzymes such as creatine phosphokinase and troponin elevate in the blood and act as biological markers in the diagnosis of a heart attack.

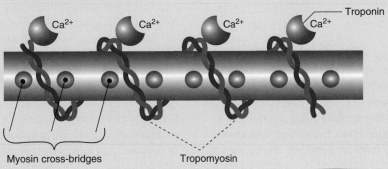

Panel B: Effect of Calcium

Re-Think

1. Why is calcium necessary for muscle contraction? (Use the words *actin*, *myosin*, *cross-bridges*, and *sliding filaments*.)
2. What is the relationship of calcium to muscle relaxation?

Sum It Up!

The three types of muscle are skeletal, smooth, and cardiac. A whole muscle is composed of many muscle fibers (muscle cells) arranged in bundles. Each muscle fiber contains actin-containing thin filaments and myosin-containing thick filaments, arranged into a series of sarcomeres. In accordance with the sliding filament mechanism, the sliding interaction of the actin and the myosin heads causes shortening of sarcomere length and muscle contraction.

SKELETAL MUSCLES AND NERVES

SOMATIC MOTOR NEURON

Skeletal muscle contraction can take place only when the muscle is first stimulated by a nerve. The type of nerve that supplies the skeletal muscle is a somatic motor nerve (Fig. 9.3A). A motor nerve, composed of many nerve cells called *motor neurons,* emerges from the spinal cord and travels to the skeletal muscle. The interaction of the motor neuron and the muscle is described in terms of the motor unit and neuromuscular junction.

Do You Know...

What the "Stiffness of Death" Is?

Both the formation of cross-bridges (muscle contraction) and the detachment of cross-bridges (muscle relaxation) depend on ATP. When a person dies, calcium leaks out of the SR, causing the muscles to contract. In addition, the production of ATP ceases. The deficiency of ATP prevents the detachment of the cross-bridges, so muscles remain contracted and become stiff. This change is called *rigor mortis,* or "stiffness of death." An assessment of rigor mortis often helps determine the exact time of death. For example, rigor begins 2 hours after death, peaks in 12 hours, and subsides in 36 hours. By assessing the degree of rigor, one can therefore determine the time of death. This fact has been used successfully in murder mysteries. By altering the environmental temperature, the murderer can alter the time course of rigor mortis and therefore make it difficult to determine the time of death.

THE MOTOR UNIT

As a motor neuron approaches the skeletal muscle, it forms many branches. Each branch innervates a single muscle fiber. The **motor unit** (see Fig. 9.3A) consists of a single motor neuron and the muscle fibers that are supplied by the motor neuron. Each muscle is innervated by many motor neurons, thereby forming many motor

units. The strength of muscle contraction can vary, depending on the number of motor units that are stimulated. A stronger force of muscle contraction develops if many motor units are stimulated at the same time; a weaker force of muscle contraction develops when fewer motor units are stimulated. For example, the muscles in the arm contract when they lift a pencil; they contract more forcefully when lifting a 100-lb weight. The consequence of activation of additional motor units is called **recruitment**.

THE NEUROMUSCULAR JUNCTION

The area where the motor neuron meets the muscle is called the **neuromuscular junction (NMJ)**. The NMJ includes the membrane at the end of the neuron, the space between the neuron and the muscle, and the receptors on the muscle membrane. What happens at the NMJ? The stimulated neuron causes the release of a chemical substance that diffuses across the NMJ and stimulates the muscle membrane. Four steps are involved in the transfer of the information from neuron to muscle at the NMJ (see Fig. 9.3B).

- Step 1. Stimulation of the neuron causes an electrical signal, or nerve impulse, to move along the neuron toward the ending of the neuron. Stored within its ending are vesicles, or membranous pouches, filled with a chemical substance called a *neurotransmitter.* The neurotransmitter at the NMJ is **acetylcholine** (ass-ee-til-KOH-leen) **(ACh).**
- Step 2. The nerve impulse causes the vesicles to move toward and fuse with the membrane at the end of the neuron. ACh is released from the vesicles into the space between the neuron and the muscle membrane.
- Step 3. ACh diffuses across the space and binds to the receptor sites on the muscle membrane.
- Step 4. The ACh stimulates the receptors and causes an electrical signal to develop along the muscle membrane. The ACh then unbinds the receptor site and is immediately destroyed by an enzyme that is found within the NMJ, near the muscle membrane. The name of the enzyme is acetylcholinesterase (ass-ee-til-koh-lin-ES-ter-ase) or cholinesterase. The free binding sites are then ready for additional ACh when the neuron is stimulated again.

THE STIMULATED MUSCLE MEMBRANE

What happens to the electrical signal that forms in the muscle membrane? It travels along the muscle membrane and triggers a series of events that result in muscle contraction (see Figs. 9.2B and C). Specifically, the electrical signal travels along the muscle cell membrane and penetrates into its interior through the T tubules. The electrical signal stimulates the SR to release calcium. The calcium floods the sarcomeres, thereby causing the thin and thick filaments to slide past one another, producing muscle contraction. Eventually, the calcium is pumped back into the SR, causing muscle relaxation.

📈 Ramp It Up!

Nicotinic Receptors (N$_M$) at the Neuromuscular Junction

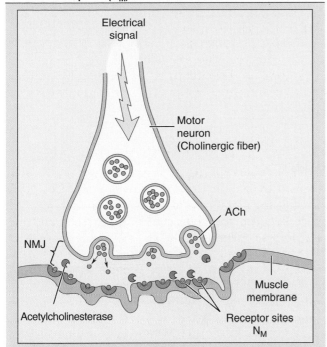

Follow the sequence of events within the neuromuscular junction (NMJ) as they are described. A nerve impulse travels along a somatic motor neuron causing the release of acetylcholine (ACh). The ACh diffuses across the NMJ and binds to the muscle membrane receptors. The receptor on the muscle membrane is a cholinergic receptor; it is called a *nicotinic receptor*. Because it is located on the muscle membrane, it is called a *nicotinic muscle (N$_M$) receptor*. Activation of the N$_M$ receptor causes a series of events that result in muscle contraction. A great deal of pharmacology involves the N$_M$ receptor. For example, curare is a skeletal muscle blocker because it blocks the N$_M$ receptors. Receptor blockade, in turn, prevents skeletal muscle contraction. What about a drug that activates the N$_M$ receptor? It stimulates muscle contraction. For example, neostigmine (Prostigmin) is a drug that inactivates acetylcholinesterase (the enzyme that destroys ACh), thereby increasing the amount of ACh that can bind to the N$_M$ receptors. (Because this drug inactivates acetylcholinesterase, it is called an *anticholinesterase agent*.) You can now understand why anticholinesterase agents improve the symptoms of myasthenia gravis and reverse postoperative sluggish intestinal activity. (Other nicotinic receptors are described in Chapter 12.)

DISORDERS OF THE NEUROMUSCULAR JUNCTION

Certain conditions affect events at the NMJ (Fig. 9.4).

Myasthenia Gravis

Myasthenia gravis is a disease that affects the NMJ. The symptoms of the disease are caused by damaged receptor sites (N$_M$ receptors) on the muscle membrane. The receptor sites are altered so that they cannot effectively bind ACh. Consequently, muscle contraction is impaired, and the person experiences extreme muscle weakness. (The word *myasthenia* means muscle weakness.) The muscle weakness first becomes noticeable as low tolerance to exercise. As the disease progresses, the person experiences difficulty in breathing because the breathing muscles are skeletal muscles.

Neuromuscular Blockade Caused by Curare

Curare is a drug classified as a skeletal muscle blocker. Skeletal muscle blockers are often used during surgery to promote muscle relaxation and paralysis. Curare works by blocking the receptor sites on the muscle membrane. Because the receptors are occupied by the drug, the ACh cannot bind with the receptor sites, and muscle contraction is prevented.

Because the respiratory muscles are also affected by curare, the patient must be mechanically ventilated until the effects of the drug disappear. Otherwise, the patient stops breathing and dies. Historically, curare was used as a paralyzing drug when hunting animals. The tip of an arrowhead was dipped in curare. When the arrow pierced the skin of the animal, the curare was absorbed and eventually caused skeletal muscle blockade and paralysis. Succinylcholine (Anectine) also blocks N$_M$ receptors and is used to induce muscle paralysis for short-term critical care situations such as intubation.

Effects of Neurotoxins on Muscle Function

Neurotoxins are chemical substances that in some way disrupt the normal function of the nervous system. Neurotoxins are produced by certain bacteria. For example, *Clostridium tetani* (a bacterium) secretes a neurotoxin that causes excessive firing of the motor nerves. This, in turn, causes excessive release of ACh, overstimulation of the muscle membrane, and severe muscle spasm and tetanic contractions—hence the name **tetanus**. Because the muscles of the jaw are the first muscles affected, the disease is often called *lockjaw*.

A second neurotoxin is secreted by the bacterium *Clostridium botulinum*. This bacterium appears most often when food has been improperly processed and canned. Infection with this organism causes botulism, a very serious form of food poisoning. The neurotoxin works by preventing the release of ACh from the ends of the neurons within the NMJ. Without ACh, the muscle fibers cannot contract, and the muscles, including the breathing muscles, become paralyzed. On a more positive note, the injection of small amounts of this "poison" (Botox) has been used successfully to treat severe muscle spasm (torticollis, cerebral palsy) and migraine headaches, as well as, for cosmetic reasons, to erase muscle-induced wrinkles.

Note that muscle paralysis can occur if there is an excess or a deficiency of ACh activity. An excess of ACh causes spastic paralysis, a state of continuous muscle contraction. A deficiency of ACh activity causes flaccid paralysis, a state in which the muscles are limp and unable to contract.

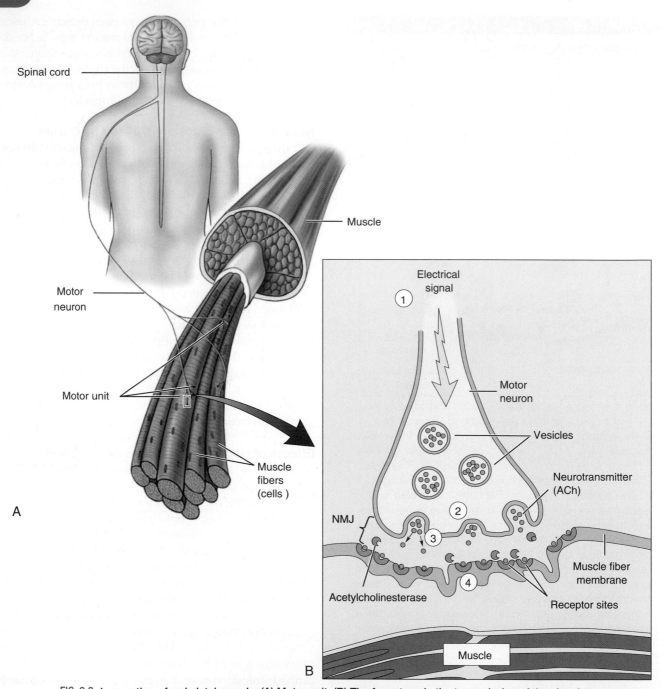

Spinal cord

Muscle

Motor neuron

Motor unit

Muscle fibers (cells)

A

Electrical signal
1

Motor neuron

Vesicles

Neurotransmitter (ACh)

NMJ

2

3

Acetylcholinesterase

4

Muscle fiber membrane

Receptor sites

 Muscle

B

FIG. 9.3 Innervation of a skeletal muscle. **(A)** Motor unit. **(B)** The four steps in the transmission of the signal at the neuromuscular junction (NMJ).

? **Re-Think**

1. Explain how the signal is passed from the nerve to the muscle at the NMJ.
2. Explain the effects of curare at the NMJ.

Sum It Up!

Fig. 9.5 summarizes the steps from the stimulation of the somatic motor, the events at the NMJ, the stimulation of the muscle membrane, and the contractile events within the sarcomeres.

Do You Know...

What the Difference Is Between Isometric Contraction and Isotonic Contraction?

An isotonic muscle contraction is a muscle contraction that causes movement, as in lifting a 20-lb object. An isometric muscle contraction is a muscle contraction that does not cause movement. For example, if you try to lift a 1000-lb object, your muscles contract but do not move the object (it is too heavy).

As you sit reading this text, you can do isometric exercises. Tighten the muscle in your thigh. Hold the tension for 30 seconds and then relax the muscle. Repetition of this type of exercise can provide you with a mini-workout without leaving your desk.

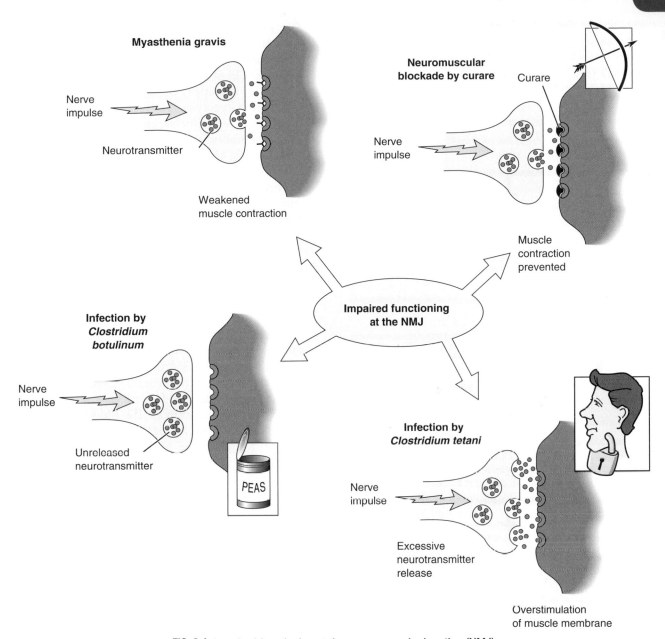

FIG. 9.4 Impaired functioning at the neuromuscular junction (NMJ).

MUSCLE RESPONSES

Muscle responses include those that characterize a single muscle fiber and responses of whole muscles (many muscle fibers bundled together):

Twitch and Tetanus. If a single electrical stimulus is delivered to a muscle fiber, the fiber contracts and then fully relaxes. This single muscle response is called a **twitch**. Twitches are not useful physiologically. However, if the muscle fiber is stimulated rapidly and repetitively, the muscle fiber has no time to relax and therefore remains contracted. Sustained muscle contraction is called *tetanus*. Tetanic muscle contraction of many muscle fibers helps maintain posture. If the muscles that maintain our upright posture merely twitched, we would be unable to stand and would instead twitch and flop around on the ground (not a pretty sight). (Do not confuse the "tetanus" described in this section with the disease called *tetanus*, or *lockjaw*.)

Recruitment. As described previously, recruitment of additional motor units increases the contractile force of a muscle. Recruitment is characteristic of the whole muscle, not a single muscle fiber.

Muscle tone. Muscle tone, or **tonus**, refers to a normal, continuous state of partial muscle contraction. Tone is caused by the contraction of different groups of muscle fibers within a whole muscle. To maintain muscle tone, one group of muscle fibers contracts first. As these fibers begin to relax, a second group contracts. This pattern of contraction and relaxation continues to maintain muscle tone. Muscle tone plays a number of important roles. For example, the tone of the skeletal muscles in the back of the neck prevents the head from falling forward.

The electrical signal (nerve impulse) travels down the nerve to the terminal and causes the release of the neurotransmitter ACh.

↓

The ACh diffuses across the neuromuscular junction and binds to the receptor sites.

↓

Stimulation of the receptor sites causes an electrical impulse to form in the muscle membrane. The electrical impulse travels along the muscle membrane and penetrates deep into the muscle through the T-tubular system.

↓

The electrical impulse stimulates the sarcoplasmic reticulum to release calcium into the sarcomere area.

↓

The calcium allows the actin, myosin, and ATP to interact, causing cross-bridge formation and muscle contraction. This process continues as long as calcium is available to the actin and myosin.

↓

Muscle relaxation occurs when calcium is pumped back into the sarcoplasmic reticulum, away from the actin and myosin. When calcium moves in this way, the actin and myosin cannot interact, and the muscle relaxes.

FIG. 9.5 Steps in the electrical stimulation of skeletal muscle and its contractile response.

 Re-Think

1. What is the difference between a twitch and tetanus?
2. Why can a whole muscle develop a greater force of contraction than a single muscle fiber?
3. What causes muscle tone?

ENERGY SOURCE FOR MUSCLE CONTRACTION

Muscle contraction requires a rich supply of energy (ATP). As ATP is consumed by the contracting muscle, it is replaced in three ways:

1. *Metabolism of creatine phosphate.* The resting muscle produces excess ATP and uses some of it to make creatine (KREE-ah-tin) phosphate. Creatine phosphate is a storage form of energy that can be used to replenish ATP quickly during muscle contraction.

For example, a brief 15-second burst of intense muscle activity is sustained by ATP and creatine phosphate. When creatine phosphate supplies are depleted (15 seconds), the muscle switches to glycolysis for its supply of ATP.

2. *Glycolysis.* Glycolysis is a series of chemical reactions that break down glucose anaerobically (without oxygen), generating ATP. The glucose is obtained from two sources: blood glucose and the glycogen that is stored in skeletal muscle. Glycolysis provides enough energy (ATP) for an additional 30 to 40 seconds of intense muscle activity. In addition to ATP production, glycolysis also produces lactic acid. Some of the lactic acid is picked up by the blood and transported to the liver, where it is used to make glucose.

3. *Aerobic (oxygen-requiring) metabolism.* After 30 to 40 seconds, the supply of ATP from glycolysis is depleted, and continued muscle activity relies on ATP production by aerobic respiration. In the presence of oxygen, pyruvic acid (formed from glycolysis) enters the mitochondria and is broken down completely to CO_2, H_2O, and ATP. Aerobic metabolism generates large amounts of ATP compared with glycolysis. The mitochondria receive their supply of oxygen from two sources: the blood (oxyhemoglobin) and myoglobin. Myoglobin is an oxygen-carrying protein found in the muscle fibers. Note the time sequence—creatine phosphate and ATP, glycolysis, and finally aerobic metabolism.

Why are your muscles sore after a heavy workout? Following a heavy workout, muscles can develop an immediate and latent soreness. Why is this? Muscles generate ATP aerobically and anaerobically through glycolysis. Lactic acid is the end-product of glycolysis, and its brief accumulation in the muscle tissue is thought to be the cause of the immediate soreness (30 to 60 minutes). The lactic acid is rapidly removed from the muscle and metabolized. The latent soreness (1 to 3 days after the workout) is attributed not to lactic acid but to tears of the connective tissue in the muscles and muscle cell membranes.

 Do You Know...

What the Good News Is About Oxygen Debt?

What's so great about oxygen debt? The payment of an oxygen debt means that you continue to expend energy long after you have come off the treadmill and have taken to your couch. In other words, you continue to exercise metabolically while recovering from your workout. When a person exercises strenuously, he or she uses up much of the oxygen available to skeletal muscles and relies more on anaerobic metabolism. Anaerobic metabolism generates lactic acid, which is normally converted to glucose in the liver. The hepatic conversion of lactic acid to glucose, however, requires oxygen. During strenuous exercise, the oxygen is used to make ATP for skeletal activity; hepatic conversion of glucose from lactic acid is delayed, creating an oxygen debt. When the person stops exercising, the skeletal muscles decrease his or her demand for oxygen. However, oxygen is required to do the exercise-induced metabolic work of converting lactic acid to glucose. So, 30 minutes of exercise is actually more than 30 minutes of exercise.

MUSCLE FATIGUE

Muscle fatigue occurs if the muscle is not allowed to rest and is defined as the inability of a muscle to contract forcefully following prolonged activity. The cause of muscle fatigue is unknown but is thought to be due to a number of factors, such as a diminishment of ATP, local changes in the electrolytes, and the accumulation of lactic acid. Occasionally muscle fatigue is accompanied by cramping, a painful condition due to sustained muscle contraction.

 Re-Think

1. What is creatine phosphate?
2. What are the three ways that muscle obtains its energy for muscle contraction?
3. Why does strenuous exercise cause an oxygen debt?

MUSCLE TERMS

ORIGIN AND INSERTION

The terms *origin* and *insertion* refer to the sites of muscle attachment. Most muscles cross or span at least one joint. When muscle contracts, one bone remains relatively stationary or immovable. The **origin** of the muscle attaches to the stationary bone, whereas the **insertion** attaches to the more movable bone (Fig. 9.6). For example, the origin of the biceps brachii is the scapula, and the insertion is on the radius. On contraction of the biceps brachii, the radius (insertion) is pulled toward the scapula (origin). Be sure that you understand *origin* and *insertion* because these terms will be used to describe muscle actions.

PRIME MOVER, SYNERGIST, AND ANTAGONIST

Although most movement is accomplished through the cooperation of groups of muscles, a single muscle is generally responsible for most of the movement. The "chief muscle" is called the **prime mover.** Assisting the prime mover are "helper muscles" called **synergists** (SIN-er-jists). Synergists are said to work with other muscles. In contrast, **antagonists** are muscles that oppose the action of another muscle. For example, contraction of the biceps brachii flexes the forearm at the elbow. The triceps brachii (posterior arm) is the antagonist. It opposes the action of the biceps brachii by extending the forearm (see Fig. 9.6).

MUSCLE OVERUSE AND UNDERUSE TERMS

HYPERTROPHY

Overused muscles increase in size. This response to overuse is called *hypertrophy*. Athletes intentionally

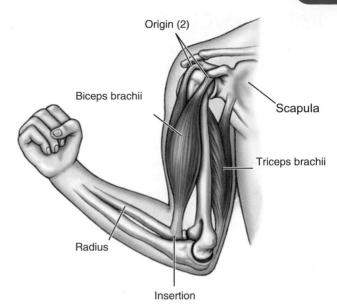

FIG. 9.6 **Origin and insertion: prime mover (biceps brachii) and antagonist (triceps brachii).**

cause their muscles to hypertrophy. Weight lifters, for example, develop larger muscles than couch potatoes.

Like skeletal muscle, cardiac muscle can also hypertrophy. Cardiac hypertrophy is undesirable and usually indicates an underlying disease, causing the heart to overwork. Hypertension, for example, causes the heart to push blood into blood vessels that are very resistant to the flow of blood. This extra work causes the heart muscle to enlarge.

ATROPHY

If muscles are not used, they will waste away, or decrease in size. A person with a broken leg in a cast, for example, is unable to exercise that leg for several months. This lack of exercise causes the muscles of the leg to atrophy, which is called *disuse atrophy*. When weight bearing and exercise are resumed, muscle size and strength can be restored. Muscle atrophy can also develop when the nerves to the muscle are severed, which is called *denervation atrophy*. Finally, muscle atrophy is part of the normal aging process; this is called *senile atrophy*. Senile atrophy can be delayed when the aging person carries out a regular exercise routine. Muscle motto: use it or lose it.

CONTRACTURE

If a muscle is immobilized for a prolonged period, it may develop a contracture, an abnormal formation of fibrous tissue within the muscle. It generally "freezes" the muscle in a flexed position and severely restricts joint mobility.

HOW SKELETAL MUSCLES ARE NAMED

The names of the various skeletal muscles are generally based on one or more of the following characteristics: size, shape, orientation of the fibers, location, number of origins, identification of origin and insertion, and muscle action.

SIZE

These terms indicate size: vastus (huge), maximus (large), longus (long), minimus (small), and brevis (short). Examples of skeletal muscles include the vastus lateralis and gluteus maximus.

SHAPE

Various shapes are included in muscle names, such as deltoid (triangular), latissimus (wide), trapezius (trapezoid), rhomboideus (rhomboid), and teres (round). Examples include the trapezius muscle, latissimus dorsi, and teres major.

ORIENTATION OF FIBERS

Fibers are oriented, or lined up, in several directions: rectus (straight), oblique (diagonal), transverse (across), and circularis (circular). Examples include the rectus abdominis and the superior oblique.

LOCATION

The names of muscles often reflect their location in the body, such as pectoralis (chest), gluteus (buttock), brachii (arm), supra (above), infra (below), sub (underneath), and lateralis (lateral). Examples include the biceps brachii, pectoralis major, and vastus lateralis.

NUMBER OF ORIGINS

A muscle may be named according to the number of sites to which it is anchored: biceps (2), triceps (3), and quadriceps (4). Examples include the biceps brachii, triceps brachii, and quadriceps femoris.

ORIGIN AND INSERTION

Some muscles are named for sites of attachment both at their origin and insertion. The sternocleidomastoid, for example, has its origin on the sternum and clavicle and its insertion on the mastoid process of the temporal bone. This information allows you to determine the function of the muscle. The sternocleidomastoid flexes the neck and rotates the head. As noted here, many muscles have multiple points of origin and insertion.

MUSCLE ACTION

The action of the muscle may be included in the name. For example, an abductor muscle moves the limb away from the midline of the body, whereas an adductor moves the limb toward the midline. In the same way, a flexor muscle causes flexion, whereas an extensor muscle straightens the limb. A levator muscle elevates a structure, and a masseter muscle enables you to chew. Examples include the adductor magnus, flexor digitorum, and levator palpebrae superioris.

 Re-Think

1. Differentiate between the origin and insertion of a muscle.
2. Differentiate between a muscle that acts synergistically and one that acts antagonistically.
3. What are the causes of muscle hypertrophy and muscle atrophy?
4. What is the basis for the naming of the following muscles: quadriceps femoris, rectus abdominis, sternocleidomastoid, and vastus lateralis?

◎ **Sum It Up!**

Contractile muscle responses are due to the characteristic of the single muscle fiber (twitch, tetanus) and whole muscle that consists of many muscle fibers (recruitment, tonus). A whole muscle contracts more forcefully than a single muscle fiber primarily because of recruitment. There are three energy sources for skeletal muscle contraction: aerobic metabolism, anaerobic metabolism, and metabolism involving creatine phosphate. Muscles are named according to their size, shape, orientation of fibers, location, number of origins, muscle action, and origin and insertion sites.

MUSCLES FROM HEAD TO TOE

Fig. 9.7 shows the major skeletal muscles of the body. Details of muscle location and function are summarized in Table 9.1.

MUSCLES OF THE HEAD

The muscles of the head are grouped into two categories: the facial muscles and the chewing muscles (Fig. 9.8).

FACIAL MUSCLES

Many of the facial muscles are inserted directly into the soft tissue of the skin and other muscles of the face. When the facial muscles contract, they pull on the soft tissue. This kind of muscular activity is responsible for our facial expressions like smiling and frowning.

- *Frontalis.* The frontalis (fron-TAL-is) is a flat muscle that covers the frontal bone. It extends from the

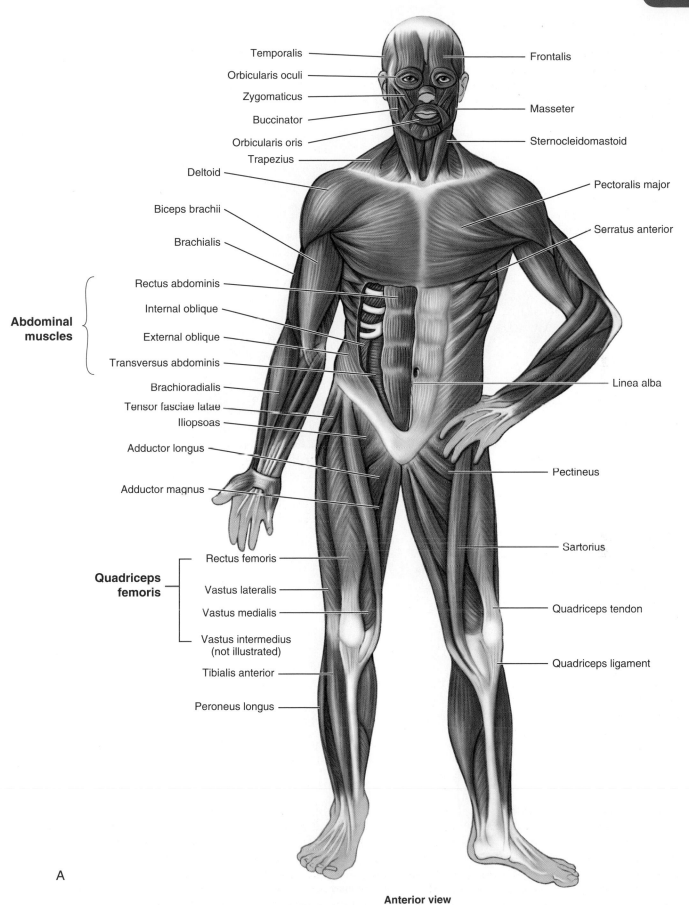

Temporalis

Orbicularis oculi

Zygomaticus

Buccinator

Orbicularis oris

Trapezius

Deltoid

Biceps brachii

Brachialis

Abdominal muscles
{
Rectus abdominis

Internal oblique

External oblique

Transversus abdominis
}

Brachioradialis

Tensor fasciae latae

Iliopsoas

Adductor longus

Adductor magnus

Quadriceps femoris
{
Rectus femoris

Vastus lateralis

Vastus medialis

Vastus intermedius (not illustrated)
}

Tibialis anterior

Peroneus longus

Frontalis

Masseter

Sternocleidomastoid

Pectoralis major

Serratus anterior

Linea alba

Pectineus

Sartorius

Quadriceps tendon

Quadriceps ligament

A

Anterior view

FIG. 9.7A Major muscles of the body. (A) Anterior view.

Continued

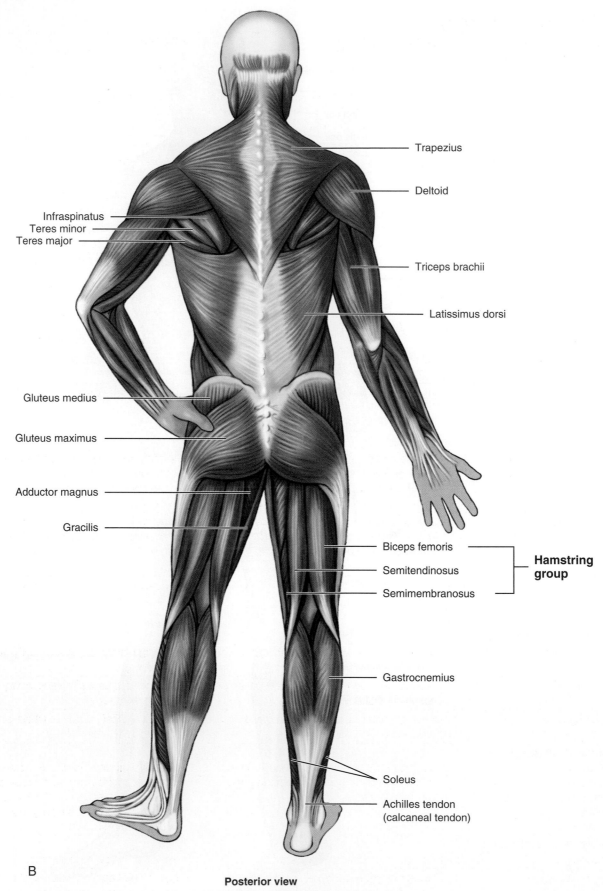

Trapezius

Deltoid

Infraspinatus
Teres minor
Teres major

Triceps brachii

Latissimus dorsi

Gluteus medius

Gluteus maximus

Adductor magnus

Gracilis

Biceps femoris
Semitendinosus
Semimembranosus

**Hamstring
group**

Gastrocnemius

Soleus

Achilles tendon
(calcaneal tendon)

B

Posterior view
FIG. 9.7B, cont'd **(B)** Posterior view.

Table 9.1   Muscles of the Body

MUSCLE	LOCATION, DESCRIPTION	FUNCTION
Head		
Muscles of Facial Expression		
Frontalis	Flat muscle covering forehead; origin on cranial aponeurosis; inserts on skin above eyebrows	Raises eyebrows; surprised look; wrinkles forehead
Orbicularis oculi	Circular muscle around eye	Closes eyes; winking, blinking, and squinting
Levator palpebrae superioris	Origin on bony orbit of eye; inserts on upper eyelid	Elevates eyelid (opens eye)
Orbicularis oris	Encircles mouth	Closes, purses lips; kissing muscle
Buccinator	Horizontal cheek muscle; origin on maxilla and mandible; inserts on orbicularis oris	Flattens cheek; trumpeter's muscle; whistling muscle; helps with chewing by positioning food between teeth
Zygomaticus	Origin on cheekbone (zygomatic bone); inserts on corner of mouth	Elevates corner of mouth; smiling muscle
Platysma	Origin in fascia of shoulder and anterior chest; inserts on mandible, angle of lower mouth, soft tissue of lower face	Pouting muscle; "open your mouth wide" muscle
Chewing Muscles		
Temporalis	Flat fan-shaped muscle over temporal bone (origin); inserts on mandible	Closes jaw; retracts jaw
Masseter	Covers lateral part of lower jaw; origin on maxilla, zygomatic process of the temporal bone; inserts on mandible	Closes jaw; retracts jaw
Neck		
Sternocleidomastoid	Extends along each side of neck; strong, narrow muscles that extend obliquely from sternum and clavicle (origin) upward to mastoid process of temporal bone (insertion)	Contraction of both muscles flexes the head at the neck; contraction of one rotates head toward opposite side
Trapezius	Large, flat, trapezoid-shaped muscle on back of neck and upper back; origin on occipital bone, C7, and all thoracic vertebrae; inserts on clavicle and scapula	Hyperextends head so as to look at sky; lateral flexion of head (see actions on shoulder)
Scalenes (3)	Origin on cervical vertebrae (C1–C7); insert on ribs 1 and 2	Act synergistically with sternocleidomastoid to flex neck
Muscles of the Trunk		
Muscles Involved in Breathing		
External intercostals	Located between ribs (intercostal space); both origin and insertion on ribs	Breathing (enlarges thoracic cavity during inhalation)
Internal intercostals	Located between ribs (intercostal space); both origin and insertion on ribs	Breathing (decreases thoracic cavity in forced exhalation)
Diaphragm	Dome-shaped muscle that separates thoracic and abdominal cavities	Breathing—chief muscle of inhalation (enlarges thoracic cavity)
Muscles of Abdominal Wall		
External oblique Internal oblique Transverse abdominis Rectus abdominis	As a group, muscles are arranged vertically, horizontally, and obliquely to strengthen abdominal wall	As a group, abdominal wall muscles compress the abdomen, thereby aiding in urination, defecation, childbirth, and forced expiration (breathing); also flex and rotate vertebral column
Muscles of Vertebral Column		
Trapezius	See trapezius above (Neck)	Helps maintain spine in extension
Erector spinae	Extends length of vertebral column from cranium to sacrum	Extends and laterally flexes vertebral column; rotates head; assists in maintenance of erect posture
Sternocleidomastoid	See above (Neck)	Flexes and rotates cervical vertebral column

Continued

Table **9.1**   **Muscles of the Body—cont'd**

MUSCLE	LOCATION, DESCRIPTION	FUNCTION
Abdominal muscles	See above (Muscles of Abdominal Wall)	Flexes and rotates vertebral column
Iliopsoas	Origin on ilium and lumbar vertebrae; inserts on femur	Flexes vertebral column
Muscles of Pelvic Floor		
	Flat muscle sheets	Support pelvic viscera; aid in urination and defecation
Muscles of Shoulder (Pectoral) Girdle and Arm		
Trapezius	See description above (Neck)	Causes shrugging and medial rotation of shoulders (by pulling shoulder blades or scapulae together)
Serratus anterior	Forms upper sides of chest wall; origin on upper ribs; inserts on scapula	Lowers shoulder and moves the arm forward as in pushing a cart
Pectoralis major	Large muscle that covers upper anterior chest; origin on clavicle, sternum, and cartilages of upper ribs; inserts on anterior humerus	Adducts and medially rotates arm across chest; flexes and extends arm at shoulder
Latissimus dorsi	Large, broad, flat muscle on mid and lower back; origin on lower vertebral column and lower ribs; inserts on the humerus	Adducts and rotates arm medially, behind the back; "swimmer's muscle"
Deltoid	Thick muscle that covers shoulder joint; origin on clavicle and scapula; inserts on humerus	Abducts arm as in "scarecrow" position; flexes, extends, and rotates arm at shoulder

Rotator cuff muscles
  Supraspinatus
  Subscapularis
  Infraspinatus
  Teres minor
	Group of four muscles that attaches humerus (insertion) to scapula (origin); tendons form cuff over proximal humerus	Adduct, extend, and rotate arm at shoulder; the "cuff" stabilizes shoulder joint

Teres major	Origin on scapula; inserts on humerus	Extends and adducts arm at shoulder; medially rotates arm at shoulder
Muscles That Move Forearm		
Biceps brachii	Major muscle on anterior surface of arm; origin on scapula; inserts on radius	Flexes and supinates forearm at elbow and flexes arm at shoulder; muscle used to "make a muscle"; acts synergistically with brachialis and brachioradialis
Triceps brachii	Origin on posterior surface of arm (scapula and humerus); inserts on ulna	Extends forearm at elbow, extends arm at shoulder; "boxer's muscle"
Brachialis	Origin on humerus; inserts on ulna	Flexes forearm at elbow
Brachioradialis	Origin on humerus; inserts on radius	Flexes forearm at elbow
Supinator	Origin on humerus and ulna; inserts on radius	Supinates forearm (palm turns upward or faces forward, as in anatomical position)
Pronator teres	Origin on humerus and ulna; inserts on radius	Pronates forearm so that palm faces downward or backward
Muscles That Move Wrist, Hand, and Fingers		
Flexor and extensor carpi group	Origin on humerus and ulna; inserts on tendon in wrist	Flex and extend hand at wrist; adduct and abduct hand at wrist
Flexor and extensor digitorum group	Origin on humerus, ulna, and radius; inserts on phalanges (fingers)	Flex and extend fingers; flex hand at wrist
Muscles That Move Thigh and Leg		
Gluteus maximus	Largest and most superficial of gluteal muscles; located on posterior surface of buttocks; origin on ilium of coxal bone, sacrum, coccyx, and local aponeurosis; inserts on femur	Forms buttocks; extends and rotates thigh laterally at hip; muscle for sitting and climbing stairs; produces backswing of leg while walking
Gluteus medius	Thick muscle partly behind and superior to gluteus maximus; origin on ilium; inserts on femur	Abducts and rotates thigh medially at hip; common site of intramuscular injections

MUSCLE	LOCATION, DESCRIPTION	FUNCTION
Gluteus minimus	Smallest and deepest of gluteal muscles; origin on ilium; inserts on femur	Abducts and rotates thigh medially at hip
Iliopsoas	Located on anterior surface of groin; origin on ilium and lumbar vertebrae; inserts on femur	Flexes and rotates thigh laterally; antagonist to gluteus maximus
Tensor fasciae latae	Located on lateral thigh; origin on ilium; inserts on tibia	Flexes and abducts thigh at hip
Adductor group Adductor longus Adductor brevis Adductor magnus	As a group, located on anteromedial surface of thigh	Adducts and medially rotates thigh; muscles used by horseback riders to stay on horse
Gracilis	Located along medial thigh; origin on symphysis pubis; inserts on proximal tibia	Adducts and medially rotates thigh at hip; flexes leg at knee
Pectineus	Located on medial thigh; origin on pubis; inserts on femur	Adducts and flexes thigh at hip
Quadriceps femoris Rectus femoris Vastus lateralis Vastus medialis Vastus intermedius	Located on anterior thigh; all insert on tibia; rectus femoris originates on ilium (coxal bone); other "quads" originate on femur	Group used to extend leg at the knee (e.g., kicking a football); rectus femoris can flex thigh at hip; vastus lateralis is common site for intramuscular injections in children
Sartorius	Long muscle that crosses obliquely over anterior thigh; origin on ilium; inserts on tibia	Allows you to sit in crossed-leg position; flexes, abducts, laterally rotates thigh at hip; flexes leg at knee
Hamstrings Biceps femoris Semitendinosus Semimembranosus	Located on posterior surface of thigh; as a group, attaches to ischium (origin) to their points of insertion on tibia. Biceps femoris also originates on femur and inserts on both tibia and fibula.	As a group, they flex leg at knee, extend thigh at hip; antagonistic to quadriceps femoris
Muscles That Move Ankle and Foot		
Tibialis anterior	Located on anterior leg; origin on tibia; inserts on tarsal and metatarsal bones	Dorsiflexes and inverts foot
Peroneus longus	Lateral surface of leg; origin on fibula and tibia; inserts on metatarsal and tarsal bones	Plantar flexion and eversion of foot; supports arch
Gastrocnemius	Posterior surface of leg; large two-headed muscle that forms calf; origin on femur; inserts on calcaneus (heel bone) by way of Achilles tendon	Plantar flexion of foot; toe dancer muscle; flexes leg at knee
Soleus	Posterior surface of leg; origin on fibula and tibia; inserts on calcaneus	Plantar flexion of foot

cranial aponeurosis (origin) and inserts in the skin above the eyebrows. Contraction of the muscle raises the eyebrows, giving you a surprised look. It also wrinkles your forehead.

• *Orbicularis oculi.* The orbicularis (or-bik-yoo-LAR-is) oculi is a sphincter muscle that encircles the eyes. A sphincter (SFINGK-ter) is a ring-shaped muscle that controls the size of an opening. Contraction of the muscle closes the eye and assists in winking, blinking, and squinting.

• *Levator palpebrae superioris.* The levator palpebrae (leh-VAH-tor PAL-peh-bray) superioris muscle has its origin in the bony orbit of the eye and inserts on the upper eyelid. As its name implies, the muscle elevates the eyelid (opens the eye).

• *Orbicularis oris.* The orbicularis oris is a sphincter muscle that encircles the mouth. Contraction of this muscle assists in closing the mouth, forming words, and pursing the lips. It is sometimes called the *kissing muscle.*

• *Buccinator.* The buccinator (BUK-si-NAY-tor) is a muscle that has its origin on the maxilla and mandible and inserts into the orbicularis oris. The buccinator is used in actions requiring compression of the cheeks, as in sucking, whistling, and playing the trumpet. The buccinator may also be considered a chewing muscle because, on contraction, it helps position the food between the teeth for chewing. The buccinator is particularly important for an infant because its contraction enables the infant

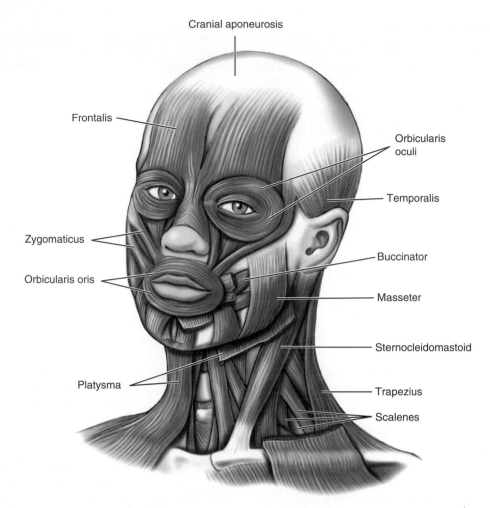

Cranial aponeurosis

Frontalis

Orbicularis oculi

Temporalis

Zygomaticus

Buccinator

Orbicularis oris

Masseter

Sternocleidomastoid

Platysma

Trapezius

Scalenes

FIG. 9.8 **Muscles of the head and neck.**

to suck; it therefore plays an important role in the nourishment and comfort of a hungry infant.

• *Zygomaticus.* The zygomaticus (zye-goh-MAT-ik-us) is a smiling muscle; it extends from the corners of the mouth to the cheekbone (zygomatic bone).

• *Platysma.* Want to pout? The platysma (plah-TIZ-mah) is your muscle. It originates in the fascia of the shoulder and anterior chest and inserts on the mandible and tissue of the mouth and lower face. In addition to pouting, it allows you to open your mouth wide, per order of your dentist. Here's another platysmal downer—with aging, there is a loss of muscle tone of the platysma, creating loose skin in the throat area and the dreaded "turkey neck" look.

CHEWING MUSCLES

The chewing muscles are also called the muscles of mastication (chewing). All of them are inserted on the mandible, or lower jaw bone, and are considered some of the strongest muscles of the body (see Table 9.1).

• *Masseter.* The masseter (MAS-eh-ter) is a muscle that has its origin on the maxilla and zygomatic process of the temporal bone and its insertion on the

mandible. It acts synergistically with the temporalis muscle to close the jaw.

• *Temporalis.* The temporalis (tem-poh-RAL-is) is a fan-shaped muscle that extends from the flat portion of the temporal bone (origin) to the mandible (insertion).

 Re-Think

1. Explain why the frontalis muscle can affect facial expression.
2. List two chewing muscles. Why may the buccinator muscles be considered chewing muscles?
3. To which facial bone must the chewing muscles insert?

 Do You Know...

About the "Droops and Drools" of Botox?

In the arsenal of anti-aging drugs, Botox is a star. It is the wrinkle-remover par excellence. Beware of Botox blunders, however. Misplaced Botox around the eyelids can cause droopy lids. Similarly, poor aim around the mouth region can cause drooling. Mercifully, the effects of Botox gradually wear off, although there may be many weeks during which you sport the droop-and-drool look. Botched batches of Botox have also caused severe, long-term paralysis.

MUSCLES OF THE NECK

Many muscles are involved in the movement of the head and shoulders and participate in throat movements.

STERNOCLEIDOMASTOID

As the name implies, the sternocleidomastoid (STERN-oh-KLYE-doh-MAS-toyd) muscle extends from the sternum and clavicle to the mastoid process of the temporal bone in the skull. Contraction of both muscles on either side of the neck causes flexion of the head. Because the head bows as if in prayer, the muscle is called the *praying muscle*. Contraction of only one of the sternocleidomastoid muscles causes the head to flex and to rotate toward the opposite direction. A spasm of this muscle can cause torticollis, or wryneck. This condition is characterized by twisting of the neck and rotation of the head to one side. Botox has been used successfully in the treatment of torticollis. Although the sternocleidomastoid muscle is the prime mover of neck flexion, three scalene (SKAY-leen) muscles act synergistically to flex the neck. The scalenes have their origin on the cervical vertebrae (C1–C7) and insert on ribs 1 and 2.

TRAPEZIUS

The trapezius (trah-PEE-zee-us) has its origins at the base of the occipital bone of the cranium and on the spines of C7 to T12 of the upper vertebral column (see Fig. 9.7B). The trapezius inserts on both the scapula and clavicle. Contraction of the trapezius allows the head to tilt back (hyperextension) so that the face looks at the sky. The trapezius works antagonistically with the sternocleidomastoid muscle, which flexes and bows the head. The trapezius also causes lateral flexion of the head and shrugs the shoulder.

MUSCLES OF THE TRUNK

The muscles of the trunk are involved in breathing, form the abdominal wall, move the vertebral column, and form the pelvic region.

MUSCLES INVOLVED IN BREATHING

The muscles of the chest include the intercostal muscles and the diaphragm. These muscles are primarily responsible for breathing (Fig. 9.9). The intercostal muscles are located between the ribs. They have their origin and insertion on the ribs and are responsible for raising and lowering the rib cage during breathing. The ribs that you barbecue are the intercostals (bone appétit!).

The diaphragm is a dome-shaped muscle that separates the thoracic cavity from the abdominal cavity. The diaphragm is the chief muscle of inhalation, or the breathing-in phase of respiration.

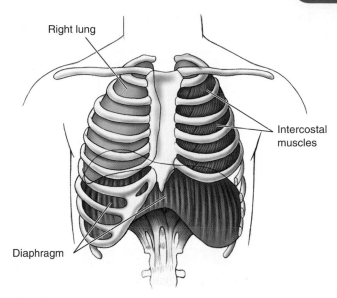

FIG. 9.9 Breathing muscles: the intercostal muscles and the diaphragm.

Without the contraction and relaxation of the intercostal muscles and diaphragm, breathing cannot occur. The breathing muscles are more fully described in Chapter 22.

MUSCLES THAT FORM THE ABDOMINAL WALL

The abdominal wall consists of four muscles (see Fig. 9.7A) in an arrangement that provides considerable strength. The muscles are layered so that the fibers of each of the four muscles run in four different directions. This arrangement enables the muscles to contain, support, and protect the abdominal organs. Contraction of the abdominal muscles performs other functions. It causes flexion and rotation of the vertebral column and compression of the abdominal organs during urination, defecation, and childbirth.

The four abdominal muscles are as follows:
* *Rectus abdominis.* As the name implies, the fibers of the rectus abdominis run in an up and down, or longitudinal, direction. They extend from the sternum to the pubic bone. Contraction of this muscle flexes the vertebral column.
* *External oblique.* Abdominal muscles called the *external oblique muscles* make up the lateral walls of the abdomen. The fibers run obliquely (slanted).
* *Internal oblique.* The internal oblique muscles are part of the lateral walls of the abdomen. They add to the strength provided by the external oblique muscles; the fibers of the internal and external oblique muscles form a crisscross pattern.
* *Transversus abdominis.* The transversus abdominis muscles form the innermost layer of the abdominal muscles. The fibers run horizontally across the abdomen.

To remember the abdominal muscles, think of that spare **TIRE:**

T	transversus abdominis
I	internal oblique
R	rectus abdominis
E	external oblique

The abdominal muscles are attached to fascia that forms a large aponeurosis along the midline of the abdominal wall. The aponeuroses of the abdominal muscles on opposite sides of the midline of the abdomen form a white line called the *linea alba*. The linea alba extends from the sternum to the pubic bone.

 Re-Think

1. Describe the movement of the head in response to contraction of the right sternocleidomastoid muscle.
2. List the muscles of respiration.
3. Explain why the arrangement of the abdominal muscles conveys added strength to the abdominal wall.

MUSCLES THAT MOVE THE VERTEBRAL COLUMN

A number of muscles attach to the vertebrae and assist in the movement of the vertebral column; the movements include flexion, extension, hyperextension, lateral flexion, and rotation of the vertebral column. Muscles that move the vertebral column include the erector spinae, sternocleidomastoid, trapezius, abdominal muscles, and iliopsoas. Deep to the trapezius and the latissimus dorsi is the erector spinae (eh-REK-tor SPIN-ay); it extends the length of the vertebral column, from the sacrum to the cranium. As the erector spinae muscle ascends, it forms three columns of muscles. The erector spinae muscle causes extension and lateral flexion of the vertebral column and rotation of the head. This muscle assists in the maintenance of an erect posture. With aging, this muscle loses contractile strength and accounts in part for the stooped posture of an older person. Hungry? The erector spinae are best known by laypersons as pork chops and T-bone steaks.

Contraction of both sternocleidomastoid muscles causes flexion of the head at the neck, whereas contraction of one muscle rotates the head in the opposite direction (causes rotation of the cervical vertebral column). The trapezius maintains the vertebral column in extension. The abdominal muscles cause flexion and rotation of the vertebral column, and the iliopsoas (see discussion later in the chapter) flexes the vertebral column at the hip.

MUSCLES THAT FORM THE PELVIC FLOOR

The pelvic floor consists primarily of two flat muscle sheets and the attached fascia. These structures support the pelvic viscera and play a role in expelling the contents of the urinary bladder and rectum.

 Do You Know...

What Is Wrong with Bulking Up?

Nothing is wrong with bulking up if it is done through weight lifting, exercise, and a healthy diet. Bulking up with the use of steroids, however, is dangerous. Steroids are thought to cause liver cancer, atrophy of the testicles in males, stunting of growth, and severe psychotic mood swings, among other health-related effects.

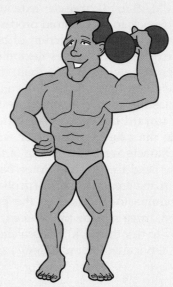

Then there is "'roid rage"—uncontrollable aggressive behavior. 'Roid rage has been implicated in many instances of serious sports-related injuries and has sent many a steroid abuser to prison for fighting, scrapping, brawling, and mauling—not a pretty picture.

MUSCLES OF THE SHOULDER (PECTORAL) GIRDLE AND ARM

Many muscles move the shoulder and the arm. The most important are the trapezius, serratus anterior, pectoralis major, latissimus dorsi, and deltoid and a group of muscles called the *rotator cuff muscles* (see Fig. 9.7A and B).

- *Trapezius.* The trapezius has its origin at the base of the occipital bone and the spines of all thoracic vertebrae; it inserts on the clavicle and scapula (shoulder blade). When contracted, the trapezius moves the clavicle and scapula and allows for a shrugging and rotating movement of the pectoral girdles. The trapezius causes medial rotation by pulling the shoulder blades (scapulae) together. The muscle gets its name because the right and left trapezius form the shape of a trapezoid.
- *Serratus anterior.* The serratus (sehr-AH-tis) anterior is located on the sides of the chest and extends from the upper ribs (origin) to the scapula (insertion). The serratus muscle has a jagged shape, much like the jagged edge of a serrated knife blade. When the serratus anterior contracts, the shoulders are lowered, and the arm moves forward as if pushing a cart. The trapezius and serratus anterior attach the scapula to the axial skeleton.

- *Pectoralis major.* The pectoralis (pek-toh-RAL-is) major is a large broad muscle that helps form the anterior chest wall. It connects the humerus (arm) with the clavicle (collarbone) and structures of the axial skeleton (ribs and sternum). Contraction of this muscle moves the arm across the front of the chest, as if pointing to an object in front of the body. (A more precise description of the function of the pectoralis major: It adducts and rotates the arm medially at the shoulder joint as well as flexes and extends the arm at the shoulder joint.) Many gym exercises are designed to hypertrophy the "pecs."

- *Latissimus dorsi.* The latissimus (LAT-iss-im-ahs) dorsi is a large broad muscle located in the middle and lower back region. Its origin is on the lower thoracic vertebrae, lumbar vertebrae, sacrum, and lower ribs; it inserts on the posterior humerus. Contraction of this muscle lowers the shoulders and brings the arm back, as if pointing to an object behind you. This same backward movement occurs in swimming and rowing. (A more precise description: The latissimus dorsi extends, adducts, and rotates the arm medially at the shoulder.) The pectoralis major and latissimus dorsi attach the humerus to the axial skeleton.

- *Deltoid.* The deltoid forms the rounded portion of the shoulder and forms the shoulder pad. The deltoid extends from its origins on the clavicle and scapula to its insertion on the humerus. Contraction of the deltoid muscle abducts the arm, raising it to a horizontal position (the scarecrow position). It also flexes, extends, and rotates the arm at the shoulder joint. Because of its size, location, and good blood supply, the deltoid is a common site of an intramuscular injection.

- *Teres major.* The teres (TER-eez) major is a long, round muscle that has its origin on the scapula and inserts on the humerus. It extends the arm at the shoulder joint and assists with the medial rotation and adduction of the arm at the shoulder joint.

- *Rotator cuff muscles.* The rotator cuff muscles are a group of four muscles that attach the humerus (insertion) to the scapula (origin). They include the subscapularis, supraspinatus, infraspinatus, and teres minor. The tendons of these muscles form a cap, or a cuff, over the proximal humerus, thus stabilizing the joint capsule. The muscles help rotate the arm at the shoulder joint. What about tennis buffs and their rotator cuffs? One of the most common causes of shoulder pain in athletes is known as *impingement syndrome*, or rotator cuff injury. It is caused by repetitive overhead motions and is commonly experienced by tennis players, swimmers, and baseball pitchers. The tendons are pinched and become inflamed, resulting in pain. If this continues, the inflamed tendon can degenerate and separate from the bone. The condition can be a career-ending sports injury.

- Note how many different movements are possible at the shoulder joint. The ball-and-socket joint and the many muscles that attach to the arm and pectoral girdle permit this freedom of movement.

> **? Re-Think**
>
> 1. Identify the origins and insertions of the following muscles: trapezius, pectoralis major, deltoid, and latissimus dorsi. Citing the origins and insertions of each, describe the movements caused by the contraction of the muscles.
> 2. Describe two exercises that would "work out" the "pecs."
> 3. Why is the latissimus dorsi called the swimmer's muscle?
> 4. Why is the deltoid a favorite site of intramuscular injections?
> 5. List the rotator cuff muscles. Explain why they are called rotator cuff muscles.

MUSCLES THAT MOVE THE FOREARM

Most of the muscles that move the forearm (ulna and radius) are located along the humerus and are classified as flexors, extensors, supinators, or pronators. The flexors, those that cause flexion at the elbow joint, include the biceps brachii, brachialis, and brachioradialis. Extension is due to contraction of the triceps brachii.

The triceps brachii (TRY-seps BRAYK-ee-eye) lies along the posterior surface of the humerus; it has its origins on the scapula and humerus and its insertion on the ulna. Contraction causes extension of the forearm at the elbow joint; it also extends the arm at the shoulder joint. The triceps brachii is the muscle that supports the weight of the body when a person does push-ups or walks with crutches. It is also the muscle that packs the greatest punch for a boxer, hence the nickname "the boxer's muscle" (see Fig. 9.7B).

The biceps brachii is located along the anterior surface of the humerus; its two heads attach to the scapula (origin), and the distal end inserts on the radius of the forearm. The biceps brachii acts synergistically with the brachialis and brachioradialis to flex the forearm. The biceps brachii and brachialis are the prime movers for flexion of the forearm. When someone is asked to "make a muscle," the biceps brachii becomes most visible.

Pronation (palm down) is achieved by two pronator muscles located along the anterior forearm (origin on the humerus and ulna, insertion on the radius). The actions of the biceps brachii and a supinator muscle (origin on the humerus and ulna, insertion on the radius) located along the posterior forearm cause supination (palm up).

MUSCLES THAT MOVE THE WRIST, HAND, AND FINGERS

More than 20 muscles move the wrist, hand, and fingers. The muscles are numerous and small, making the wrist, hand, and fingers capable of delicate movements. The muscles are generally located along the forearm and consist of flexors and extensors. The flexors are located on the anterior surface of the forearm, and the extensors are located on the posterior surface. The tendons of these muscles pass through the wrist into the hand and fingers. The flexor carpi radialis and the flexor carpi ulnaris flex the hand at the wrist joint; they also adduct and abduct the hand at the wrist. Contraction of the flexor digitorum muscle (in the forearm) pulls on the tendons of the phalanges, thereby moving the fingers (like puppet strings). Imagine how fat your fingers would be if they were filled with muscle rather than tendons—your ring size would double or triple!

The puppet string setup, with the muscles in the forearm and tendons in the wrists and fingers, is responsible for another clinical mishap. If the tendons in the wrist are accidentally severed, the muscles in the forearm pull the tendons up into the forearm. The tendons "disappear" from the injured site. If the surgeon merely patches up the wrist injury and fails to retrieve and reattach the tendons, finger movement is lost.

The extensors of the wrist, hand, and fingers lie along the posterior forearm. The extensor carpi radialis longus extends and abducts the hand at the wrist. The extensor carpi ulnaris extends and adducts the hand at the wrist. The extensor digitorum extends the hand at the wrist and extends the fingers.

The flexors of the fingers are stronger than the extensors so that in a relaxed hand, the fingers are slightly flexed. If a person is unconscious for an extended period, the fingers remain in a flexed position. In response to inactivity, the tendons of the fingers shorten, thereby preventing extension of the fingers, which gives a clawlike appearance to the hand. This problem can be prevented by an exercise program that includes passive exercises of the hands and fingers.

THE CARPAL TUNNEL

Most of the tendons of the muscles that supply the hand pass through a narrow tunnel created by transversely oriented carpal ligaments (flexor retinaculum) and the carpal (wrist) bones (Fig. 9.10). The flexor tendons in the carpal tunnel are encased in tendon sheaths and normally slide back and forth very easily. However, repetitive motion of the hand and fingers can cause the tissues within the carpal tunnel to become inflamed and swollen. The swelling puts pressure on the median nerve, which is also located in the carpal tunnel. The irritated nerve causes tingling, weakness, and pain in the hand and arm. The condition, carpal tunnel syndrome, is a major cause of disability in persons who must perform repetitive wrist motion (e.g., pianists, machinists, butchers, and keyboard operators).

Carpal Tunnel Syndrome

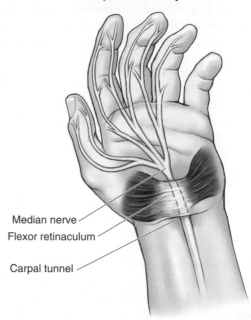

Median nerve
Flexor retinaculum
Carpal tunnel

FIG. 9.10 Carpal tunnel.

❓ Re-Think

1. Identify the origins and insertions of the following muscles: biceps brachii, brachialis, triceps brachii, and supinators. Citing the origins and insertions of each, describe the movements caused by the contraction of the muscles.
2. Identify the muscles responsible for flexion of the forearm at the elbow.
3. Which arm muscle supports body weight while walking with crutches?
4. What are the actions of supinator and pronator muscles?
5. What is the location of the muscles that move the fingers?

MUSCLES THAT MOVE THE THIGH, LEG, AND FOOT

The muscles that move the thigh, leg, and foot are some of the largest and strongest muscles in the body. These muscles not only move the lower extremities but also provide stability for the joints and help maintain posture.

MUSCLES THAT MOVE THE FEMUR (THIGH BONE)

The muscles that move the thigh at the hip all attach to some part of the pelvic girdle (coxal bones) and the femur (thigh bone). These include the gluteal muscles, the iliopsoas, the tensor fascia latae, and a group of adductor muscles. Contraction of these muscles causes movement at the hip joint (see Fig. 9.7).

The gluteal muscles are located on the posterior surface and include the gluteus maximus, gluteus medius, and gluteus minimus. The gluteus maximus is the largest muscle in the body; it forms the area of the buttocks and is the muscle on which you sit.

The gluteus maximus has its origins on the ilium (coxal bone) and sacrum and inserts on the femur. It rotates the thigh laterally and extends the thigh at the hip, as in climbing stairs or walking. It produces the backswing of the leg while walking. The gluteus medius and gluteus minimus have their origins on the ilium (coxal bone) and insert on the femur. They abduct and rotate the thigh medially at the hip joint. Both the gluteus maximus and gluteus medius are commonly used sites for intramuscular injections.

The iliopsoas (il-ee-OHP-so-us) is located near the groin; it has its origins on the lower vertebrae and ilium (coxal bone) and its insertion on the femur. Contraction of this muscle flexes and rotates the thigh laterally.

The tensor fasciae latae (TEN-sor FASH-ee-ah LAT-ah) is on the lateral thigh; it has its origin on the ilium (coxal bone) and inserts on the tibia. Contraction of this muscle flexes and abducts the thigh at the hip joint.

The adductor muscles are located on the medial surface of the thigh; they have their origin on the lower coxal bones and insert on the medial and posterior surfaces of the femurs. This group of muscles adduct the thighs, pressing them together. These are the muscles that a horse rider uses to stay on the horse. The adductor muscles include the adductor longus, adductor brevis, adductor magnus, gracilis (GRAH-sil-is), and pectineus (pek-TIN-ee-us). In addition to adduction, most of the adductor muscles rotate the thigh. (See Table 9.1.)

The quadriceps femoris, sartorius, and hamstring muscles (described later) also move the thigh. The quadriceps femoris flexes the thigh at the hip, whereas the hamstrings extend the thigh at the hip. The sartorius allows you to sit cross-legged on the floor.

Note the many types of movement that occur at the hip, a ball-and-socket joint.

MUSCLES THAT MOVE THE LEG

The muscles that move the leg are located in the thigh. The extensor muscles lie along the anterior and lateral surfaces of the leg, whereas the flexors lie along the posterior and medial surfaces. Muscles that move the legs include the quadriceps femoris, sartorius, hamstring group, and the gastrocnemius.

The quadriceps femoris is located on the anterior thigh, is the most powerful muscle in the body, and has four heads as its origin. All four parts of the muscle insert on the tibia by the quadriceps ligament. (The quadriceps tendon extends distally to the tibial tuberosity as the quadriceps ligament.) The "quads" straighten, or extend, the leg at the knee, as in kicking a football. The four heads of the muscle give rise to four parts of the quadriceps femoris muscle, each

of which has its own name: the vastus lateralis, vastus intermedius, vastus medialis, and rectus femoris. The vastus lateralis is frequently used as an injection site for children because it is more developed than the gluteal muscles.

The sartorius allows you to sit cross-legged on the floor. It assists in knee and hip flexion, abduction, and lateral rotation of the thigh. At one time tailors used to sit cross-legged as they worked. The Latin word for tailor is *sartor*, so this muscle was named the sartorius.

The hamstrings are a group of muscles located on the posterior surface of the thigh. All the muscles extend from the ischium (coxal bone) to the tibia. They flex the leg at the knee and are therefore antagonistic to the quadriceps femoris. Because these muscles also span the hip joint, they extend the thigh. The strong tendons of these muscles can be felt behind the knee. The tendons form the pit behind the knee called the *popliteal fossa*. These same tendons are found in hogs. In times past, butchers used these tendons to hang the hams for smoking and curing—hence the name *hamstrings*. The hamstring muscles include the biceps femoris, semimembranosus, and semitendinosus. An athlete often pulls a hamstring or experiences a groin injury.

Because the gastrocnemius has its origin on the distal femur, it also flexes the leg at the knee. This large calf muscle is described later.

Do You Know...
What a Wolf Knows About the Hamstrings?

Hungry wolves spot their prey—and the chase is on. The wolf will often attack the knee joint of its prey, severing the tendons of the hamstrings. Once the tendons are severed, the victim's legs are useless. Dinner is served!

MUSCLES THAT MOVE THE FOOT

The muscles that move the foot are located on the anterior, lateral, and posterior surfaces of the leg. See Fig. 8.21 for movements of the foot. The tibialis anterior is located on the anterior surface. It has its origin on the tibia (shin bone) and inserts on the tarsal and metatarsal bones. It causes dorsiflexion and inversion of the foot. There are a number of muscles that cause plantar flexion. The peroneus (per-oh-NEE-us) longus muscle is on the lateral surface. It everts (turns outward) the foot, supports the arch of the foot, and assists in plantar flexion. The gastrocnemius (GAS-trok-NEE-mee-us) and soleus are the major muscles on the posterior surface of the leg and form the calf of the leg. They attach to the calcaneus (heel bone) by the calcaneal tendon, or Achilles tendon. Contraction of these muscles causes plantar flexion. The tibialis posterior also assists in plantar flexion and inverts the foot.

Plantar flexion aids in walking and allows a person to stand on tiptoes. For this reason the gastrocnemius is sometimes called the *toe dancer's muscle*. Runners, especially sprinters, occasionally tear or rupture the Achilles tendon. Because the heel then cannot be lifted, this injury severely impedes the ability of the runner to perform.

Finally, there are the toes. Like the fingers, some of the toes are tugged on by tendons whose muscles (flexors and extensors) lie in the leg. Other muscles have their origin in the tarsal and metatarsal bones.

Some muscles have acquired rather interesting names. Fig. 9.11 shows the many interesting movements we are able to make.

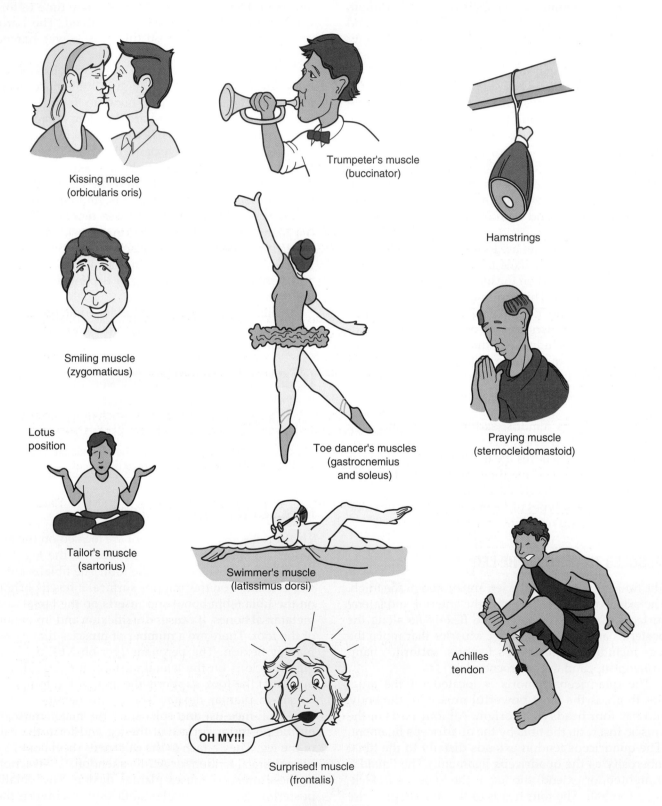

FIG. 9.11 A medley of special muscles.

Re-Think

Identify the origins and insertions of the following muscles: gluteus maximus, quadriceps femoris, biceps femoris, tibialis anterior, soleus, and gastrocnemius. Citing the origins and insertions of each, describe the movements caused by the contraction of these muscles.

 Sum It Up!

The skeleton is stabilized and covered with muscle. The ability of the muscles to contract and relax allows the skeleton to move about and engage in all the activities that make life so enjoyable. The location and function of the major muscles of the body are summarized in Table 9.1.

 As You Age

1. At about the age of 40, the number and diameter of muscle fibers decrease. Muscles become smaller, dehydrated, and weaker. Muscle fibers are gradually replaced by connective tissue, especially adipose or fat cells. By the age of 80, about 50% of the muscle mass has been lost.
2. Mitochondrial function in muscles decreases, especially in muscles that are not exercised regularly.
3. Motor neurons are gradually lost, resulting in muscle atrophy.
4. These changes lead to decreased muscle strength and slowing of muscle reflexes.

Medical Terminology and Disorders   Disorders of the Musculoskeletal System

MEDICAL TERM	WORD PARTS	WORD PART MEANING OR DERIVATION	DESCRIPTION
Words			
adduction/ abduction	ad-	to, toward, or near	Adduction of the thigh indicates that the thigh is moving toward the midline of the body, whereas abduction means it is moving away from the midline of the body.
	ab-	away from	
	-duction	From the Latin word *ducere*, meaning "to lead"	
myalgia	my/o-	muscle	**Myalgia** means *muscle pain,* a characteristic of many musculoskeletal disorders.
	-algia	pain	
myopathy	my/o-	muscle	A **myopathy** is *a muscle disease where the primary defect is within the muscle itself and not in the neuromuscular junction or brain.*
	-path/o-	disease	
	-y	process or condition	
osteocyte	oste/o-	bone	**Osteocytes** are *bone cells.* Osteoblasts (-blast = immature) mature into osteocytes *(bone cells),* while osteoclasts (-clast = breakdown) break down osseous (bone) tissue.
	-cyte	cell	
periosteum	peri-	around	The **periosteum** is *the membrane around a bone.*
	-osteon	bone	
synergist	syn-	together	Refers to *muscles that work together to generate a movement.* Several muscles may work synergistically to flex the forearm.
	-erg-	From a Greek word meaning "to work"	
	-ist	one that specializes in	
Disorders			
arthralgia	arthr/o-	joint	**Arthralgia,** also called noninflammatory joint pain, has multiple causes: injury, infection, many diseases, or a reaction to medications.
	-algia	pain	
arthritis	arthr/o	joint	**Arthritis** is *inflammation of a joint.* There are over 25 types of arthritis; two common types are **osteoarthritis** and **rheumatoid arthritis. Osteoarthritis** is called *degenerative or "wear-and-tear" arthritis,* most frequently seen in older persons. It affects primarily the weight-bearing joints, but may also affect the hands. Bony nodules may develop in the interphalangeal joints. **Rheumatoid arthritis** (RA)—*the most debilitating type of arthritis*—is an autoimmune disease characterized by inflammation of the joints and systemic symptoms such as fever, fatigue, and anemia. Joint disease progresses from *thickening of joint tissue,* called **pannus formation,** to cartilage destruction and finally to deformity and fusion of the joints.
	-itis	inflammation	

Continued

Medical Terminology and Disorders   Disorders of the Musculoskeletal System—cont'd

MEDICAL TERM	WORD PARTS	WORD PART MEANING OR DERIVATION	DESCRIPTION
bursitis	burs-	bursa	**Bursitis** is *the inflammation of one or more bursae, causing pain, swelling, and restriction of movement.* Common forms include subacromial bursitis (painful shoulder), olecranon bursitis (student's elbow, water on the elbow), and prepatellar bursitis (housemaid's knee, carpet layer's knee).
	-itis	inflammation	
fibromyalgia	fibr/o-	fiber	**Fibromyalgia** is *a syndrome characterized by pain in the muscles, tendons, and soft tissues.* Although the joints are not affected, the pain is experienced as originating in the joints. The musculoskeletal symptoms are accompanied by generalized feelings of fatigue, depression, headache, and anxiety.
	-my/o-	muscle	
	-algia	pain	
fracture		From a Latin word meaning "to break"	**Fracture** refers to *a broken bone.* Most fractures are due to traumatic injuries; a small number are a result of another disease and are called **pathological fractures.** There are numerous ways to classify fractures: open/closed; stable/unstable; spiral, comminuted; transverse; stress.
luxation	lux-	From a Latin word meaning "to dislocate"	**Luxation** refers to *the displacement of a bone from its joint, with tearing of ligaments, tendons, and articular capsule.* The shoulder joint is a commonly dislocated joint. *A partial dislocation* is called a **subluxation**.
	-ation	condition or state	
multiple myeloma	myel/o-	bone marrow	Also called plasma cell myeloma, **multiple myeloma** refers to *malignant tumors of the bone marrow in which there are collections of abnormal plasma cells.* **CRAB** is a mnemonic that indicates the characteristic tetrad (four parts) of multiple myeloma: calcium (hypercalcemia), renal failure, anemia, and bone lesions.
	-oma	tumor	
muscular dystrophy	dys-	painful, difficulty, or faulty	**Muscular dystrophy** (MD) is *a group of inherited muscle disorders that cause progressive muscle weakness and degeneration of muscle tissue.* Numerous disorders are included in this category, with Duchenne MD being the most common.
	-troph/o-	nourishment or development	
	-y	condition or process of	
neoplasms (bone)	neo-	new	Osteogenic sarcoma or osteosarcoma is a highly malignant and rapidly metastasizing neoplasm. Osteoclastoma (tumor originating from osteoclasts) or giant cell tumor is most often nonmalignant, but highly destructive; it occurs in the long bones of the lower extremities. Ewing's sarcoma is a common malignancy of bone and soft tissue. Its rapid growth occurs within the pelvis and the medullary cavities of long bones of the extremities. Pathological fractures develop in response to the cancer-inducing osteonecrosis.
	plas/o-	formation	
osteomalacia	oste/o-	bone	**Osteomalacia** refers to *softening of the bones.* The loss of calcium and phosphorus is caused by vitamin D deficiency. The bone softening results in skeletal deformities and fractures. Osteomalacia in the growing bones of children is called *rickets.*
	-malacia	softening	
osteomyelitis	oste/o-	bone	**Osteomyelitis** is *a serious infection of the bone, bone marrow, and surrounding tissue.* It can be caused by many pathogens, the most common being *Staphylococcus aureus.* Infection can occur by direct (open wound) or indirect (hematogenous) entry.
	-myel/o-	bone marrow	
	-itis	inflammation	
osteoporosis	oste/o-	bone	A loss of bone mass that makes the bones so porous that they crumble under the ordinary stress of moving about. Osteoporosis is related to the loss of estrogen in older women, a dietary deficiency of calcium and vitamin D, and low levels of exercise. Osteopenia (-penia = abnormal reduction) is indicative of early osteoporosis.
	-por/os-	From a Greek word meaning "pore" or "passage"	
	-osis	condition of	
Plantar fasciitis	fasci/o-	fascia	**Plantar fasciitis** is *inflammation of the plantar fascia on the bottom of the foot.* It is usually exercise-induced and painful.
	-itis	inflammation of	

Medical Terminology and Disorders   Disorders of the Musculoskeletal System—cont'd

MEDICAL TERM	WORD PARTS	WORD PART MEANING OR DERIVATION	DESCRIPTION
rhabdomy-olysis	rhabd/o-	rod-shaped or striated (skeletal)	**Rhabdomyolysis** *is the breakdown of muscle with the release of myo-globin into the blood.* It is a consequence of conditions in which muscle activity is excessive (seizures, drugs) or injurious (crush injuries).
	-my/o-	muscle	
	-lysis	breakdown	
strains and sprains			The two most common musculoskeletal injuries, usually as a result of twisting forces associated with physical activity. A **sprain** is *an injury or tearing of the ligaments of a joint.* A **strain** is *excess stretching of a muscle and its surrounding fascia.*
tendonitis	tend/o-	tendon	*Inflammation of a tendon causing pain and tenderness just outside the joint.* The joints most often affected are the elbows (tennis elbow, golfer's elbow), shoulders (pitcher's shoulder, swimmer's shoulder), wrists, and heels (Achilles tendonitis).
	-itis	inflammation	

Get Ready for Exams!

Summary Outline

The purpose of muscle is to contract and to cause movement.

I. **Muscle Function: Overview**
   A. Types and functions of muscles
      1. Skeletal muscle is striated and voluntary; its primary function is to produce movement.
      2. Smooth (visceral) muscle is nonstriated and involuntary; it helps the organs perform their functions.
      3. Cardiac muscle is striated and involuntary; it is found only in the heart and allows the heart to function as a pump.
   B. Structure of the whole muscle
      1. A large muscle consists of thousands of single muscle fibers (muscle cells).
      2. Connective tissue binds the muscle fibers (cells), blood vessels, and nerves together and attaches muscle to bone and other tissue by tendons and aponeuroses.
   C. Structure and function of a single muscle fiber
      1. The muscle fiber (cell) is surrounded by a cell membrane (sarcolemma). The cell membrane penetrates to the interior of the muscle as the transverse tubule (T tubule).
      2. An extensive sarcoplasmic reticulum (SR) stores calcium.
      3. Each muscle fiber consists of a series of sarcomeres. Each sarcomere contains thin filaments (actin and troponin–tropomyosin complex) and thick filaments (myosin).
   D. How muscles contract
      1. Electrical signals run along the muscle membrane.
      2. Electrical signal enters the T-tubular system and stimulates the SR to release calcium.

3. Muscles shorten or contract as the actin and myosin (in the presence of calcium and ATP) interact through cross-bridge formation, according to the sliding filament mechanism.
      4. Calcium is pumped back into the SR and the muscles relax.
   E. Skeletal muscles and nerves: for a skeletal muscle to contract, it must be stimulated by a motor nerve.
      1. Motor unit: formed by a motor neuron and the muscle fibers that it innervates (forms the basis of recruitment)
      2. Neuromuscular junction (NMJ): the nerve terminal (ending) containing neurotransmitter (ACh), the space between the nerve terminal and muscle membrane, and the muscle membrane with its receptors
   F. Muscle responses
      1. Twitch and tetanus, a characteristic of the single muscle fiber
      2. Recruitment engages many muscle fibers as additional motor units are stimulated. A whole muscle increases its force of contraction primarily by recruitment.
   G. Energy for muscle contraction can be obtained from three sources: burning fuel aerobically, burning fuel anaerobically, and metabolizing creatine phosphate.
   H. Terms that describe muscle movement
      1. Origin and insertion: the attachments of the muscles
      2. Prime mover: the muscle most responsible for the movement achieved by the muscle group
      3. Synergist or antagonist: works with or has an opposing action

II. **Muscles from Head to Toe**
   A. Skeletal muscles are named according to size, shape, orientation of fibers, location, number of origins, place of origin and insertion, and muscle action.
   B. See Table 9.1 for a list of the body's muscles.

Review Your Knowledge

Matching: Muscle Terms

Directions: Match the following words with their descriptions. Some words may be used more than once and others not at all.

a. origin
b. sarcoplasmic reticulum
c. smooth muscle
d. aponeurosis
e. actin
f. sarcomere
g. insertion
h. atrophy
i. synergist
j. skeletal muscle
k. myosin
l. tendon

1. ___ Cordlike structure that attaches muscle to bone
2. ___ Type of muscle classified as striated and voluntary
3. ___ Type of muscle that must be stimulated by a somatic motor nerve
4. ___ Flat, sheetlike fascia that attaches muscle to muscle or muscle to bone
5. ___ The head of this contractile protein binds to actin; forms a cross-bridge
6. ___ Calcium is stored within this muscle structure
7. ___ Series of contractile units that make up each myofibril: extends from Z line to Z line
8. ___ The muscle attachment to the movable bone
9. ___ Use it or lose it
10. ___ A helper muscle

Matching: Names of Muscles

Directions: Match the following words with their descriptions. Some words may be used more than once and others not at all.

a. quadriceps femoris
b. gastrocnemius
c. masseter
d. hamstrings
e. triceps brachii
f. deltoid
g. pectoralis major
h. latissimus dorsi
i. gluteus maximus
j. biceps brachii
k. diaphragm

1. ___ A muscle of mastication
2. ___ The major breathing muscle
3. ___ Major muscle of the anterior chest; attaches to the humerus
4. ___ The shoulder pad; pulls the arm into the scarecrow position
5. ___ A muscle that flexes the arm at the elbow
6. ___ A muscle that lies along the anterior thigh; flexes the thigh at the hip and extends the leg
7. ___ The muscle group that lies along the posterior thigh; flexes the leg at the knee
8. ___ The large muscle on which you sit
9. ___ Contraction of this muscle causes plantar flexion
10. ___ This muscle attaches to the calcaneus by the Achilles tendon

Multiple Choice

1. When the electrical signal travels along the T tubule and stimulates the sarcoplasmic reticulum (SR),
   a. calcium is released, causing cross-bridge formation between actin and myosin.
   b. acetylcholine (ACh) is released into the neuromuscular junction (NMJ).
   c. calcium is pumped into the SR from the sarcomere.
   d. ACh binds to the receptor on the muscle membrane.

2. Which of the following does *not* occur within the neuromuscular junction (NMJ)?
   a. ACh is released from the motor nerve terminal.
   b. ACh diffuses across the junction.
   c. Actin and myosin "slide."
   d. ACh is inactivated by an enzyme.

3. When skeletal muscle is stimulated quickly and repetitively,
   a. ACh within the NMJ is depleted.
   b. the muscle tetanizes, and the force of contraction increases.
   c. the sarcoplasmic reticulum is depleted of calcium, and the muscle becomes flaccid.
   d. the muscle merely twitches.

4. Which of the following pairs slides?
   a. ACh and cholinesterase
   b. Calcium and ATP
   c. Troponin and tropomyosin
   d. Actin and myosin

5. Which of the following happens when calcium is pumped back into the sarcoplasmic reticulum?
   a. The muscle relaxes.
   b. ACh binds to the muscle membrane receptors in the NMJ.
   c. ACh is destroyed by cholinesterase.
   d. Actin and myosin slide.

6. Which of the following must occur to achieve flexion of the forearm?
   a. The triceps brachii contracts.
   b. The biceps brachii and brachialis contract.
   c. The brachioradialis relaxes.
   d. The deltoid and brachioradialis relax.

7. Which of the following does *not* characterize the quadriceps femoris?
   a. Has four heads, or points of attachment
   b. Is the prime mover for extension of the leg
   c. Inserts on the proximal tibia at the tibial tuberosity
   d. Causes plantar flexion, as in toe dancing

8. Which of the following is true of the hamstrings?
   a. Located along the anterior thigh
   b. Is the prime mover for flexion of the leg
   c. Acts synergistically with the gastrocnemius to cause dorsiflexion
   d. Attaches to the Achilles tendon and inserts on the calcaneus

9. Which of the following is *least* descriptive of the masseter and temporalis muscles?
   a. Insert on the mandible
   b. Muscles of mastication
   c. Nonstriated and involuntary
   d. Innervated by somatic motor neurons

10. This muscle is best viewed on an anterior view of the body.
    a. Biceps femoris
    b. Pectoralis major
    c. Latissimus dorsi
    d. Gastrocnemius

11. Which of the following is descriptive of myosin, actin, and the troponin–tropomyosin complex?
    a. Depolarization, repolarization
    b. Thick filaments/thin filaments
    c. Dendrites, axons
    d. Voluntary, involuntary

12. The muscles that move the fingers
    a. have their origins on the distal metacarpals.
    b. have their origins on the bones of the forearm.
    c. insert on the humerus.
    d. are called pronators and supinators.

13. Which of the following moves the thigh toward the midline of the body?
    a. Abductors
    b. Flexors
    c. Supinators
    d. Adductors

14. Contraction of the soleus and gastrocnemius causes
    a. abduction of the thigh.
    b. extension of the leg.
    c. dorsiflexion.
    d. plantar flexion.

15. Which of the following muscles act synergistically?
    a. Trapezius, sternocleidomastoid, quadriceps femoris
    b. Biceps brachii, brachioradialis, and brachialis
    c. Gastrocnemius, anterior tibialis, and sternocleidomastoid
    d. Temporalis, trapezius, and masseter

Go Figure

1. Which of the following is correct according to Fig. 9.1?
   a. Visceral muscle is nonstriated and voluntary.
   b. The heart is primarily comprised of visceral or smooth muscle.
   c. Skeletal muscle is striated and voluntary.
   d. Cardiac muscle is smooth and involuntary.

2. Which of the following is correct according to Fig. 9.2?
   a. Panel C compares sarcomere length in the contracted and relaxed muscle.
   b. Panel C illustrates the location of the sarcoplasmic reticulum and T-tubular system.
   c. Panel A uses the biceps brachii to illustrate skeletal muscle function at the sarcomere level.
   d. Panel B illustrates the relationship of the thin and thick filaments within the sarcomere.

3. Which of the following is correct according to Fig. 9.3?
   a. The motor unit is located within the spinal cord.
   b. Acetylcholine (ACh) is the neurotransmitter within the NMJ.
   c. Acetylcholinesterase is stored within the vesicles of the nerve terminal.
   d. The somatic motor neuron innervates only one muscle fiber (cell).

4. Which of the following is correct according to Fig. 9.4?
   a. Curare induces muscle paralysis because it blocks the release of acetylcholine (ACh) from the nerve terminal.
   b. *C. botulinum* induces paralysis because its toxin blocks muscle receptors.
   c. Myasthenia gravis is caused by the inability of the neuron to synthesize ACh.
   d. Curare induces paralysis because it blocks the muscle membrane receptors.

5. According to Fig. 9.5, which event occurs first?
   a. Calcium is released from the sarcoplasmic reticulum.
   b. The electrical signal runs along the T tubule.
   c. ACh is released from the terminal of the somatic motor neuron.
   d. ACh binds to the receptors on the muscle membrane.

6. Which of the following is correct according to Fig. 9.6?
   a. The triceps brachii acts synergistically with the biceps brachii.
   b. Contraction of the biceps brachii causes extension of the arm at the elbow.
   c. The heads of the biceps brachii attach to the proximal humerus.
   d. The biceps brachii lies across the elbow joint.

7. According to Fig. 9.7 and Table 9.1, contraction of the pectoralis major causes
   a. abduction of the arm at the shoulder.
   b. internal or medial rotation of the arm at the shoulder, as if pointing to an object in front of you.
   c. flexion of the forearm at the elbow and external rotation of the arm, as if pointing behind you.
   d. movement of the arm into a "scarecrow" position.

8. According to Fig. 9.7 and Table 9.1, the sartorius
   a. is visible only on the posterior view of the body.
   b. works synergistically with the muscles of the pectoral girdle.
   c. lies obliquely across the anterior thigh.
   d. inserts on the Achilles tendon.

9. Which muscles are not illustrated in Figs. 9.8 and 9.9?
   a. Sternocleidomastoid, buccinator, and masseter
   b. Diaphragm, trapezius, and intercostals
   c. Latissimus dorsi, trapezius, and sartorius
   d. Frontalis, orbicularis oris, and platysma

10. Which of the following is correct according to Fig. 9.8?
    a. The platysma is the smiling muscle.
    b. The sternocleidomastoid has its origin on the cranial aponeurosis.
    c. The sternocleidomastoid flexes the head.
    d. The scalenes are muscles of mastication.

11. Which of the following is correct according to Fig. 9.9?
    a. The diaphragm is located between the ribs.
    b. The intercostals insert on the clavicle.
    c. The diaphragm is a dome-shaped muscle that separates the thoracic and abdominal cavities.
    d. The diaphragm has its origins on the sternum.

12. Which of the following is correct according to Fig 9.10?
    a. Carpal tunnel syndrome is characterized by an inability to flex the forearm at the elbow.
    b. The medial nerve runs through the carpal tunnel; pressure on the nerve causes tingling and pain

c. The flexor retinaculum is the somatic neuron that innervates the muscles of the fingers.

d. The flexor retinaculum forms a tunnel through which the flexor carpi radialis and the flexor carpi ulnaris attach to the fingers.

13. Which of the following is correct according to Fig 9.11?

a. The hamstrings are called the toe dancer's muscles.

b. The surprised look is caused by contraction of the frontalis muscle.

c. Contraction of the buccinator muscles allows one to sit in the lotus position.

d. The zygomaticus enables one to flex the head, as in praying.

Nervous System: Nervous Tissue and Brain

Objectives

1. Define the two divisions of the nervous system.
2. List three general functions of the nervous system.
3. Discuss the cellular composition of the nervous system, including the following:
   - Compare the structure and functions of the neuroglia and neuron.
   - Explain the function of the myelin sheath.
   - Explain how a neuron transmits information.
4. Describe the structure and function of a synapse.
5. Describe the functions of the four major areas of the brain and the four lobes of the cerebrum.
6. Describe how the skull, meninges, cerebrospinal fluid, and blood–brain barrier protect the central nervous system.

Key Terms

action potential (p. 177)	depolarize (p. 177)	nodes of Ranvier (p. 176)
association areas (p. 187)	fissure (p. 185)	occipital lobe (p. 187)
axon (p. 176)	frontal lobe (p. 185)	parietal lobe (p. 187)
blood–brain barrier (p. 175)	ganglion (p. 177)	peripheral nervous system (PNS)
brain (p. 173)	gyrus (p. 184)	(p. 173)
brain stem (p. 188)	hypothalamus (p. 188)	repolarize (p. 177)
central nervous system (CNS) (p. 173)	interneuron (p. 176)	resting membrane potential (p. 177)
cerebellum (p. 189)	limbic system (p. 190)	reticular formation (p. 190)
cerebrospinal fluid (CSF) (p. 191)	medulla oblongata (p. 189)	subarachnoid space (p. 191)
cerebrum (p. 183)	meninges (p. 191)	sulcus (p. 185)
choroid plexus (p. 191)	myelin sheath (p. 176)	synapse (p. 181)
convolution (p. 184)	neuroglia (p. 174)	temporal lobe (p. 187)
corpus callosum (p. 183)	neuron (p. 175)	thalamus (p. 188)
dendrite (p. 176)	neurotransmitters (p. 182)	threshold potential (p. 177)

THE NERVOUS SYSTEM: STRUCTURE AND FUNCTION

Thinking great thoughts, feeling, moving, seeing, hearing, responding, planning, remembering, being aware of environmental cues, and so much more are functions performed by the nervous system. No small feat!

DIVISIONS OF THE NERVOUS SYSTEM

The structures of the nervous system are divided into two parts: the central nervous system and the peripheral nervous system. The **central nervous system (CNS)** includes the **brain** and the spinal cord. The CNS is located in the dorsal cavity. The brain is located in the cranial cavity; the spinal cord is enclosed in the spinal cavity. The **peripheral nervous system (PNS)** is located outside the CNS and consists of the nerves that connect the CNS with the rest of the body (Fig. 10.1).

FUNCTIONS OF THE NERVOUS SYSTEM

The nervous system performs three general functions: a sensory function, an integrative function, and a motor function (Fig. 10.2).

SENSORY FUNCTION

Sensory nerves gather information from inside the body and from the outside environment. The nerves then carry the information to the CNS. For example, information about a cat is picked up by special cells in the boy's eye and transmitted to the brain.

INTEGRATIVE FUNCTION

Sensory information brought to the CNS is interpreted. The brain not only sees the cat but also does much more. It recalls very quickly how a cat behaves. It may determine that the cat is acting hungry or is distressed and ready to attack. The brain integrates, or

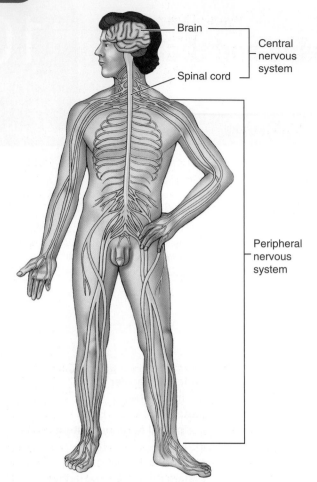

FIG. 10.1 Nervous system: central nervous system and peripheral nervous system.

puts together, everything it knows about cats and then makes its plan.

MOTOR FUNCTION

Motor nerves convey information from the CNS toward the muscles and glands of the body. Motor nerves carry out the plans made by the CNS. For example, the boy decides to feed the hungry cat. Information must travel along the motor nerves from the CNS to all the skeletal muscles needed to feed the cat. The motor nerve converts the plan into action.

> **? Re-Think**
>
> 1. State the two divisions of the nervous system.
> 2. Differentiate between sensory, integrative, and motor function; provide an example of each.

CELLS THAT MAKE UP THE NERVOUS SYSTEM

Nervous tissue is composed of two types of cells: the neuroglia and the neurons.

NEUROGLIA

Neuroglia (noo-ROHG-lee-ah), or glial cells, are the nerve glue. Neuroglia are the most abundant of the nerve cells; most glial cells are located in the CNS. Glial cells support, protect, insulate, nourish, and generally care for the delicate neurons. Some of the glial cells

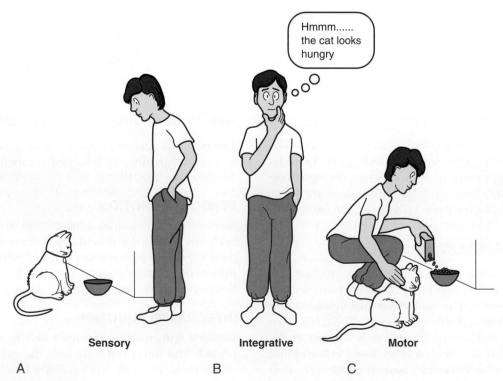

FIG. 10.2 Three functions of the nervous system. (A) Sensory function. (B) Integrative function. (C) Motor function.

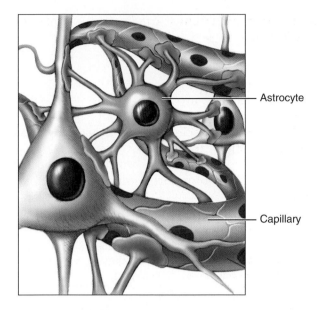

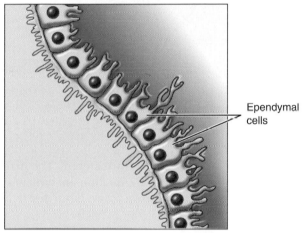

FIG. 10.3 Neuroglia: astrocytes and ependymal cells.

Table 10.1   Types of Neuroglia

CELL NAME	FUNCTION
Astrocytes	Star-shaped cells present in blood–brain barrier; also anchor or bind blood vessels to nerves for support, act as phagocytes, and secrete nerve growth factors
Ependymal cells	Line the ventricles as part of the choroid plexus; involved in the formation of cerebrospinal fluid
Microglia	Protective role; phagocytosis of pathogens and damaged tissue
Schwann cells	Produce myelin sheath for neurons in the peripheral nervous system; assist in regeneration of damaged fibers
Oligodendrocytes	Produce myelin sheath for neurons in the central nervous system

Do You Know...
The Good News About the Polio Virus and Brain Cancer?

Many years ago, poliomyelitis, an infection caused by poliovirus, was terrifying because it often resulted in life-long severe paralysis (infantile paralysis). Recently, however, the poliovirus has been modified by scientists in a way that not only prevents its ability to cause poliomyelitis but enables it to be used in the treatment of glioblastoma, a common and lethal type of brain cancer. Here's the link. Cancer cells often surround themselves with a protective shield that covers their surface antigens and protects them from the host's immune system. When injected, the modified poliovirus removes the shield surrounding the cancer cells, thereby exposing their surface antigens. The immune system of the host recognizes the antigens as foreign, mounts an immune attack against the cancer cells, and destroys the tumor. The result of this therapy is both encouraging and enlightening. It offers hope for a cure and also sheds light on the role of the immune system in cancer biology.

participate in phagocytosis; others assist in the secretion of cerebrospinal fluid. Glial cells, however, do not conduct nerve impulses.

Two of the more common glial cells are the astrocytes and the ependymal cells (Fig. 10.3). The star-shaped astrocytes (ASS-troh-sytes) are the most abundant of the glial cells and have the most diverse functions; they support the neurons structurally, cover the entire surface of the brain, and help form a protective barrier, called the **blood–brain barrier**. This barrier helps prevent toxic substances in the blood from entering the nervous tissue of the brain and spinal cord. Astrocytes also secrete nerve growth factors that promote neuron growth and enhance synaptic development. A second glial cell is the ependymal (eh-PEN-di-mal) cell. These cells line the inside cavities of the brain and assist in the formation of cerebrospinal fluid. Other glial cells are listed in Table 10.1. Because glial cells undergo mitosis, most primary CNS tumors are composed of glial cells, such as astrocytomas.

NEURON

The second type of cell within the nervous system is the neuron. Of the two types of nerve cells, the **neuron** (NOO-ron) is the most important in the transmission of electrical signals. The neuron enables the nervous system to act as a vast communication network. Neurons have many shapes and sizes. Some neurons are extremely short; others are very long, with some measuring 4 feet in length. Unlike glial cells, neurons are nonmitotic and therefore do not replicate or replace themselves when injured. Because they are nonmitotic, neurons generally do not give rise to primary malignant brain tumors.

As indicated in Fig. 10.2, neurons are functionally classified as follows:

- Sensory neurons: they carry information to the CNS.

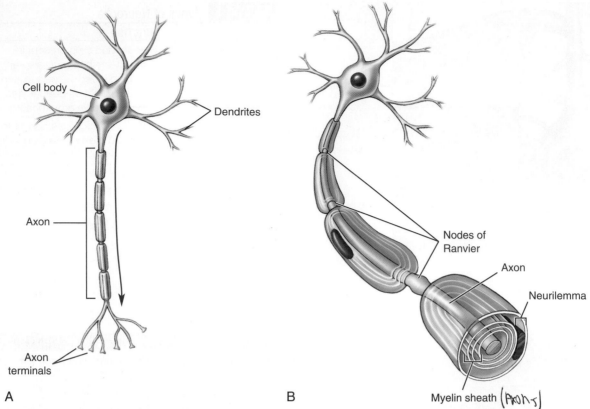

FIG. 10.4 Structure of a neuron. (A) Dendrites, cell body, axon, and axon terminals. (B) Structure surrounding the axon, showing the myelin sheath, the nodes of Ranvier, and the neurilemma.

- Motor neurons: they carry information away from the CNS.
- **Interneurons**: they are found only in the CNS. They form connections between sensory and motor neurons within the CNS. They play an important role in integrating all sensory information and the appropriate motor responses (not shown).

PARTS OF A NEURON

Three Parts

The three parts of the neuron are the dendrites, cell body, and axon (Fig. 10.4).

- **Dendrites** are treelike structures that receive signals from other neurons and then transmit the signals toward the cell body. One neuron may have thousands of dendrites, whereas other neurons have fewer dendrites. The neuron with the greater number of dendrites can receive signals from many other neurons.
- The cell body contains the nucleus and is essential for the life of the cell. The cell body usually receives thousands of signals from the dendrites and "decides" on the signal it wants to send to the axon.
- The **axon** is a long extension that transmits signals away from the cell body. The end of the axon undergoes extensive branching to form many axon terminals; it is within the axon terminals that the

chemical neurotransmitters are stored. The arrow in Fig. 10.4 indicates the direction in which signal travels over the neuron: from dendrites to cell body to axon.

The Axon: A Special Structure

What is so special about the axon? An enlarged view of the axon shows several unique structures: the myelin sheath, the neurilemma, and the **nodes of Ranvier** (see Fig. 10.4). Most long nerve fibers of both the peripheral and central nervous systems are encased by a layer of white fatty material called the myelin sheath. Myelin (MY-eh-lin) protects and insulates the axon. Nerve fibers covered by myelin are said to be myelinated. Some neurons are not encased in myelin and are called *unmyelinated neurons*. Myelination begins during the fourth month of fetal life and continues into the teenage years. Because some axons of immature motor neurons lack myelination, the movements of an infant are slower and less coordinated than those of an older child. Severely restricting the fat intake of an infant or young child is unwise, because the child is still laying down myelin.

The formation of myelin sheath differs in the peripheral and central nervous systems. Surrounding the axon of a neuron in the peripheral nervous system is a layer of special cells called *Schwann* (shwon) *cells*. The Schwann cells form the myelin sheath that surrounds the axon. The nuclei and cytoplasm of the Schwann cells lie outside the myelin sheath and are called the *neurilemma*. The neurilemma (NUR-ih-LEM-uh) is important in the regeneration of a severed nerve.

In the CNS, the myelin sheath is formed not by Schwann cells but by oligodendrocytes (ohl-i-go-DEN-droh-sytes), a type of glial cell (see Table 10.1). Because there are no Schwann cells, there is no neurilemma. The lack of the neurilemma surrounding the axons accounts, in part, for the inability of the CNS neurons to regenerate. Failure of the neurons of the CNS to regenerate, however, is not fully explained by the lack of neurilemma; other factors include the formation of scar tissue and the lack of critical nerve growth factors.

Nodes of Ranvier, axonal areas not covered by myelin, appear at regular intervals along the myelinated axon.

 Re-Think

1. What is the biggest functional difference between glial cells and the neuron?
2. List the three main parts of a neuron.
3. What are the nodes of Ranvier?

WHITE MATTER VERSUS GRAY MATTER

The tissue of the CNS is white or gray. White matter is white because of the myelinated axons, whereas gray matter is made up of unmyelinated axons, cell bodies, interneurons, and synapses.

Sometimes cell bodies appear in small clusters and are given special names. Clusters of cell bodies located in the CNS are generally referred to as *nuclei*. Small clusters of cell bodies in the peripheral nervous system are called *ganglia* (sing., **ganglion**). For example, patches of gray called the *basal nuclei* are located in the brain. (Sometimes, these patches of gray are called *basal ganglia*, despite their location in the CNS.)

 Sum It Up!

The nervous system plays a crucial role in allowing us to interact with our environment, both internal and external—and to think great thoughts! The nervous system has two divisions: the central nervous system and the peripheral nervous system. The nervous system performs three major functions: sensory, integrative, and motor. There are two types of cells in the nervous system: the neuroglia and the neurons. The neuron is responsible for the rapid communication of electrical signals. The three parts of the neuron are the dendrites, cell body, and axon. The nodes of Ranvier are well-spaced unmyelinated areas along the axon.

THE NEURON CARRYING INFORMATION

Neurons allow the nervous system to convey information rapidly from one part of the body to the next. A stubbed toe makes itself known almost immediately. Think of how fast the information travels from your toe, where the injury occurred, to your brain, where the injury is interpreted as pain. Information is carried along the neuron in the form of a nerve impulse.

THE NERVE IMPULSE: WHAT IT IS

The nerve impulse is an electrical signal that conveys information along a neuron. The nerve impulse is called the **action potential**. There are two phases of an action potential: depolarization and repolarization. Follow Fig. 10.5 through the events of the action potential, from its resting state (resting membrane potential) to depolarization to repolarization.

- **Resting membrane potential** refers to the electrical charge difference across the membrane of the resting neuron. The inside of a resting neuron is more negative (−) than the outside (+). The resting cell is said to be polarized. As long as the neuron is polarized, no nerve impulse is being transmitted. The cell is quiet, or resting.
- Depolarization. When the neuronal membrane is stimulated, a change occurs in the cell's electrical state. In the resting (polarized) state, the inside of the cell is negative. When the cell membrane is stimulated, the inside becomes positive. As the inside of the cell changes from negative to positive, it is said to **depolarize.**
- Repolarization. Very quickly, however, the inside of the cell again becomes negative; in other words, it returns to its resting state, or **repolarizes.** Unless the cell repolarizes, it cannot be stimulated again.

Fig. 10.6 shows a recording of an action potential. Note the negative (−) 90 millivolt (mv) reading inside the unstimulated neuron (resting membrane potential). When stimulated, the cell depolarizes, that is, the inside of the cell becomes positive (+ 20 mv). Immediately the cell repolarizes, that is the inside of the cell returns to its (−) resting membrane potential. Also shown is the threshold potential. The **threshold potential** is the degree of depolarization that must be attained for the neuron to completely fully depolarize to +20 mv. If threshold potential is not achieved by the stimulus, the signal decays, and the cell returns to the resting membrane potential. Under this condition the action potential fails to fire.

 Re-Think

1. What is the meaning of the resting membrane potential, polarization, depolarization, and repolarization?
2. Describe the relationship of the threshold potential to the action potential.

THE NERVE IMPULSE: WHAT CAUSES IT

The changes associated with the action potential, or nerve impulse, are caused by the movement of specific ions across the cell membrane of the neuron. This

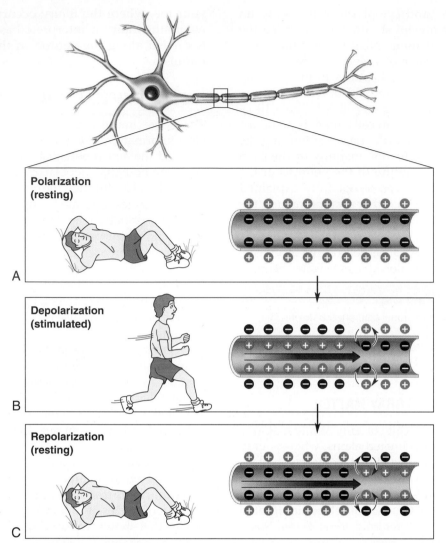

FIG. 10.5 Nerve impulse (action potential). (A) Polarization. (B) Depolarization. (C) Repolarization.

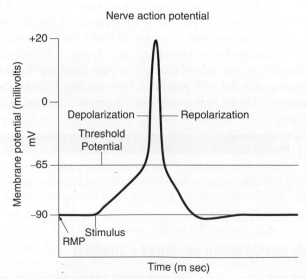

FIG. 10.6 Nerve impulse (action potential) illustrating the resting membrane potential (RMP), threshold potential, depolarization, and repolarization.

is called the ionic basis of the action potential. To understand the diffusion of ions across the axonal membrane, you must remember the following: the chief intracellular cation is potassium (K⁺) and the chief extracellular cation is sodium (Na⁺). If the membrane is or becomes permeable to K⁺, it diffuses outwardly. If the membrane is permeable to Na⁺, it diffuses inwardly. The flow of ions is thus dependent on two factors: the concentration gradients of K⁺ and Na⁺ and the permeability characteristics of the membrane. Follow the movement of the ions in Fig. 10.7.

RESTING MEMBRANE POTENTIAL

What makes the inside of the cell negative in the resting state? The resting state is the result of the numbers and types of ions, both positive (cations) and negative (anions), located inside the neuron.

How do these ions get into the cell in such high concentrations? They are pumped in by ATP-driven

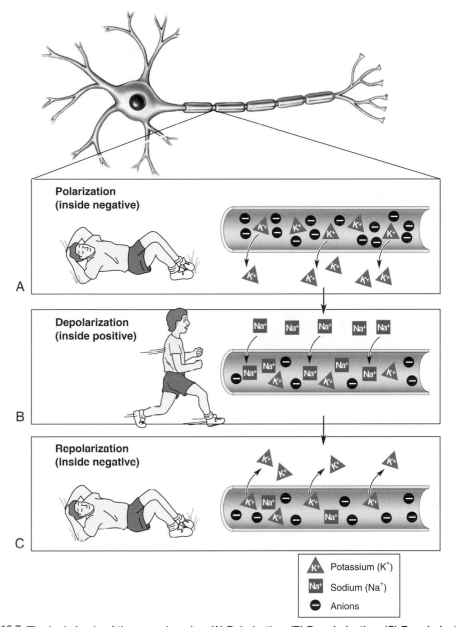

FIG. 10.7 The ionic basis of the nerve impulse. (A) Polarization. (B) Depolarization. (C) Repolarization.

pumps in the cell membrane. The chief intracellular cation is K^+. In the resting state, however, some of the K^+ ions leak out of the cell, taking with them the positive charge. The lost positive charge and the excess anions trapped in the cell make the inside of the cell negative (−90 mv). Remember: it is the outward leak of K^+ that is responsible for the resting membrane potential!

DEPOLARIZATION

Why does the interior of the cell become positive when stimulated? When the neuron is stimulated, the permeability of the neuronal membrane changes in a way that allows sodium ions (Na^+) to diffuse rapidly across the membrane into the cell, carrying with it a positive (+) charge. Thus, it is the rapid inward diffusion of Na^+ that causes depolarization.

REPOLARIZATION

Why does the inside of the cell quickly return to its resting negative state? Soon after the cell depolarizes, the neuronal membrane undergoes a second change. The change in the membrane permeability does two things: (1) it stops additional diffusion of Na^+ into the cell, and (2) it allows K^+ to rapidly diffuse out of the cell. The outward diffusion of K^+ decreases the positive charge from the inside of the cell, leaving behind the negatively charged anions. Thus, the outward movement of K^+ causes repolarization and a return to the resting state.

Eventually, membrane pumps restore intracellular ion concentrations; Na^+ is pumped out of the cell, while K^+ is pumped into the cell. Note that the repolarizing phase of the nerve impulse is not caused by the active transport pumps. Repolarization is caused by the rapid outward diffusion of K^+.

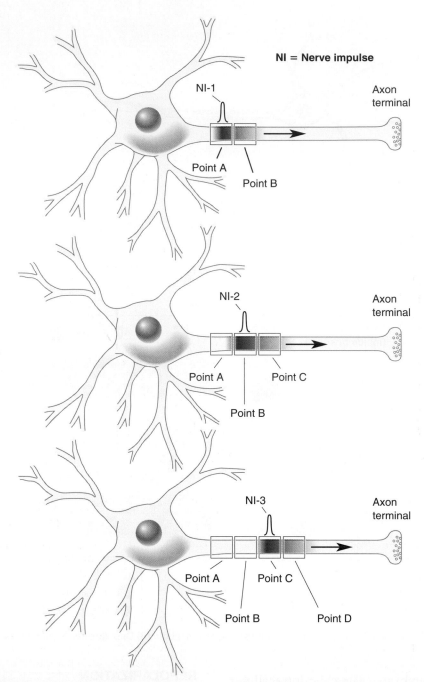

NI = Nerve impulse

FIG. 10.8 **What causes the nerve impulse to move from the cell body to the axon terminals?**

❓ Re-Think

1. What is the ionic basis of the resting membrane potential (polarization)?
2. What is the ionic basis of depolarization?
3. What is the ionic basis of repolarization?

THE NERVE IMPULSE: WHAT CAUSES IT TO MOVE

To convey information, a nerve impulse (action potential) must move the length of the neuron, from the cell body to the axon terminal. Fig. 10.8 shows that when nerve impulse one (NI-1) forms at point A, it also depolarizes the next segment of the membrane (point B), causing nerve impulse two (NI-2) to form. Nerve impulse 2 then depolarizes the next segment of the membrane at point C, causing the formation of nerve impulse three (NI-3).

Because of the ability of each nerve impulse to depolarize the adjacent membrane, the nerve impulse moves toward the axon terminal much like a wave. Note also in Fig. 10.8 that the height or amplitude of each nerve impulse along the axon is the same. This is important because it ensures that the nerve impulse does not weaken as it travels the length of a long axon.

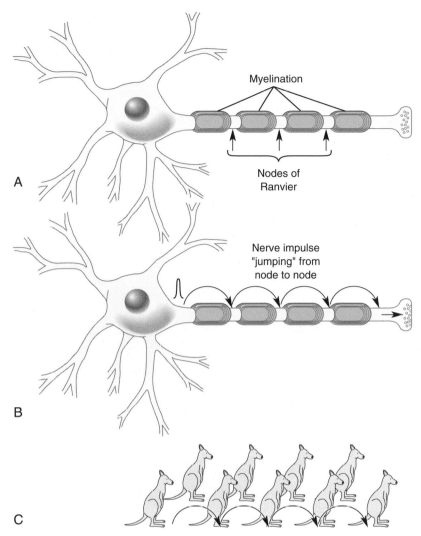

FIG. 10.9 Jumping from node to node (saltatory conduction). (A) A myelinated axon and the nodes of Ranvier. (B) The nerve impulse jumps from node to node toward the axon terminal. (C) The jumping of the nerve impulse resembles the jumping of a kangaroo.

THE NERVE IMPULSE: WHAT CAUSES IT TO MOVE QUICKLY

We understand why the nerve impulse moves, but why does it move so quickly? Myelination increases the movement of the nerve impulse along the axonal membrane. Recall that the axons of most nerve fibers are wrapped in myelin, a fatty material. At the nodes of Ranvier, the axonal membrane is bare or unmyelinated.

The nerve impulse arrives at the axon from the cell body but cannot develop on any part of the membrane covered with myelin. The nerve impulse can, however, develop at the nodes of Ranvier, the bare axonal membrane. Thus in a myelinated fiber, the nerve impulse jumps from node to node, much like a kangaroo, to the end of the axon (Fig. 10.9). This "jumping" from node to node is called *saltatory conduction* (from the Latin word *saltare*, meaning "to leap"). Saltatory conduction increases the speed with which the nerve impulse travels along the nerve fiber. For this reason, myelinated fibers are considered fast-conducting nerve fibers.

? Re-Think

1. What is the function of the nodes of Ranvier?
2. Explain how myelination and the nodes of Ranvier affect the rate of nerve impulse (action potential) conduction.

SYNAPSE ACROSS NEURONS

The nerve impulse travels the length of the axon. However, the signal does not jump from one neuron to the next. A **synapse** helps information move chemically from one neuron to the next. The big question is how.

PARTS OF A SYNAPSE

Follow Fig. 10.10 as the synaptic structures in the following list are described.

- *Synaptic cleft.* The synaptic (si-NAP-tik) cleft is a space (much like the neuromuscular junction in Chapter 9). The space exists because the axon terminal of neuron A (presynaptic neuron) does not physically touch the dendrite of neuron B (postsynaptic neuron).

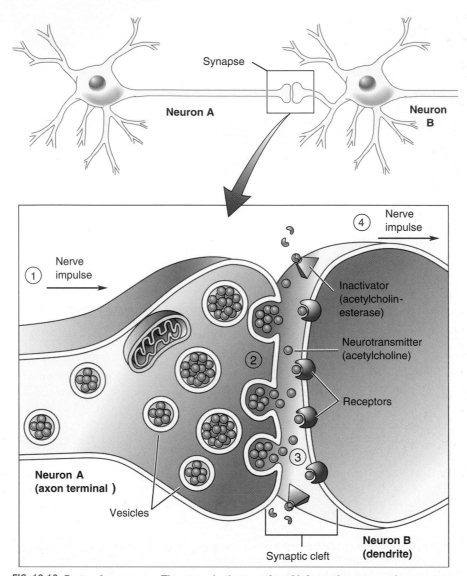

FIG. 10.10 Parts of a synapse. The steps in the transfer of information across the synapse..

- *Receptors.* The dendrite of neuron B contains receptor sites. Receptor sites are places on the membrane to which the neurotransmitters bind. For example, acetylcholine (ACh) binds to the receptors on dendrite B. Each receptor site has a specific shape and accepts only those neurotransmitters that "fit" its shape.
- *Neurotransmitters.* The axon terminal of neuron A contains thousands of tiny vesicles that store chemical substances called **neurotransmitters** (noo-roh-TRANS-mit-ters). The most common neurotransmitters are ACh and norepinephrine (NE). Other CNS transmitters include epinephrine, serotonin, glutamate, dopamine, gamma-aminobutyric acid (GABA), and endorphins.
- *Inactivators.* These are substances that terminate the activity of the neurotransmitters when they have completed their task. For example, the neurotransmitter ACh is terminated by acetylcholinesterase. Acetylcholinesterase is an enzyme located in the

same area as the receptor sites on neuron B. Once ACh has completed its task, it is inactivated by acetylcholinesterase.

EVENTS AT THE SYNAPSE

The following details the events at the synapse (see Fig. 10.10):

1. The nerve impulse travels along neuron A to its axon terminal.
2. The nerve impulse causes the vesicles to fuse with the membrane of the axon terminal. The vesicles open and release the neurotransmitter into the synaptic cleft.
3. The neurotransmitter diffuses across the synaptic cleft and binds to the receptor site. The binding of the neurotransmitter to the receptor site causes a change in the membrane potential of the dendrite of neuron B, thereby developing a nerve impulse. The neurotransmitter then vacates the receptor and is degraded.

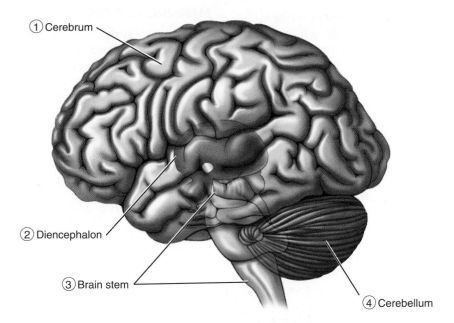

① Cerebrum

② Diencephalon

③ Brain stem

④ Cerebellum

FIG. 10.11 Four major areas of the brain: cerebrum, diencephalon, brain stem, and cerebellum.

4. Electrical information travels toward the cell body and axon of neuron B. What has happened at the synapse? Information from neuron A has been chemically transmitted chemically to neuron B.

? Re-Think

1. List the parts of a synapse.
2. How does the nerve impulse (action potential) of the first neuron stimulate the dendrite of a second neuron?

◎ Sum It Up!

The electrical signal that travels along the neuron is called the *nerve impulse* or *action potential*. The nerve impulse has two phases: depolarization and repolarization. The resting membrane potential and the phases of the nerve impulse are caused by the movement of ions, particularly Na^+ and K^+. The resting membrane potential is due to the outward leak of K^+. Depolarization is due to the influx of Na^+. Repolarization is due to the rapid efflux of K^+. Initial depolarization must reach threshold potential in order for the nerve impulse to develop. The nerve impulse travels along the neuron from the dendrites to the cell body to the end of the axon. Many of the axons are myelinated to increase the speed of the nerve impulse. During saltatory conduction, the nerve impulse jumps from node to node, thereby rapidly moving along the axon. The nerve impulse stimulates the release of neurotransmitters into the synaptic cleft; the transmitter diffuses across the synaptic cleft, binds to the postsynaptic receptor, and stimulates the dendrites of the second neuron. The synapse allows for the chemical transmission of information from neuron to neuron.

BRAIN: STRUCTURE AND FUNCTION

The brain is located in the cranial cavity. It is a pinkish-gray, delicate structure with a soft consistency. The surface of the brain appears bumpy, much like a walnut. The "boss of it all" weighs only 3 lb!

The blood supply to the brain is unique and is described in Chapter 18. Despite the fact that the brain weighs only 2% of the total body weight, it requires 20% of the body's oxygen supply. The primary source of energy for the brain is glucose. When blood glucose levels get very low (hypoglycemia), the person experiences mental confusion, dizziness, seizures, loss of consciousness, and death. No wonder that many of the body's hormones are concerned with making glucose available to the brain.

The brain is divided into four major areas: the cerebrum, the diencephalon, the brain stem, and the cerebellum (Fig. 10.11).

CEREBRUM

The **cerebrum** (seh-REE-brum) is the largest part of the brain. It is divided into the right and left cerebral hemispheres. The cerebral hemispheres are joined together by bands of white matter that form a large fiber tract called the **corpus callosum**. The corpus callosum (cah-LOH-sum) allows the right and left sides of the brain to communicate with each other. Each cerebral hemisphere has four major lobes: frontal, parietal, temporal, and occipital (Fig. 10.12). These four lobes are named for the overlying cranial bones.

GRAY ON THE OUTSIDE, WHITE ON THE INSIDE

The cerebrum contains both gray and white matter. A thin layer of gray matter, called the *cerebral cortex*, forms the outermost portion of the cerebrum. The cerebral cortex is composed primarily of cell bodies and interneurons and is therefore gray. The gray matter of the cerebral cortex allows us to perform higher mental tasks such as learning, reasoning, language, and memory.

The bulk of the cerebrum is composed of white matter located directly below the cortex. The white matter is composed primarily of myelinated axons that form connections between the parts of the brain and spinal cord. Scattered throughout the white matter are patches of gray matter called *nuclei*.

MARKINGS OF THE CEREBRUM

The bumpy surface of the cerebrum has numerous markings with special names. The surface of the cerebrum is folded into elevations that resemble speed bumps on a road. The elevations are called **convolutions**, or *gyri* (sing., **gyrus**).

Do You Know...

If You Are a Left-Brain or a Right-Brain Person?

Some years ago, a surgeon severed the corpus callosum in the brain of a patient with severe epilepsy. This surgical procedure eliminated all communication between the left and right cerebral hemispheres. From these and other experiments, neuroscientists learned that there is a left brain and a right brain and that these two brains have different abilities. The difference in function between the two cerebral hemispheres is called *cerebral lateralization*. The left brain is more concerned with language and mathematical abilities; it is the reasoning and analytical side of the brain. The right side of the brain is far superior with regard to spatial relationships, art, music, and the expression of emotions. The right brain is intuitive; it is the poet and the artist. Many of us are predominantly left-brain or right-brain persons. How much richer our lives are when we use both sides of our brains!

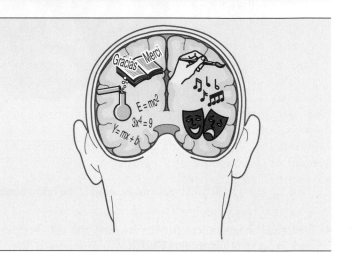

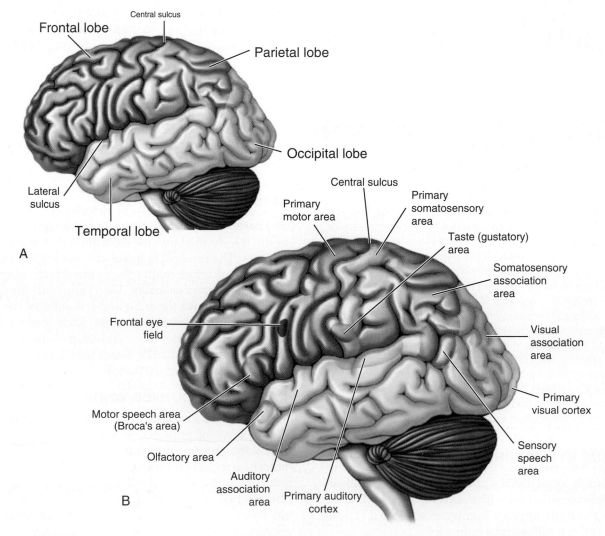

FIG. 10.12 (A) Lobes of the cerebrum: frontal lobe, parietal lobe, temporal lobe, and occipital lobe. (B) Functional areas of the cerebrum.

This extensive folding arrangement increases the amount of cerebral cortex, or thinking tissue. It is thought that intelligence is related to the amount of cerebral cortex and therefore to the numbers of convolutions or gyri. The greater the numbers of convolutions in the brain, the more intelligent the species. For example, the cerebral cortex of the human brain has many more convolutions than the brain of an elephant (except in the memory part of the brain).

Gyri are separated by grooves called *sulci* (sing., **sulcus**). A deep sulcus is called a **fissure**. Sulci and fissures separate the cerebrum into lobes. Fig. 10.12 illustrates two of the numerous sulci and fissures: the central sulcus and the lateral sulcus. (Identify each structure on the diagram as it is described in the text.)

The central sulcus separates the frontal lobe from the parietal lobe. The central sulcus is an important landmark, separating the precentral and postcentral gyri. The precentral gyrus is located in the frontal lobe, directly in front of the central sulcus, and the postcentral gyrus is located in the parietal lobe, directly behind the central sulcus. The lateral sulcus separates the temporal lobe from the frontal and the parietal lobes. The longitudinal fissure separates the left and right cerebral hemispheres (not shown).

Re-Think

1. What is the major source of energy for the brain?
2. What are the four major divisions of the brain?
3. What is the role of the corpus callosum?
4. In what cerebral lobe is the precentral gyrus? The postcentral gyrus?

LOBES OF THE CEREBRUM

What does each cerebral lobe do? (See Table 10.2.)

Frontal Lobe

The **frontal lobe** is located in the front of the cranium under the frontal bone (see Fig. 10.12). The frontal lobe plays a key role in voluntary motor activity, personality development, emotional and behavioral expression, and performance of high-level tasks such as learning, thinking, and making plans; these are sometimes called *executive functions*. The frontal lobe also contains the primary motor area (cortex). Nerve impulses that originate in the primary motor cortex control voluntary muscle movement. When you decide to move your leg, the nerve impulse originates in the precentral gyrus, or primary motor cortex, of the frontal lobe. The axons of these motor neurons form the voluntary motor tracts that descend down the spinal cord.

The function of the precentral gyrus of the frontal lobe is illustrated by a homunculus, meaning "little man"

Table 10.2 Brain Structure and Function

STRUCTURE	FUNCTIONS
Cerebrum	
Frontal lobe	Motor area, personality, behavior, emotional expression, intellectual functions ("executive" functions), memory storage
Parietal lobe	Somatosensory area (especially from skin and muscle; taste; speech; reading)
Occipital lobe	Vision, vision-related reflexes and functions (reading, judging distances, seeing in three dimensions)
Temporal lobe	Hearing (auditory area), smell (olfactory area), taste, memory storage, part of speech area
Diencephalon	
Thalamus	Relay structure and processing center for most sensory information going to the cerebrum
Hypothalamus	Integrating system for the autonomic nervous system; regulation of temperature, water balance, sex, thirst, appetite, and some emotions (pleasure and fear); regulates the pituitary gland and controls endocrine function
Brain Stem	
Midbrain	Relays information (sensory and motor); associated with visual and auditory reflexes
Pons	Relays information (sensory and motor); plays a role in respiration
Medulla oblongata	Vital function (regulation of heart rate, blood flow, blood pressure, respiratory centers); reflex center for coughing, sneezing, swallowing, and vomiting
Cerebellum	Smoothes out and coordinates voluntary muscle activity; helps in the maintenance of balance and muscle tone
Other Structures	
Limbic system	Experience of emotion and behavior (emotional brain)
Reticular formation	Alerts the cerebrum of incoming sensory signals; regulates muscle tone in the resting body; includes the reticular activating system (RAS) and regulates the sleep–wake cycle
Basal nuclei	Smooths out and coordinates skeletal muscle activity

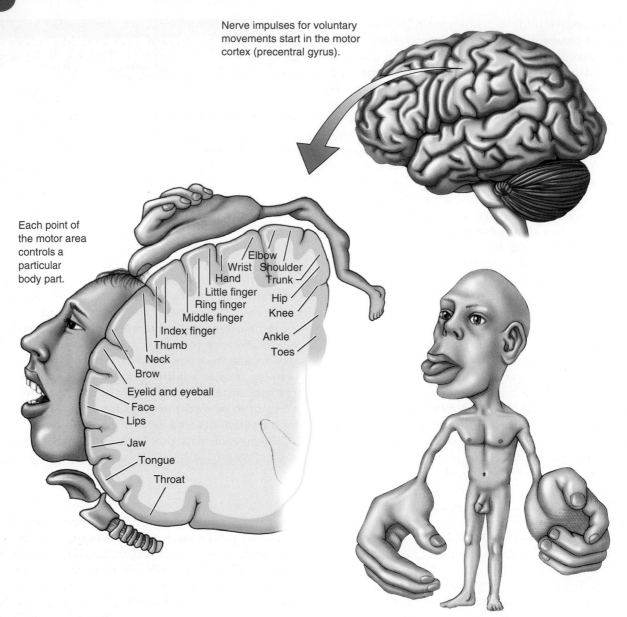

Nerve impulses for voluntary movements start in the motor cortex (precentral gyrus).

Each point of the motor area controls a particular body part.

Elbow
Wrist Shoulder
Hand   Trunk
Little finger   Hip
Ring finger   Knee
Middle finger
Index finger   Ankle
Thumb   Toes
Neck
Brow
Eyelid and eyeball
Face
Lips
Jaw
Tongue
Throat

FIG. 10.13 Motor area of the frontal lobe (precentral gyrus), illustrated with a homunculus.

(Fig. 10.13). The homunculus represents the amount of brain tissue that corresponds to a function of a particular body part. The homunculus shows two important points; each part of the body is controlled by a specific area of the cerebral cortex of the precentral gyrus, and the complicated nature of certain movements requires large amounts of brain tissue. (Locate the specific points for the toe, foot, leg, trunk, hand, and face.)

For example, the movements of the hand are much more delicate and complicated than the movements of the foot. Therefore, the amount of brain tissue devoted to hand and finger movement is much greater than the amount devoted to foot and toe movement. Consequently, the homunculus has huge hands and small feet. Note also the amount of brain tissue required to run your mouth.

In addition to its role in voluntary motor activity, the frontal lobe plays a key role in motor speech.

Motor speech refers to the movements of the mouth and tongue necessary for the formation of words to express your thoughts. The part of the frontal lobe concerned with motor speech is called *Broca's area*. In most persons, Broca's area is in the left hemisphere (see Fig. 10.12). What happens when Broca's area is broken? If damaged, as commonly happens with a stroke or brain attack, the person develops a type of aphasia. The person knows what he or she wants to say but cannot say it. Just above Broca's area is an area called the *frontal eye field*. It controls voluntary movements of the eyes and the eyelids. Your ability to scan this paragraph is a function of this area.

? Re-Think

1. What are the functions of the frontal lobe? Of Broca's area? Of the frontal eye fields?
2. What information is conveyed by a homunculus?

Parietal Lobe

The **parietal lobe** is located posterior to the central sulcus (see Fig. 10.12). The parietal lobe, particularly the postcentral gyrus, is primarily concerned with receiving general sensory information from the body. Because it receives sensations from the body, the parietal lobe is called the *primary somatosensory area*. This area receives information primarily from the skin and muscles and allows you to experience the sensations of temperature, pain, light touch, and proprioception (a sense of where your body is). The parietal lobe is also concerned with reading, speech, and taste. Like the motor homunculus in the precentral gyrus, a sensory homunculus can be drawn along the postcentral gyrus (not shown). Remember! The precentral gyrus is located in the frontal lobe and is the primary motor area. The postcentral gyrus is located in the parietal lobe and is the primary somatosensory area.

Temporal Lobe

The **temporal lobe** is located inferior to the lateral fissure in an area just above the ear. The temporal lobe contains an area called the *primary auditory cortex*. It receives sensory information from the ears and allows you to hear. Damage to the temporal lobe causes cortical deafness. The temporal lobe also receives sensory information from the nose; this area is called the *olfactory area*, the area that senses smell. Sensory information from the taste buds in the tongue is interpreted in both the temporal and parietal lobes. A broad region called *Wernicke's area* (not shown) is located in the parietal and temporal lobes; it is concerned with the translation of thought into words. Damage to this area, as occurs with chronic alcohol abuse, can result in severe deficits in language comprehension.

Occipital Lobe

The **occipital** (ok-SIP-it-al) **lobe** is located in the posterior part of the cerebrum, underlying the occipital bone. The occipital lobe contains the visual cortex. Sensory fibers from the eye send information to the primary visual cortex of the occipital lobe, where it is interpreted as sight. The occipital lobe is also concerned with many visual reflexes and vision-related functions such as reading (through the visual association area). Damage to the primary visual cortex of the occipital lobe causes cortical blindness.

FUNCTIONS INVOLVING MANY CEREBRAL LOBES

Speech Area

Although specific functions can be attributed to each cerebral lobe, most functions depend on more than one area of the brain. The speech area, for example, is located in an area that includes the temporal, parietal, and occipital lobes. In most people, the speech area is located in the left hemisphere. The speech area allows you to understand words, whether written or spoken. When you have gathered your thoughts, Broca's area in the frontal lobe directs the muscles of the larynx, tongue, cheeks, and lips to speak.

 Do You Know...

Why a Person Might "Neglect" Half of His Face?

A person with a lesion in the parietal lobe may become unaware of the opposite side of his body. For example, he may not recognize his left leg as his own. When shaving, he may shave only one side of his face. When dressing, he may dress only one side of his body. When eating, he may eat only foods on one side of his plate. This neurological condition is called *contralateral neglect syndrome*.

Other functions require input from more than one brain structure. The ability to read, for example, requires interpretation of the visual information by the occipital lobe. It also requires understanding of the words and the coordination of the eyes as they scan the page. A vast amount of brain tissue beyond the occipital lobe is involved in vision and vision-related functions such as reading.

 Re-Think

1. Identify the cerebral lobes concerned with these functions: vision, hearing, taste, smell, and speech.
2. Identify one consequence of damage to Wernicke's area.

ASSOCIATION AREAS

Large areas of the cerebral cortex are called **association areas** (see Fig. 10. 12). These areas are concerned primarily with analyzing, interpreting, and integrating information. For example, a small area of the temporal lobe, called the *primary auditory cortex*, receives sensory information from the ear. The surrounding area, called the *auditory association area*, uses a large store of knowledge and experience to identify and give meaning to the sound. In other words, the auditory cortex hears the noise, and the auditory association area interprets the noise. The brain contains receiving and association areas for other sensations as well (e.g., visual association area, somatosensory association area).

PATCHES OF GRAY

Scattered throughout the cerebral white matter are patches of gray matter called *basal nuclei* (sometimes called *basal ganglia*). The basal nuclei help regulate body movement and facial expression. The neurotransmitter dopamine is largely responsible for the activity of the basal nuclei.

A deficiency of dopamine within the basal nuclei is called *Parkinson's disease*. It is a movement disorder or dyskinesia (dis-kin-EE-see-ah). Because of the characteristic shaking (tremors), Parkinson's disease is sometimes called *shaking palsy*. Dopamine-producing drugs are usually prescribed to treat this condition.

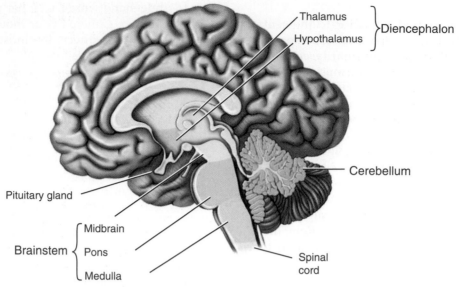

FIG. 10.14 Diencephalon, brain stem, and cerebellum.

DIENCEPHALON

The diencephalon (dye-en-SEF-ah-lon) is the second main area of the brain. It is located beneath the cerebrum and above the brain stem. The diencephalon includes the thalamus and the hypothalamus (Fig. 10.14).

The **thalamus** serves as a relay station for most of the sensory fibers traveling from the lower brain and spinal cord region to the sensory areas of the cerebrum. The thalamus sorts out the sensory information, gives us a hint of the sensation we are to experience, and then directs the information to the specific cerebral areas for more precise interpretation. For example, pain fibers coming from the body to the brain pass through the thalamus. At the level of the thalamus, we become aware of pain, but we are not yet aware of the type of pain or the exact location of the pain. Fibers that transmit pain information from the thalamus to the cerebral cortex provide us with that additional information.

The **hypothalamus** is the second structure in the diencephalon. It is situated directly below the thalamus and helps regulate many body processes, including body temperature (thermostat), water balance, and metabolism. Because the hypothalamus helps regulate the function of the autonomic (involuntary) nerves, it exerts an effect on heart rate, blood pressure, and respiration.

Located under the hypothalamus is the pituitary gland. The pituitary gland directly or indirectly affects almost every hormone in the body. Because the hypothalamus controls pituitary function, the widespread effects of the hypothalamus are obvious. (The relationship of the hypothalamus to endocrine function is described in Chapter 14.)

? Re-Think

1. What roles do the visual and auditory association areas play?
2. What is the function of the basal nuclei?
3. What is the relationship of the hypothalamus to the pituitary gland?
4. What functions are influenced by the hypothalamus?

BRAIN STEM

The **brain stem** connects the spinal cord with higher brain structures. It is composed of the midbrain, pons, and medulla oblongata (see Fig. 10.14). The white matter of the brain stem includes tracts that relay both sensory and motor information to and from the cerebrum. Scattered throughout the white matter of the brain stem are patches of gray matter called *nuclei*. These nuclei exert profound effects on functions such as blood pressure and respiration.

MIDBRAIN

The midbrain extends from the lower diencephalon to the pons. Like the rest of the brain-stem structures, the midbrain relays sensory and motor information. The midbrain also contains nuclei that function as reflex centers for vision and hearing.

PONS

The pons (bridge) extends from the midbrain to the medulla oblongata. It is composed primarily of tracts that act as a bridge for information traveling to and from several brain structures. The pons also plays an important role in the regulation of breathing rate and rhythm.

MEDULLA OBLONGATA

The **medulla oblongata** (meh-DUL-ah oh-blohn-GAHT-ah) connects the spinal cord with the pons. The medulla acts as a relay for sensory and motor information. Several important nuclei within the medulla control the vital functions: heart rate, blood pressure, and respiration. Because of its importance with regard to these life-sustaining functions, the medulla oblongata is called the *vital center*.

The medulla oblongata is sensitive to certain drugs, especially opioids such as morphine. An overdose of an opioid causes depression of the medulla oblongata and death because the person stops breathing. This danger is the reason for assessing respiratory rate before giving a patient an opioid.

 Do You Know...

How the Brain Tranquilizes Itself?

The brain produces natural morphine-like substances called *endorphins* (endogenous morphine) and *enkephalins* (meaning "in the head"). Like morphine, these substances bind to opiate receptors in the CNS, moderating pain, relieving anxiety, and producing a sense of well-being. The "high" experienced by joggers may be caused by endorphins and enkephalins.

Vomiting Center

The medulla oblongata contains the vomiting center, or emetic center (emesis refers to vomiting). The vomiting center can be activated directly or indirectly. Direct activation includes stimuli from the cerebral cortex (fear), stimuli from sensory organs (distressing sights, bad odors, pain), and signals from the equilibrium apparatus of the inner ear (spinning). Indirect stimulation of the vomiting center comes from the chemoreceptor trigger zone (CTZ) located in the floor of the fourth ventricle. The CTZ can be stimulated by emetogenic compounds, such as anticancer drugs and opioids. Signals from the digestive tract, especially the stomach, travel via the vagus nerve to the CTZ. The CTZ, in turn, activates the vomiting center. Antiemetic agents can work on both the CTZ and medullary vomiting center to relieve nausea and vomiting. The pharmacological management of vomiting is a common clinical problem. Another interesting point is that nausea, which often precedes vomiting, is derived from the Greek word for "ship," as in seasickness.

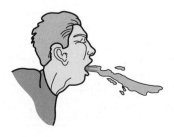

1. List the three parts of the brain stem.
2. Why is the medulla oblongata called the "vital center"?
3. Differentiate between the vomiting center and the CTZ.

CEREBELLUM

The **cerebellum** (sair-eh-BELL-um), the fourth major area, is the structure that protrudes from under the occipital lobe (see Fig. 10. 14). The interior of the cerebellum is composed largely of white tracts. Notice the appearance of the tracts; the cerebellum looks like a tree and is therefore called the *arbor vitae* or literally the "living tree." The cerebellum is connected to the brain stem by three pairs of cerebellar peduncles (sair-eh-BELL-ahr peh-DUN-kuls); these connections allow the cerebellum to receive, integrate, and deliver information to many parts of the brain and spinal cord. The cerebellum is concerned with the coordination of voluntary muscle activity and maintaining equilibrium and posture. Damage to the cerebellum produces jerky muscle movements, staggering gait, and difficulty maintaining balance. The person with cerebellar dysfunction may appear intoxicated. To help diagnose cerebellar dysfunction, the physician may ask the person to touch the tip of his or her nose with a finger. Why? The cerebellum normally coordinates skeletal muscle activity. In attempting to touch the nose, a patient with cerebellar dysfunction may overshoot, first to one side and then to the other.

The cerebellum also plays an important role in the evaluation of sensory input. For example, the cerebellum allows a person to evaluate the texture of different fabrics without seeing the fabric. It also "times" events, thereby allowing the person to predict where a moving object will be in the next few seconds. For example, a basketball player has a keen sense of where the ball is and should be in the next dribble or two. And, most of us can rhythmically drum our fingers on a desk—a task that is impaired in someone with cerebellar dysfunction.

 Do You Know...

Where and Why There Is a Tent in Your Brain?

At several areas in the brain, the dura mater forms rigid membranes that separate and support parts of the brain. One such membrane is the tentorium cerebelli; it forms a tentlike membrane over the cerebellum, separating it from the upper cerebral structures. The tentorium also functions as a common landmark in the brain. Brain tumors are classified according to their locations; those that occur in structures located above the tentorium are called *supratentorial brain tumors*, and those occurring below the tentorium are called *infratentorial brain tumors*. An increase in intracranial pressure can force the brain downward past the tentorium, causing life-threatening symptoms. The displacement is called *tentorial herniation*.

Re-Think

1. Locate and list two functions of the cerebellum.
2. Why is a "staggering gait" characteristic of cerebellar dysfunction?

STRUCTURES ACROSS DIVISIONS OF THE BRAIN

Three important structures are not confined to any of the four divisions of the brain because they "overlap" several areas. These structures are the limbic system, the reticular system, and the memory areas.

LIMBIC SYSTEM: THE EMOTIONAL BRAIN

Parts of the cerebrum and the diencephalon form a wishbone-shaped group of structures called the *limbic system*. The **limbic system** functions in emotional states and behavior. For example, when the limbic system is stimulated by electrodes, states of extreme pleasure or rage can be induced. Because of these responses, the limbic system is called the *emotional brain*.

RETICULAR FORMATION

Extending through the entire brain stem and diencephalon, with numerous connections to the cerebral cortex, is a special mass of gray matter called the **reticular formation**.

The reticular formation has both a sensory and motor function. Its primary sensory function is to alert the cerebral cortex of incoming sensory information. Its primary motor function is to regulate muscle tone, the mild state of muscle contraction while the body is at rest.

Other nuclei within the reticular formation include the gaze centers (allow the eyes to track an object) and special groups of cells that rhythmically send signals to the muscles that control breathing and swallowing. The reticular formation is also concerned with habituation, the process whereby the brain learns to ignore repetitive background information. For example, a parent may ignore the background noise of children playing and horns honking, but responds immediately to a crying child. Similarly, while driving a car, you ignore much of the background visual information but are aware of traffic signals, nearby cars and, hopefully, any oncoming vehicles.

Reticular Activating System (RAS): Wakefulness, Sleep, and Coma

A portion of the reticular formation, the reticular activating system (RAS) is concerned with the sleep–wake cycle. Signals passing up to the cerebral cortex from the RAS stimulate us, keeping us awake and tuned in. Diminished activation of the RAS produces sleep, a state from which one can be aroused. What causes sleep? In the 6th century BC, it was believed that sleep was caused by a temporary retreat of blood from the brain. Death was attributed to the permanent retreat of blood from the brain. As to the cause of sleep today? We still do not know. What we do know is that neurotransmitters are replenished during sleep. We also know that most Americans do not get enough sleep (most adults require 7 to 8 hours of sleep) and that sleep deprivation is linked to numerous health problems, such as obesity, diabetes mellitus, and hypertension.

Coma is a hyporesponsive state with several stages, ranging from light to deep coma. In the lightest stages of coma, some reflexes are intact; the patient may respond to light, sound, touch, and painful stimuli. As the coma deepens, however, these reflexes are gradually lost, and the patient eventually becomes unresponsive to all stimuli. Many clinical conditions affect level of consciousness (LOC) or awareness. As a clinician, you must be able to assess the patient's LOC.

 Re-Think

1. Locate the limbic system, and explain why it is called the "emotional brain."
2. State a major role of the reticular activating system.
3. List two ways that you would evaluate LOC.

Stages of Sleep

The two types of sleep are non–rapid eye movement (NREM) sleep and rapid eye movement (REM) sleep. The four stages of NREM sleep progress from light to deep. In a typical 8-hour sleep period, a person regularly cycles through the various stages of sleep, descending from light to deep sleep and then ascending from deeper sleep to lighter sleep.

REM sleep is characterized by fluctuating blood pressure, respiratory rate and rhythm, and pulse rate. The most obvious characteristic of REM sleep is rapid eye movements, for which the sleep segment is named. REM sleep totals 90 to 120 minutes per night; most dreaming occurs during REM sleep. For unknown reasons, REM sleep deprivation is associated with mental and physical distress. Most sedatives and CNS depressants adversely affect REM sleep, perhaps accounting for that "hangover" feeling that often follows their use.

 Do You Know...

About Chemo Fog?

We all know that many drugs exert profound effects on the brain. There is the euphoria of opioids, the hallucinogenic effects of LSD, the "buzz" of methamphetamines, the sedation of antihistamines, and the list goes on. For many years, breast cancer survivors have complained of the lingering effects of their cancer chemotherapy. Many noted difficulty with memory, attention span, retrieving words, multitasking, and clarity of thought. (One woman filled the water glasses with turkey gravy at a Thanksgiving Day dinner.) They complained of "living in a fog"—hence, the term *chemo fog* or *chemobrain*. Chemo fog is real and lingers for many months, even years, after the chemo has ended! Today it has a new, respectable name: *postchemotherapy cognitive impairment*, or *postchemotherapy cognitive dysfunction*.

MEMORY AREAS

Memory is the ability to recall thoughts and images. Many areas of the brain are concerned with memory. There are three categories of memory: immediate memory, short-term memory, and long-term memory. Immediate memory lasts for a few seconds. An example of your immediate memory is your ability to remember the words in the first part of the sentence so that you can get the thought of the entire sentence. Short-term memory lasts for a short period (seconds to a few hours). It allows you to recall bits of information, such as the price of those new jeans or a phone number that you looked up. Unfortunately, cramming for exams falls into this category—short-term memorization, 5-second retention, and then: BLANK. Long-term memory lasts much longer—years, decades, or a lifetime. If you continuously use the new address or phone number, you will enter that information into your long-term memory. The same effect is achieved when you study over a longer period. Another interesting point: although memory is important, forgetting is also important. Imagine all the trivial information that you take in every second. Think of the many stones, trees, birds, street signs, and other things that you pass on your way to work. Persons who have difficulty in forgetting trivia have a great deal of difficulty in comprehension and in remembering things that need to be remembered.

 Re-Think

1. What is REM sleep?
2. List the three categories of memory. Explain why "cramming" for an exam is an ineffectual learning process.

 Do You Know...

Why People in Ancient Times Bored Holes in the Skull?

Trephination refers to the drilling of holes into the skull for the purpose of reducing intracranial pressure. Today, it is performed in the operating room under sterile conditions; the surgically drilled holes are called *burr holes*. People in ancient times also performed trephination procedures. The patient sat on a log while the priest chipped a hole in the skull using a sharp stone. Ouch! It was thought that trephination could relieve headaches and release the devils of madness.

PROTECTING THE CENTRAL NERVOUS SYSTEM

The tissue of the CNS (brain and spinal cord) is very delicate. Injury to CNS neuronal tissue cannot be repaired. Thus, the CNS has an elaborate protective system that consists of four structures: bone, meninges, cerebrospinal fluid, and the blood–brain barrier.

BONE: FIRST LAYER OF PROTECTION

The CNS is protected by bone. The brain is encased in the cranium, and the spinal cord is encased in the vertebral column.

MENINGES: SECOND LAYER OF PROTECTION

Three layers of connective tissue surround the brain and spinal cord (Fig. 10.15). These tissues are called the **meninges** (meh-NIN-jeez). The outermost layer is a thick, tough, connective tissue called the *dura mater,* literally meaning "hard mother." Inside the skull, the dural membrane splits to form the dural sinuses. These sinuses are filled with blood. Beneath the dura mater is a small space called the *subdural space.* The middle meningeal layer is the arachnoid (ah-RAK-noyd) mater (meaning "spider-like"), so named because the membrane looks like a spider web.

The pia mater is the innermost layer and literally means "soft or gentle mother." The pia mater is a very thin membrane that contains many blood vessels and lies delicately over the brain and spinal cord. These blood vessels supply the brain with much of its blood. Between the arachnoid layer and the pia mater is a space called the **subarachnoid space.** A fluid called the **cerebrospinal fluid (CSF)** circulates within this space and forms a cushion around the brain and spinal cord. If the head is jarred suddenly, the brain first bumps into this soft cushion of fluid. Specialized projections of the arachnoid membrane, called the *arachnoid villi* (sing., villus), protrude up into the blood-filled dural sinuses and are involved in the drainage of the CSF (described in the next section).

Remember—the meninges form a brain **PAD** (noting that the brain is closer to pia, the softer mother):

P	**p**ia mater
A	**a**rachnoid mater
D	**d**ura mater

The meninges can become inflamed or infected, causing meningitis. Meningitis is serious because the infection can spread to the brain, sometimes causing serious, irreversible brain damage. The bacterial or viral organism causing the meningitis can often be found in a sample of CSF obtained by lumbar puncture.

CEREBROSPINAL FLUID: THIRD LAYER OF PROTECTION

The CSF forms a third protective layer of the CNS. CSF is formed from the blood within the brain. It is a clear fluid that looks like clear soda and is similar in composition to plasma. The CSF is composed of water, glucose, protein, and several ions, especially Na^+ and Cl^-. An adult circulates about 130 mL of CSF; 500 mL is formed every 24 hours, so CSF is replaced every 8 hours. In addition to its protective function, CSF also delivers nutrients to the CNS and removes waste.

Where is CSF formed? CSF is formed within the ventricles of the brain by a structure called the **choroid plexus** (Fig. 10.16). The four ventricles are two lateral ventricles and a third and fourth ventricle. The choroid plexus, a grapelike collection of blood vessels and

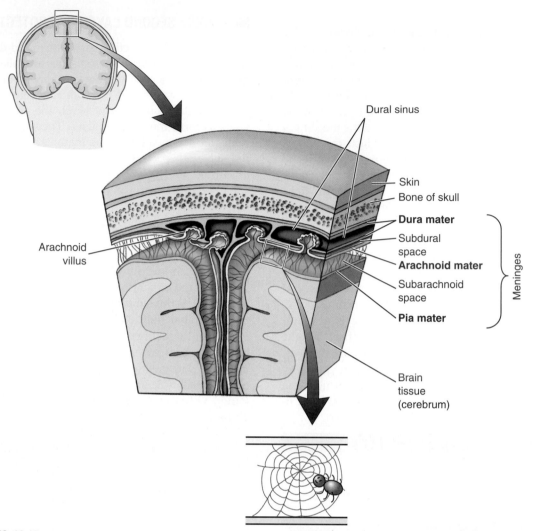

FIG. 10.15 **Three layers of meninges: the dura mater, arachnoid mater, and pia mater. Note the subarachnoid space, arachnoid villi, and dural sinuses.**

ependymal cells (see Table 10.1), is suspended from the roof of each ventricle. Water and dissolved substances are transported from the blood across the walls of the choroid plexus into the ventricles (see Fig. 10.16).

Where does the CSF flow? As CSF leaves the ventricles, it follows two paths. Some of the CSF flows through a hole in the center of the spinal cord called the *central canal*. The central canal eventually drains into the subarachnoid space at the base of the spinal cord. The rest of the CSF flows from the fourth ventricle laterally through tiny holes, or foramina, into the subarachnoid space that encircles the brain.

How does the CSF leave the subarachnoid space? Eventually, CSF flows into the arachnoid villi; water and waste diffuse from CSF in the arachnoid villi into the blood of the dural sinuses. Blood then flows from the dural sinuses into the cerebral veins and back to the heart. Remember that the CSF is formed across the walls of the choroid plexus within the ventricles, circulates throughout the subarachnoid space around the brain and spinal cord, and then drains into the dural sinuses. The rate at which CSF is formed must equal the rate at which it is drained. If excess CSF is formed or drainage is impaired, CSF will accumulate in the ventricles of the brain, increasing the pressure within the skull. If the flow of CSF occurs before the sutures in the skull fuse, the child may develop hydrocephalus, increased intracranial pressure, and brain damage. Fortunately, shunting procedures restore the flow of CSF by surgically creating a detour around the blocked pathway.

Do You Know...

What a Little Red Worm's Doing in Your Brain?

In the 1300s, an anatomist claimed that mental function was controlled by a red worm. The worm referred to the fleshy choroid plexus of the ventricles of the brain. The plexi allegedly controlled brain functions by wiggling back and forth and modifying the flow of cerebrospinal fluid (CSF), which was supposed to contain the animal spirit. Several things have since been cleared up; mental function is the result of neuronal activity and not the flow of animal spirit, and the choroid plexus secretes CSF and does not wiggle and shake. There is, however, a little red worm—the choroid plexus—and it is located in the ventricles of your brain, where it secretes CSF.

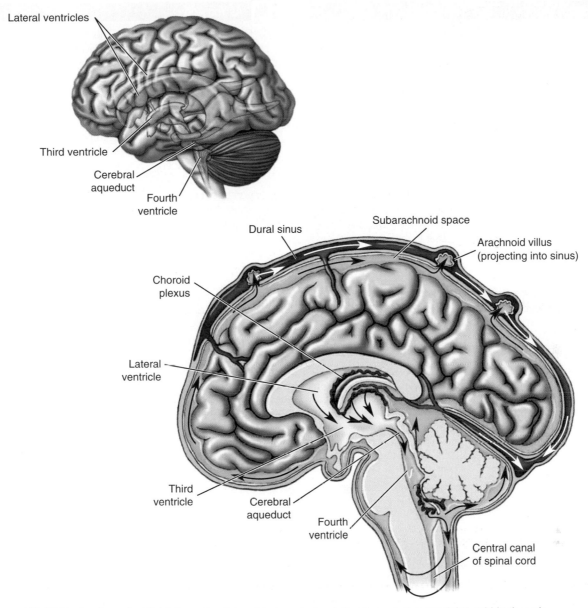

FIG. 10.16 Cerebrospinal fluid: formation (choroid plexus); circulation through the ventricles, within the sub-arachnoid space, and in the central canal; and drainage through the arachnoid villi and dural sinuses.

BLOOD–BRAIN BARRIER: FOURTH LAYER OF PROTECTION

The blood–brain barrier is an arrangement of cells, particularly the glial astrocytes and the selectively permeable capillary cells; they act as a barrier to the movement of potentially harmful chemicals into the CNS. The astrocytes and the capillary cells select the substances allowed to enter the CNS from the blood. For example, oxygen, glucose, and certain ions readily cross the membrane. However, if a potentially harmful substance is present in the blood, the cells of the blood–brain barrier prevent that substance from entering the brain and the spinal cord.

Although the blood–brain barrier is successful in screening many harmful substances, not all toxic substances are blocked. Alcohol, for example, crosses the blood–brain barrier and affects brain tissue.

The blood–brain barrier may present a problem in the pharmacological treatment of infections within the CNS. Most antibiotics, for example, cannot cross the blood–brain barrier and therefore cannot reach the site of infection. Given this problem, how is an infection of the CNS treated? The two options are to select an antibiotic that does cross the blood–brain barrier or inject the antibiotic directly into the subarachnoid space; this mode of drug delivery is called an *intrathecal injection*.

? Re-Think

1. Trace the formation, flow, and drainage of CSF.
2. What is the consequence of obstructed drainage of CSF?
3. What is the blood–brain barrier?
4. What effect may the blood–brain barrier have on drug distribution?

Sum It Up!

The brain makes us humans—that is, thinking, sensing, doing, caring, feeling, remembering persons. It also coordinates the various organ systems of the body efficiently, with fine precision. The brain is divided into four regions: the cerebrum, diencephalon, brain stem, and cerebellum. The cerebrum is the largest part of the brain and has four lobes: frontal, parietal, temporal, and occipital. The diencephalon is composed of the thalamus and the hypothalamus. The brain stem is composed of the midbrain, pons, and medulla oblongata. The medulla oblongata is considered the vital structure in that it affects basic functions such as respiration, cardiac function, and blood vessel tone. Three other areas are the reticular formation, which keeps us awake; the limbic system (emotional brain); and the memory areas. Because of the crucial role played by the CNS, it is afforded excellent protection—that is, bone, three layers of meninges, a soft cushion of fluid, and a blood–brain barrier.

 As You Age

1. Beginning at the age of 30, the number of neurons decreases. The number lost, however, is only a small percentage of the total number of brain cells and does not cause mental impairment. Although a decrease in short-term memory may cause some forgetfulness, most memory, alertness, intellectual functioning, and creativity remain intact. Severe alteration of mental functioning is generally caused by age-related diseases such as arteriosclerosis.
2. Impulse conduction speed decreases along an axon, amounts of neurotransmitters are reduced, and the number of receptor sites decreases at the synapses. These changes result in progressive slowing of responses and reflexes.

Medical Terminology and Disorders   Disorders of the Brain

MEDICAL TERM	WORD PARTS	WORD PART MEANING OR DERIVATION	DESCRIPTION
Words			
meninges		From a Latin word meaning "membrane"	The **meninges** are *the three membranes that form the outer lining of the brain and spinal cord.* The Arabians referred to these membranes as *mater* (mother) because they believed these membranes were the "mother" of all membranes.
neurology	neur/o-	nerve	**Neurology** is *the study of the structure, function, and organic disorders of the nervous system.*
	-logy	study of	
Polarize		From a French word meaning a "division within a group"	*Refers to a separation of electrical charge.* A **polarized** nerve cell has a negative charge on the inside of the cell membrane and a positive charge on the outside of the cell membrane. The electric charge of a **depolarized** (*de* = away from) cell becomes positive. A **repolarized** (*re* = again) cell has returned to an internal negative charge.
Synapse	syn-	together	A **synapse** is *a junction or meeting place for two neurons.* The axon of one neuron interacts chemically at a **synapse** with the dendrite of a second neuron.
	-apse	From a Greek word, *haptein,* meaning "to clasp"	
Disorders			
cephalgia	cephal/o-	Head	*Pain in the head or headache.* An example is the **migraine headache,** a severe, recurring headache that usually affects only one side of the head. (*Migraine* comes from the Latin *hemicranium,* meaning "one side of the head.") A simple **tension headache** may develop when a person is anxious or tense. Headaches may also develop secondarily in response to increased intracranial pressure (e.g., brain tumor), irritation of the meninges, or spasm of the cerebral blood vessels. **Cluster headaches** occur in cyclical patterns and are called "alarm clock headaches" because they often awaken the person with intense and sharp pain in and around one eye.
	-algia	Pain	
cerebrovascular accident (CVA)			Called a **CVA, stroke,** or **brain attack.** A CVA is caused by a sudden lack of blood, causing oxygen deprivation and brain damage. Depending on the location and severity of the brain damage, a CVA can result in loss of sensory and motor function and speech impairment. The patient often experiences **hemiparalysis** (hemi- = half) and **hemiparesis.** In addition to loss of motor function, the patient experiences various types of **aphasia** (a- = without; phas/o = speech), *an impairment of language.* Before suffering a stroke, many persons will have experienced a **transient ischemic attack** (TIA), or *mini stroke.* During a TIA, blood flow to the brain is temporarily stopped or diminished.

Medical Terminology and Disorders   Disorders of the Brain—cont'd

MEDICAL TERM	WORD PARTS	WORD PART MEANING OR DERIVATION	DESCRIPTION
dementia	de-	without	Originally from the Latin meaning "madness." **Dementia** is not a single disease, but *a group of symptoms affecting intellectual and social abilities to the extent that daily living is impaired.* There is a serious loss of cognitive ability, with impairment of language, problem solving, memory, attention, and judgment. Behavior may be disorganized, restless, and inappropriate. **Static dementia** is commonly caused by traumatic brain injury. **Progressive dementia** refers to a long-term decline and is caused by chronic conditions such as Alzheimer's disease, multiple sclerosis, and small or mini-strokes **(vascular dementia).**
	-ment/o-	mind	
	-ia	condition of	
dyskinesias	dys-	difficulty	*Any medical disorder that is characterized by diminished voluntary muscle control (a movement disorder).* This broad term includes Parkinson's disease, Tourette's syndrome (muscle tics, verbal outbursts, sometimes profanity), chorea ("dancelike" muscle contractions that begin in one part of the body [toe] and work their way to another part [leg]), athetosis (graceful but purposeless movements primarily of the extremities), and asterixis ("flapping tremor" of the wrists). The term **dyskinesia** also includes many dystonias (impaired muscle tone), sustained muscle contractions that twist or contort the body. Some types of dyskinesias are localized, as in torticollis (lateral flexion of the neck caused by muscle spasm), whereas others are generalized, as in epileptic seizures. Tardive dyskinesias (TDs), often a result of antipsychotic drug therapy and dopaminergic antagonists, are characterized by involuntary movement of the lips (lip smacking), tongue (tongue rolling, protrusions), face, trunk, and extremities. Drug-induced TDs are usually irreversible.
	-kinesi/o-	movement	
	-ia	condition of	
encephalopathy	en-	within	*A broad term that refers to disease, damage, or dysfunction of the brain.* There are more than 150 types. The term **encephalopathy** is often described by its cause. **Anoxic encephalopathy** is due to a lack of oxygen, whereas **hepatic encephalopathy** is a response to liver disease. Chronic and excessive ingestion of alcohol causes irreversible injury to the nervous system. The result is mental deterioration, loss of memory, inability to concentrate, irritability, and uncoordinated movement. **Wernicke–Korsakoff syndrome** is an alcohol-related type of encephalopathy.
	-cephal/o-	Head	
	-path/o-	disease	
	-y	condition or process	
Epilepsy	epi-	Upon	Historically referred to as the "sacred disease" by the ancients because they believed that epilepsy was a punishment for offending the gods. Epilepsy is a group of neurological disorders that all present with spontaneous seizure activity. Neurons in the brain fire suddenly, unpredictably, and repetitively, creating "electrical storms" in the brain. Although most cases of epilepsy are idiopathic (arising spontaneously; unknown) in origin, many underlying conditions cause seizure activity: brain tumors, toxins, trauma, fever **(febrile seizures),** and emotional stress. Epileptic seizures are classified as primarily generalized seizures (widespread electrical storm including both sides of the brain) and partial seizures (more limited brain involvement and localized responses). There are many types of seizures, two of which are **tonic-clonic seizures** (grand mal) and **absence seizures** (petit mal). The tonic phase of a grand mal seizure occurs when the motor areas fire repetitively, causing muscle stiffening, and loss of consciousness. The clonic phase is characterized by jerking activity. **Status epilepticus,** a medical emergency, refers to the failure of the seizures to resolve or to the rapid succession of seizure activity. Absence seizures occur when sensory areas are affected, causing a brief period (5–15 sec) of altered consciousness. They are not accompanied by generalized stiffening or prolonged unconsciousness and are often unnoticed. Epileptic seizures are described by the term **ictus.**
		From a Latin word meaning "seized upon" (by the gods)	
Glioma	gli/o-	Glue	**Glioma** is *the most common type of primary brain tumors in adults.* They arise from glial tissue, most commonly astrocytic (star-shaped) tissue (astrocytoma). The second most common brain tumor is a **meningioma,** arising from the meninges. Brain tumors can be malignant or benign.
	-oma	Tumor	

Continued

Medical Terminology and Disorders   Disorders of the Brain—cont'd

MEDICAL TERM	WORD PARTS	WORD PART MEANING OR DERIVATION	DESCRIPTION
head injury			*Due to trauma of the head, and may or may not involve the brain.* A **traumatic brain injury** (TBI) occurs when an external force traumatically injures the brain. TBI is a major cause of death and disability worldwide. Initially, brain injury is due to direct impact or by acceleration/deceleration alone; additional injury is sustained secondarily by injury-induced diminishment of blood flow and increases in intracranial pressure. A mechanism-related classification system divides TBIs into closed and penetrating head injuries. A **closed head injury** occurs when the brain is not exposed, as in blunt trauma. A **penetrating (open) head injury** occurs when the penetrating object pierces the dura mater. Depending on its severity and location, TBI causes numerous deficits: physical, emotional, social, and cognitive. Trauma to the head can cause bleeding and the formation of a **hematoma,** *a swelling or tumor formed by a collection of blood.* An **epidural hematoma** forms between the dura mater and the skull. A **subdural hematoma** forms under the dura mater.
hydrocephalus	hydro-	Water	Called "water on the brain." There is an abnormal accumulation of cerebrospinal fluid (CSF) within the cerebral ventricles that can cause enlargement of the cranium. The clinical presentation is dependent on chronicity and age. There is also a **normal pressure hydrocephalus** (NPH), which develops more gradually in the elderly and is characterized by intermittent episodes of increased intracranial pressure.
	-cephal/o-	Head	
infection		From the Latin word *inficere,* meaning transmission of disease by agency of air or water	The brain can be infected by a large number of microorganisms, most commonly bacteria and viruses. The pathogens cause inflammation of the surrounding tissue. **Encephalitis** is *inflammation of the brain itself.* **Meningitis** is *inflammation of the meninges.* A **brain abscess** is *a collection of infectious material within the brain.* Globally, bacterial meningitis is a major health concern in children. African children living in the "meningitis belt" are particularly vulnerable.
neurotoxin	neur/o-	Nerve	*Any natural or artificial substance that is toxic or harmful to nervous tissue.* Commonly encountered neurotoxins include chemotherapeutic drugs, organic solvents, pesticides, cosmetics, heavy metals, alcohol ingestion, and exposure to radiation. There are some naturally occurring neurotoxins, including beta-amyloid and glutamate.
	-tox/o-	Poison	
Palsy			A generalized term that refers to a loss of motor function. Three types of palsy are cerebral palsy, Bell's palsy, and brachial palsy (Erb's palsy). **Cerebral palsy** (CP), also called **spastic paralysis,** is a consequence of brain injury most often occurring in response to anoxic conditions around birth. All persons with CP experience muscle tightness and spasm causing limitations in muscle movement. **Bell's palsy** is due to inflammation or injury to the facial nerve (CN VII). **Brachial palsy** is usually caused by damage to the brachial plexus during a traumatic birth experience.
Parkinson's disease		Named after J. Parkinson, an English professor who wrote extensively about the disease	Called "shaking palsy." **Parkinson's disease** (PD) is *a dyskinesia that is classified as a movement disorder; it is due to diminished dopaminergic cell activity in the basal ganglia.* PD is characterized by tremors (rest tremors) or shaking of the extremities, especially the hands and jaw; rigidity (muscle stiffness), **akinesia** (inability to initiate voluntary movement), **bradykinesia** (slow voluntary movement), stooped posture, shuffling or freezing gait, poor balance, slow speech, and drooling. Cognitive abilities are generally preserved. **Parkinsonism** is a broad term that refers to disorders that present with similar symptoms. For instance, prolonged use of antipsychotic drugs and brain injuries sustained by boxers cause symptoms similar to PD.

Ready for Exams!

Summary Outline

The purpose of the nervous system is to bring information to the central nervous system, interpret the information, and enable the body to respond to the information.

I. The Nervous System: Overview
  A. Divisions of the nervous system
    1. The central nervous system (CNS) includes the brain and the spinal cord.
    2. The peripheral nervous system includes the nerves that connect the CNS with the rest of the body.
  B. Cells that make up the nervous system
    1. Neuroglia (glia) support, protect, and nourish the neurons.
    2. Neurons conduct the nerve impulse.
    3. The three parts of a neuron are the dendrites, cell body, and axon.
  C. Types of neurons
    1. Sensory, or afferent, neurons carry information toward the CNS.
    2. Motor, or efferent, neurons carry information away from the CNS toward the periphery.
    3. Interneurons are located in the CNS (make connections).
  D. White matter and gray matter
    1. White matter is the result of myelinated fibers.
    2. Gray matter is composed primarily of cell bodies, interneurons, and unmyelinated fibers.
    3. Clusters of cell bodies (gray matter) are called *nuclei* and *ganglia*.

II. The Neuron Carrying Information
  A. Nerve impulse
    1. The electrical signal is called the *action potential* or *nerve impulse*.
    2. The nerve impulse is caused by the following changes in the neuron: polarization, depolarization, and repolarization.
    3. Initial depolarization must reach threshold potential in order for the neuron to become fully depolarized.
    4. The nerve impulse results from the flow of ions: polarization (outward leak of K^+), depolarization (influx of Na^+), and repolarization (outward flux of K^+).
    5. The nerve impulse jumps from node to node as it travels along a myelinated fiber. Myelination increases the speed of the nerve impulse.
    6. The nerve impulse causes the release of the neurotransmitter at the synapse.
  B. Synapse
    1. The synapse is a space between two neurons.
    2. The nerve impulse of the first (presynaptic) neuron causes the release of neurotransmitter into the synaptic cleft. The neurotransmitter diffuses across the synaptic cleft and binds to the receptors on the second (postsynaptic) membrane. The activation of the receptors stimulates a nerve impulse in the second neuron.

III. Brain: Structure and Function
  A. Cerebrum
    1. The right and left hemispheres are joined by the corpus callosum.
    2. The four main cerebral lobes are the frontal, parietal, temporal, and occipital lobes. Functions of each lobe are summarized in Table 10.2.
    3. Large areas of the cerebrum, called *association areas,* are concerned with interpreting, integrating, and analyzing information.
  B. Diencephalon
    1. The thalamus is a relay station for most sensory tracts traveling to the cerebrum.
    2. The hypothalamus controls many body functions such as water balance, temperature, and the secretion of hormones from the pituitary gland. It exerts an effect on the autonomic nervous system.
  C. Brain stem
    1. Brain stem: midbrain, pons, and medulla oblongata
    2. The medulla oblongata is called the *vital center* because it controls the heart rate, blood pressure, and respirations (the vital functions).
    3. The vomiting center is located in the medulla oblongata; it receives input directly and indirectly from activation of the chemoreceptor trigger zone (CTZ).
  D. Cerebellum
    1. The cerebellum is sometimes called the *little brain.*
    2. The cerebellum is concerned primarily with the coordination of voluntary muscle activity.
  E. Structures involving more than one lobe
    1. The limbic system is sometimes called the *emotional brain.*
    2. The reticular formation alerts the cerebral cortex of sensory signals and regulates muscle tone in the resting state.
    3. The reticular activating system (RAS) is a specialized area of the reticular formation and is concerned with the sleep–wake cycle. It keeps us awake.
    4. Decreased activity of the RAS induces sleep.
    5. There are two types of sleep: REM and NREM.
    6. The memory areas handle immediate, short-term, and long-term memory.

IV. Protection of the CNS
  A. Bone: cranium and vertebral column
  B. Meninges: pia mater, arachnoid mater, and dura mater
  C. Cerebrospinal fluid (CSF): forms across the choroid plexus, circulates throughout the subarachnoid space, and drains from the arachnoid villi into the blood of the dural sinuses
  D. Blood–brain barrier

Review Your Knowledge

Matching: Nerve Cells
Directions: Match the following words with their descriptions.

a. neurons
b. ganglia
c. CNS
d. neuroglia
e. axon terminal
f. axon
g. nodes of Ranvier
h. Schwann cell
i. dendrite
j. myelin

1. ___ Storage site for neurotransmitters
2. ___ Nerve glue—astrocytes and ependymal cells
3. ___ Part of the neuron that carries the action potential away from the cell body
4. ___ Nerve cells that transmit information by way of electrical signals called action potentials
5. ___ Composed of the brain and the spinal cord
6. ___ Clusters of cell bodies located outside of the CNS
7. ___ White insulating material that surrounds the axon; increases the speed at which the electrical signal travels along the axon
8. ___ Short segments of an axon that are not covered with myelin; allow for saltatory conduction
9. ___ A glial cell that makes myelin
10. ___ Treelike structure of the neuron that receives information from another neuron and transmits that information to the cell body

Matching: Brain
Directions: Match the following words with their descriptions. Some words can be used more than once.

a. medulla oblongata
b. frontal
c. occipital
d. parietal
e. hypothalamus
f. temporal

1. ___ Cerebral lobe that performs the "executive functions" and contains the primary motor cortex
2. ___ Part of the brain stem that is called the *vital center*
3. ___ Part of the diencephalon that controls body temperature (thermostat) and endocrine function by its influence on the pituitary gland
4. ___ Location of the somatosensory area
5. ___ Cerebral lobe that contains the primary visual area
6. ___ Considered part of the diencephalon
7. ___ This structure descends through the foramen magnum as the spinal cord
8. ___ Considered part of the brain stem
9. ___ Cerebral lobe that contains the primary auditory area

Multiple Choice

1. The precentral gyrus is
   a. located in the parietal lobe.
   b. the primary motor cortex.
   c. the primary visual cortex.
   d. a brain-stem structure.

2. Which of the following is *not* descriptive of Broca's area?
   a. Located in the frontal lobe
   b. Concerned with motor speech
   c. Most often located in the left cerebral hemisphere
   d. Concerned only with sensory functions

3. Which of the following statements is true?
   a. The medulla oblongata is a cerebral structure.
   b. The hypothalamus is a brain-stem structure.
   c. The medulla oblongata descends as the spinal cord.
   d. The midbrain, pons, and medulla oblongata are supratentorial structures.

4. Which of the following is *not* descriptive of the medulla oblongata?
   a. It is a brain-stem structure.
   b. It is called the *vital center.*
   c. It is sensitive to the effects of narcotics (opioids).
   d. It performs the "executive" functions.

5. The postcentral gyrus
   a. is located in the parietal lobe.
   b. controls all voluntary motor activity.
   c. is the home of Broca's area.
   d. contains the primary visual cortex.

6. Cerebrospinal fluid (CSF)
   a. drains out of the subarachnoid space into the choroid plexus.
   b. circulates within the subarachnoid space.
   c. looks like blood.
   d. flows up the central canal into the fourth, third, and lateral ventricles.

7. Which of the following relationships is accurate?
   a. Temporal lobe: vision
   b. Frontal lobe: somatosensory (touch, pressure, pain)
   c. Occipital lobe: vision
   d. Parietal lobe: hearing

8. Neuroglia
   a. are classified as sensory and motor.
   b. include astrocytes, oligodendrocytes, Schwann cells, and ependymal cells.
   c. fire action potentials when stimulated.
   d. contain dendrites and axons.

9. Depolarization and repolarization
   a. are both caused by the movement of Na^+ into the neuron.
   b. are phases of the action potential.
   c. occur only in the neuroglia.
   d. are both caused by the movement of K^+ out of the neuron.

10. Activation of the emetic center or CTZ
    a. elevates blood pressure.
    b. lowers body temperature.
    c. causes diaphoresis.
    d. induces vomiting.

11. Characteristics of the hypothalamus include which of the following?
    a. Part of the diencephalon
    b. Synthesizes hormones (antidiuretic hormone and oxytocin)
    c. Controls pituitary gland activity
    d. All of the above

12. Schwann cells
    a. line the ventricles and help in the secretion of cerebrospinal fluid.
    b. are found in all glial cells.
    c. produce myelin sheath for neurons located within the peripheral nervous system.
    d. secrete cerebrospinal fluid.

13. The nodes of Ranvier
    a. are cells that secrete cerebrospinal fluid.
    b. are glial cells.
    c. are axonal sites covered by fatty insulation.
    d. are areas of the axonal membrane that are not covered by a myelin sheath.

14. Which of the following is true with regard to the nerve impulse?
    a. The outward leaky diffusion of K+ and trapped anions within the cell are responsible for the resting membrane potential.
    b. The rapid efflux of K+ from the neuron is responsible for depolarization.
    c. The rapid influx of Na+ is responsible for repolarization.
    d. The rapid efflux of Na+ is responsible for repolarization.

15. Which of the following describes the precentral and postcental gyri?
    a. Right and left hemispheres
    b. Motor and sensory
    c. Supratentorial and infratentorial
    d. Vision and hearing

Go Figure

1. Which of the following is correct according to Fig. 10.2?
    a. Panel A represents the brain making a decision to feed Kitty.
    b. Panel B represents the activation of sensory receptors in the eye enabling the boy to see the cat and the bowl.
    c. Panel B represents the decision-making ability of the CNS.
    d. Panel C represents activation of the touch receptors of the boy's right hand.

2. Which of the following is correct according to Fig. 10.4?
    a. The electrical signal runs from the axon terminals, along the axon, to the cell body and dendrites.
    b. The electrical signal runs from the cell body, along the axon, to the axon terminals.
    c. Nodes of Ranvier are myelinated axonal membranes.
    d. All dendrites are myelinated.

3. Which of the following is correct according to Fig. 10.5?
    a. Repolarization is characterized by a return of the membrane potential to its resting state.
    b. The inside of the repolarized neuron is (+).
    c. The inside of the depolarized neuron is (–).
    d. Depolarization is characterized by a return of the membrane potential to its resting state.

4. Which of the following is correct according to Fig. 10.6?
    a. The action potential only refers to attainment of threshold potential.
    b. The action potential refers to the depolarization and repolarization of the cell.
    c. The inside of the cell becomes more negative as the membrane potential moves from –90 mV to –60 mV.
    d. The threshold potential is a characteristic of the repolarizing phase of the resting membrane potential.

5. Which of the following is correct according to Fig. 10.7?
    a. Panel B illustrates the influx of Na+ and depolarization.
    b. Panel B illustrates the influx of Na+ and repolarization.
    c. Panel C illustrates the influx of K+ and depolarization.
    d. Panel C illustrates the efflux of K+ and depolarization.

6. Which of the following is correct according to Fig. 10.8?
    a. The action potential travels from the axon terminal to the cell body.
    b. The action potential (NI-1) at point A depolarizes the adjacent membrane, thereby causing NI-2 at point B.
    c. The electrical events at point C cause an action potential to form at point A.
    d. The electrical events at point D cause an action potential to form at point B.

7. Which of the following is illustrated in Fig. 10.9?
    a. The formation of a nerve impulse at each node
    b. The effect of myelination on conduction velocity (the speed at which the nerve impulse travels along the axon)
    c. Saltatory conduction
    d. All of the above

8. Which of the following is correct according to Fig. 10.10?
    a. Acetylcholine (ACh) is an enzyme that inactivates acetylcholinesterase.
    b. Acetylcholinesterase inactivates ACh immediately after its release from the axon terminal.
    c. The receptors on the membrane of neuron B are activated by ACh.
    d. Both acetylcholine and acetylcholinesterase are stored within the vesicles of the axon terminal.

9. Which of the following is correct according to Fig. 10.11?
    a. The diencephalon is a cerebral structure.
    b. The cerebellum is a brain-stem structure.
    c. The cerebrum is the largest and most superior of the areas of the brain.
    d. The brain stem is separated from the spinal cord by the cerebellum.

10. Which of the following is correct according to Fig. 10.12?
    a. The primary somatosensory area is located in the precentral gyrus.
    b. The primary motor area is located in the postcentral gyrus.
    c. Broca's area is concerned with motor speech and is located in the frontal lobe.
    d. The primary auditory cortex and the auditory association area are located in the occipital lobe.

11. According to Fig. 10.13, the homunculus
    a. is a sensory homunculus.
    b. lies over the cerebellum.
    c. depicts the function of the brain-stem structures.
    d. indicates that most of the precentral gyrus is dedicated to the motor activity of the face and hands.

12. Which of the following is correct according to Fig. 10.14?
    a. The pituitary gland is a brain-stem structure.
    b. The thalamus and hypothalamus are cerebral structures.
    c. The midbrain, pons, and medulla oblongata are brain-stem structures.
    d. The thalamus extends downward as the spinal cord.

13. Which of the following is correct according to Fig. 10.15?
    a. The arachnoid villi protrude into the dural sinuses.
    b. Cerebrospinal fluid circulates within the subarachnoid space.
    c. The dural sinuses are filled with blood.
    d. All of the above.

14. Which of the following is correct according to Fig. 10.16?
    a. Cerebrospinal fluid is secreted by the arachnoid villi and drained by the choroid plexus.
    b. The arachnoid villi protrude into the lateral ventricles, where they are bathed in cerebrospinal fluid.
    c. Cerebrospinal fluid is secreted by the choroid plexus into the dural sinuses.
    d. The cerebral aqueduct drains cerebrospinal fluid from the third ventricle.

Nervous System: Spinal Cord and Peripheral Nerves

Objectives

1. Describe the anatomy of the spinal cord, and list its three functions.
2. Discuss reflexes, and list four components of the reflex arc.
3. List and describe the functions of the 12 pairs of cranial nerves.
4. Do the following regarding the peripheral nervous system:
   - Identify the classification of spinal nerves.
   - List the functions of the three major plexuses.
   - Describe a dermatome.
   - Provide the functional classification of the peripheral nervous system.

Key Terms

afferent nerve (p. 215)
ascending tract (p. 202)
cranial nerves (p. 207)
decussate (p. 203)
dermatome (p. 212)
descending tract (p. 203)
efferent nerve (p. 215)

gray matter (p. 202)
mixed nerves (p. 207)
motor nerves (p. 207)
nerve (p. 207)
peripheral nervous system (p. 207)
plexus (p. 211)
reflex arc (p. 205)

sensory nerves (p. 207)
spinal cord (p. 201)
spinal nerves (p. 210)
tract (p. 207)
white matter (p. 202)

The brain, spinal cord, and peripheral nervous system work together as an intricate communication system. The spinal cord continuously carries information to and from the brain. In the absence of spinal cord function, no sensory activity is present, and the person cannot feel. The person also lacks voluntary motor activity and cannot move. The spinal cord also plays a crucial role in reflex activity, and many of our rapid and patterned responses are processed by the spinal cord.

WHAT THE SPINAL CORD IS

LOCATION AND SIZE

The **spinal cord** is a continuation of the brain stem. It is a tubelike structure located within the spinal cavity. The diameter of the spinal cord is similar to the thickness of your thumb. The spinal cord is about 17 inches (43 cm) long and extends from the foramen magnum of the occipital bone to the level of the first lumbar vertebra (L1), just below the bottom rib. Like the brain, the spinal cord is well protected by bone (vertebrae), meninges, cerebrospinal fluid (CSF), and the blood–brain barrier (Fig. 11.1).

An infant's spinal cord extends the full length of the spinal cavity. As the infant grows, however, the vertebral column grows faster than the cord. Because of the different rates of growth, the spinal cavity eventually becomes longer than the spinal cord, with the cord extending only to L1 in the adult. The meningeal membranes, however, extend the length of the spinal cavity.

This anatomical arrangement forms the basis for the site of a *lumbar puncture* (see Fig. 11.1B and C). In this procedure, a hollow needle is inserted into the subarachnoid space, between L3 and L4, at about the level of the top of the hip bone. A sample of CSF is withdrawn from the subarachnoid space. The CSF is then examined for pathogens, blood, or other abnormal signs. Because the spinal cord ends at L1, there is no danger of injuring the cord with the needle.

> **? Re-Think**
>
> 1. Describe the length and location of the adult spinal cord.
> 2. List the structures that protect the spinal cord.
> 3. Why is a lumbar puncture performed between L3 and L4?

GRAY ON THE INSIDE, WHITE ON THE OUTSIDE

GRAY MATTER

A cross-section of the spinal cord shows an area of gray matter and an area of white matter (Fig. 11.2). The

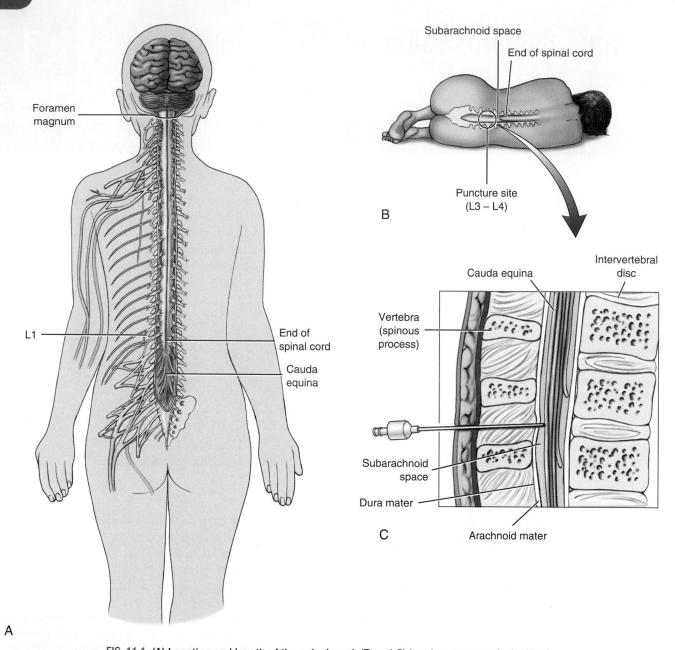

FIG. 11.1 (A) Location and length of the spinal cord. (B and C) Lumbar puncture (spinal tap).

gray matter is located in the center and is shaped like a butterfly. It is composed primarily of cell bodies, interneurons, and synapses. Two projections of the gray matter are the dorsal (posterior) horn and the ventral (anterior) horn. In the middle of the gray matter is the central canal. The central canal is a hole that extends the entire length of the spinal cord. It is open to the ventricular system in the brain and to the subarachnoid space at the bottom of the spinal cord. CSF flows from the ventricles in the brain down through the central canal into the subarachnoid space at the base of the spinal cord. The CSF then circulates throughout the subarachnoid space surrounding the spinal cord and brain.

WHITE MATTER

The **white matter** of the spinal cord is composed of myelinated and unmyelinated axons. These neuronal

axons are grouped together into sensory and motor tracts.

Sensory tracts carry information from the periphery, up the spinal cord, and toward the brain (see Fig. 11.2). They are therefore called **ascending tracts**. The spinothalamic (spy-no-thah-LAM-ik) tract is an example of an ascending tract. It carries sensory information for touch, pressure, and pain from the spinal cord to the thalamus in the brain. Note that the name of the tract (spinothalamic) often indicates its origin (spinal cord) and destination (thalamus). Where did the sensory information originate? From activation of receptors in the periphery. For instance, you accidentally injured your finger, thereby activating pain receptors in the finger. This information is carried by a sensory nerve to the spinal cord and brain where it is interpreted as pain. A peripheral sensory

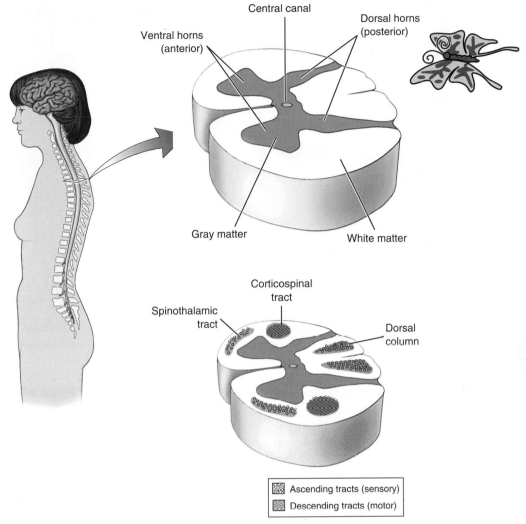

FIG. 11.2 **Cross section of the spinal cord: inner gray matter ("butterfly") and outer white matter.**

nerve is also called an afferent nerve (from the Latin meaning "to bring toward"). Remember: sensory, afferent, and ascending...all words referring to sensory information and transfer!

Motor tracts carry information from the brain, down the spinal cord, and toward the periphery. They are called **descending tracts**. The major descending tracts are the pyramidal and extrapyramidal tracts. The pyramidal tract, or corticospinal tract, is the major motor tract, originating in the precentral gyrus of the frontal lobe of the cerebrum. As its name (corticospinal) implies, motor information is carried from the cortex (origin) of the brain to the spinal cord Motor information is then carried from the spinal cord toward the periphery. For instance, the intent to move your leg originates in the brain; the signal travels down the spinal cord in a motor tract and along motor nerves to the muscles of the lower extremities causing movement. A motor nerve is called an efferent nerve. (from the Latin meaning to carry away). Remember: motor, efferent, and descending. all words referring to motor information and transfer. Additional information concerning tracts and their functions is in Table 11.1.

Table 11.1	Major Spinal Cord Tracts
TRACTS	**FUNCTIONS**
Ascending	
Spinothalamic	Temperature, pressure, pain, light touch
Dorsal column	Touch, deep pressure, vibration
Spinocerebellar	Proprioception
Descending	
Pyramidal (corticospinal)	Skeletal muscle tone, voluntary muscle movement
Extrapyramidal	Skeletal muscle activity, primarily involuntary reflexes and movement (balance and posture)

Decussation

Most tracts **decussate** (de-KUS-ate), or cross over, from one side to the other. For example, a corticospinal tract that originates in the left frontal lobe descends to the medulla oblongata, in the brain stem. The fibers then decussate, descend down the right side of the spinal cord, and innervate the right side of the body. Stated in more clinical terms, the corticospinal

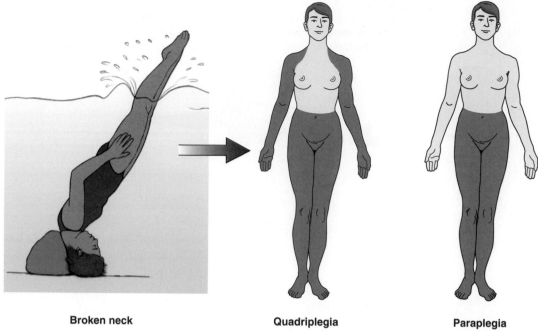

Broken neck   **Quadriplegia**   **Paraplegia**

FIG. 11.3 Spinal cord injuries. Diving into a shallow pool can result in a damaged spinal cord (quadriplegia and paraplegia).

tract decussates within the medulla oblongata and descends on the contralateral (opposite) side. Decussation accounts for the right-sided paralysis (hemiparalysis) in a person who has experienced a stroke on the left side of the brain. Some motor fibers do not decussate and therefore descend on the same (ipsilateral) side. Thus, a patient who has sustained a stroke in the left brain may experience both a right-sided paralysis and left-sided weakness. Whereas most motor tracts decussate at the level of the brain stem, most sensory tracts decussate in the spinal cord and ascend contralaterally to the brain.

If injured, the neurons of the brain and spinal cord do not regenerate. If the neck is broken, the spinal cord might be severed. If the spinal cord is severed at the neck region, the trunk and all four extremities are paralyzed. This condition is called *quadriplegia*. This type of spinal cord injury is common in automobile, football, and diving accidents in which the neck is either compressed or bent excessively (Fig. 11.3). If the spinal cord injury is lower, involving only the lumbar region of the spinal cord, the person has full use of the upper extremities but is paralyzed from the waist down. Paralysis of the lower extremities is called *paraplegia*.

 Re-Think

1. Differentiate between ascending and descending tracts.
2. Differentiate between afferent and efferent nerves
3. What clue identifies the corticospinal tract as a motor tract?
4. What clue identifies the spinothalamic tract as a sensory tract?

Sum It Up!

The spinal cord and the peripheral nervous system allow the brain to communicate with the body and external environment. The spinal cord transmits information up and down the cord. Sensory information is brought to the brain from the lower cord region along ascending tracts whereas motor information is transmitted from the brain, down the spinal cord in descending tracts. Afferent nerves bring sensory information toward the central nervous system, whereas efferent nerves carry motor information away from the central nervous system. Major spinal cord tracts are identified in Table 11.1. Most spinal tracts decussate or cross over. Varying degrees of paralysis, such as quadriplegia and paraplegia, are experienced if the spinal cord is severed.

WHAT THE SPINAL CORD DOES

The spinal cord serves three major functions: sensory pathway, motor pathway, and reflex center.

- **Sensory pathway.** The spinal cord provides pathways for sensory information traveling from the periphery to the brain.
- **Motor pathway.** The spinal cord provides pathways for motor information coming from the brain and going to the periphery.
- **Reflex center.** The spinal cord acts as a major reflex center. Read on.

REFLEXES

WHAT REFLEXES ARE

What is a reflex? A reflex is an involuntary response to a stimulus. Many of the activities that we engage in every day occur very rapidly and without any conscious

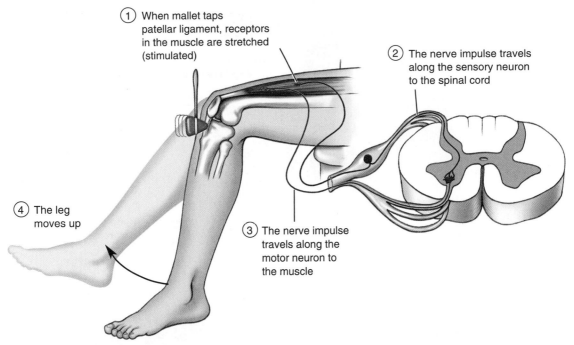

① When mallet taps patellar ligament, receptors in the muscle are stretched (stimulated)

② The nerve impulse travels along the sensory neuron to the spinal cord

④ The leg moves up

③ The nerve impulse travels along the motor neuron to the muscle

FIG. 11.4 Reflex arc. The knee-jerk reflex illustrates the components of the reflex arc.

control. In other words, they happen reflexively. Many of the reflexes occur at the level of the spinal cord and are called *spinal reflexes*. If you touch a hot surface, for example, you very quickly remove your hand (withdrawal reflex). Your hand is safely away from the source of injury long before you consciously say, "This is hot. I must remove my hand!" Similarly, your ability to walk and maintain your balance requires hundreds of reflex movements. For example, you don't have to think about swinging your arms as you walk.

A typical reflex response is demonstrated by the patellar tendon, or knee-jerk, reflex (Fig. 11.4). During a physical examination, the doctor taps the quadriceps ligament below your kneecap. In response to the tap, your leg quickly and involuntarily pops up. The physician has elicited the patellar tendon reflex. How does this reflex help you? If you are standing erect and your knee bends, even slightly, the patellar reflex is stimulated. In response to the bending, the quadriceps muscle in the thigh contracts, thereby straightening the leg and helping you maintain an upright position.

 Do You Know...
How Anesthesia Affects the Spinal Cord?

Anesthetic agents such as the "-caine" drugs may be injected into the subarachnoid space to achieve spinal anesthesia. When injected into the subarachnoid space, these drugs deaden, or anesthetize, the lumbar and sacral sensory nerves. Pain sensation from the areas innervated by these deadened nerves is temporarily lost.

How is epidural anesthesia used in childbirth? During the last, uncomfortable phase of childbirth, anesthetic agents may be continuously infused into the epidural space. The nerves that are deadened by the anesthesia supply the lower pelvic region of the body, thereby relieving the pain of childbirth.

THE REFLEX ARC

The knee-jerk reflex illustrates the four basic components of the reflex arc (see Fig. 11.4). The **reflex arc** is the nerve pathway involved in a reflex. The four basic components of the reflex arc include the following:

1. *A sensory receptor.* By tapping the patellar ligament, the mallet stimulates sensory receptors in the anterior thigh muscles (quadriceps femoris).
2. *An afferent or sensory neuron.* The nerve impulse is carried from the receptors along a sensory neuron to the spinal cord. The gray matter of the spinal cord most often contains interneurons that determine the motor response to the sensory input. This is referred to as the *integrating center.* In the simplest reflex arc (knee-jerk reflex), there is a single synapse with no interneuron and therefore no integrating center. All other reflexes require two or more interneurons and have an integrating center.
3. *An efferent or motor neuron.* The nerve impulse is carried by a motor nerve to the muscles of the thigh.
4. *An effector organ.* The muscles of the thigh, the quadriceps femoris, are effector organs for this reflex. In response to the motor nerve impulse, the muscles contract and extends the leg at the knee.

MANY, MANY REFLEXES

OUCH! THE WITHDRAWAL REFLEX

There are many spinal reflexes. The withdrawal reflex (Fig. 11.5A) helps protect you from injury. For example, this reflex quickly moves your finger away from a hot iron, thereby preventing a severe burn. The "ouch" occurs after your finger is safely away from the hot iron.

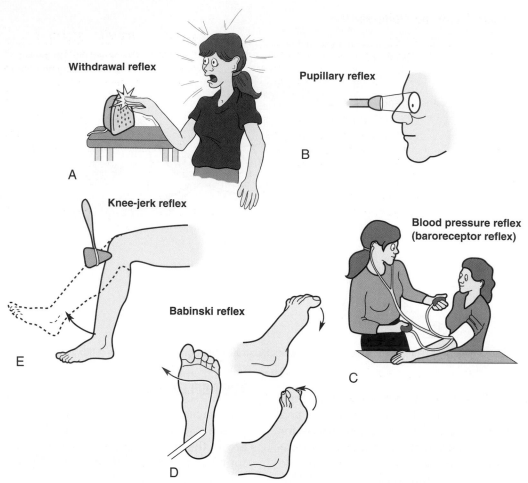

FIG. 11.5 Many reflexes. **(A)** Withdrawal reflex. **(B)** Pupillary reflex. **(C)** Blood pressure, or baroreceptor, reflex. **(D)** Babinski reflex. **(E)** Knee-jerk reflex.

Organ Reflexes

Reflexes also help regulate organ function. Fig. 11.5B and C illustrates some of the reflexes that regulate body function. The pupillary reflex, for example, regulates the amount of light that enters the eye. When a bright light is directed at the eye, the muscles that control pupillary size constrict. The size of the pupil diminishes, thereby restricting the amount of additional light entering the eye. Blood pressure is also under reflex control. When blood pressure changes abruptly, the baroreceptor reflex causes the heart and blood vessels to respond in a way that restores blood pressure to normal.

In addition to performing important physiological functions, some reflexes are used diagnostically to assess nerve function. Abnormal findings may indicate central nervous system (CNS) lesions, tumors, and other neurological diseases such as multiple sclerosis. You may have observed a physician elicit the Babinski reflex (Fig. 11.5D) by stroking the lateral sole of the foot in the direction of heel to toe with a hard, blunt object. In the adult, the Babinski reflex is normal, or negative, if the response to the stroking is plantar flexion, or a curling of the toes. An abnormal, or positive,

Babinski reflex is dorsiflexion of the big toe, sometimes with fanning of the other toes. An infant normally dorsiflexes the big toe, an indicator of the immaturity of the infant's nervous system. Some clinically significant reflexes and their functions are listed in Table 11.2.

◎ Sum It Up!

The spinal cord and the peripheral nervous system allow the brain to communicate with the body and the external environment. The spinal cord transmits sensory and motor information to and from the brain. It also acts as a reflex center. A reflex is an involuntary response to a stimulus. A reflex arc has four components: sensory receptor, afferent neuron, efferent neuron, and effector organ. Clinically significant reflexes are identified in Table 11.2.

? Re-Think

1. What are the three functions of the spinal cord?
2. Use the steps of the reflex arc to describe the withdrawal reflex in response to sticking your finger on a sharp tack.

Table 11.2	Clinically Significant Reflexes	
REFLEX	**DESCRIPTION**	**MEANING OF ABNORMAL RESPONSE**
Abdominal	With stroking of the lateral abdominal wall, the abdominal wall contracts and moves the umbilicus toward the stimulus.	Impaired in lesions of peripheral nerves Impaired in lesions of spinal cord (thoracic) and in patients with multiple sclerosis
Achilles tendon (ankle-jerk reflex)	A stretch reflex. The mallet strikes the Achilles tendon, causing plantar flexion.	Impaired in damage to nerves involved in the reflex Impaired in damage to lower spinal cord (L5–S2)
Babinski	With stroking of the lateral sole of the foot from heel to toe, the toes curl, with slight inversion of the foot (see text).	Impaired in lesions or damage of the spinal cord In children younger than 2 years old, the Babinski reflex appears positive.
Patellar tendon (knee-jerk reflex)	A stretch reflex. The mallet strikes the patellar ligament below the knee; in response, the leg is extended.	Impaired in damage to nerves involved in the reflex Impaired in damage to lumbar region of spinal cord Impaired in patients with diseases that affect the nerves and spinal cord (e.g., diabetes mellitus, neurosyphilis, and chronic alcoholism)

PERIPHERAL NERVOUS SYSTEM

The **peripheral nervous system** consists of the nerves and ganglia located outside the CNS.

NERVES

Before classifying the nerves, you need to differentiate between a nerve and a neuron (see Chapter 10). A neuron is a single nerve cell. The **nerve** contains many neurons bundled together with blood vessels and then wrapped in connective tissue (Fig. 11.6). Nerves are located outside the CNS. Within the CNS, bundles of nerve axons are called **tracts**. Nerves are classified as the following:

- **Sensory nerves,** composed only of sensory neurons
- **Motor nerves,** composed only of motor neurons
- **Mixed nerves,** containing both sensory and motor neurons

Most nerves are mixed, and all spinal nerves are mixed.

CLASSIFYING THE PERIPHERAL NERVOUS SYSTEM

The peripheral nervous system can be classified in two ways: structurally (by the anatomy) or functionally (according to what they do).

STRUCTURAL CLASSIFICATION OF THE PERIPHERAL NERVOUS SYSTEM

The structural classification of the peripheral nervous system divides the nerves into cranial and spinal nerves. The classification is based on the origin of the fiber (where it originates).

Cranial Nerves

Names and Numbers of Cranial Nerves. Cranial nerves exit the brain and generally supply the head, neck and shoulder areas. Twelve pairs of **cranial nerves** are shown in Fig. 11.7. Each cranial nerve has a specific number, always designated by a Roman

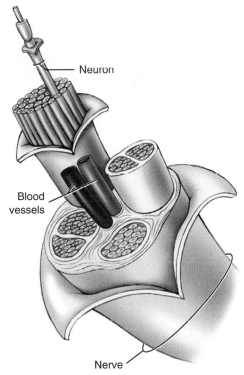

FIG. 11.6 **Difference between a neuron and nerve. The nerve includes neurons, connective tissue, and blood vessels.**

Labels: Neuron; Blood vessels; Nerve

numeral, and a name. The numbers indicate the order in which the nerves exit the brain from front to back. Ten of the twelve cranial nerves originate in the brain stem.

In general, the name of the nerve indicates the specific anatomical area served by the nerve. For example, the optic nerve serves the eye. While the cranial nerves primarily serve the head, face, and neck region, one pair—the vagus—branches extensively and extends throughout the thoracic and abdominal cavities.

A common mnemonic used to memorize the cranial nerves in proper order is shown in Table 11.3: On Old Olympus Towering Tops A Finn Viewed Germans Vaulting And Hopping. The first letter of each word

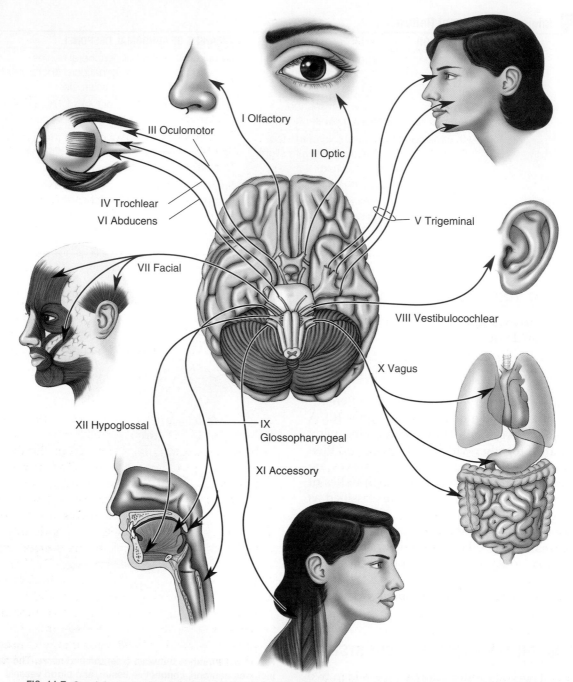

FIG. 11.7 Cranial nerves. Cranial nerves (12 pairs) are known by their numbers (Roman numerals) and names.

is the same as the first letter of each cranial nerve. (My personal mnemonic is Oh! Oh! Oh! Tough, Tricky Anatomy Final … Very Grave Vibes … Aching Head.) Try to develop your own creative mnemonic, or search the Web for others. Unfortunately, you must know the name and Roman numeral of each cranial nerve. For instance, the vestibulocochlear nerve is CN VIII.

Functions of Cranial Nerves. Cranial nerves perform four general functions that carry different types of information:

- Sensory information for the special senses: smell, taste, vision, hearing, and balance

- Sensory information for the general senses: touch, pressure, pain, temperature, and proprioception.
- Motor information that results in contraction of skeletal muscles
- Motor information that results in the secretion of glands and the contraction of cardiac and smooth muscle

Cranial nerve function is summarized in Table 11.3. Locate each cranial nerve on Fig. 11.7 as it is described below.

CN I, olfactory nerve. A sensory nerve that carries information from the nose to the olfactory areas of the temporal and parietal lobes of the cerebrum.

Table 11.3   Cranial Nerves

MNEMONIC	NUMBER/NERVE	TYPE	FUNCTION
On	I/Olfactory	Sensory	Sense of smell
Old	II/Optic	Sensory	Sense of sight
Olympus	III/Oculomotor	Mixed (mostly motor)	Movement of eyeball, raising of eyelid, change in pupil size
Towering	IV/Trochlear	Mixed (mostly motor)	Movement of eyeball
Tops	V/Trigeminal	Mixed	Chewing of food; sensations in face, scalp, cornea (eye), and teeth
A	VI/Abducens	Mixed (mostly motor)	Movement of eyeball
Finn	VII/Facial	Mixed	Facial expressions, secretion of saliva and tears, taste, blinking
Viewed	VIII/Vestibulocochlear	Sensory	Sense of hearing and balance
Germans	IX/Glossopharyngeal	Mixed	Swallowing, secretion of saliva, taste, sensory for the reflex regulation of blood pressure, part of the gag reflex
Vaulting	X/Vagus	Mixed	Visceral muscle movement and sensations, especially movement and secretion of the digestive system; sensory for reflex regulation of blood pressure
And	XI/Accessory	Mixed (mostly motor)	Swallowing, head and shoulder movement, speaking
Hopping	XII/Hypoglossal	Mixed (mostly motor)	Speech and swallowing

The olfactory nerve is concerned with the sense of smell. A person who damages the olfactory nerve may lose the sense of smell (anosmia). In addition, the person may complain of loss of taste because the appeal of food is determined by both taste and smell.

CN II, *optic nerve.* A sensory nerve that carries visual information from the eye to the primary visual cortex of the occipital lobe of the cerebrum. Damage to the optic nerve causes diminished vision or blindness in the affected eye.

CN III, *oculomotor nerve.* Primarily a motor nerve that causes contraction of most of the extrinsic eye muscles, thereby moving the eyeball in its socket. The oculomotor nerve also raises the eyelid and constricts the pupil of the eye.

Because the oculomotor nerve is located close to the hard tentorium within the cranium, it is easily compressed by brain tumors or by increased intracranial pressure. Compression of the nerve interferes with the ability of the pupil of the eye to respond to light (sluggish pupillary response). With more severe compression, the pupils may become dilated and fixed. Compression of CN III also interferes with raising the eyelid; the person experiences ptosis (TOH-sis) of the eyelid. Observation of the eyes provides excellent clinical clues to neurological status.

CN IV, *trochlear nerve.* Primarily a motor nerve that innervates one of the extrinsic muscles of the eyeball, thereby helping move the eyeball. Damage may cause double vision and an inability to rotate the eye properly.

CN V, *trigeminal nerve.* A mixed nerve with three branches supplying the facial region. The sensory branches carry information from the face, scalp, eye, and teeth to the brain. One of the sensory branches, the ophthalmic branch, detects sensory information from the cornea. For example, if you touch the surface of the cornea, the ophthalmic branch is stimulated and sends information to the brain. In response to the corneal irritation, motor fibers of the facial nerve (CN VII) respond by eliciting blinking and the secretion of tears. Thus, both the trigeminal and facial nerves help to relieve the irritation. The motor branch of the trigeminal nerve innervates the muscles of mastication (chewing). Nerve damage causes a loss of sensation and impaired movement of the mandible (lower jaw).

CN VI, *abducens nerve.* Primarily a motor nerve that, like the trochlear, controls eye movement by innervating only one of the extrinsic eye muscles. Nerve damage prevents a lateral rotation of the eye; at rest, the eye drifts medially (toward the nose).

CN VII, *facial nerve.* A mixed nerve that performs mostly motor functions. It is called the nerve of facial expression and allows you to smile, frown, and "make other faces." It also stimulates the secretion of saliva and tears. The facial nerve innervates the orbicularis oculi, the muscle involved in blinking. Blinking not only protects the eye from foreign objects, such as dust, but also washes tears over the cornea, thereby keeping the cornea moist and preventing corneal ulceration. Its sensory function is taste.

If the facial nerve is damaged, facial expression is absent on the affected side of the face. This condition is called *Bell's palsy.* Cosmetically, this condition is very distressing because one side of the face may smile and look alive, but the other side of the face sags, drools, and is expressionless. In addition, salivation and the secretion of tears are diminished, thereby requiring the use of moistening eyedrops to protect the cornea. Fortunately, Bell's palsy most often responds well to steroid therapy.

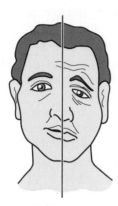

Bell's palsy

CN VIII, vestibulocochlear nerve. A sensory nerve that carries information for hearing and balance from the inner ear to the brain. The vestibular branch of this nerve is responsible for equilibrium, or balance, and the cochlear branch is responsible for hearing. Damage to this nerve may cause loss of hearing or balance or both (see Chapter 13).

CN IX, glossopharyngeal nerve. A mixed nerve that carries taste sensation from the posterior tongue to the brain. Motor fibers stimulate the secretion of salivary glands in the mouth. Other motor fibers innervate the throat and aid in swallowing. The glossopharyngeal nerve is also associated with the gag reflex. The gag reflex plays an important role in preventing food and water from entering the respiratory passages. Normally, when something goes down the wrong way, you gag and cough until the airway is cleared. Gagging is a good thing—and clinically important when depressed. A second sensory function of this nerve involves the regulation of blood pressure via the baroreceptor reflex (see Chapter 19).

CN X, vagus nerve. A mixed nerve that innervates the tongue, pharynx (throat), larynx (voicebox), and many organs in the thoracic and abdominal cavities (lungs, stomach, intestines). Nerve damage causes hoarseness or loss of voice, impaired swallowing, and diminished motility of the digestive tract. Damage to both vagus nerves can be fatal. The word *vagus* literally means "wanderer"; the name refers to the far-reaching distribution of this nerve. The sensory fibers of the vagus

nerve also participate in the regulation of blood pressure via the baroreceptor reflex (see Chapter 19).

CN XI, accessory nerve. Primarily a motor nerve that supplies the sternocleidomastoid and the trapezius muscles, thereby controlling movement of the head and shoulder regions. Nerve damage impairs your ability to shrug your shoulders and rotate your head.

CN XII, hypoglossal nerve. Primarily a motor nerve that controls movement of the tongue, thereby affecting speaking and swallowing activities. Nerve damage causes the tongue to deviate toward the injured side.

A neurological assessment includes simple procedures that test the ability of each cranial nerve to perform these functions. Table 11.4 illustrates some methods used to test cranial nerve function. The table also includes common disorders and abnormal findings involving the cranial nerves.

 Do You Know...

About the "Wandering" Characteristics of the 10th Cranial Nerve ?

Check the local jail, and you will find a couple of unsavory characters locked up on charges of vagrancy—the habit of wandering around and generally getting into trouble. (The word *vagrant* means "someone who wanders about.") The vagus nerve, the 10th cranial nerve (CN X), is also a wanderer. Unlike the other cranial nerves that are confined to the head and shoulder area, the vagus nerve leaves the head and wanders, or makes its way through, the thoracic and abdominal cavities. The vagus nerve is named for these vagrant or wandering characteristics.

 Re-Think

1. CNs II, III, IV, and VI all innervate eye structures. What is the difference in function of each?
2. Describe the cranial nerve response to corneal irritation/blinking.
3. List two effects of a damaged CN VIII.
4. Why is the vagus nerve called the "wanderer" nerve?

SPINAL NERVES ATTACHED TO THE SPINAL CORD

Attached to the spinal cord are the **spinal nerves**. Each nerve is attached to the spinal cord by two roots: the dorsal root and the ventral root (Fig. 11.8). Sensory nerve fibers from the periphery travel to the cord through the dorsal root. The cell bodies of the sensory fibers are gathered together in the dorsal root ganglia. The ventral root is composed of motor fibers. These motor fibers are distributed to muscles and glands. The dorsal(sensory) and ventral(motor) roots are packaged together to form a spinal nerve. (All spinal nerves are mixed.)

Table 11.4	Cranial Nerves: Assessment and Disorders	
NERVE	**ASSESSMENT**	**SOME DISORDERS**
I Olfactory	Person is asked to sniff and identify various odors (e.g., vanilla).	Inability to smell (anosmia)
II Optic	Examination of the interior of the eye by ophthalmoscopic visualization. Use of eye charts and tests of peripheral vision.	Diminished, or loss of, vision
III Oculomotor	Observation of eyelids. Test the ability of the eyes to follow a moving object. Examination of pupils for size, shape, and size equality. Pupillary reflex is tested with a penlight (the pupils should constrict). Test the ability of the eyes to converge.	Drooping upper eyelids (ptosis) Difficulty in focusing eyes on an object Absence of pupillary reflex (e.g., dilated and fixed pupils that may indicate an increase in intracranial pressure)
IV Trochlear	Test ability of the eyes to follow a moving object.	Inability to move eyeball in a particular direction
V Trigeminal	Sensations (pain/touch/temperature) are tested with sharp pin and hot/cold objects. Corneal reflex (sensory) is tested with a cotton wisp. Motor function is tested by asking the person to open the mouth (against resistance) and to move the jaw from side to side.	Loss of sensation (pain/touch); paresthesias (tingling, itching, and numbness) Pain, tearing, and blinking Shift of jaw to side of lesion when opened Difficulty in chewing
VI Abducens	Test ability of the eyes to follow a moving object.	Inability to move eyes laterally
VII Facial	Person is asked to cause facial muscle movement (e.g., smile, close eyes, wrinkle forehead, whistle). Test anterior two-thirds of tongue for sweet, salty, sour, and bitter taste. Ability to secrete tears is tested by asking person to sniff ammonia fumes.	Bell's palsy (expressionless face, drooping mouth and drooling, inability to close eyes and blink) Loss of taste on anterior two-thirds of tongue on side of lesion
VIII Vestibulocochlear	Hearing is checked by air and bone conduction (use of tuning fork).	Loss of hearing, noises in ear (tinnitus) Loss of balance (vertigo)
IX Glossopharyngeal	Check gag and swallowing reflex. Test posterior two-thirds of tongue for taste. Person is asked to speak and cough.	Loss of gag reflex Difficulty in swallowing (dysphagia) Loss of taste on posterior two-thirds of tongue Decreased salivation Hoarseness of voice
X Vagus	Similar to testing for CN IX (because they both innervate throat).	Sagging of soft palate Hoarseness of voice resulting from paralysis of vocal fold
XI Accessory	Ask person to rotate head from side to side and to shrug shoulders (against resistance).	Drooping shoulders Inability or difficulty in rotating head (wryneck)
XII Hypoglossal	Person is asked to stick out tongue—note any deviation in position of the protruded tongue.	Some difficulty in speaking (dysarthria), chewing, and swallowing (dysphagia)

Names and Numbers of Spinal Nerves

Thirty-one pairs of spinal nerves emerge from the spinal cord (Fig. 11.9). Each pair is numbered according to the level of the spinal cord from which it arises. The 31 pairs are grouped as follows: 8 pairs of cervical nerves, 12 pairs of thoracic nerves, 5 pairs of lumbar nerves, 5 pairs of sacral nerves, and 1 pair of coccygeal nerves. The lumbar and sacral nerves at the bottom of the cord extend the length of the spinal cavity before exiting from the vertebral column. These nerves are called the *cauda equina* because they look like a horse's tail. The nerves exit from the bony vertebral column through tiny holes in the vertebrae called *foramina*.

Spinal Nerve Plexuses

As the spinal nerves exit from the vertebral column, they divide into many fibers. At various points, most nerve fibers converge, or come together again, into nerve **plexuses** (PLEX-sus-ez), or networks. The three major nerve plexuses are the cervical plexus, the brachial plexus, and the lumbosacral plexus (see Fig. 11.9). Each plexus sorts out the many fibers and sends them to a specific part of the body. The three plexuses and the major nerves that emerge from each plexus are listed in Table 11.5 and described as follows. The results of damage to major peripheral nerves are listed in Table 11.6.

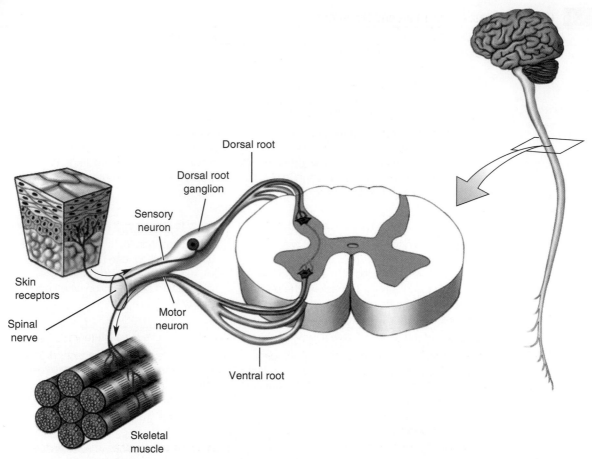

FIG. 11.8 **Attachment of the spinal nerves to the spinal cord. Note the dorsal root ganglia (sensory) and ventral root (motor). All spinal nerves are mixed nerves.**

Cervical plexus (C1 to C4). Fibers from the cervical plexus supply the muscles and skin of the neck. Motor fibers from this plexus also pass into the phrenic nerve. The phrenic nerve stimulates the contraction of the diaphragm, the major breathing muscle (Fig. 11.10; see Fig. 11.9).

If the spinal cord is severed below the C5 level, the person is paralyzed but can breathe without ventilator assistance. If the level of injury is higher, at C2, the phrenic nerve is injured, motor impulses to the diaphragm are interrupted, and the person cannot breathe normally. This person generally needs the assistance of a ventilator in order to breathe.

Brachial plexus (C5 to C8, T1). The nerves that emerge from the brachial plexus supply the muscles and skin of the shoulder, arm, forearm, wrist, and hand. The axillary nerve emerges from this plexus and travels through the shoulder into the arm.

The axillary nerve in the shoulder region is susceptible to damage. For example, a person using crutches should be taught to bear the weight of the body on the hands and not on the armpit, or axillary region. The weight of the body can damage the axillary nerve, causing crutch palsy (Fig 11-10).

The radial and ulnar nerves, which serve the forearm, wrist, and hand, also emerge from the brachial plexus. Damage to the radial nerve can cause a wristdrop, and injury to the ulnar nerve causes the hand to appear clawlike; the person is unable to spread the fingers apart.

Lumbosacral plexus (T12, L1 to L5, S1 to S4). The lumbosacral plexus gives rise to nerves that supply the muscles and skin of the lower abdominal wall, external genitalia, buttocks, and lower extremities. The sciatic nerve, the longest nerve in the body, arises from this plexus. The sciatic nerve supplies musculature of the thigh, leg, and foot. The sciatic nerve can become inflamed and cause intense pain in the buttock and posterior thigh region. A common cause of sciatica is a ruptured or herniated vertebral disc (see Fig. 11.10).

What a Dermatome Is

A dermatome is a sensory thing. Each dorsal root of a spinal nerve innervates a particular area of the skin; this distribution of nerves is called a **dermatome** (DER-mah-tohm). Fig. 11.11 illustrates the dermatomes for the entire body. Each dermatome is named for the particular nerve that serves it. For example, the C4 dermatome is innervated by the C4 spinal nerve.

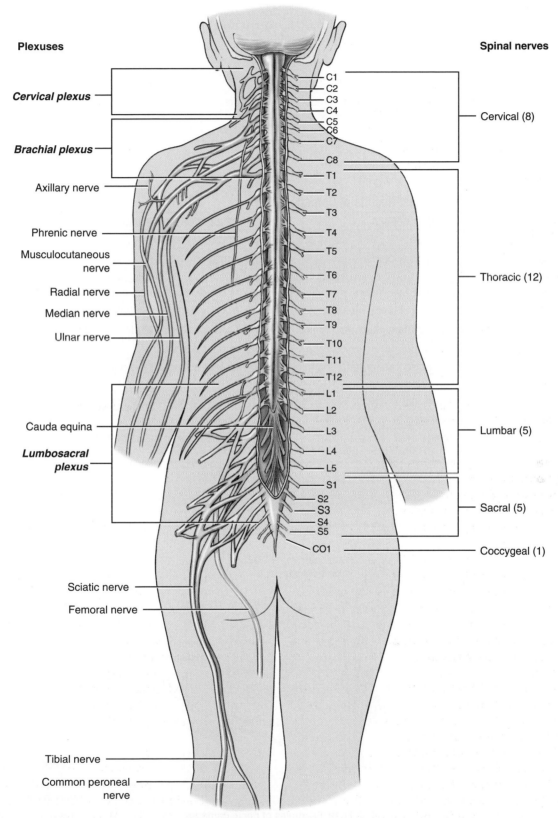

Plexuses

Cervical plexus

Brachial plexus

Axillary nerve

Phrenic nerve

Musculocutaneous
nerve

Radial nerve

Median nerve

Ulnar nerve

Cauda equina

*Lumbosacral
plexus*

Sciatic nerve

Femoral nerve

Tibial nerve

Common peroneal
nerve

Spinal nerves

C1
C2
C3
C4
C5
C6
C7
C8
T1
T2
T3
T4
T5
T6
T7
T8
T9
T10
T11
T12
L1
L2
L3
L4
L5
S1
S2
S3
S4
S5
CO1

Cervical (8)

Thoracic (12)

Lumbar (5)

Sacral (5)

Coccygeal (1)

FIG. 11.9 Spinal nerves: cervical, thoracic, lumbar, sacral, and coccygeal. Nerve plexuses: cervical, brachial, and lumbosacral plexuses.

Table 11.5 Spinal Nerve Plexuses

PLEXUS	SPINAL NERVE ORIGIN	REGION INNERVATED	MAJOR NERVES EMERGING FROM PLEXUS
Cervical	C1–C4	Skin and muscles of the neck and shoulder, diaphragm	Phrenic
Brachial	C5–C8, T1	Skin and muscles of the upper extremities	Axillary Radial Median Musculocutaneous Ulnar
Lumbosacral	T12, L1–L5, S1–S4	Skin and muscle of lower torso and lower extremities	Femoral Obturator Sciatic

Table 11.6 Major Peripheral Nerves: Results of Damage

NERVE	BODY AREA SERVED	RESULTS OF NERVE DAMAGE
Phrenic	Diaphragm	Impaired breathing
Axillary	Muscles of shoulder	Crutch palsy
Radial	Posterior arm, forearm, hand; thumbs and first two fingers	Wristdrop, also radial nerve palsy (inability to lift or extend hand at wrist, inability to extend fingers)
Median	Forearm and some muscles of the hand	Inability to pick up small objects
Ulnar	Wrist and many muscles in hand	Clawhand—inability to spread fingers apart
Intercostal	Rib cage	Impaired breathing
Femoral	Lower abdomen, anterior thigh, medial leg, foot	Inability to extend leg and flex hip
Sciatic	Lower trunk; posterior thigh and leg	Inability to extend hip and flex knee
Common peroneal	Lateral area of leg and foot	Footdrop—inability to dorsiflex foot
Tibial	Posterior area of leg and foot	Shuffling gait caused by inability to invert and dorsiflex foot

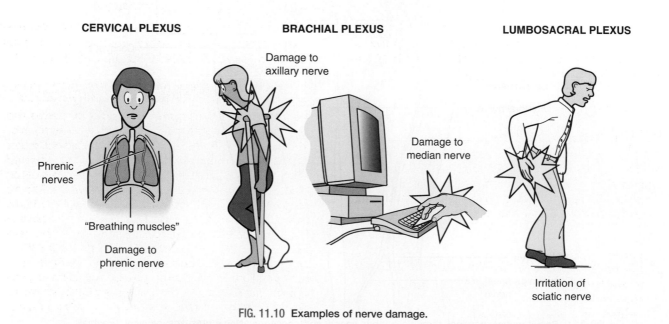

CERVICAL PLEXUS

BRACHIAL PLEXUS

LUMBOSACRAL PLEXUS

Damage to axillary nerve

Phrenic nerves

"Breathing muscles"

Damage to phrenic nerve

Damage to median nerve

Irritation of sciatic nerve

FIG. 11.10 **Examples of nerve damage.**

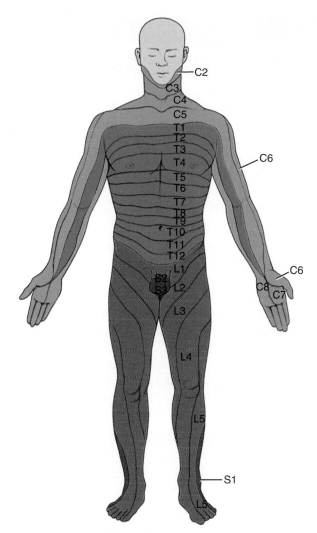

FIG. 11.11 **Dermatomes.**

Dermatomes are useful clinically; for example, if the skin of the shoulder region is stimulated with the tip of a pin and the person cannot feel it, the clinician has reason to believe that the C4 nerve is impaired.

 Do You Know...

About Tingling Thigh Syndrome?

Although tight, low-slung jeans are "in," your thigh nerves are on edge about this fashion craze. The snug jeans are compressing the nerves in your thighs, causing a tingling sensation. The "tingling thigh syndrome" is easily cured, but the jeans have to go—or go higher.

 Re-Think

1. Explain the difference between a cranial nerve and a spinal nerve.
2. What happens at a nerve plexus?
3. Explain why a quadriplegic with a C2 injury is ventilator-dependent, whereas a quadriplegic with a C5 injury is not ventilator-dependent.

 Do You Know...

What Was on Dr. Herby Zoster's Shingle?

The doctor's shingle indicates that he specializes in chickenpox, shingles, and postherpetic neuralgia; all three are caused by the herpes zoster virus. Following a chickenpox infection, the herpes virus "hides out" in nerves and often reactivates in later life, causing shingles. Clusters of vesicles develop along cranial or spinal dermatomes. The painful lesions eventually crust over. For months after the "crusting over period," a significant number of patients with shingles develop a persistent and painful neuralgia, called *postherpetic neuralgia.* The term *shingles* comes from a word meaning "girdle," a reference to the usual appearance of lesions around the waist.

Any pharmacological help for shingles? Yes! Analgesics are prescribed for pain. Antiviral drugs may be used if the shingles is diagnosed quickly. On a preventive note, a shingles vaccine is now available.

Are shingles contagious? No! However, a person with shingles can transmit chickenpox to a person with no immunity to the disease. Also, a child with chickenpox can activate the dormant herpes virus in a person who has had chickenpox in the past.

FUNCTIONAL CLASSIFICATION OF THE PERIPHERAL NERVOUS SYSTEM

The functional classification explains where the nerves go and what they do. The functional classification of the peripheral nervous system includes the following:
- The somatic **afferent nerves,** which bring sensory information from the different parts of the body, particularly the skin and muscles, to the CNS (see Chapter 13).
- The somatic **efferent nerves,** which bring motor information from the CNS to the skeletal muscles throughout the body (see Chapter 9).
- The autonomic nervous system (ANS) is composed of nerves that supply the organs (viscera), smooth muscle, and glands. The ANS is the topic of Chapter 12.

 Sum It Up!

The peripheral nervous system consists of the nerves and ganglia located outside the CNS. Nerves are sensory, motor, or mixed. Mixed nerves carry both sensory and motor neurons. The peripheral nervous system can be classified structurally and functionally. The structural classification divides the nerves into cranial and spinal nerves. The 12 pairs of cranial nerves contain fibers that originate in the brain (see Fig. 11.7 and Table 11.3). There are 31 pairs of spinal nerves; their fibers originate in the spinal cord (see Fig. 11.9 and Tables 11.5 and 11.6). Most spinal nerve fibers converge into nerve plexuses, or networks. The three major nerve plexuses are the cervical plexus, brachial plexus, and lumbosacral plexus. The functional classification of nerves includes somatic afferent nerves, somatic efferent nerves, and autonomic nerves.

Note: The As You Age box and the Medical Terminology and Disorders table appear in Chapter 12.

Get Ready for Exams!

Summary Outline

The brain, spinal cord, and peripheral nerves act as a vast communication system. The spinal cord transmits information to and from the brain. The peripheral nervous system brings information to the CNS (its sensory role) and delivers information from the CNS to the periphery (its motor role).

I. **What the Spinal Cord Is**
  A. The spinal cord is a tubelike structure located in the spinal cavity, extending from the foramen magnum (occipital bone) to L1.
  B. Arrangement of nervous tissue
    1. The gray matter is a butterfly-shaped area located centrally; it is composed primarily of cell bodies, interneurons, and synapses.
    2. The white matter is composed of myelinated and unmyelinated fibers arranged in tracts. Ascending tracts are sensory tracts; descending tracts are motor tracts.

II. **What the Spinal Cord Does: Functions**
  A. The spinal cord relays sensory information (ascending tracts).
  B. The spinal cord relays motor information (descending tracts).
  C. The spinal cord acts as a major reflex center.

III. **Reflexes**
  A. A reflex is an involuntary response to a stimulus.
  B. The four components of a reflex are a sensory receptor, an afferent neuron, an efferent neuron, and an effector organ.
  C. Many reflexes involving skeletal muscle and organ function.

IV. **Peripheral Nervous System**
  A. Nerve
    1. A nerve is a group of neurons, blood vessels, and connective tissue.
    2. There are sensory nerves, motor nerves, and mixed nerves.
  B. Structural classification of nerves
    1. A classification of nerves on the basis of structure (anatomy) divides nerves into cranial nerves and spinal nerves. There are 12 pairs of cranial nerves (see Table 11.3) and 31 pairs of spinal nerves (see Fig. 11.9).
    2. Spinal nerves are sorted out at nerve plexuses. The three major plexuses are the cervical plexus, the brachial plexus, and the lumbosacral plexus.
    3. A dermatome is the area of skin innervated by each spinal nerve; a dermatome is purely sensory.
  C. Functional classification of nerves
    1. Somatic afferent nerves carry sensory information to the CNS.
    2. Somatic efferent nerves carry motor information to skeletal muscles.
    3. Autonomic nerves carry motor information to the organs (viscera).

Review Your Knowledge

Matching: Reflexes
Directions: Match the following words with their descriptions.
a. gag reflex
b. baroreceptor reflex
c. withdrawal reflex
d. Achilles tendon reflex
e. corneal reflex
f. pupillary reflex
g. patellar tendon reflex

1. ___ Helps you maintain balance; also called the *knee-jerk reflex*
2. ___ Regulates blood pressure
3. ___ Controls the amount of light that enters the eye
4. ___ When you pull your finger away from a sharp object
5. ___ Helps prevent food and water from entering the respiratory passages
6. ___ Tapping of the calcaneal tendon; causes plantar flexion
7. ___ Involves CN V (sensory) and VII (motor) resulting in blinking and tearing

Matching: Nerves
Directions: Match the following words with their descriptions. Some words may be used more than once.
a. oculomotor
b. optic
c. vagus
d. facial
e. sciatic
f. olfactory
g. phrenic
h. vestibulocochlear

1. ___ Innervates the skeletal muscles that move the eyeball
2. ___ Carries sensory information to the primary visual cortex of the occipital lobe
3. ___ Carries sensory information for hearing and balance
4. ___ Innervates the diaphragm, causing it to contract
5. ___ Innervates muscles of the thigh
6. ___ "Wanderer" nerve that is distributed throughout the thoracic and abdominopelvic cavities
7. ___ The "smell" nerve
8. ___ The nerve of facial expression
9. ___ Ototoxicity refers to this damaged nerve
10. ___ "Fixed and dilated" describes this injured nerve

Multiple Choice

1. Which of the following does *not* describe the oculomotor nerve?
  a. It is also CN III.
  b. It innervates the skeletal muscles that move the eyeball.
  c. It is the carrier of information to the primary visual cortex in the occipital lobe.
  d. It innervates skeletal muscle that raises the eyelids.

2. Characteristics of the trigeminal nerve include which of the following?
   a. Is CN V
   b. Has both sensory and motor fibers
   c. Affects chewing
   d. All of the above

3. The sciatic nerve
   a. is a motor nerve that innervates thigh muscles.
   b. is a cranial nerve.
   c. enters the cervical plexus for distribution to the periphery.
   d. travels within the spinothalamic tract.

4. Which of the following is descriptive of the spinothalamic tract?
   a. It carries sensory information regarding touch, pressure, and pain.
   b. It is the major motor tract.
   c. It is also called the *pyramidal tract.*
   d. It is a descending tract.

5. Which of the following is *least* descriptive of the corticospinal tract?
   a. Descending tract
   b. Major motor tract
   c. Pyramidal tract
   d. Carries information from the spinal cord to the thalamus

6. What is the final step in the reflex arc?
   a. Response of the effector organ(s)
   b. Activation of the sensory receptor
   c. Communication of the sensory neuron with an interneuron within the spinal cord
   d. Traveling of the nerve impulse along the motor neuron

7. Which of the following is *not* true of the gag reflex?
   a. It is impaired in a paraplegic person.
   b. It is associated with CN IX.
   c. It is associated with the glossopharyngeal nerve.
   d. It prevents food and water from entering the respiratory passages.

8. Damage to the phrenic nerve
   a. interferes with the pupillary response to light.
   b. impairs breathing.
   c. eliminates the gag reflex.
   d. causes dysphagia.

9. CN IX, CN X, and the baroreceptor reflex are concerned with the regulation of
   a. the amount of light that enters the eye.
   b. facial expression.
   c. the movement of the eyeballs and elevation of the eyelids.
   d. blood pressure.

10. The olfactory nerve
    a. is CN III.
    b. is concerned with the sense of smell.
    c. travels through the cervical plexus from the nose to the brain.
    d. has two branches: cochlear and vestibular.

11. A person suffers a stroke to the left cerebral hemisphere and develops a right-sided hemiparalysis. Which of the following words describes the paralysis of the right side of the body?
    a. Cerebral lateralization
    b. Decussation
    c. Saltatory conduction
    d. Repolarization

12. Stimulation of the ophthalmic branch of which cranial nerve detects painful irritation of the cornea?
    a. Optic
    b. Oculomotor
    c. Trigeminal
    d. Trochlear

13. Damage to which nerve causes the tongue to deviate toward the injured side and impairs swallowing and speaking?
    a. Vagus (CN X)
    b. Hypoglossal (CN XII)
    c. Accessory (CN XI)
    d. Facial (CN VII)

14. Which of the following is *least* descriptive of the cauda equina?
    a. Lumbar and sacral nerves
    b. Spinal nerves
    c. Brachial plexus
    d. Innervation of the lower extremities

15. Which of the following is most descriptive of a dermatome?
    a. Motor and muscle
    b. Sensory and skin
    c. Autonomic and visceral
    d. Cranial and spinal

Go Figure

1. Which of the following is correct according to Fig. 11.1?
   a. The spinal cord fills the entire adult spinal cavity.
   b. The usual lumbar puncture site is between L6 and L7.
   c. The cauda equina exits from the distal end of the spinal cord.
   d. The subarachnoid space ends at L1.

2. Which of the following is correct according to Fig. 11.2?
   a. The corticospinal tract, spinothalamic tract, and dorsal columns ascend and descend in the gray matter.
   b. The corticospinal tract runs only on the left side of the spinal cord.
   c. The ventral and posterior horns are composed of white matter.
   d. All tracts ascend and descend in white matter.

3. Which of the following is correct according to Table 11.1?
   a. The spinothalamic tract is ascending and motor.
   b. The pyramidal and extrapyramidal tracts are concerned with motor activity.
   c. The corticospinal tract is descending and sensory.
   d. The dorsal columns, spinocerebellar tract, and corticospinal tract are ascending and motor.

4. Which of the following is correct according to Fig. 11.4?
   a. The effector organ of the patellar tendon reflex is the patellar tendon.
   b. A sensory neuron carries information to the gray matter in the spinal cord.
   c. The response to the patellar tendon reflex is flexion of the leg at the knee.
   d. A motor neuron carries information from the patellar tendon to the spinal cord.

5. Which of the following is correct according to Fig. 11.5?
   a. The pupillary reflex is stimulated by corneal irritation.
   b. The Babinski reflex is elicited by tapping the patellar tendon.
   c. The baroreceptor reflex maintains body temperature.
   d. The reflex response to the stretching of the receptors in the quadriceps femoris muscle is extension of the leg.

6. According to Table 11.2, the Babinski reflex is
   a. elicited by tapping the patellar tendon.
   b. also called the Achilles tendon or ankle-jerk reflex.
   c. elicited by shining light at the pupil of the eye.
   d. elicited by stroking the lateral sole of the foot.

7. Which of the following is correct according to Fig. 11.6?
   a. A neuron is the same as a nerve.
   b. A nerve is composed of many neurons, a blood supply, and connective tissue.
   c. *Neuron* is the name given to nerves bundled together by connective tissue.
   d. A nerve contains a single neuron and its blood supply.

8. Which of the following is correct according to Fig. 11.7 and Table 11.3?
   a. The vagus nerve is restricted to thoracic organs.
   b. The facial nerve is CN V.
   c. The extrinsic eye muscles are innervated only by CN III.
   d. CN VIII has two branches: the cochlear and vestibular.

9. Which of the following is correct according to Fig. 11.7 and Table 11.3?
   a. CNs I, II, and VIII are sensory.
   b. The optic nerve (CN II) innervates the extrinsic eye muscles, causing the eyeballs to move.
   c. The olfactory nerve (CN I) is primarily responsible for taste and swallowing.
   d. CN VIII arises from the precentral gyrus of the frontal lobe.

10. Which of the following is correct according to Fig. 11.8?
    a. Spinal nerves are mixed, containing both sensory and motor fibers.
    b. Sensory fibers travel to the spinal cord through the dorsal root.
    c. Motor fibers travel from the spinal cord to the periphery through the ventral root.
    d. All of the above are true.

11. Which of the following is correct according to Fig. 11.9?
    a. The cauda equina emerges from the brachial plexus.
    b. The phrenic nerve emerges from the cervical plexus.
    c. The sciatic and femoral nerves are classified as sensory.
    d. There are eight cervical nerves, all of which extend to and emerge from the cervical plexus.

12. Which of the following is correct according to Fig. 11.9?
    a. The sciatic and femoral nerves innervate the thoracic cavity.
    b. The phrenic nerve exits the spinal cord at the level of T6.
    c. The radial, median, and ulnar nerves exit from the lumbosacral plexus.
    d. Transection of the spinal cord at C2 causes quadriplegia and impaired ventilation (breathing).

Objectives

1. Describe the function and pathway of autonomic (visceral) reflexes.
2. Do the following regarding the autonomic nervous system:
   - Describe the function of the autonomic nervous system.
   - Identify the two divisions of the autonomic nervous system.
   - State the anatomical and functional differences between the sympathetic and parasympathetic nervous systems.

- Define autonomic terminology used in pharmacology.
- Differentiate between autonomic tone and vasomotor tone.

3. Discuss autonomic nervous system neurons, including the following:
   - Define *cholinergic* and *adrenergic* fibers.
   - Name the major neurotransmitters of the autonomic nervous system.
   - Name and locate the cholinergic and adrenergic receptors.

4. Explain the terms used to describe the effects of neurotransmitters and drugs on autonomic receptors.

Key Terms

acetylcholine (ACh) (p. 224)
adrenergic fiber (p. 224)
alpha-adrenergic receptor (p. 226)
autonomic nervous system
   (ANS) (p. 219)
beta-adrenergic receptor (p. 226)
cholinergic fiber (p. 224)
craniosacral outflow (p. 223)
dual innervation (p. 220)

feed-and-breed division (p. 221)
fight-or-flight division (p. 220)
ganglion (p. 222)
muscarinic receptors (p. 225)
nicotinic receptors (p. 225)
norepinephrine (NE) (p. 224)
parasympathetic nervous
   system (p. 221)
paravertebral ganglia (p. 223)

postganglionic fiber (p. 222)
preganglionic fiber (p. 222)
sympathetic nervous system
   (p. 220)
thoracolumbar outflow (p. 223)
vagolytic (p. 222)
vagomimetic (p. 222)
visceral reflex (p. 219)

Throughout the day, you are busy doing various things. You walk across a room, run up the stairs, write, tie your shoes, and chew your food. You perform all these activities voluntarily and consciously. Your body, however, performs many more activities automatically. For example, when you eat, you don't think, "I am eating. Therefore, I should increase the flow of my digestive enzymes and then increase the rate of contraction of my intestinal muscles to enhance the digestive process." Instead, your body automatically makes these decisions and carries them out for you. This automatic response is the function of the **autonomic nervous system (ANS)**. Autonomic = automatic!

AUTONOMIC (VISCERAL) REFLEXES

WHAT THEY DO

Mention the word *reflex* and what comes to mind is the knee-jerk reflex. Tap the patellar ligament and up pops the leg. The knee-jerk reflex is mediated by somatic nerves. There are also visceral reflexes. These reflexes are mediated by the ANS. As the name implies, visceral reflexes regulate organ function. Visceral reflexes control such things as heart rate, blood pressure, body temperature, digestion, airflow through respiratory passages, elimination, and pupillary (eye) responses. Note the wide variety of functions controlled by autonomic activity. It takes a load off your mind!

PATHWAY

A **visceral reflex** is mediated in a manner similar to the knee-jerk reflex: activation of a receptor, transmission of sensory information to the central nervous system (CNS), the processing of the information by the CNS, and the motor response sent to the effector organ(s). For example, a sudden decrease in blood pressure activates pressure receptors (baroreceptors). The information about the low blood pressure is carried to the medulla oblongata in the brain stem by sensory nerves. The medulla oblongata determines that the blood pressure

Table **12.1**	Autonomic Nervous System: Organ Responses	
ORGAN	**SYMPATHETIC RESPONSE**	**PARASYMPATHETIC RESPONSE**
Heart	Increases rate and strength of contraction	Decreases rate: no direct effect on strength
Bronchial tubes	Dilates (↑ airflow)	Constricts (↓ airflow)
Iris of eye	Dilates (pupil enlarges)	Constricts (pupil becomes smaller)
Blood vessels	Constricts	No innervation
Sweat glands	Stimulates	No innervation
Intestine	Inhibits motility and secretion	Stimulates motility and secretion
Uterus	Relaxes muscle	No effect
Adrenal medulla	Stimulates secretion of epinephrine and norepinephrine	No effect
Salivary glands	Stimulates thick secretion	Stimulates watery secretion
Urinary system		
Bladder wall	Relaxes muscle	Contracts muscle
Internal sphincter	Closes sphincter	Opens sphincter

is low and sends motor signals to the visceral effector organs (heart and blood vessels). The motor response results in changes in the heart and blood vessels that elevate blood pressure. What has been accomplished? A sudden decrease in blood pressure stimulates a visceral reflex that restores blood pressure to normal. All this has been accomplished without conscious input.

 Do You Know...

What Pinocchio and Your Autonomic Nervous System Have in Common?

Although Pinocchio's nose was a dead giveaway to his lying ways, most of us do not do "the nose thing" in response to fibbing. But fibbers beware! Your ANS can act like the puppet's nose. Lying, even those little white lies, activates the sympathetic nervous system and causes physiological responses that are readily found by a polygraph machine. A modern-day Gepetto knew that we are generally unable to control the ANS and so invented the lie detector.

Why does 007 wear shades? The ANS is constantly adjusting our innards to environmental stresses. The adjustments are noticeable in our eye responses, particularly in the changes in pupil size. Bored, you say? Pupils constrict. Got your eye on a "person of interest"? Pupils dilate. James Bond certainly doesn't want to give away any of his autonomic cues and therefore wears his shades—as do poker players.

ORGANIZATION AND FUNCTION OF THE AUTONOMIC NERVOUS SYSTEM

DIVISION OF THE AUTONOMIC NERVOUS SYSTEM

The ANS is the part of the peripheral nervous system that supplies motor activity to the effector organs: glands, smooth muscles within organs and tubes, and the heart.

The two divisions of the ANS are the sympathetic (sim-pah-THET-ik) and parasympathetic (pair-ah-sim-pah-THET-ik) nervous systems. The distribution of sympathetic and parasympathetic nerves to the viscera

varies. A single organ most often receives fibers from both divisions of the ANS; this is called **dual innervation**. Because of dual innervation, the effects of autonomic stimulation are either antagonistic or cooperative. In most instances, stimulation of one division of the ANS causes a specific effect, whereas stimulation by the other division causes an antagonistic or opposing effect. For example, the cells of the heart that determine heart rate receive both sympathetic and parasympathetic fibers. Stimulation of the sympathetic fibers increases heart rate, whereas stimulation of the parasympathetic fibers decreases heart rate. There are exceptions to this arrangement. In a few organs that receive dual innervation, the effects of sympathetic and parasympathetic activity are cooperative rather than antagonistic. For example, in the male, erectile activity is regulated by the parasympathetics, whereas ejaculation is regulated by the sympathetics. The sympathetics and parasympathetics work in a cooperative way to achieve the desired effect: penetration of the female and ejection of the sperm. Finally, not all organs have dual innervation. For example, the blood vessels are innervated only by the sympathetic nervous system. Regulation of blood vessel diameter is achieved through an adjustment of sympathetic activity. Increased sympathetic activity causes constriction of the blood vessels, and decreased sympathetic activity causes the blood vessels to dilate.

Table 12.1 indicates the effects of sympathetic and parasympathetic stimulation on some major organs of the body.

SYMPATHETIC NERVOUS SYSTEM: FIGHT OR FLIGHT

In general, the **sympathetic nervous system** is activated during periods of stress or times when a person feels threatened in some way (Fig. 12.1). For this reason, the sympathetic nervous system is called the **fight-or-flight division** of the ANS. In other words, the sympathetic nervous system causes you to be prepared either to confront (fight) or to remove yourself from the threatening

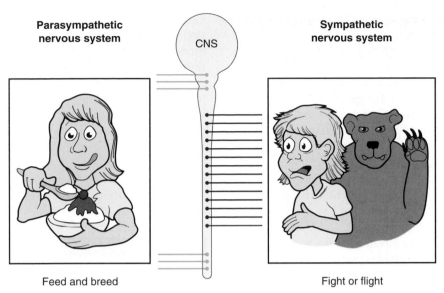

Parasympathetic nervous system

CNS

Sympathetic nervous system

Feed and breed

Fight or flight

FIG. 12.1 Autonomic nervous system: parasympathetic nervous system and sympathetic nervous system. Craniosacral outflow (green fibers), thoracolumbar outflow (red fibers).

situation (flight). Recall a time when you were frightened. Your heart raced and pounded in your chest. The pupils of your eyes opened wide. You breathed more quickly and more deeply. The palms of your hands became wet with perspiration, and your mouth became so dry you could hardly speak. The easiest way to remember the sympathetic responses is to recall your personal response to your own worst nightmare. You can check Table 12.1 to see if your responses matched the sympathetic column.

Although the sympathetic nervous system is activated during periods of stress, these periods are normally short-lived. If you keep yourself stressed out, however, the sympathetic nervous system keeps the body in a state of high alert. Over time, this state takes its toll on the body through stress-induced illnesses. Laughter, play, rest, and relaxation diminish sympathetic outflow and are good buffers against stress. So relax and be happy!

 Do You Know...

About the Sympathetic Nervous System Gone Wild?

Several clinical conditions are caused by out-of-control sympathetic activity. One condition is called *autonomic dysreflexia*. Autonomic dysreflexia is experienced by a person who has sustained a high cervical spinal cord injury (e.g., C4 transection and quadriplegia). With this condition, the quadriplegic patient develops a distended urinary bladder, usually from a kinked urinary catheter. The distended bladder sends signals to the spinal cord, setting off massive thoracolumbar (sympathetic) discharge. The intense sympathetic activity severely elevates blood pressure, sometimes to the point of causing a cerebral hemorrhage (stroke). The sympathetic stimulation continues as long as the bladder remains distended. The ANS cannot counteract the sympathetic firing because of the spinal cord injury. Immediate treatment is to remove the stimulus (distended bladder), which then lowers the blood pressure. Out-of-control sympathetic activity is life threatening and is always taken seriously.

PARASYMPATHETIC NERVOUS SYSTEM: FEED AND BREED

The **parasympathetic nervous system** is most active during quiet, nonstressful conditions. It has a calming effect on the body. The parasympathetic nervous system plays an important role in the regulation of digestion and in reproductive function. For this reason, it is sometimes referred to as the **feed-and-breed division** of the ANS. Another descriptive term for the parasympathetic nervous system is *resting and digesting*.

What is "paradoxical fear"? Although the sympathetics are usually associated with fear reactions, the parasympathetics can be activated in situations that are perceived as hopeless and where fight or flight seems futile. The massive parasympathetic discharge can result in uncontrolled urination and defecation. It can also cause the heart rate to decrease so severely that the person faints or experiences a potentially lethal electrical disturbance of the heart. Clinically, this type of cardiac stress reaction is described as "bradying down," a reference to severe bradycardia (dangerously slow heart rate). Yes, one can die of fright!

 Re-Think

1. Name the two divisions of the autonomic nervous system.
2. Explain the antagonistic and cooperative effects of dual innervation.
3. Explain why sympathetic activity is called the fight-or-flight division.
4. Explain why parasympathetic activity is called the feed-and-breed division.

AUTONOMIC TERMINOLOGY AND PHARMACOLOGY

Many drugs work by altering autonomic activity. Thus, many pharmacology terms refer to the autonomic nervous system. In fact, you cannot understand pharmacology without knowing ANS terminology. So get ready for some challenging words.

If a drug causes effects similar to the activation of the sympathetic nervous system, it is called a *sympathomimetic* (sim-pah-thoh-mim-ET-ik) (as in mimicking) drug. A sympathomimetic agent increases heart rate, force of cardiac contraction, and blood pressure. If the drug causes effects that are similar to a situation where the sympathetic nervous system cannot be activated, the drug is called a *sympatholytic* (sim-pah-thoh-LIT-ik) drug (*-lytic* means "inhibiting"). The administration of a sympatholytic drug prevents an increase in cardiac activity when the sympathetic nerves are fired.

If a drug causes effects similar to the activation of the parasympathetic nervous system, it is called a *parasympathomimetic* (pair-ah-sim-pah-thoh-mim-ET-ik) drug. A parasympathomimetic agent decreases heart rate and increases digestive activity. The administration of a *parasympatholytic* (pair-ah-sim-pah-thoh-LIT-ik) agent prevents activation of the parasympathetic nervous system. As if this isn't confusing enough! Most parasympathetic fibers travel with the vagus nerve (CN X). If a drug causes effects similar to parasympathetic activity, it is also called **vagomimetic.** If a drug slows parasympathetic activity, it is called **vagolytic.** The vagomimetic and vagolytic terminology is more commonly used in clinical situations. If an organ, such as the heart, is being driven excessively by the parasympathetic nervous system, the heart rate becomes dangerously slow (bradycardia). The administration of a parasympatholytic or vagolytic drug, such as atropine, blocks the parasympathetic effect on the heart, thereby allowing the heart rate to increase.

AUTONOMIC TONE AND VASOMOTOR TONE

The sympathetics and parasympathetics are active at the same time, creating a background (continuous, low-level) firing of the ANS. This background autonomic activity is called *autonomic tone*. In the resting state, parasympathetic activity is generally stronger. For example, parasympathetic tone maintains the resting heart rate at around 72 beats per minute. When physical activity increases, however, the sympathetic nerves fire more intensely, whereas parasympathetic activity decreases. The shift to sympathetic discharge during exercise results in an increase in heart rate, thereby supplying more oxygen and energy to the exercising muscles. The balance between sympathetic and parasympathetic activity is maintained by the hypothalamus and parts of the brain stem.

A second example of autonomic tone involves the blood vessels. Blood vessels are innervated only by the sympathetic nerves; there is no parasympathetic innervation. Thus, the autonomic tone of the blood vessels is determined by the sympathetic nervous system. Background sympathetic firing keeps the blood vessels somewhat constricted. This sympathetically induced continuous state of blood vessel constriction is called *vasomotor tone* or *sympathetic tone*. Additional sympathetic firing causes blood vessels to constrict, thereby elevating blood pressure. A decrease in sympathetic firing causes blood vessels to dilate, thereby lowering blood pressure. A change in vasomotor tone is clinically very important. For example, loss of vasomotor tone can dangerously lower blood pressure, plunging a person into a lethal shock.

 Re-Think

1. What is a sympathomimetic effect? A parasympathomimetic effect?
2. What is the effect of a vagomimetic drug on heart rate? What is the effect of a vagolytic drug on heart rate?

 Sum It Up!

The ANS regulates visceral (organ) functions such as blood pressure. There are two divisions of the ANS: the sympathetic (fight or flight) and parasympathetic (feed and breed) nervous systems. Most organs receive dual innervation by both the sympathetic and parasympathetic nervous systems. Because of dual innervation, the effects of autonomic stimulation are either antagonistic or cooperative. Background firing of the sympathetic nervous system to the blood vessels is responsible for vasomotor or sympathetic tone that, in turn, plays a crucial role in the maintenance of normal blood pressure.

AUTONOMIC NERVOUS SYSTEM NEURONS

NUMBERS AND GANGLIA

The numbers and arrangement of the neurons of the ANS are important. The pathways of the ANS use two neurons with a **ganglion** between each neuron (Fig. 12.2A). The cell body of neuron 1 is located in the CNS, in the brain or the spinal cord. The axon of neuron 1 leaves the CNS and extends to the ganglion where it synapses on neuron 2. The axon of neuron 1 is called the **preganglionic fiber** (because it comes before [*pre*] the ganglion). The axon of neuron 2 leaves the ganglion and extends to the effector or target organ. This axon is called the **postganglionic fiber** (because it comes after [*post*] the ganglion). Pay particular attention to the postganglionic fibers; they are key to understanding autonomic function. The postganglionic fibers of the sympathetic and parasympathetic nervous systems secrete different neurotransmitters. These different neurotransmitters account for the different effects caused by the sympathetic and parasympathetic nervous systems.

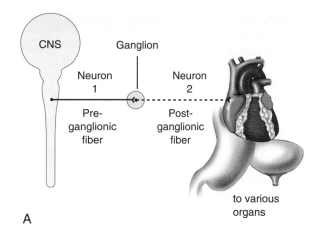

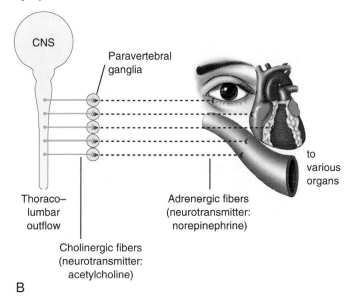

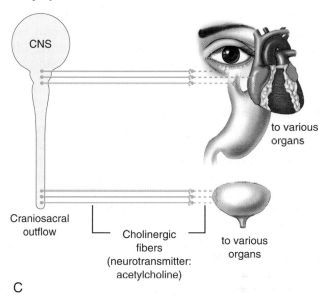

FIG. 12.2 (A) Arrangement of autonomic fibers. (B) Sympathetic nervous system. (C) Parasympathetic nervous system.

NEURONS OF THE SYMPATHETIC NERVOUS SYSTEM

The neurons of the sympathetic nervous system leave the spinal cord at the thoracic and lumbar levels (T1 to L2) (see Fig. 12.2B). The sympathetic nervous system is therefore called the **thoracolumbar outflow.** Most preganglionic sympathetic fibers travel a short distance and synapse within ganglia located close to the spinal cord. The sympathetic ganglia form a chain that runs parallel to the vertebral column. This chain is called the **paravertebral ganglia** or *sympathetic chain ganglia.* Postganglionic fibers leave the ganglia and extend to the various target organs.

The location of the paravertebral ganglia is important. The paravertebral ganglia provide a site where each preganglionic fiber synapses with multiple postganglionic fibers. Why is this important? The firing of a single sympathetic neuron is capable of providing a generalized, widespread sympathetic response; many organs respond to sympathetic firing. This makes sense—if you are confronted with an emergency situation, you want the entire body to respond immediately!

The adrenal gland (adrenal medulla) acts as a modified sympathetic ganglion. Preganglionic sympathetic fibers supply the adrenal medulla, causing it to secrete hormones (epinephrine and norepinephrine) that resemble the neurotransmitters of the sympathetic nervous system. These hormones circulate in the blood throughout the body. Thus, the sympathetic nervous system and the adrenal medulla function together to achieve a sustained response.

NEURONS OF THE PARASYMPATHETIC NERVOUS SYSTEM

The neurons of the parasympathetic nervous system leave the CNS at the level of the brain stem and sacrum (S2 to S4; see Fig. 12.2C). The parasympathetic nervous system is therefore called the **craniosacral outflow.**

Because the ganglia of the parasympathetic nervous system are located close to or within the target organs, the parasympathetic nerves do not have a chain of ganglia running parallel to the spinal cord. The preganglionic fibers are long because the ganglia of the parasympathetic nervous system are located near the target organ. Short postganglionic fibers run from the ganglia to the smooth muscle or glands within the organ. Because of the location of the ganglia close to the target organs, parasympathetic activity generates a more localized response (as opposed to the generalized sympathetic response). Table 12.2 compares the anatomical arrangement of the sympathetic and parasympathetic nervous systems.

RUNNING WITH CRANIAL NERVES

Parasympathetic fibers travel from the brain stem with four cranial nerves (CNs): oculomotor (CN III), facial (CN VII), glossopharyngeal (CN IX), and vagus (CN X).

Oculomotor Nerve (CN III)

The oculomotor nerve innervates most of the extrinsic eye muscles (skeletal muscles) that move the eyeball. The oculomotor nerve also carries parasympathetic fibers to two intrinsic eye muscles: the constrictor muscle of the eye, which causes pupillary constriction, and the ciliary muscle, which controls the shape of the lens of the eye.

Facial Nerve (CN VII)

The facial nerve carries parasympathetic fibers to the tear glands (eyes), salivary glands (mouth), and nasal glands (nose).

Glossopharyngeal Nerve (CN IX)

The glossopharyngeal nerve (with the assistance of the trigeminal nerve) carries parasympathetic fibers to the salivary glands in the mouth.

Vagus Nerve (CN X)

The vagus nerve (the "wanderer" nerve) carries over 80% of the parasympathetic fibers. It travels from the brain stem to organs within the thoracic and abdominal cavities. Thus, the terms parasympathomimetic/parasympatholytic are used synonymously with vagomimetic/vagolytic.

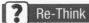 **Re-Think**

1. State the difference between a preganglionic and postganglionic fiber.
2. Why is the preganglionic fiber of the sympathetic nervous system shorter than that of the parasympathetic nervous system?
3. Why are the sympathetic nerves referred to as thoracolumbar outflow?
4. Why are the parasympathetic nerves referred to as the craniosacral outflow?
5. List the four cranial nerves that carry parasympathetic fibers.

 Sum It Up!

The sympathetic nervous system is called the *thoracolumbar outflow*; the parasympathetic nervous system is called the *craniosacral outflow*. Each system has preganglionic and postganglionic fibers. The ganglia of the sympathetic nerves are located in the paravertebral ganglia, and the ganglia of the parasympathetics are located near the target organ. Parasympathetic fibers travel from the brain stem with four cranial nerves: oculomotor, facial, glossopharyngeal, and vagus nerves.

NAMING FIBERS AND NEUROTRANSMITTERS

The key to understanding autonomic function and autonomic pharmacology is based on knowledge of the autonomic neurotransmitters and their receptors. The two major neurotransmitters of the ANS are **acetylcholine (ACh)** and **norepinephrine** (nor-ep-i-NEF-rin) **(NE)**.

The neurotransmitter is used to name the fibers of the ANS. For example, a fiber that secretes NE as its neurotransmitter is called an **adrenergic fiber** (NE is also called nor*adrenaline*). A fiber that secretes ACh (acetyl*choline*) as its neurotransmitter is called a **cholinergic fiber**.

Now, here's the challenging part. Remember, we are concerned with four fibers (two preganglionic and two postganglionic fibers...sympathetic and parasympathetic). All preganglionic fibers secrete ACh and are therefore cholinergic fibers. The postganglionic fibers of the parasympathetic nervous system secrete ACh and are also cholinergic. The postganglionic sympathetic nervous system fibers, however, secrete NE and are called *adrenergic fibers*. Refer to

Table 12.2   Autonomic Nervous System: Comparison

CHARACTERISTIC	SYMPATHETIC	PARASYMPATHETIC
Origin of fibers	Thoracolumbar	Craniosacral
Functions	Fight or flight	Feed and breed
Ganglia	Paravertebral ganglia	Located near or in target organ
Effects	Generalized, widespread	Localized
Neurotransmitter	Norepinephrine (postganglionic)	Acetylcholine

Fig. 12.2B and C, and note the color coding that differentiates the adrenergic from the cholinergic fibers. The cholinergic fibers are colored green, whereas the adrenergic fibers are colored red. You absolutely need this fiber-neurotransmitter information to learn autonomic pharmacology.

NEUROTRANSMITTERS: TERMINATION OF ACTIVITY

ACh is secreted by cholinergic fibers and diffuses to its receptor. After ACh exerts its effect on its receptor, it is quickly degraded by acetylcholinesterase (AChE), an enzyme found in the synapse.

NE is secreted by adrenergic fibers. The effects of NE are more prolonged because of the manner in which NE is terminated. Most of the NE is reabsorbed by the adrenergic nerve terminals themselves. The termination of NE is called *reuptake*. Note that its termination differs from that of ACh. The NE taken up by the nerve terminal is processed in two ways. Most of the NE is simply reused. Excess NE can be degraded by an enzyme located within the adrenergic nerve terminal and is called *monoamine oxidase* (MAO). Some of the NE is merely "washed away" from the synapse and is degraded by another enzyme found in surrounding tissue. The name of this enzyme is *catechol-O-methyltransferase* (COMT).

Do You Know...

Why You Might Have to "Hold the Beer and Sausage" If You Are Taking an MAO Inhibitor?

Monoamine oxidase (MAO) is an enzyme that breaks down norepinephrine in the CNS. An MAO inhibitor drug prevents the breakdown of NE and is used in the treatment of depression. Although the drug relieves the depression by increasing NE in the CNS, it can also cause serious adverse effects such as a dangerously elevated blood pressure. Certain foods (e.g., beer, cheese, sausage) contain an amino acid that is used in the synthesis of NE. The combination of the drugs and food increases NE and blood pressure and the possibility of a stroke. Some herbals such as St. John's wort have MAO inhibitor activity and may also dangerously elevate blood pressure. Taking an MAO inhibitor? Hold the beer and sausage!

Sum It Up!

The two major neurotransmitters of the ANS are acetylcholine (ACh) and norepinephrine (NE). ACh is secreted by cholinergic fibers. The effects of ACh are short lived; the ACh is degraded by acetylcholinesterase located in the synapse. NE is secreted by adrenergic fibers. The effects of the sympathetic nervous system are primarily caused by NE. The effects of NE are more prolonged because of how NE is terminated (through reuptake). Excess NE is degraded by monoamine oxidase (MAO). Some NE is simply washed away and degraded at distal sites by another enzyme.

Re-Think

1. What is the difference between a cholinergic and adrenergic fiber?
2. Explain how neurotransmitter activity is terminated.

RECEPTORS OF THE AUTONOMIC NERVOUS SYSTEM

The neurotransmitters of the ANS—ACh and NE—bind to receptors on target cells (cardiac muscle, smooth muscle, and glands). A receptor is any site on the cell to which a neurotransmitter binds, causing an alteration in cellular function. For example, ACh binds to a receptor on a heart cell and causes the heart rate to decrease. NE binds to a different receptor on the heart cell and causes the heart rate to increase. The ANS has two receptor types: cholinergic and adrenergic receptors.

CHOLINERGIC RECEPTORS

Cholinergic receptors are activated by ACh. There are two types of cholinergic receptors: **muscarinic** (mus-kar-IN-ik) **receptors** and **nicotinic receptors.** The different types of cholinergic receptors explain the variety of effects of cholinergic receptor activation by ACh.

Where are these receptors located? Muscarinic receptors are located on the effector or target organs (cardiac muscle, smooth muscle, and glands) of the parasympathetic nerves (Fig. 12.3A). Thus, activation of the parasympathetic nervous system releases ACh and stimulates muscarinic receptors. Refer to Table 12.3 and note several of the effects of muscarinic activation. For example, activation of the muscarinic receptors on the constrictor muscle of the iris causes pupil size to decrease. Activation of the muscarinic receptors in the heart (sinoatrial node) causes the heart rate to decrease. Muscarinic activation of the urinary bladder causes the bladder muscle to contract and the outlet sphincter muscle of the urinary bladder to relax; these coordinated muscarinic responses of the bladder promote urination.

There are two types of nicotinic receptors in the peripheral nervous system. The nicotinic neural (N_N) receptors are located within the ganglia of the ANS (see Fig. 12.3A and B). Because these nicotinic receptors are located in both the sympathetic nervous system and parasympathetic nervous system, the responses to N_N activation are difficult to predict. Nicotinic receptors are also located outside the ANS. For example, the receptors located on skeletal muscles in the neuromuscular junction are nicotinic muscle receptors (N_M; see Fig. 12.3C). Activation of the N_M receptors in the neuromuscular junction causes skeletal muscle contraction. Remember, the N_N receptors are part of the ANS; the N_M receptors are part of the somatic motor nervous system and skeletal muscle. The cholinergic receptor subtypes are important in pharmacology and are worthwhile learning. However, in this chapter, we will refer only to the muscarinic receptors.

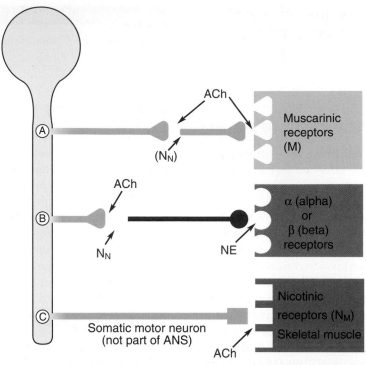

FIG. 12.3 Receptors and neurotransmitters: adrenergic (NE) and cholinergic (ACh).

Table **12.3**	Cholinergic Receptors and Responses*	
ORGAN	**RECEPTOR**	**ACTIVATION RESPONSE**
Heart	Muscarinic	Decreases heart rate
Bronchial tubes	Muscarinic	Constricts (↓ airflow)
Iris of eye	Muscarinic	Constricts (pupil becomes smaller)
Urinary system		
Bladder wall	Muscarinic	Contracts
Internal sphincter	Muscarinic	Relaxes and opens sphincter

*Muscarinic receptors that are commonly targeted by pharmacological agents are listed in this table.

 ## Do You Know...

About "Green Tobacco Sickness" and Your Nicotinic Receptors?

Here's the scenario. A young child of migrant farm workers is harvesting tobacco leaves in the early morning. The tobacco leaves are laden with nicotine-rich morning dew, which quickly saturates the child's clothing. The dermal absorption of nicotine from the surface of wet tobacco leaves is rapid, and the child experiences nausea, abdominal pain, excess salivation, tachycardia, hypertension, and headache. As the nicotine level in the blood further increases, the child develops muscle twitching and generalized muscle weakness that may progress to skeletal muscle paralysis and respiratory arrest. The child is experiencing "green tobacco sickness" (GTS), which is, no doubt, complicated by exposure to pesticides and a vomiting-induced dehydration. His family attempts to prevent the most severe symptoms of GTS by wearing

plastic trash bags on their arms until the blistering sun eventually dries the tobacco leaves and slows the absorption of nicotine.

What has happened physiologically? The nicotine in the child's blood has saturated the nicotinic receptors (N_M) within the neuromuscular junction, causing twitching and extreme muscle weakness/paralysis/respiratory arrest. In addition, the nicotine has saturated the nicotinic receptors (N_N) within the autonomic ganglia; this causes a release of catecholamines, such as the fight-or-flight epinephrine and dopamine, from the adrenal medulla. The catecholamines cause the tachycardia (racing heart) and hypertension (high blood pressure). Activation of nicotinic receptors within the CNS intensifies these responses and causes additional cognitive symptoms. One can only speculate about the long-term developmental effects.

In some parts of the world, child labor laws are lax or nonexistent, and the incidence of GTS is high. But, closer to home...in the United States, it is illegal for a child younger than 18 years of age to purchase cigarettes and other tobacco-containing products. However, it is not illegal for children under 18 years of age to work in the tobacco fields, where they commonly experience serious nicotinic poisoning. Go figure!

ADRENERGIC RECEPTORS

There are two main types of adrenergic receptors: **alpha- (α) adrenergic** and **beta- (β) adrenergic receptors** (see Fig. 12.3B). There are subtypes of the adrenergic receptors: alpha₁-, alpha₂-, beta₁-, and beta₂-adrenergic receptors. Adrenergic receptors are located on the target organs of the sympathetic nerves, so that stimulation of the sympathetic nervous system causes activation

Table 12.4 Adrenergic Receptors and Responses*

ORGAN	RECEPTOR†	ACTIVATION RESPONSE
Heart	β_1	Increases heart rate and strength of contraction
Bronchial tubes	β_2	Dilates (↑ airflow)
Iris of eye	α_1	Dilates (pupil enlarges)
Blood vessels	α_1	Constricts
Uterus	β_2	Relaxes

*Adrenergic receptors commonly targeted by pharmacological agents are listed in this table.
†α, Alpha; β, beta.

of adrenergic receptors. See Table 12.4 for the effects of adrenergic receptor activation. Note that activation of the alpha$_1$ receptors of the blood vessels of the mucous membrane causes constriction, thereby decreasing blood flow and shrinking swollen membranes to relieve the discomfort of a stuffy nose. Activation of the alpha$_1$ receptors on blood vessels causes vasoconstriction, thereby elevating blood pressure. These drugs are used in the treatment of conditions that involve low blood pressure, such as shock. Activation of the beta$_1$ receptors in the heart increases heart rate and the strength of cardiac muscle contraction. Activation of the beta$_2$ receptors dilates the breathing tubes, thereby increasing airflow; this action is the basis of the bronchodilators used in the treatment of asthma. Activation of the alpha$_1$ receptors in the iris (eye) causes the radial muscle to contract and the pupil to dilate. Finally, activation of the beta$_2$ receptors in the pregnant uterus causes the uterine muscles to relax, thereby preventing the premature delivery of the fetus. The adrenergic receptors are activated by NE and other natural catecholamines, such as epinephrine and dopamine.

There is a small number of dopamine receptors (also classified as adrenergic receptors) located in the blood vessels of the kidney. Activation of the dopamine receptors causes the blood vessels in the kidney to dilate, thereby increasing blood flow to the kidneys. Dopamine is often administered clinically to maintain blood flow to the kidneys during shocklike episodes that would normally diminish blood flow to the kidneys.

 Re-Think

1. Name and locate the cholinergic receptors. Name the neurotransmitter that activates cholinergic receptors.
2. Name and locate the adrenergic receptors. Name a neurotransmitter that activates adrenergic receptors.

AUTONOMIC TERMINOLOGY: "DOING" AUTONOMIC PHARMACOLOGY

Autonomic pharmacology classifies drugs according to their receptors. For example, a beta$_1$-adrenergic agonist is a drug that activates the beta$_1$-adrenergic receptors. (An agonist is a drug that activates a receptor.) A beta$_1$-adrenergic antagonist is a drug that blocks the effect of beta$_1$-adrenergic activation. (An antagonist or blocker is a drug that prevents receptor activation.) A muscarinic agonist activates the muscarinic receptor, whereas a muscarinic antagonist blocks muscarinic receptor activation. The same terminology (agonist/antagonist) is applied to drugs that interact with cholinergic and adrenergic receptors.

Let's see if you can figure out some autonomic physiology and pharmacology.

- **Question 1.** Mr. T was admitted to the ER, experiencing respiratory distress caused by asthma. Why was he given a beta$_2$-adrenergic agonist (albuterol)? Check Table 12.4 for the respiratory effects of beta$_2$-adrenergic activation. **Answer.** Activation of the beta$_2$-adrenergic receptors on the bronchioles (airways) causes the airways to dilate (open up), thereby improving the flow of air and relieving the respiratory distress of asthma.

- **Question 2.** A very anxious Mr. Q was admitted with a rapid heart rate. Why was he given a beta$_1$-adrenergic blocker (propranolol)? Check Table 12.4 for the cardiac (heart) effects of beta$_1$-adrenergic response. **Answer.** Mr. Q's heart rate was elevated because of excess sympathetic stimulation (an anxiety effect). A beta$_1$-adrenergic blocker prevents activation of the beta$_1$-adrenergic receptors on the heart, thereby reducing heart rate.

- **Question 3.** A patient has had a heart attack and is experiencing a very slow heart rate caused by excessive parasympathetic (vagal) activity. Why was he given a muscarinic antagonist (atropine)? Check Table 12.3 for the effects of muscarinic activation on heart rate. **Answer.** Muscarinic activation (caused by excess parasympathetic activity) slows heart rate. By blocking muscarinic receptors with atropine, heart rate increases.

- **Question 4.** Ms. S is diagnosed with hypertension (high blood pressure). Why did her physician prescribe an alpha$_1$-adrenergic blocker? Check Table 12.4 for the effect of an alpha$_1$-adrenergic response on blood vessels. **Answer.** The alpha$_1$-adrenergic antagonist blocks the alpha$_1$ receptors in the blood vessels, causing them to dilate. Blood vessel dilation decreases blood pressure.

- **Question 5.** A postoperative patient is unable to urinate because of the anticholinergic drugs used during the perioperative period. Why was she given a muscarinic agonist such as bethanechol? **Answer.** Activation of the muscarinic receptors stimulates contraction of the urinary bladder and relaxation of the bladder sphincter. Both actions facilitate urination.

- **Question 6.** A patient goes to his eye doctor for an eye exam. Why did the physician put anticholinergic eyedrops in his eyes (see Table 12.3)? **Answer.** Activation of the muscarinic receptor on the pupillary muscles causes pupillary constriction. By using anticholinergic (antimuscarinic) eyedrops, the muscarinic receptors are blocked, and the pupil dilates. The dilated pupils facilitate the eye exam.

- **Question 7.** A canine friend (Dillon) routinely "bradys down" in response to general anesthesia and is therefore premedicated with atropine. What happens to Dillon without and with the atropine? **Answer.** The general anesthesia causes sustained vagal discharge to the heart and a significant decrease in heart rate (bradycardia). By premedicating with a vagolytic or antimuscarinic drug (see Table 12.3), atropine, the decline in heart rate is prevented.

This is how to analyze autonomic function and "do" autonomic pharmacology. Learn the receptors and the consequences of receptor activation (agonist) and blockade (antagonist).

 Do You Know...

About the Parasympathetics, Nitric Oxide, Erections ... and, by the Way, Viagra?

In response to sexual stimulation, parasympathetic fibers stimulate the endothelial cells of the blood vessels of the penis to secrete nitric oxide, a gas that triggers a series of reactions that produce cyclic guanosine monophosphate (cGMP). cGMP relaxes the smooth muscle of the blood vessels, thereby increasing blood flow to the penis. Hence, the erection. Having done its job, the cGMP is degraded by an enzyme called *phosphodiesterase.* Most men with erectile dysfunction have difficulty sustaining their erections. Enter Viagra (sildenafil)! Viagra inhibits the activity of phosphodiesterase, thereby prolonging the life of cGMP and sustaining the erection.

 Sum It Up!

The neurotransmitters, ACh and NE, bind to receptors. There are two types of autonomic receptors: cholinergic and adrenergic. Cholinergic receptors are activated by ACh. There are two types of cholinergic receptors: muscarinic and nicotinic. The muscarinic receptors are located on the target organs of the parasympathetic nerves. The adrenergic receptors are activated by NE. There are two types of adrenergic receptors: alpha- and beta-adrenergic receptors. The adrenergic receptors are located on the target organs of the sympathetic nervous system.

 As You Age

1. Aging causes an increase in synaptic delay and a 5% to 10% decrease in the speed of nerve conduction. Consequently, nerve reflexes become slower.
2. Aging causes a loss of the sense of vibration at the ankle after the age of 65. This change is accompanied by a decrease of the ankle-jerk reflex and may affect balance, increasing the chance of falling.
3. An aging ANS causes many changes. For example, a less efficient sympathetic nervous system may cause transient hypotension and fainting. A decreased responsiveness of the baroreceptor reflex contributes to the fainting episodes.
4. Decreased autonomic nerve activity supplying the eyes causes changes in pupil size and pupillary reactivity. There is some decline in function of the cranial nerves mediating taste and smell.

Medical Terminology and Disorders — Disorders of the Somatic Efferent and Autonomic Nervous Systems

MEDICAL TERM	WORD PARTS	WORD PART MEANING OR DERIVATION	DESCRIPTION
Words			
autonomic	auto-	self	**Autonomic** means *automatic.* In response to changing body needs, the autonomic nervous system (ANS) automatically helps regulate organ function, such as heart rate. The sympathetic division increases heart rate, whereas the parasympathetic division lowers heart rate.
	-nom(os)-	law	
	-ic	pertaining to	
contralateral	contra-	opposite	*A reference to the opposite side of the body.* For example, a patient suffered a brain attack on the left side of her brain and experienced hemiparalysis on the contralateral side (right) of her body.
	-later/o-	side	
	-al	pertaining to	
decussate		From a Latin word meaning "to mark with a cross"	Means *to cross over.* For example, the pyramidal tract decussates at the medulla oblongata and descends on the contralateral side of the spinal cord.
ipsilateral	ipse-	same	*A reference to the same side of the body.* For example, a patient suffered a brain attack (left brain) and suffered right-sided hemiparalysis and ipsilateral paresis (left side of the body).
	-lateral	side	
Disorders			
amyotrophic lateral sclerosis	a-	without	Also called **ALS** or **Lou Gehrig disease**. ALS refers to *progressive deterioration of motor nerve cells resulting in a progressive loss of muscle control.* Muscle atrophy is caused by hardening of nerve tissue on the lateral columns of the spinal cord. Disability increases from muscle weakness in the extremities, muscles of speech and swallowing, and muscles of respiration to total paralysis and death.
	-myo-	muscle	
	-throph/o-	nourishment	
	later/o	side	
	scler/o-	hardening	
	-osis	condition of	

| Medical Terminology and Disorders | | | Disorders of the Somatic Efferent and Autonomic Nervous Systems—cont'd |

MEDICAL TERM	WORD PARTS	WORD PART MEANING OR DERIVATION	DESCRIPTION
autonomic dysreflexia	dys-	difficult or faulty	See the "Do You Know" feature on p. 220.
	-reflexia	reflex	
meningocele	mening/o-	meninges	*Protrusion of the meninges through a defect in the skull or vertebra (spina bifida).* A **myelomeningocele** is *a protrusion of the spinal cord and meninges through a defect in the vertebrae. Disability is related to the location and size of the protruding spinal cord and nervous tissue.*
	-cele	protrusion, hernia	
multiple sclerosis	scler/o-	hardening	**Multiple sclerosis** (MS) is *a progressive demyelination of the neurons, especially the oligodendrocytes; the demyelination produces sclerotic lesions along the neurons, thereby interfering with nerve conduction.* The most common form of MS is called *relapsing-remitting MS,* in which the symptoms appear and disappear (exacerbations and remissions). Degenerative changes affect cognitive, sensory, and motor activity. Fatigue, weakness, paresthesias, ataxia (a- = without; -tax/o- = coordination), and optic neuritis are common. Optic neuritis causes a variety of visual disturbances: diplopia, nystagmus, diminished vision, and blindness.
	-osis	condition of	
neuralgia	neur/o-	nerve	**Neuralgia** is *pain that involves a nerve.* Sciatica is a form of neuralgia; pain moves along the sciatic nerve and its branches through the buttocks and into the thigh and leg. Shingles or herpes zoster sometimes causes postherpetic neuralgia, a severe pain that persists long after the lesions have healed. Pain and a vesicular rash progress along the course of one or more spinal nerves, usually the intercostal nerves and sometimes the trigeminal nerve. Trigeminal neuralgia is due to inflammation of the trigeminal nerve (CN V); it causes excruciating pain in the facial area.
	-algia	pain	
paralysis	para-	alongside of or abnormal	**Paralysis** refers to *the complete loss of muscle function in one or more muscle groups.* Paralysis (-plegia) may be accompanied by loss of sensation. Most episodes of paralysis in adults are due to CVA and spinal cord injury. Paralysis may be described as being flaccid or spastic. Flaccid paralysis is described as flabby or lack of muscle control and is caused by damaged nerves. With spastic paralysis there is stiff and poorly coordinated muscle control. It is due to CNS disorders such as cerebral palsy. Infantile paralysis or polio is a contagious viral infection that destroys the motor neurons in the gray matter (polio means "gray") of the brain stem and the spinal cord. Bell's palsy is a weakness or paralysis of one side of the face in response to inflammation of the facial nerve (CN VII). The word part *paresis* means "slight paralysis," as in hemiparesis (slight paralysis or weakness of the right or left half of the body). Gastroparesis causes weak stomach (gastr/o- = stomach) muscle contractions and delayed gastric emptying. Vocal cord paresis causes diminishment in voice quality and volume.
	-lysis	breakdown	
paresthesia	para-	alongside of or abnormal	*Refers to abnormal sensation such as burning, numbness, prickling, or tingling.* Paresthesias can be caused by lesions of both the central and peripheral nervous system and often are symptomatic of other disorders such as multiple sclerosis and diabetes mellitus. **Anesthesia** is *a lack of sensation* and hyperesthesia is *an increased sensitivity to a sensory stimulus (skin/touch).*
	-esthesia	sensation or feeling	
peripheral neuropathy	neur/o-	nerve	*A loss of normal sensation caused by peripheral nerve damage.* There are many causes of neuropathies. The pain has different intensities (severe to mild), multiple distribution patterns (hands, foot, pain), and a variety of descriptions (numbness, burning, tingling, prickly, akin to electric shock).
	-path/o-	disease	
	-y	condition of	
spinal cord injury			*Any condition or event that damages the spinal cord.* Complete transection of the cord produces quadriplegia or paraplegia, depending on the level of injury. Immediately after the injury, the person experiences spinal shock that may last from several hours to several weeks.

Get Ready for Exams!

Summary Outline

I. Autonomic or Visceral Reflexes
  A. What they do: autonomic nerves reflexively regulate organ function.
  B. Pathway: the sequence is receptor activation, sensory input (→ CNS), motor neuron response, and effector response.

II. Organization and Function of the Autonomic Nervous System
  A. Divisions of the ANS: two divisions
    1. Sympathetic nervous system, called *fight or flight*
    2. Parasympathetic nervous system, called *feed and breed*
  B. Autonomic terminology and autonomic pharmacology
    1. Drugs that affect the sympathetic nervous system are called *sympathomimetic* and *sympatholytic.*
    2. Drugs that affect the parasympathetic nervous system are called *parasympathomimetic* (vagomimetic) and *parasympatholytic* (vagolytic).
  C. Autonomic tone and vasomotor tone
    1. Background firing of the ANS causes autonomic tone.
    2. Background sympathetic stimulation of the blood vessels causes vasomotor or sympathetic tone.

III. Autonomic Nervous System: Neurons
  A. Numbers and ganglia
    1. Preganglionic fibers are fibers that extend from the CNS to the ganglia.
    2. Postganglionic fibers are fibers that extend from the ganglia to the effector or target organ.
  B. Neurons of the sympathetic nervous system
    1. The sympathetic nervous system is called the *thoracolumbar outflow.*
    2. The sympathetic ganglia are located in a chain close to the spinal cord; the chain is called *paravertebral ganglia.*
    3. The adrenal medulla secretes hormones that mimic the sympathetic nervous system.
  C. Neurons of the parasympathetic nervous system
    1. The parasympathetic nervous system is called the *craniosacral outflow.*
    2. Some parasympathetic fibers travel with cranial nerves; most parasympathetics run with the vagus nerve (CN X).
  D. Naming fibers and neurotransmitters
    1. Cholinergic fibers secrete acetylcholine (ACh).
    2. Adrenergic fibers secrete norepinephrine (NE).
  E. Neurotransmitters: termination of activity
    1. ACh is degraded immediately by acetylcholinesterase.
    2. NE activity is ended primarily by reuptake of the NE into the nerve terminal and by MAO activity in the nerve terminal. Distally, NE is degraded by COMT.

IV. Receptors of the Autonomic Nervous System
  A. Cholinergic receptors
    1. Activated by ACh
    2. Two types: muscarinic and nicotinic (and subtypes)
  B. Adrenergic receptors
    1. Activated by NE
    2. Two types: alpha and beta (and subtypes)
  C. Receptor activation and blockade can be determined by examining Tables 12.1, 12.3, and 12.4.
  D. Autonomic receptors—doing autonomic pharmacology
    1. Clinical examples where drugs target autonomic receptors

Review Your Knowledge

Matching: Sympathetic or Parasympathetic
Directions: Indicate if the following statements describe the sympathetic nervous system (S) or the parasympathetic nervous system (P).

1. ____ Paravertebral ganglia
2. ____ Feed-and-breed function
3. ____ Thoracolumbar outflow
4. ____ Postganglionic fiber is adrenergic.
5. ____ The target organs are stimulated by norepinephrine (NE).
6. ____ Fight-or-flight function
7. ____ The postganglionic fiber is cholinergic.
8. ____ The target organs are stimulated by acetylcholine (ACh).
9. ____ Craniosacral outflow
10. ____ The effects of this system are more widespread and prolonged.

Matching: Norepinephrine or Acetylcholine
Directions: Indicate if the statements are descriptive of norepinephrine (NE) or acetylcholine (ACh).

1. ____ Secreted by adrenergic fibers
2. ____ Causes activation of alpha-adrenergic receptors
3. ____ Secreted by the postganglionic fibers of the parasympathetic nervous system
4. ____ Causes activation of muscarinic receptors
5. ____ Action terminated by acetylcholinesterase, an enzyme located within the synapse
6. ____ Action terminated by reuptake of the neurotransmitter and MAO
7. ____ Causes activation of beta-adrenergic receptors
8. ____ Causes activation of nicotinic receptors, including the N_M receptors in the neuromuscular junction of skeletal muscle
9. ____ Mediates fight or flight (postganglionic)
10. ____ Mediates feed and breed

Multiple Choice

1. Which of the following is *least* related to the sympathetic nervous system?
   a. Includes the paravertebral ganglia
   b. Is also called the *fight-or-flight* response
   c. Is also called *craniosacral outflow*
   d. Uses norepinephrine as a transmitter

2. Which of the following is most related to the parasympathetic nervous system?
   a. Uses norepinephrine as a postganglionic transmitter
   b. Mediates feed-and-breed activities
   c. Is also called the *fight-or-flight* response
   d. Adrenergic postganglionic fiber

3. What is the role of monoamine oxidase (MAO)?
   a. Destroys norepinephrine
   b. Activates the muscarinic receptors
   c. Activates the beta$_1$-adrenergic receptors
   d. Inactivates acetylcholine

4. Activation of the beta$_2$-adrenergic receptors
   a. is a response to the binding of ACh.
   b. causes wheezing.
   c. dilates the breathing passages.
   d. slows the heart rate.

5. Activation of the muscarinic receptors
   a. dilates the breathing passages.
   b. slows the heart rate.
   c. dilates the pupil.
   d. is a response to norepinephrine.

6. Blockade of the alpha$_1$-adrenergic receptors is the basis for what group of drugs?
   a. Hypoglycemic agents
   b. Blood-pressure-lowering drugs
   c. Cardiac stimulants
   d. Bronchodilators

7. Pupillary dilation, an increase in heart rate, and an inability to urinate are effects of
   a. alpha$_1$-adrenergic activation.
   b. beta$_2$-adrenergic activation.
   c. muscarinic blockade.
   d. vagomimetic activity.

8. A vagolytic drug exerts the same effects as
   a. a sympathomimetic agent.
   b. a beta$_1$-adrenergic agonist.
   c. a muscarinic agonist.
   d. an antimuscarinic agent.

9. Fight or flight, paravertebral ganglia, and norepinephrine are most related to
   a. cholinergic fibers.
   b. sympathetic nervous system.
   c. nicotinic and muscarinic receptors.
   d. craniosacral outflow.

10. Feed and breed, craniosacral outflow, and ACh are most related to the
    a. sympathetic nervous system.
    b. adrenergic fibers.
    c. nicotinic and muscarinic receptors.
    d. paravertebral ganglia.

Go Figure

1. Which of the following is correct according to Fig. 12.1?
   a. The sympathetic nervous system is called the *craniosacral outflow.*
   b. The parasympathetic nervous system is called the *thoracolumbar outflow.*
   c. Activation of the craniosacral outflow mediates a calming effect.
   d. The fight-or-flight response best describes craniosacral outflow.

2. Which of the following is correct according to Fig. 12.2?
   a. All preganglionic fibers secrete ACh.
   b. All postganglionic fibers secrete ACh.
   c. Cholinergic fibers are restricted to the parasympathetic nervous system.
   d. Adrenergic fibers are restricted to the parasympathetic nervous system.

3. Which of the following is correct according to Fig. 12.2?
   a. The postganglionic fibers of the sympathetic nervous system are longer than those of the parasympathetic nervous system.
   b. All fibers of the sympathetic nervous system secrete norepinephrine.
   c. Paravertebral ganglia are found only within the parasympathetic nervous system.
   d. The ganglia of sympathetic fibers are found near or in the organ of innervation.

4. Which of the following is correct according to Fig. 12.3?
   a. ACh activates muscarinic receptors.
   b. Discharge of the parasympathetic nervous system activates muscarinic receptors.
   c. Discharge of the sympathetic nervous system activates alpha- and beta-adrenergic receptors.
   d. All of the above are true.

5. According to Fig. 12.3, the red postganglionic fibers
   a. secrete ACh.
   b. are present only in the parasympathetic nervous system.
   c. are adrenergic.
   d. innervate skeletal muscle.

6. According to Fig. 12.3, N$_M$ receptors are found
   a. only in the autonomic ganglia.
   b. on skeletal muscles.
   c. only in the parasympathetic nervous system.
   d. only in the sympathetic nervous system.

7. According to Fig. 12.3, muscarinic receptors are located on/in
   a. skeletal muscles.
   b. autonomic ganglia.
   c. all end organs of parasympathetic nerves.
   d. all end organs of sympathetic nerves.

8. Which of the following is correct according to Tables 12.3 and 12.4?
   a. Activation of the muscarinic receptors decreases heart rate.
   b. Activation of the nicotinic receptors on skeletal muscle is an autonomic effect.
   c. Activation of the adrenergic receptors decreases heart rate and dilates all blood vessels.
   d. All of the above are true.

Sensory System

Objectives

1. State the functions of the sensory system.
2. Define the five types of sensory receptors.
3. Describe the four components involved in the perception of a sensation and two important characteristics of sensation.
4. Describe the five general senses.
5. Describe the special senses of smell and taste.
6. Describe the sense of sight, including the following:
   - Describe the structure of the eye.
   - Explain the movement of the eyes.
   - Describe how the size of the pupils changes.
7. Describe the sense of hearing, including the following:
   - Describe the three divisions of the ear.
   - Describe the functions of the parts of the ear involved in hearing.
   - Explain the role of the ear in maintaining the body's equilibrium.

Key Terms

accommodation (p. 246)
chemoreceptors (p. 232)
cochlea (p. 251)
cornea (p. 241)
equilibrium (p. 237)
eustachian tube (p. 250)
extrinsic eye muscles (p. 241)
general senses (p. 234)
hearing (p. 249)
intrinsic eye muscles (p. 243)
lacrimal apparatus (p. 240)
mechanoreceptors (p. 233)
nociceptors (p. 232)

olfactory receptors (p. 237)
optic chiasm (p. 248)
ossicles (p. 250)
pain (p. 234)
perception (p. 233)
photoreceptors (p. 233)
pressure (p. 236)
proprioception (p. 237)
referred pain (p. 235)
refraction (p. 245)
retina (p. 241)
sclera (p. 241)
semicircular canals (p. 251)

sensation (p. 233)
smell (p. 237)
special senses (p. 234)
taste (p. 238)
temperature (p. 236)
thermoreceptors (p. 232)
touch (p. 236)
vestibule (p. 251)
vision (p. 239)
visual accessory organs (p. 239)
visual pathway (p. 247)

The sensory system allows us to experience the world. Senses let you see the trees, hear the voices of your friends and family, feel the heat of the sun, and taste your favorite foods. When the external environment becomes threatening, the sensory system also acts as a warning system. For example, if you place your hand on a hot surface, the sensory system experiences the episode as pain. The pain is a danger signal indicating that the body must make an adjustment to remove the harmful stimulus.

In addition to sensing outside information, the sensory system also allows us to keep track of what is happening within our bodies. For example, when the stomach fills with food, sensory information is carried to the central nervous system (CNS). In response to this information, the stomach is told to digest the food.

RECEPTORS AND SENSATION

CELLS THAT DETECT STIMULI

Sensory neurons transmit information to the CNS (Table 13.1). A receptor is a specialized area of a sensory neuron that detects a specific stimulus. For example, the receptors in the eye respond to light, whereas the receptors on the tongue respond to chemicals in food. The five types of sensory receptors are as follows:

- **Chemoreceptors** (kee-moh-ree-SEP-tors): Receptors stimulated by changes in the chemicals such as hydrogen ion (H^+), calcium, and food
- Pain receptors, or **nociceptors** (noh-see-SEP-tors): Receptors stimulated by tissue damage or distention
- **Thermoreceptors**: Receptors stimulated by changes in temperature

Table 13.1 Types of Sensory Receptors

RECEPTOR	STIMULUS	EXAMPLE
Chemoreceptors	Changes in chemical concentrations of substances	Taste and smell
Pain receptors (nociceptors)	Tissue damage or distortion	Pain
Thermoreceptors	Changes in temperature	Heat and cold
Mechanoreceptors	Changes in pressure or movement of fluids	Hearing and equilibrium
Photoreceptors	Light	Sight

- **Mechanoreceptors:** Receptors stimulated by changes in pressure or movements of body fluids
- **Photoreceptors:** Receptors stimulated by light

SENSATION AND PERCEPTION

A **sensation** is the conscious or unconscious awareness of incoming sensory information. A **perception** refers to conscious awareness of a sensation. Yelling, "Ouch, that knife is sharp," for example, indicates that you have become aware of a painful stimulus and what caused it.

EXPERIENCING A SENSATION

FOUR COMPONENTS

Four components are involved in sensation. Using the sense of sight as an example, these four components are illustrated in Fig. 13.1 and described as follows:

- Stimulus: Light is the stimulus for the sense of sight. In the absence of light, you cannot see.
- Receptor: Light waves stimulate the photoreceptors in the eye, producing a nerve impulse.
- Sensory nerve: The nerve impulse is conducted by a sensory nerve (optic nerve) to the occipital lobe of the brain.
- Special area of the brain: The sensory information is interpreted as sight in the occipital lobe of the brain. This is an important point; the sensation is experienced by the brain and not by the sensory receptor. For example, you see an object, hear a voice, or feel pain because the sensory information has stimulated a part of the brain.

As you study each sensation, identify the stimulus, type of receptor, name of the sensory nerve, and specific area of the brain that interprets the sensation.

TWO CHARACTERISTICS OF SENSATION

Two important characteristics of sensation are projection and adaptation. Projection describes the process whereby the brain, after receiving a sensation, refers that sensation back to its source. You see with

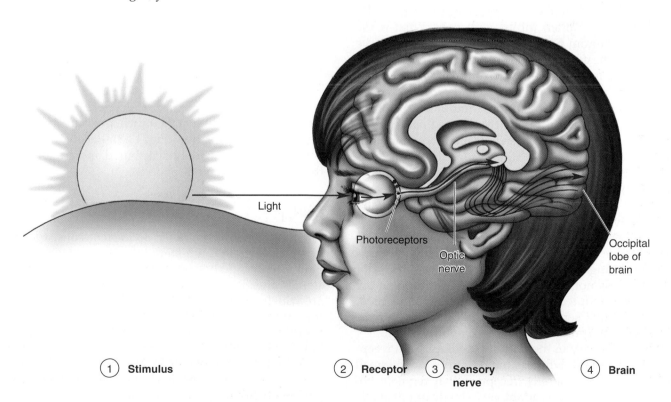

① **Stimulus**   ② **Receptor** ③ **Sensory nerve**   ④ **Brain**

Light

Photoreceptors

Optic nerve

Occipital lobe of brain

FIG. 13.1 Four components of sensation.

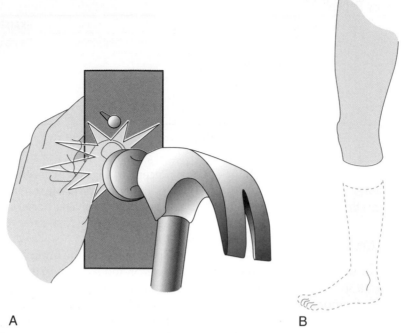

A   B

FIG. 13.2 (A) Projection...ouch! (B) Phantom limb. The *dashed line* represents the amputated part.

your eyes, hear with your ears, and feel pain in your injured finger because the cortex of your brain receives the sensation and projects it back to its source. Projection answers the question, "If pain is experienced by the brain, why does my injured finger hurt?" (Fig. 13.2A).

The experience of "phantom limb pain" is another example of projection. If a leg is amputated, the person may still feel pain in the amputated leg (see Fig. 13.2B). The missing leg often throbs with pain. What is the cause of phantom limb sensation? The severed nerve endings of the amputated leg continue to send sensory information to the parietal lobe of the brain. The brain interprets the information as pain and projects the feeling back to the leg area. For most amputees, the phantom limb pain diminishes as the severed nerves heal, but the person often experiences a phantom limb presence. The amputated leg still feels as though it is attached. There is some good news about phantom limb sensation—the sensation often "locates" the amputated limb and helps a patient learn to use an artificial limb.

Sensory adaptation is another characteristic of sensation; it is illustrated by the sense of smell. When you enter a room with a strong odor, the odor at first seems overwhelming. After a short time, however, the odor becomes less noticeable. The sensory receptors in the nose have adapted. When continuously stimulated, these receptors send fewer signals to the area of the brain that interprets sensory information as smell.

Receptors vary in their ability to adapt. Pain receptors do not adapt, whereas the receptors for the smell adapt rapidly. Generally, receptors that regulate homeostatic mechanisms adapt very slowly or not at all.

There are two groups of senses: general and special senses. **General senses** are called *general*, or

somatic, because their receptors are widely distributed throughout the body. The **special senses** are localized within a particular organ in the head. The special senses include taste, smell, sight, hearing, and balance.

 Re-Think

1. List five types of sensory receptors.
2. Differentiate between sensation and perception.
3. Define *projection* and *adaptation.* Provide an example of each.

THE GENERAL SENSES

General senses include pain, touch, pressure, temperature, and proprioception (Fig. 13.3). Receptors for the general senses are widely distributed and are found in the skin, muscles, joints, and viscera.

PAIN

The receptors for **pain**, called *nociceptors*, consist of free nerve endings that are stimulated by tissue damage. Pain receptors do not adapt and may continue to send signals after the stimulus is removed. Pain receptors are widely distributed throughout the skin and other internal tissues. Oddly enough, the nervous tissue of the brain lacks pain receptors. Tissues surrounding the brain, like the meninges and the blood vessels, however, do contain pain receptors. You can feel a headache.

Pain serves a protective function. Being unpleasant, pain motivates the person to remove its cause. The failure of the pain receptors to adapt is also protective. For example, if a person complains of right lower quadrant

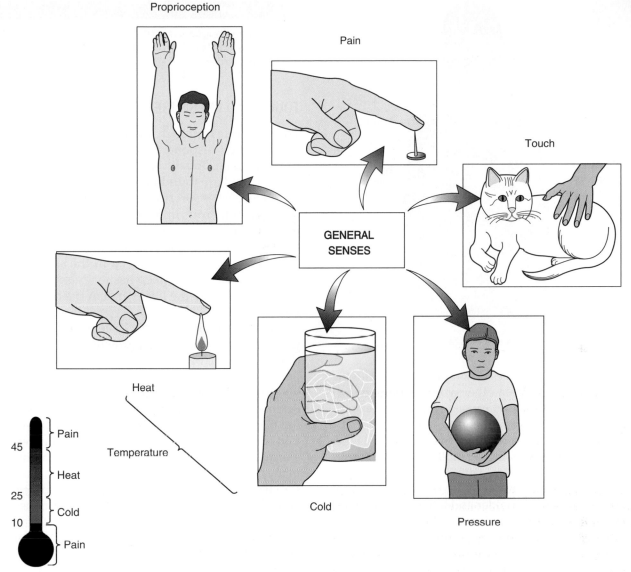

Proprioception

Pain

Touch

GENERAL SENSES

Heat

Temperature

Pain
45
Heat
25
Cold
10
Pain

Cold

Pressure

FIG. 13.3 **General senses.**

(RLQ) abdominal pain, the pain is used as a valuable clue about what is wrong. In this example, the pain is indicative of acute appendicitis, requiring an appendectomy (surgical removal of the appendix). Once the diagnosis is made, the pain is treated. If the physician merely relieved the pain, surgical intervention might have been delayed, resulting in a ruptured appendix and life-threatening peritonitis. Although unpleasant and undesirable, pain serves the body well.

Some patients are at risk because of a diminishment or alteration in the sensation of pain. Patients with diabetes mellitus, for example, often develop nerve damage in their legs and feet; the nerve damage is called *diabetic neuropathy*. Because of the distortion in the sensation of pain, diabetic persons may ignore the discomfort of ill-fitting shoes and may develop blisters on their feet. The blistered site continues to expand and eventually becomes infected and gangrenous, requiring amputation. This is a common experience among diabetic persons and is the reason for meticulous attention to their foot care.

What causes pain? The specific signals that stimulate pain are not well understood. Three pain triggers have been identified. First, tissue injury promotes the release of chemicals that stimulate pain receptors. Second, a deficiency of oxygen stimulates pain receptors. For example, if the blood supply to an internal organ is diminished, a condition called *ischemia,* the tissue is deprived of oxygen, and the person experiences pain. The pain of a heart attack is caused in part by the oxygen deprivation experienced by the cardiac muscle. The administration of oxygen helps relieve pain. Third, pain may be experienced when tissues are stretched or deformed. The stimulus is mechanical distortion rather than chemical. For example, if the intestine becomes distended, the person will often experience a severe cramping pain.

Why is pain originating in the heart (visceral pain) often experienced in the shoulder and left arm? When pain feels as if it is coming from an area other than the site where it originates, it is called **referred pain** (Fig. 13.4). Patients with heart disease often complain of pain or an aching sensation that starts in the

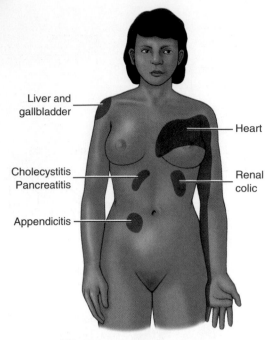

Liver and
gallbladder

Heart

Cholecystitis
Pancreatitis

Renal
colic

Appendicitis

FIG. 13.4 **Sites of referred pain.**

shoulder region and moves down the left arm into the fourth and fifth fingers. In other words, stimulation of pain receptors in the heart causes pain that is experienced as being away from the heart.

What is the explanation for referred pain? The occurrence of referred pain is the result of shared sensory nerve pathways. The nerve pathways that carry information from the heart are the same pathways that carry information from the shoulder and left arm. As a result, the brain interprets heart pain as shoulder and arm pain.

Once the pain receptors are stimulated, where does the information go? Pain impulses for most of the body travel up the spinal cord in a sensory nerve tract called the *spinothalamic tract*. The information is then transmitted to the thalamus, where the person first becomes aware of the pain, and then to the parietal lobe. The parietal lobe can identify the source of the pain and judge its intensity and other characteristics.

You will spend much time assessing pain. You will determine the location of the pain, its duration, and what the pain "feels like"—sharp, dull, deep, superficial, burning, throbbing, cramping, aching, gnawing, stabbing, and a host of other descriptive terms. You will also use a pain scale that will help you evaluate the intensity of pain. For example, you may ask your patient to rate his or her pain from 1 (pain-free) to 5 (horrible pain). Create your own pain scale (1 to 5) using the following "smiley face" approach.

No pain

Horrible
pain

◯ ◯ ◯ ◯ ◯

 Re-Think

1. List three triggers for pain.
2. List five words used to describe pain.
3. Provide an example of referred pain.

TOUCH AND PRESSURE

The receptors for touch and **pressure** are mechanoreceptors; they respond to forces that press, move, or deform tissue. **Touch** receptors are also called *tactile receptors* and are found mostly in the skin; they allow us to feel a cat's soft fur (see Fig. 13.3). They are particularly numerous in the lips and tips of the fingers, toes, tongue, penis, and clitoris. Fingers have the highest concentration of touch receptors. Receptors for heavy pressure are located in the skin, subcutaneous tissue, and the deep tissue. Pressure receptors are stimulated by the heavy ball in the boy's arms in Fig. 13.3.

Touch is the first sensory system to develop in the fetus and is essential to its growth and development. The importance of touch extends throughout the lifespan. If an infant is not touched, it does not thrive and will likely die (failure-to-thrive syndrome). An appreciation of touch in the health of a preterm infant forms the basis of "kangaroo care"; the tiny, diaper-clad infant is placed in the blouse or shirt of its parent. The warmth and physical contact with the parent cause many neurobiological changes that calm the infant, stabilize its temperature, and improve feeding. Sadly, you will often encounter infants or "warehoused" elderly persons who have been diagnosed with failure to thrive. They are generally the untouched and ignored. Touch is life-sustaining!

TEMPERATURE

The receptors for **temperature** are called *thermoreceptors*. The two types of thermoreceptors are heat and cold receptors. Thermoreceptors are found on free nerve endings and are scattered widely throughout the body. Note the temperature scale in Fig. 13.3. The cold receptors are stimulated at between 50° and 76°F (10° and 25°C). Heat receptors are stimulated between 76° and 112°F (25° and 45°C). At both ends (extremes) of the temperature scale, pain receptors are stimulated, producing a freezing or burning sensation. Both heat and cold thermoreceptors display adaptation so that the sensation of heat or cold fades rapidly. Immerse your hand in warm water and note how quickly the feeling of warmth disappears, even though the temperature of the water has not decreased. Your heat receptors have adapted.

Remember that pain receptors do not adapt. If you place your hand in boiling water, you will feel intense continuous pain. Sensory information regarding temperature is sent to the parietal lobe.

Table 13.2 Special Senses

TYPE OF SENSE	ORGAN	SPECIFIC RECEPTOR	STIMULUS	RECEPTOR
Smell	Nose	Olfactory cell	Changes in chemical concentrations of substances	Chemoreceptor
Taste	Tongue	Gustatory cell	Changes in chemical concentrations of substances	Chemoreceptor
Sight	Eye	Rods and cones	Light	Photoreceptor
Hearing	Inner ear: cochlea	Organ of Corti (hair cells)	Movement of fluids	Mechanoreceptor
Balance	Inner ear, vestibular apparatus	Hair cells	Movement of fluids	Mechanoreceptor

PROPRIOCEPTION

Proprioception (proh-pree-oh-SEP-shun) is the sense of orientation, or position. This sense allows you to locate a body part without looking at it. In other words, if you close your eyes, you can still locate your arm in space; you do not have to see your arm to know that it is raised over your head (see Fig. 13.3). Proprioception plays an important role in maintaining posture and co-ordinating body movements.

The receptors for proprioception, called *propriocep-tors,* are located in muscles, tendons, and joints. Proprioceptors are also found in the inner ear, where they function in balance or **equilibrium**. The cerebellum, which plays a major role in coordinating skeletal muscle activity, receives sensory information from these receptors. Sensory information regarding movement and position is also sent to the parietal lobe of the cerebrum. Think how busy the proprioceptors are in the midst of a basketball game!

 Re-Think

1. What receptors are stimulated when you immerse your hand in boiling water?
2. Name three triggers that activate nociceptors.
3. What information is conveyed by the sense of proprioception?

 Sum It Up!

The sensory system is designed to detect information from within and outside the body and to convey that information to the CNS for interpretation. Receptors located on sensory neurons respond to specific stimuli. There are five types of receptors: chemoreceptors, pain receptors (nociceptors), thermoreceptors, mechanoreceptors, and photoreceptors. There are four components necessary for experiencing a sensation: stimulus, receptor, sensory nerve, and special area of the brain. Two characteristics of a sensation are adaptation and projection. Senses are classified as general or special. The general senses include pain, touch, pressure, temperature, and proprioception.

THE SPECIAL SENSES

The five special senses are smell, taste, sight, hearing, and balance (Table 13.2). The receptors for the special senses are located in the head.

SENSE OF SMELL: THE NOSE

The sense of **smell**, olfaction, is associated with sensory structures located in the upper nose (Fig. 13.5). These **olfactory** (ol-FAK-tor-ee) **receptors** are very sensitive and classified as chemoreceptors, meaning that they are stimulated by chemicals that dissolve in the moisture of the nasal tissue. Once the olfactory receptors have been stimulated, the sensory impulses travel along the olfactory nerve (CN I). The sensory information is eventually interpreted as smell within the olfactory area of the temporal and frontal lobes. Faint odor? Sniff harder, because the olfactory receptors are located high in the nose where the air circulation is poor.

WHAT A SMELL CAN TELL

Think of the many pleasant "smell experiences" you have each day: food, flowers, home, fragrant candles, your child, a pet—the list goes on, as do the functions served by the sense of smell. Food odors can stimulate the digestive tract secretions, literally causing you to drool and ingest necessary nutrients. The sense of smell can function as a protective warning, telling you of spoiled food and threatening environments, such as a room filled with leaking gas. Other familiar odors pack an emotional punch, often eliciting memories (pleasant and not-so pleasant). Aromatherapy uses the sense of smell for its healing and calming effects on the body. And, of course, Mr. and Ms. Rover, in the heat of the moment, illustrate well the role of pheromones (sex odors) in mating and reproduction. By the way, each person has a unique odor as distinctive as fingerprints.

Some odors are harsh and unpleasant. For example, ammonia fumes activate both the olfactory receptors and the trigeminal nociceptors. Thus, "smelling salts"

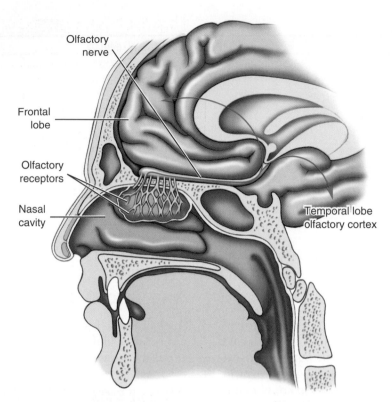

Olfactory nerve

Frontal lobe

Olfactory receptors

Nasal cavity

Temporal lobe olfactory cortex

FIG. 13.5 Sense of smell: olfactory receptors, olfactory nerve, and olfactory cortex of temporal and frontal lobes.

quickly and uncomfortably revive a semiconscious person. Unpleasant odors can trigger distressing visceral responses. For example, putrid odors can stimulate the emetic center, causing the person to vomit in response to the noxious stimulus.

Some persons experience an olfactory aura, meaning that they smell an odor that is not present. Olfactory auras most often occur before seizure activity or before the onset of a migraine headache. The person may "smell" chicken soup, bleach, rotting flesh, or worse. Sometimes, the aura is a distortion of an odor. For example, a person may experience body odor as a smell of beer. These strange smell events are called *olfactory hallucinations*.

Your sense of smell is also a valuable diagnostic tool. You can smell the acetone breath of a person in diabetic ketoacidosis, the putrid odor of an infected wound, and the odor of alcohol on the breath of an intoxicated person. Think that's good? Rover can smell the presence of melanoma, and his ears perk right up when he smells the breath of a person with pulmonary tuberculosis. Cranial nerve (CN I) assessment? Have the person identify various odors such as vanilla; an intact olfactory nerve identifies the vanilla odor. Clearly, the olfactory receptors that hang out in the nose are very busy and do much more than just smell perfume.

SENSE OF TASTE: THE TONGUE

The sense of **taste** is often called the *social sense*, as in "let's do lunch"; it is also called the *gustatory*

(GUS-tah-tor-ee) *sense* or *gustation*. Taste buds are the special organs of taste. The taste receptors are located primarily on the tongue and are classified as chemoreceptors, meaning that they are activated by the chemicals in our food. A small number of taste buds are also located on the palate, tonsils, and throat. Rover, of course, has many taste buds in his throat. So not to worry when he gulps his treat; he is tasting and thoroughly enjoying it despite its rapid disappearance. The four basic taste sensations are salty, sweet, sour, and bitter. Each sensation is concentrated on a particular area of the tongue, as illustrated in Fig. 13.6. The tip of the tongue is most sensitive to sweet and salty substances. Sour sensations are found primarily on the sides of the tongue, and bitter substances are most strongly tasted on the back part of the tongue.

When the taste receptors are stimulated, the taste impulses travel along three cranial nerves (facial, glossopharyngeal, and vagus nerves) to various parts of the brain, eventually arriving in the temporal and frontal lobes of the cerebral cortex. Note that because the taste sensation is carried by three cranial nerves, when assessing cranial nerve function, you will be asking the patient to detect specific tastes and stimulating only parts of the tongue. For example, a person with damage to the facial nerve may experience loss of taste only on the anterior two-thirds of the left side of the tongue.

SOME TASTEFUL COMMENTS

- The salty receptors can trigger a "salt craving." For example, as her blood volume expands during

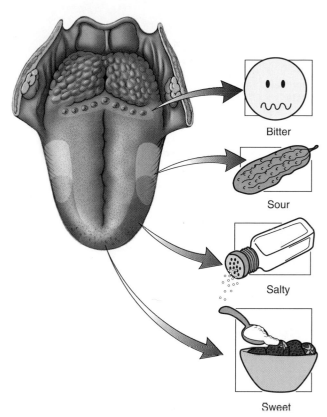

FIG. 13.6 **Sense of taste. The four taste sensations are bitter, sour, salty, and sweet.**

Bitter

Sour

Salty

Sweet

? Re-Think

1. Locate and classify olfactory receptors.
2. Define the words *olfactory* and *gustatory.*
3. List the cranial nerves and cerebral lobes concerned with the sensation of smell and taste.
4. Why does food taste different when you have a cold?

◎ Sum It Up!

The special senses include smell, taste, sight, hearing, and balance. The nose houses the receptors for smell, the olfactory receptors. CN I (olfactory nerve) carries information from the nose to the temporal and frontal lobes of the cerebrum. Distortions in the sense of smell are common and include anosmia and olfactory auras/hallucinations. The sense of taste is called the *gustatory sense.* Sensory information from the taste buds is carried by three cranial nerves (CN VII, IX, and X) to the parietal lobe of the cerebrum.

pregnancy, the woman's taste buds may sense a decrease of salt in her blood, causing her to increase her intake of salt. Because salt plays a crucial role in blood volume regulation, the salt craving has an important survival role. Ever notice the gathering of deer around a salt lick?

- Taste receptors seem especially sensitive to bitter-tasting substances. This sensitivity serves a protective role because the poisonous substances in plants are often bitter.
- Food often tastes differently when you have a cold. The senses of taste and smell are closely related. When interpreted in the cerebral cortex, information from both senses may combine to produce a different taste sensation. Therefore, food often tastes different when you have a cold or stuffy nose.
- The sense of taste can be lost or altered. Drugs and radiation used in the treatment of cancer often change or destroy the sensation of taste. Obviously, the loss of taste affects appetite and nutrition.
- Two other tastes have been suggested. A metallic taste has been attributed to the effects of certain drugs. A second taste has been described by a Japanese word, *umami,* which means "yummy" or "delicious" and refers to a meaty flavor.
- There is also some evidence that the tongue can taste the texture and shape of food.

SENSE OF SIGHT: THE EYE

The sense of sight (**vision**) is one of our most cherished senses. Think of all that you see that brings so much joy to your life—the smiles of children, the faces of your friends and pets, and the beautiful colors of the trees and flowers. The eyes are the organs of vision; they contain the visual receptors. Assisting the eyes in their function and protecting them from injury are the visual accessory organs. The study of the eye is called *ophthalmology.*

VISUAL ACCESSORY ORGANS

The **visual accessory organs** include the eyebrows, eyelids, conjunctiva, eyelashes, lacrimal apparatus, and extrinsic eye muscles (Fig. 13.7).

Eyebrows

The eyebrows, patches of hair located above the eyes, perform a protective role. They keep perspiration out of the eyes and shade the eyes from glaring sunlight. Eyebrows also perform a cosmetic role and participate in your facial expression, as in the "raised eyebrow" look.

Eyelids

The eyelids, called *palpebrae,* protect the eyes. They prevent the entrance of foreign objects and wash tears over the surface of the eye. The upper and lower eyelids meet at the corners of the eyes. The corners are called the *medial (inner) canthus* and *lateral (outer) canthus.* The eyelids are composed of four layers: skin, skeletal muscle (orbicularis oculi), connective tissue, and an inner lining called the *conjunctiva.* The margin of the eyelids contains tarsal or meibomian glands, special types of sebaceous glands that secrete an oil that coats the surface of the eye and reduces evaporation of the tears. Skeletal muscles open and close the eyelids. The levator palpebrae superioris muscle

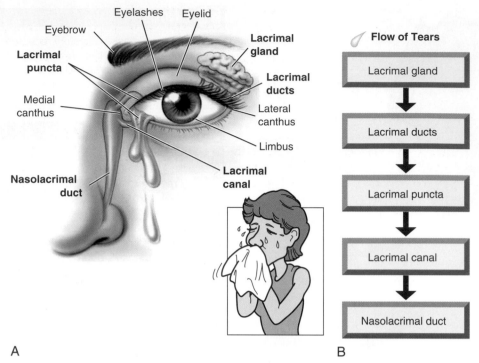

FIG. 13.7 (A) Visual accessory organs and lacrimal apparatus. (B) Flow of tears from the lacrimal gland to the nasolacrimal duct

(*levator* means "to raise," like an elevator) is attached to the eyelid and the upper bony orbit; contraction of this muscle opens the eye. Contraction of the orbicularis oculi muscle closes it.

Look in the mirror. Lid levels matter. Your eyelid normally covers a small part of the upper iris (colored part of your eye); it should not cover the pupil (hole). Sometimes, a patient cannot lift the eyelid completely, giving the person a sleepy look. This condition is called *ptosis of the eyelid*. The upper eyelid of a person with an overactive thyroid may appear to be pulled up too high, thereby exposing the white sclera above the iris. This is called "lid lag." Thus, the eyelids often provide diagnostic clues about underlying diseases or disorders. While you are looking in the mirror, pull down your lower lid and note its inner lining; it forms a sac (the conjunctival sac). Eyedrops are temporarily held in this sac until the blinking eyelids wash the medication over the surface of the eye.

Occasionally, a hair follicle at the edge of the lid becomes infected, usually by *Staphylococcus*. This infection is called a *stye*, or *hordeolum*; it is red, swollen, and painful.

Conjunctiva

The conjunctiva (kon-junk-TIE-vah) is a thin mucous membrane that lines the inner surface of the eyelids. The conjunctiva also folds back to cover a portion of the sclera on the anterior surface of the eyeball; this part of the sclera is called the *white of the eye*. The conjunctiva does not cover the cornea. It secretes a thin mucous film that moistens the surface of the eye. The anterior surface of the eye must be kept moist;

otherwise, it will ulcerate and scar. Fig. 13.7 identifies the limbus, the meeting place of the white of the eye with the cornea that overlies the colored iris.

The conjunctiva is very vascular, meaning that it has many blood vessels. Evidence of its rich vascularity is its bloodshot appearance when the blood vessels are dilated. Eyedrops that claim to "get the red out" cause the blood vessels of the conjunctiva to constrict, thereby decreasing the amount of blood. Pink eye, also associated with dilated blood vessels, is a highly contagious bacterial or viral conjunctivitis. It is commonly seen in groups of children in whom it is difficult to maintain good hygienic conditions. Conjunctivitis can also be caused by irritation and allergies.

Eyelashes

Eyelashes line the edges of the eyelid and help trap dust. Touching the eyelashes stimulates blinking—a mascara challenge! Interestingly, the camel has three eyelids and two layers of eyelashes to deal with its sandy environment. Imagine how long it would take to get out of the house with so many lids and lashes to paint!

Lacrimal Apparatus

The **lacrimal** (LAK-ri-mal) **apparatus** is concerned with the secretion, distribution, and drainage of tears. It is composed of the lacrimal gland and a series of ducts called *tear ducts* (see Fig. 13.7). The lacrimal gland is located in the upper lateral part of the orbit. The lacrimal gland secretes tears, which flow across the surface of the eye toward the nose. The tears drain through small openings called *lacrimal puncta* and then into the lacrimal canals and nasolacrimal duct. The naso-lacrimal duct eventually empties into the nasal cavity. Normally, tears flow to the back of the throat and are swallowed. However, if the secretion of tears increases, as in crying, the nose begins to run. The excess tears may overwhelm the drainage system and spill onto the cheeks. Similarly, the nasolacrimal ducts can become swollen and close when a person has a cold. The tears cannot drain and thus spill out onto the cheeks.

Tears perform several important functions. They moisten, lubricate, and cleanse the surface of the eye. Tears also contain an enzyme called *lysozyme,* which helps destroy pathogens and prevents infection. Blinking stimulates lacrimation and helps spread the tears over the surface of the eye. Historically, tears were assumed to have been literally squeezed out of the brain by a force caused by grief. Interestingly, the chemical composition of tears that are shed in response to grief differs from those elicited by joy. Mind–body interaction!

Extrinsic Eye Muscles

Extrinsic eye muscles also function as visual accessory organs (see "Muscles of the Eye" later in this chapter).

 Re-Think

1. List the visual accessory organs.
2. Locate the conjunctiva, and explain how it forms the "white of the eye" and the limbus.
3. Trace the flow of tears from their origin to their destination.

THE EYEBALL

The eyeball has a spherical shape and is approximately ¾ to 1 inch (2 to 3 cm) in diameter (Fig. 13.8A). Most of the eyeball sits within the bony orbital cavity of the skull, partially surrounded by a layer of orbital fat. Thus, the eyeball is recessed and well protected. Interestingly, our eyes are the same size from infancy to adulthood. Think about it: the large eyeballs in young animals are what make them so stinkin' cute!

The eyeball is composed of three layers: the sclera, the choroid, and the retina. Identify the structures in Fig. 13.8 as they are described in the following text.

Layers of the Eyeball

Sclera. The outermost layer is called the **sclera** (SKLEH-rah). The sclera is a tough fibrous connective tissue that covers most of the eyeball. The sclera helps contain the contents of the eye; it also shapes the eye and is the site of attachment for the extrinsic eye muscles. The sclera extends toward the front of the eye. The anterior sclera is covered by conjunctiva and, as indicated earlier, is called the *white of the eye.* A transparent extension of the sclera is called the **cornea** (KOR-nee-ah). The cornea covers the area over the iris (the colored portion of the eye).

The cornea is avascular (contains no blood vessels) and transparent, meaning that light rays can go through this structure. Because light enters the eye first through the cornea, it is called *the window of the eye.* The cornea has a rich supply of sensory nerve fibers and therefore is sensitive to touch (see "Corneal reflex" in the Ramp It Up!: Commonly Assessed Eye Reflexes box later in the chapter).

Choroid. The middle layer of the eye is the choroid (KOH-royd). The choroid layer is highly vascular and is attached to the innermost layer, the retina. The choroid performs two functions: (1) it provides the retina with a rich supply of blood, and (2) dark pigments located in the choroid absorb any excess light to prevent glare.

The choroid extends toward the front of the eyeball to form the ciliary body and the iris. Collectively, the middle layer (choroid, ciliary muscle, and iris) is called the *uvea.* The ciliary body secretes a fluid called *aqueous humor* and gives rise to a set of intrinsic eye muscles called the *ciliary muscles.* The most anterior portion of the choroid is the iris, the colored portion of the anterior eye.

The opening, or hole, in the middle of the iris is called the *pupil.* The size of the pupil is determined by two sets of intrinsic eye muscles located in the iris. The iris regulates the amount of light entering the eye (see "Photopupillary reflex" in the Ramp It Up!: Commonly Assessed Eye Reflexes box later in the chapter).

 Do You Know...

Why the "Beautiful Lady" Can't See?

A group of drugs, including atropine and scopolamine (muscarinic receptor antagonists), belongs to a drug classification called *belladonna,* or "beautiful lady." Why beautiful? When belladonna is placed in the eyes of the young lady, the pupils dilate, becoming wide, dark, and very seductive. Dilated pupils may indeed be beautiful, but they do not promote acute vision. "Beautiful lady" may be beautiful, but she needs an escort because she certainly cannot see.

Today, belladonna drugs are still used, primarily for their mydriatic and cycloplegic effects in eye examinations and surgical procedures. Interestingly, atropine is still used by photographers to create pictures of "beautiful ladies."

Retina. The innermost layer of the eyeball is the **retina** (RET-i-nah). It lines the posterior two-thirds of the eyeball. The retina is the nervous layer containing the visual receptors, which are sensitive to light and are therefore called *photoreceptors.* The two types of photoreceptors are rods and cones. The rods are scattered throughout the retina but are more abundant along its periphery. The rods are sensitive to dim light and provide us with black-and-white vision. The cones are most abundant in the central portion of the retina and provide us with color vision. The area of the retina that contains the highest concentration of cones is called the *fovea centralis,* an area in the center of a yellow spot called the *macula lutea* (see Fig. 13.8A). Because the fovea centralis contains so many cones, it is considered the area of most acute vision.

A second small circular area of the retina is in the back of the eye. The neurons of the retina converge

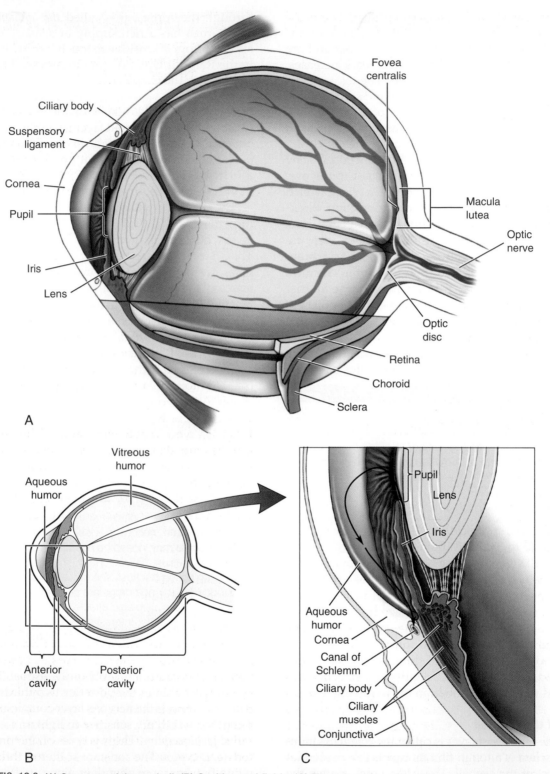

FIG. 13.8 (A) Structure of the eyeball. (B) Cavities and fluids. (C) Flow of aqueous humor from the ciliary body to the canal of Schlemm *(arrow).*

there to form the optic nerve; it contains no rods or cones. This area is called the *optic disc*. Because there are no photoreceptors on the optic disc, images that focus on this area are not seen. The optic disc is therefore called the *blind spot*. You can locate your own blind spot. Draw a rectangle with a small X on the left side and a dot on the right. On a piece of paper, draw an X on the left side, and a large dot 5 inches to the right. Cover your left eye and hold it in front of you, looking at the X with your right

eye. Move the paper slowly around you and notice the dot will disappear from your vision at your blind spot.

Here's another interesting fact about the optic disc. A head-injured person may develop increased intracranial pressure as the brain swells. This increased pressure pushes the optic disc forward. The bulging optic disc seen on ophthalmic examination is called a *choked disc* or *papilledema*. The eyes can provide a wealth of information about a patient with a head injury.

Re-Think

1. List the three layers of the eyeball.
2. Name the anterior extensions of the choroid and the sclera.
3. List the two types of photoreceptors and their retinal locations.
4. Why is the optic disc called the blind spot?

Cavities and Fluids

There are two cavities in the eyeball: the posterior and anterior cavities (see Fig. 13.8B). The posterior cavity is larger and is located between the lens and the retina. The posterior cavity is filled with a gel-like substance called the *vitreous humor*. The vitreous humor gently pushes the retina against the choroid layer, thereby ensuring that the retina receives a good supply of oxygenated blood. For the forensic sleuths: Immediately after death, the concentration of potassium ion (K$^+$) in the vitreous humor increases slowly and consistently. Thus, its measurement is used to determine time of death and is considered more accurate than the onset of rigor mortis.

 Do You Know...

Why We Sometimes See Spots in Front of Our Eyes?

The spots are called *floaters* or *muscae volitantes*, meaning "flying flies." They are either particles or red blood cells that have escaped from the capillaries in the eye. These substances float through the vitreous humor, occasionally getting in our line of vision. The presence of these substances is usually considered normal and harmless. However, the sudden appearance of floaters or an increase in the number of floaters may indicate that a hole has formed in the retina. The development of a retinal tear often precedes retinal detachment and demands immediate professional attention.

The anterior cavity is located between the lens and the cornea. The anterior cavity is filled with a watery fluid called aqueous humor. Aqueous humor is produced by the ciliary body and circulates through the pupil into the space behind the cornea (see Fig. 13.8B). The aqueous humor performs two functions: (1) it maintains the shape of the anterior portion of the eye, and (2) it provides nourishment for the cornea. The aqueous humor leaves the anterior cavity by way of tiny canals located at the junction of the sclera and the cornea. These outlet canals are called venous sinuses or the canals of Schlemm (see Fig. 13.8C).

Drainage of aqueous humor through the canals of Schlemm may become impaired. Consequently, aqueous humor accumulates in the eye and elevates the pressure in the eye. An elevated intraocular pressure is called glaucoma. Glaucoma is serious because the elevated pressure compresses the choroid, chokes off the blood supply to the retina, and damages the optic nerve.

 Re-Think

1. Locate the vitreous humor, and describe its function.
2. Locate the aqueous humor, and describe its function.
3. Trace the origin, path, and drainage of aqueous humor.

◎ Sum It Up!

The eyeball has three layers: sclera, choroid, and retina. The sclera extends anteriorly as the cornea. The choroid extends anteriorly as the ciliary body and iris. (The middle layer and its extensions are called the *uvea*.) The inner retinal layer contains the photoreceptors, the rods and cones. There are two cavities: the posterior cavity that contains vitreous humor, and the anterior cavity that contains aqueous humor. Aqueous humor is secreted by the ciliary body, flows anteriorly through the pupil, and is drained through the canal of Schlemm. Impaired drainage of aqueous humor increases intraocular pressure (glaucoma), leading to blindness.

MUSCLES OF THE EYE

The two groups of muscles associated with the eye are the extrinsic and intrinsic eye muscles. The extrinsic eye muscles move the eyeball in its bony orbit. The **intrinsic eye muscles** move structures within the eyeball.

Extrinsic Eye Muscles

How do you move your eyes? The extrinsic eye muscles are skeletal muscles located outside the eye (Fig. 13.9A). Six extrinsic eye muscles attach to the bone of the eye orbit and the sclera, the tough outer connective tissue layer of the eyeball. There are four rectus muscles and two oblique muscles:

- Superior rectus
- Inferior rectus
- Medial rectus
- Lateral rectus
- Superior oblique
- Inferior oblique

The extrinsic eye muscles move the eyeball in various directions. You can move your eyes up, down, and sideways because of the rectus muscles. You can also roll your eyes because of the oblique muscles. The extrinsic eye muscles are innervated by three cranial nerves, with the most important being the oculomotor nerve (CN III). Then there is LR$_6$SO$_4$, which sounds like a nasty chemical formula. However, it helps you remember that the lateral rectus (LR) muscle is innervated by the abducens nerve (CN VI), whereas the superior oblique (SO) muscle is innervated by the trochlear nerve (CN IV). Cranial nerve assessment of CN III, IV, and VI: observe movement of the eyeballs up, down, medial, lateral, and around.

Back to the mirror. Note that both eyes move together in a coordinated way; when one eye moves, the other eye moves. Both eyes focus on the same object. In the event of a traumatic injury to an eye, you may need to immobilize the injured eye, usually by applying a loose covering over it. However, because both eyes move in a coordinated way, if you want to immobilize the injured eye, you must cover both eyes. Then it is off to the ophthalmologist for treatment.

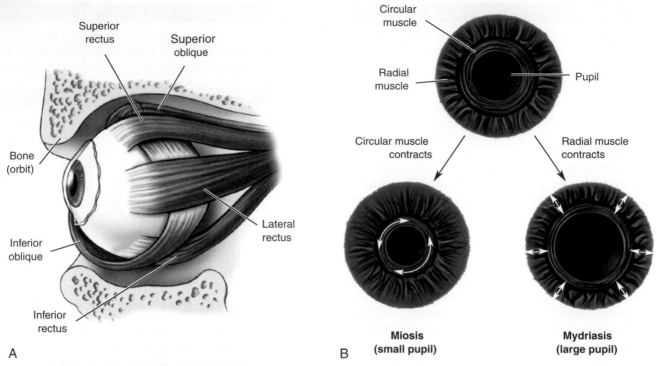

FIG. 13.9 **(A)** Extrinsic muscles: four rectus muscles and two oblique muscles (only five are shown). **(B)** Intrinsic eye muscles: iris (circular and radial muscles).

 Do You Know...

About Lazy Eye?

Normally, both eyes work together and focus on one object; in response, the brain forms a single image. Sometimes, both eyes do not focus on the same object, usually because the muscles of one eye are weak (lazy) and therefore are unable to move the affected eye into position. The occipital lobe is then presented with different information from each eye. The occipital lobe, however, can't process both signals; it receives information from one eye and suppresses information from the lazy eye. If uncorrected, the "lazy" eye will become nonfunctional (blind). Loss of vision resulting from lazy eye is called *suppression amblyopia*. It is common and preventable; treatment, however, must begin early.

 Do You Know...

That Your Eyeballs "Dance" as Blood Alcohol Levels Increase?

Yes! Dancing eyeballs can earn the intoxicated driver a DUI. The dancing eyeballs in question refer to an alcohol-induced nystagmus, an involuntary jerking or oscillation of the eyeballs. It is the basis of the horizontal gaze nystagmus (HGN) test, one of the most reliable of the field sobriety tests.

The HGN test specifically refers to a lateral or horizontal jerking movement of the eyeballs when the intoxicated driver looks toward the side. Here's how it is done. The law enforcement officer positions an object such as a finger or pen about 1 foot in front of the driver's face. The officer moves the object from side to side and observes the movement of the eyeballs. In particular, the officer notes the angle of the eyeball at which the oscillation begins. The higher the blood alcohol level, the earlier the dancing begins. Also noted is the stability of the eyeball when the driver is asked to move the eyeball as far to the side as it can go; it dances away. Although the most common cause

of a positive HGN test is alcohol intoxication, other drugs that depress the CNS, such as phencyclidine (PCP), can also induce nystagmus.

DUI is suspected in response to the barroom odor, slurred speech, elevated breathalyzer readings, and "falling off the straight line" balance test. Added to this evidence are the telltale dancing eyeballs.

Intrinsic Eye Muscles

The intrinsic muscles are smooth muscles located in the eyeball, specifically in the iris and the ciliary body. There are three intrinsic eye muscles. Read on.

Muscles of the Iris. The iris is composed of two eye muscles: the radial muscle and the circular muscle (see Fig. 13.9B). These muscles control the size of the pupil and therefore regulate the amount of light that enters the eye. The muscle fibers of the radial muscle are arranged like the spokes of a wheel. Just as the spokes radiate from the center of the wheel, the radial muscle fibers radiate from the area of the pupil. Contraction of the radial muscle causes the pupil to dilate, thereby increasing the amount of light entering the eye. Sympathetic nerve fibers supply the radial muscles. Thus, sympathetic nerve stimulation causes pupillary dilation, or mydriasis (mi-DRY-ah-sys). Drugs that dilate the pupil are called *mydriatic agents*.

The second muscle located in the iris is the circular muscle. Contraction of the circular muscles causes the pupil to constrict, thereby decreasing the amount of light entering the eye. The circular muscle is supplied by parasympathetic nerve fibers in the oculomotor nerve (CN III). Parasympathetic nerve stimulation causes pupillary constriction, or miosis (see Fig. 13.9B).

📈 **Ramp It Up!**

Pupil Size and Drugs That Affect the Autonomic Receptors on the Iris

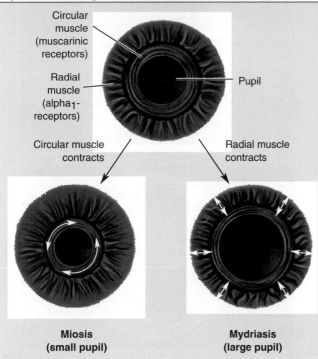

Miosis
(small pupil)

Mydriasis
(large pupil)

Many drugs affect pupillary size, and you must understand these effects so that you can make sound clinical judgments. The effects of drugs on pupil size are described in terms of autonomic receptor terminology. (You may need to review cholinergic and adrenergic receptors in Chapter 12.)

The radial muscle of the iris is innervated by sympathetic fibers and contains alpha₁-adrenergic receptors. Activation of the alpha₁ receptor by norepinephrine (NE) causes pupillary

dilation or mydriasis. The circular muscle of the iris is innervated by parasympathetic fibers and contains muscarinic receptors. Activation of the muscarinic receptors causes pupillary constriction or miosis. There are several clinical important implications.

1. An ophthalmologist may want to examine the interior of the eye; dilation of the pupils and paralysis of the muscles of accommodation (ciliary muscles) facilitates the exam. Eyedrops containing an antimuscarinic drug (e.g., atropine, other drugs included in the belladonna drug class) achieve mydriasis and cycloplegia (paralysis of the muscles of accommodation). Remember that muscarinic activation causes pupillary constriction, so muscarinic blockade causes pupillary dilation, or mydriasis.

2. Patients with glaucoma (increased intraocular pressure) are advised to avoid taking drugs that cause mydriasis because mydriasis diminishes the drainage of aqueous humor and further elevates intraocular pressure. Patients often take a number of drugs. Many commonly used drugs, such as antidepressants, have antimuscarinic effects. Therefore, while treating the primary problem of depression, you must also consider other secondary clinical conditions, such as glaucoma. Otherwise, the depression may improve in response to the antidepressant drug, but the glaucoma may worsen because of its antimuscarinic effect on the eye.

3. A neurological assessment includes the response of the photopupillary reflex. Drugs that activate or block the receptors on the iris affect the pupillary response and interfere with the neurological assessment.

Pupillary size is also affected by drugs that do not affect the autonomic receptors. For example, opioids, such as morphine, cause miosis; the pupils may be described as pinpoint pupils. The eyes reveal much about the patient.

Drugs that constrict the pupils are called *miotic agents*. Some drugs, such as opioids (narcotics), constrict the pupils so intensely that the pupils are described as pinpoint. (An easy way to remember the difference between mydriasis and miosis is that the words *dilate* and *mydriasis* both contain the letter *d*.)

Ciliary Muscle. The third intrinsic eye muscle is the ciliary muscle. Locate the ciliary muscles in Fig. 13.8C. The ciliary muscles arise from the ciliary body. The ciliary muscles attach to the suspensory ligaments, which, in turn, tug on the lens, causing the lens to change its shape. Why tug? Read on.

? **Re-Think**

1. List the extrinsic eye muscles, and state their functions.
2. List the intrinsic eye muscles, and state their functions. Define mydriasis and miosis.

PATHWAY OF LIGHT

For us to see, light waves must enter the eye (cornea) and focus on the retina. Fig 13.10 illustrates the path

of light as it moves from the cornea to the photoreceptors in the retina. Each structure of this pathway must retain its ability to allow for the passage of light. For instance, light must pass through the lens; a clouded lens, or cataract, prevents light from reaching the retina and stimulating the photoreceptors. Therefore, cataracts impair vision. The same holds true for a scarred cornea.

REFRACTION AND ACCOMMODATION

In addition to following an unimpeded path, light waves must bend to focus on the retina. The bending of light waves is called **refraction**. Let's see how this happens. Although the cornea and aqueous humor are both capable of refracting light, the lens can change its shape and its refracting power, thereby enabling the eye to continuously adjust to near and far vision. The need for refraction by the lens is illustrated in Fig. 13.11A. The light waves are shown traveling in a straight line toward the retina. Light wave 2 focuses on point X, with no need for refraction. However, unless light waves 1 and 3 are bent, they will not focus on point X.

Pathway of Light

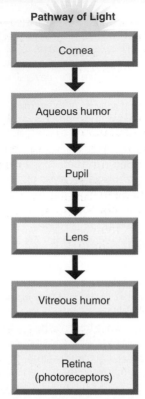

FIG. 13.10 **Pathway of light: from cornea to photoreceptors in the retina.**

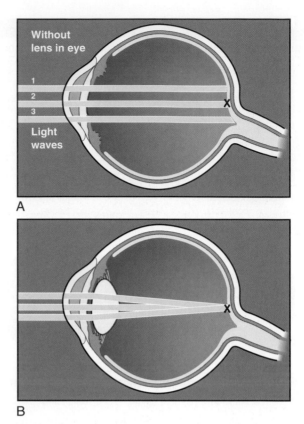

FIG. 13.11 **Refraction. (A) Path that the light waves travel (without lens). (B) Refraction of the first and third light waves (with lens).**

How does the lens bend light waves (see Fig. 13.11B)? The bottom part of light wave 1 hits the lens first and is slowed before penetrating it. The top of the light wave continues to travel until it hits the lens. For a split second, the top of the light wave travels faster than the bottom. The light wave therefore bends. The same is true for light wave 3. The top of light wave 3 hits the lens first and is slowed, while the bottom continues to travel faster until it, too, hits the lens. For a split second the bottom of light wave 3 travels faster than the top. The light wave therefore bends. It illustrates how the lens bends several light waves. For sharp vision, light waves must be refracted to focus on one particular area of the retina.

Why and how does the lens change its shape? The lens can change its shape, becoming fatter or thinner. The lens is an elastic structure held in place by the suspensory ligaments attached to ciliary muscles (see Fig. 13.8A). When the ciliary muscles contract and relax, the changes in tension cause a change in the shape of the lens. The lens either thins out or becomes fatter. The change in shape affects how much the light is bent. For example, if the lens becomes fatter, the light wave is bent at a sharper angle. If the lens thins, the degree of refraction lessens, and the light wave is not bent as much.

The ability of the lens to change its shape allows the eye to focus objects close up or at a distance. For example, if you hold a pencil 6 inches in front of your eyes, you will be able to see it clearly. The focusing of the close-up object (pencil) on the retina is caused primarily by the lens. The lens becomes fatter and bends the light waves more acutely so as to focus them on the retina. This ability of the lens to change its shape to focus on a close object is called **accommodation**.

Accommodation is accompanied by pupillary constriction and by convergence, the movement of the eyes medially toward the nose. Accommodation, pupillary constriction, and convergence all work together to focus both eyes on one object.

Emmetropia (em-eh-TROHP-ee-ah) refers to the ability of the eye to refract light without the assistance of a corrective lens. With advancing age, the lens loses some of its ability to change shape, thereby diminishing the ability to accommodate for close objects. This condition, which is often evident after age 40, is called *presbyopia* (pres-bee-OH-pee-ah) (*presbyter* means "an old man"). Persons with presbyopia have difficulty adjusting to close objects. Presbyopia accounts for the tendency of older persons to hold the newspaper at arm's length. You may have heard older persons comment good-naturedly on how their arms have gotten shorter as they have gotten older!

Do You Know...

What Is Meant by 20/20 Vision?

The ability of the eye to focus an image on the retina is assessed by use of the Snellen chart. This chart is composed of lines of letters arranged in decreasing size. The person is placed at a distance 20 feet away from the chart and is asked to cover one eye and read a line of letters. A score of 20/20 means that the person can see at 20 feet what a person with normal eye function can see. Thus, 20/20 vision is considered normal. A score of 20/40 means that a person can see at 20 feet what a person with normal vision can see at 40 feet. Thus, 20/40 vision is less perfect than 20/20 vision. A score of 20/200 indicates severely impaired vision, and the person is considered legally blind.

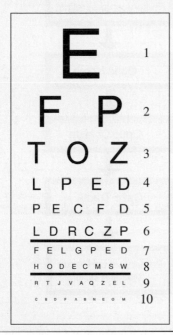

 Re-Think

1. List the structures through which light passes from the cornea to the retina.
2. Define *refraction*, and explain how the lens refracts light.
3. Define *accommodation* and *convergence*.
4. Why do scarred corneas and cataracts diminish vision?
5. With regard to refraction, why does a person with presbyopia move his or her arms to see a newspaper more clearly?

 Sum It Up!

There are two groups of muscles associated with the eyeball: extrinsic eye muscles and intrinsic eye muscles. The extrinsic eye muscles move the eyeball and are innervated by CN III, IV, and VI. The intrinsic eye muscles control pupillary size and the shape of the lens. By changing pupillary size, the iris regulates the amount of light that enters the posterior cavity. Light penetrates the following structures to stimulate the retinal photoreceptors: cornea, aqueous humor, pupil, lens, and vitreous humor. Light must be bent or refracted to focus on the retina. The curvature of the lens can be adjusted so as to refract light.

STIMULATION OF THE PHOTORECEPTORS

Once the light penetrates the various eye structures, it must stimulate the photoreceptors (rods and cones) of the retina. Why do you see black and white at night and color during daylight?

Night Vision

The rods are widely scattered throughout the retina but are more abundant in the periphery. In low-light conditions the pupil dilates, thereby allowing more light to enter the eye. The dilated pupil also allows the light rays to scatter along the periphery of the retina, thereby stimulating the rods. The image produced by the stimulation of rods is black and white and somewhat fuzzy. Because rods respond to dim light, stimulation of rods is often called *night vision*.

 Do You Know...

What Night Blindness Is?

Stimulation of the rods (night vision photoreceptors) by light waves causes the breakdown of a chemical substance called *rhodopsin*. This chemical breakdown, in turn, stimulates nerve impulses. As nerve impulses are formed, the amount of rhodopsin is used up and must be replaced. The synthesis of additional rhodopsin requires vitamin A. Because night vision depends on an adequate supply of rhodopsin, a deficiency of vitamin A can cause night blindness.

Color Vision

Cones are the photoreceptors for color vision. Cones are most abundant in the central portion of the retina, especially in the macula lutea. When in a well-lit environment, the pupil is constricted and directs the light toward the central cone-rich part of the retina. The image produced by the stimulation of cones is colored and sharp. Why colored? There are three types of cones, each with a different visual pigment (a light-sensitive chemical). One type of cone produces a green color, another produces blue, and a third produces red. Stimulation of combinations of these cones produces the many different colors and shades of colors that we enjoy.

INFORMING THE BRAIN: THE VISUAL PATHWAY

Nerve impulses that arise from the photoreceptors leave the eye (retina) by way of the optic nerve (CN II). The nerve impulses travel along the fibers of the optic nerves and optic tracts to the occipital lobe of the brain. This pathway from the retina to the brain is called the **visual pathway.**

Fig. 13.12 A and B illustrates the pathways of the optic nerves as each leaves the eye. Note that half of the fibers from the left eye cross over and travel to the right side of the brain, and half of the fibers from the right eye cross over and travel to the left side

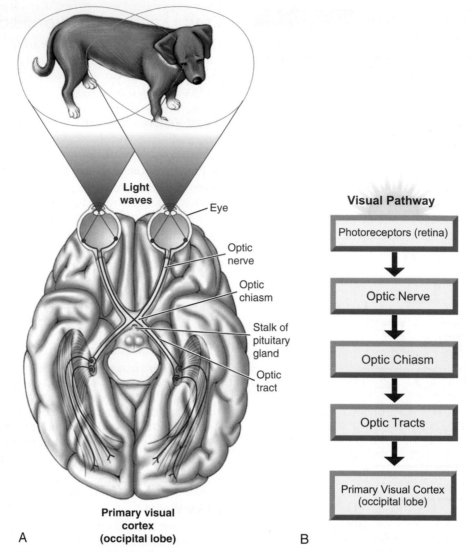

FIG. 13.12 Visual pathway. (A) From retina to primary visual cortex (occipital lobe). Note the optic chiasm and the pituitary gland (behind the optic chiasm). (B) From retina to primary visual cortex (occipital lobe).

of the brain. The crossing over of the fibers allows the occipital lobe to integrate the information from both eyes and produce only one image. The point at which the fibers from the left and right eyes crisscross is called the **optic chiasm** (KYE-ass-im). The optic chiasm is located directly in front of the pituitary gland. After passing through the optic chiasm, the nerve impulses follow the optic tracts, eventually reaching the primary visual cortex of the occipital lobe.

VISION LOSS—WHEN ALL IS NOT RIGHT

When all the parts of the eye, visual pathway, and the primary visual cortex of the brain are working correctly, you can see.

However, when the parts of the eye, visual pathway, and primary visual cortex do not work normally, a person may experience diminished vision or blindness. Any defect along this pathway from the cornea to the brain can interfere with vision. Certain conditions may prevent the entrance of light into the eye. For example, a scarred cornea or a cloudy lens (cataract) may block the entrance of light, thereby preventing the stimulation of the rods and cones. Errors of refraction such as nearsightedness and farsightedness can adversely affect the focusing of light on the retina. Light waves are focused either in front of the retina (nearsightedness) or beyond the retina (farsightedness). These "errors of refraction" can diminish vision. The more serious and often untreatable conditions affect the retina; some conditions destroy retinal tissue, injure the optic nerve, or deprive the retina of its blood supply from its underlying choroid layer. Of particular concern is diabetic retinopathy. Over time retinal blood vessels develop microaneurysms that rupture causing bleeding and the formation of scar tissue. Scar tissue eventually replaces retinal tissue leading to blindness. Last, vision loss can result from injury to the primary visual cortex in the occipital lobe.

Ramp It Up!

Commonly Assessed Eye Reflexes

There are many reflexes involving the eye (ocular reflexes). Two reflexes of clinical concern are the corneal reflex and the photopupillary reflex. Pay particular attention to the sensory input and motor responses of these reflexes.

Corneal reflex. The corneal reflex is also called the *blink reflex*; it is an involuntary blinking of the eyelids elicited by stimulation of the cornea and serves a protective function. The cornea has a rich supply of sensory nerve fibers and is therefore sensitive to touch. If the surface of the cornea is touched lightly, the eye tears and blinks to remove the source of irritation. The corneal reflex involves two cranial nerves. The ophthalmic branch of the trigeminal nerve (CN V) provides sensory fibers to the surface of the cornea. Information travels to the parietal lobe where it is interpreted as pain. The motor response is transmitted by the facial nerve (CN VII); motor fibers result in tearing and blinking. Think of how your eye responds to a piece of dust—through pain, tearing, and blinking.

Photopupillary reflex. The photopupillary reflex is a reflex that controls the diameter of the pupil of the eye in response to light. When the eye is exposed to light, the pupil immediately constricts, thereby restricting the amount of light entering the eye. The reflex has an afferent or sensory limb and an efferent or motor limb. The sensory limb includes photosensitive retinal cells associated with the optic nerve (CN II). When light stimulates these cells, the information is transmitted to and is analyzed by a specialized area in the midbrain (brain stem). In response to the retinal stimulation by light, parasympathetic fibers carried within the oculomotor nerve (CN III) provide the motor response; they stimulate the circular muscles of the iris to contract, thereby causing pupillary constriction.

In addition to the response of the light-stimulated pupil, the pupil of the other eye also constricts even if no light is directed at it. The second eye is said to constrict consensually; it consents to constrict when the photopupillary reflex is stimulated in the opposite eye. Both of these effects are assessed when an eye exam is performed. Keep in mind that many commonly used drugs affect this reflex.

Who is PERRLA? Pupillary function is evaluated by noting the size, shape, and reactivity to light. PERRLA is an assessment term for pupillary function: Pupils Equal, Round, React to Light, and Accommodation.

 Do You Know...

About High Concentrations of Oxygen and Blindness?

The administration of oxygen is generally beneficial and often lifesaving. Oxygen (O_2) therapy, however, must be delivered with care, particularly in preterm infants. In "preemies" younger than 32 weeks' gestation, the administration of very high concentrations of oxygen can cause blindness. The oxygen is usually administered to a severely hypoxemic infant. While relieving the hypoxemia, the high concentration of O_2 also causes constriction of the developing blood vessels of the retina. Deprived of its blood supply, the retina dies and is replaced by a retrolental membrane of fibrous tissue. The O_2-induced blindness is called *retrolental fibroplasia* (classified as a retinopathy of prematurity).

 Re-Think

1. Differentiate between the locations and roles of the rods and cones.
2. Differentiate between night and color vision.
3. What is the optic chiasm?
4. Describe the visual pathway of the nerve impulses (action potentials) generated in the photoreceptors to the primary visual cortex in the occipital lobe.

 Sum It Up!

Light stimulates the photoreceptors, rods (black and white) and cones (color), generating nerve impulses or electrical signals (action potentials) that are carried by the optic nerve (CN II) and visual pathway to the primary visual cortex of the occipital lobes. The optic chiasm is a "crossing over" of some of the optic nerve fibers of each eye. Thus, the primary visual cortex processes information of an object that is seen by both eyes. By tracing these pathways of light and action potentials, you can understand the sequence of events in seeing.

SENSE OF HEARING: THE EAR

Listen to the sounds around you. Perhaps some of it is background noise that you mostly ignore. Other sounds provide you with information. Most important, you can hear sounds that you enjoy, such as the voices of friends and sounds of music. The ear is the organ of the sense of **hearing**.

Refer to Fig. 13. 13 to identify the structures described as follows.

STRUCTURE OF THE EAR

The ear is divided into three parts: the external ear, the middle ear, and the inner ear.

External Ear

The external ear is the part of the ear you can see. It is composed of the auricle and the external auditory canal. The auricle, or pinna (Latin for "wing"), is composed of cartilage covered by a layer of loose-fitting skin. The auricle functions like a satellite dish gathering sound waves. The auricle opens into the external auditory canal, a passageway for sound waves to enter the ear. The external auditory canal is hollowed out of the temporal bone. It is about 1 inch long (2.5 cm) and ½ inch (1.25 cm) wide and extends to the tympanic membrane, or eardrum. The tympanic membrane separates the external ear from the middle ear.

The external auditory canal is lined with tiny hairs and glands that secrete cerumen, a yellowish waxy substance also known as *earwax*. The hairs and cerumen help prevent dust and other foreign objects from entering the external ear. Cerumen tends to be a victim of our cleanliness fetish; we insert hairpins, toothpicks, and other sharp objects into the canal in an attempt to dig out the wax. These objects may damage

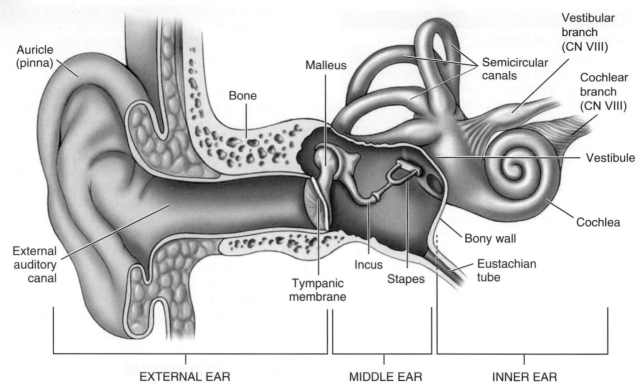

FIG. 13.13 **Three divisions of the ear: external, middle, and inner ear. Structures within the ear.**

the tympanic membrane. Cotton-tipped applicators, although appearing safer, actually remove very little wax and can push any accumulated wax up against the eardrum and impair hearing. It is best not to insert *any* objects into the ear canal. The ear canal is also a common target for the young child, who may insert an object such as a bean into the external canal; over time, the bean accumulates moisture and swells, making it difficult to remove. Off to the ear doctor for bean removal!

Middle Ear

The middle ear is a small, air-filled chamber located between the tympanic membrane at one end and a bony wall at the other end. The middle ear contains several structures: the tympanic membrane, three tiny bones, several small muscles, and the eustachian tube (also called the *pharyngotympanic tube*).

The tympanic membrane is composed primarily of connective tissue and has a rich supply of nerves and blood vessels. The tympanic membrane vibrates in response to sound waves entering the ear through the external auditory canal. The vibration of the tympanic membrane is passed on to the tiny bones in the middle ear.

The middle ear contains three tiny bones, or **ossicles**, which are the tiniest bones in the body—the malleus (hammer), incus (anvil), and stapes (stirrup). The ossicles transmit vibration from the tympanic membrane to the oval window, a membranous structure that separates the middle ear from the inner ear.

The middle ear has a passageway connecting it to the pharynx, or throat. This passageway is called the *auditory tube,* or the **eustachian tube**. The purpose of the eustachian tube is to equalize the pressure on both sides of the tympanic membrane by permitting air to pass from the pharynx into the middle ear. If the pressures across the membrane become unequal, the tympanic membrane bulges. As the tympanic membrane is stretched, pain receptors are stimulated. Pain caused by stretched tympanic membranes is why your ears sometimes hurt when you take off and land in an airplane. Hints to prevent a pressure difference across the tympanic membrane include chewing gum, drinking water through a straw, yawning, and swallowing. Babies can suck on a nipple or pacifier.

Inner Ear

The inner ear consists of an intricate system of tubes, or passageways, hollowed out of the temporal bone. This coiled network of tubes is called a *bony labyrinth* (Fig. 13.14). Inside the bony labyrinth is a similarly shaped *membranous labyrinth*. The bony labyrinth is filled with a fluid called *perilymph*. The membranous labyrinth is surrounded by perilymph and is itself filled with a thick fluid called *endolymph*. (For our purposes, the endolymph is the more important fluid.) The inner ear has three parts: the vestibule, the semicircular canals, and the cochlea. The cochlea is concerned with hearing. The vestibule and semicircular canals are concerned with balance.

Do You Know...

Why Children Tend to Outgrow Ear Infections?

The size and position of the eustachian tube in a child are different than in an adult. The eustachian tube of a child is shorter and lies in a more horizontal position than the adult eustachian tube. The child who develops a cold will often sniffle, thereby forcing the nasal drainage from the throat region into the eustachian tubes and middle ear. This drainage results in a middle ear infection called *otitis media*.

As the child grows, the eustachian tube grows longer and becomes more vertical. There is less chance for bacteria to enter the middle ear from the throat. In this sense, children are said to outgrow ear infections.

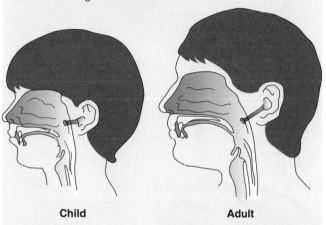

Child   **Adult**

The **cochlea** is a snail-shaped part of the bony labyrinth. Sitting on a membrane within the cochlea and immersed in endolymph are the receptors for hearing (see Fig. 13.14B). The receptors are cells that contain tiny hairs; these are called the *organ of Corti*. When the hairs on the receptor cells are bent, a nerve impulse is sent by the cochlear branch of the vestibulocochlear nerve (CN VIII) to the primary auditory cortex of the temporal lobe of the brain, where the sensation is interpreted as hearing. Note that the receptors are stimulated by the bending of the hairs; hence, the receptors are classified as mechanoreceptors.

HEARING HAPPENS WHEN...

How do we hear the sounds of music? As Fig. 13.15 illustrates, the vibrating guitar strings disturb the air, causing sound waves. The sound waves are gathered by the auricle, travel through the external auditory canal, and hit the tympanic membrane, causing the tympanic membrane to vibrate. This vibration, in turn, causes the middle ear bones (malleus, incus, and stapes) to vibrate. The stapes, sitting within the oval window, then causes the fluid in the inner ear to move. Because the hairs (organ of Corti) are sitting within the endolymph, movement of the fluid causes the hairs to bend. The bending of the hairs triggers a nerve impulse carried by the cochlear branch of the vestibulocochlear nerve (CN VIII) to the primary auditory cortex of the temporal lobe, where it is interpreted as sound.

HEARING DOESN'T HAPPEN WHEN...

What happens when the parts do not work? Following the steps listed in Fig. 13.15, consider the number of ways our hearing may become impaired. For example, the vibration of the tympanic membrane may become blunted if a plug of cerumen (earwax) becomes lodged against the tympanic membrane. The sound waves may then be unable to vibrate the eardrum. Or, the problem may involve the ossicles causing a bone conduction deafness. The bones may fuse together or fuse with the oval window. Or, the problem may involve the nerves and/or brain. The cochlear branch of CN VIII in the inner ear may be damaged causing nerve conduction deafness. The damaged nerve cannot conduct nerve impulses from the ear to the brain. Cochlear nerve damage develops for several reasons. Chronic exposure to loud noise will do it. For example, "rock and roll deafness" is hearing loss associated with loud music. Nerve damage also occurs in response to certain drugs, especially antibiotics. Drugs that cause damage to the vestibulocochlear nerve are called *ototoxic agents*. Nerve conduction deafness is commonly experienced by the elderly (presbycusis). Finally, deafness may develop in response to injury to the primary auditory cortex of the temporal lobe.

? Re-Think

1. List the three parts of the ear.
2. Describe the pathway of hearing, from the collection of sound waves in the external ear to the primary auditory cortex in the temporal lobe of the cerebrum.
3. Locate and explain the function of the eustachian tube.

SENSE OF BALANCE: THE EAR

We all appreciate our ears as organs of hearing, but we may not realize that our ears play an important role in equilibrium or balance. Damage to the inner ear, for example, may make it impossible for us to stand without losing balance.

As mentioned earlier, the inner ear has three parts: the vestibule, the semicircular canals, and the cochlea (Fig. 13.14 C). The cochlea is concerned with hearing. The **vestibule** and **semicircular canals**, collectively called the *vestibular apparatus*, are concerned with equilibrium or balance. The receptors for balance are mechanoreceptors and are located within the semicircular canals and vestibule.

There are two types of equilibrium or balance: static and dynamic equilibrium. Static equilibrium senses the position of the head and maintains the posture when the body makes no sudden movement. Dynamic equilibrium detects sudden movements of the head and maintains posture while the body is moving or rotating.

STATIC EQUILIBRIUM

The vestibule contains the organs of static equilibrium, called *maculae* (not shown). The maculae contain hair cells. The upward-projecting hairs are embedded in a jellylike substance that contains otoliths. The otoliths are stony particles made of calcium carbonate and add weight to the gel. When the head is tilted in any

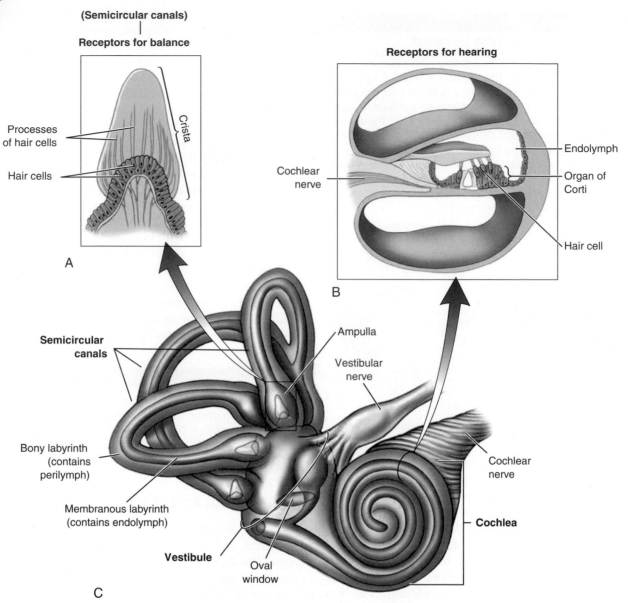

FIG. 13.14 Inner ear. (A) The receptors for balance. (B) The receptors for hearing (organ of Corti). (C) Structures of the inner ear.

direction, the otolith-containing gel moves and bends the tiny hairs. The bent hairs (mechanoreceptors) initiate a nerve impulse, which travels along the vestibulocochlear nerve (CN VIII) to the brain. The brain analyzes the information and sends motor information to the skeletal muscles to maintain balance and posture.

DYNAMIC EQUILIBRIUM

The three semicircular canals are the organs of dynamic equilibrium and respond to sudden movement. (Fig. 13.14A). They are located at right angles to each other so that any rapid change of head position or accelerating/decelerating motion can be detected. At the base of each of the semicircular canals is an ampulla; at the base of each ampulla is small elevation called a *crista*. The crista contains hair cells. The upward-projecting tiny hairs are embedded within a jellylike substance and sit within endolymph-containing ducts. When the head suddenly moves, the cristae also move, but the endolymph does

not move. In response to this disparity in movement, the hairs (mechanoreceptors) bend, thereby initiating a nerve impulse. The nerve impulse travels along the vestibular branch of CN VIII to different parts of the brain, particularly the cerebellum. The cerebellum analyzes the input from CN VIII and sends information to the skeletal muscles to maintain balance and posture.

In addition to the inner ear receptors, there are other mechanoreceptors scattered throughout the body (proprioceptors in skeletal muscle) that send information to the brain to maintain equilibrium. Visual information also participates in equilibrium. Many elderly patients, in particular, rely heavily on visual input for their balance. Vestibular dysfunction leads to balance disorders and motion sickness that appear as vertigo, nausea, and vomiting. Although the exact cause of the symptoms is unclear, it is thought to be due to the conflicting signals sent by the inner ear, mechanoreceptors (proprioceptors) in skeletal muscle and visual signals.

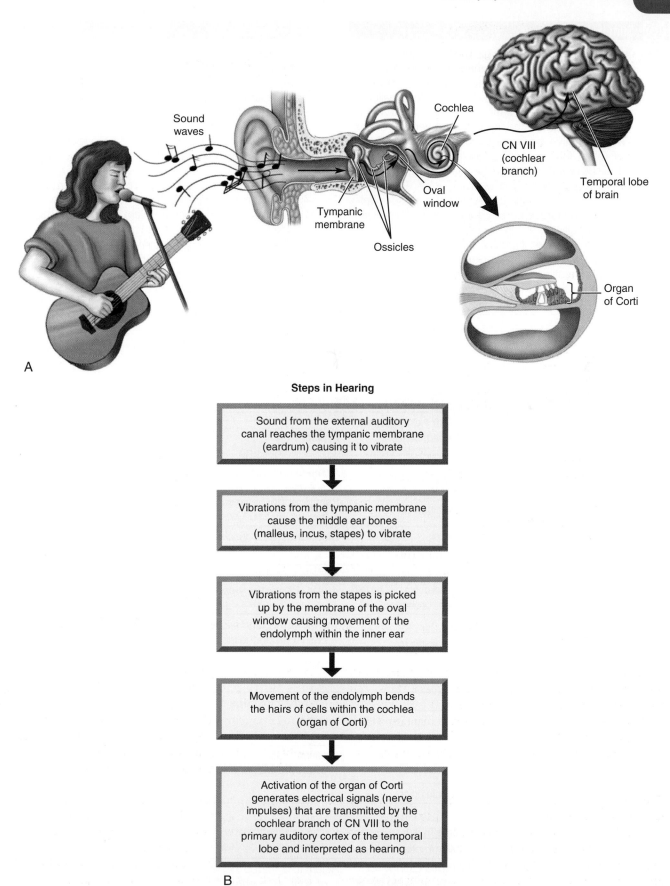

FIG. 13.15 Steps in hearing: from external ear to the primary auditory cortex of the temporal lobe.

Sum It Up!

The ear is the organ of hearing. There are three parts of the ear: external, middle, and inner ear. Sound waves enter the external ear, vibrate the tympanic membrane, which in turn vibrates the middle ear ossicles (malleus, incus, stapes). The stapes, sitting in the oval window, vibrates the endolymph in the inner ear. Movement of the endolymph activates the hearing mechanoreceptors, the organ of Corti, forming nerve impulses. The nerve impulses travel along the cochlear branch of CN VIII to the primary auditory cortex in the temporal lobe. The ear is also the organ that contains the sense receptors for balance. The mechanoreceptors are located within the inner ear and specifically within the semicircular canals and vestibule. There are two types of equilibrium: static and dynamic equilibrium. Activation of the receptors causes nerve impulses that are carried by the vestibular branch of CN VIII to various parts of the brain, particularly the cerebellum.

As You Age

1. The general senses diminish with age. A decrease in the number and sensitivity of sensory receptors, dermatomes, and neurons results in dulling of pain, touch, and tactile sensation.
2. A gradual loss of taste and smell begins around the age of 50 years.
3. Cumulative damage to hair cells in the organ of Corti occurs after the age of 60. Older adults can lose the ability to hear high-pitched sounds and the consonants *ch, f, g, s, sh, t, th,* and *z.* Also, 25% of older adults are hearing impaired.
4. Vision diminishes by the age of 70, primarily because of a decrease in the amount of light that reaches the retina and impaired focusing of the light on the retina.
5. The muscles of the iris become less efficient, so the pupils usually remain somewhat constricted.
6. The lacrimal glands become less active, and the eyes become dry and more susceptible to bacterial infection and irritation.

Medical Terminology and Disorders — Disorders of the Senses: Eyes and Ears

MEDICAL TERM	WORD PARTS	WORD PART MEANING OR DERIVATION	DESCRIPTION
Eye			
aphakia	a-	without	**Aphakia** refers to *the absence of the lens when the cataract is extracted.*
	-phak/o-	lens	**Pseudoaphakia (pseudo = false or fake)** refers to *an eye that has an artificial lens.*
	-ia	condition of	
blepharitis	blephar/o-	eyelid	**Blepharitis** is *an inflammation of the eyelid.*
	-itis	inflammation	
cataracts		From a Latin word meaning "waterfall" or "broken water"	*Clouding of the lens, thereby diminishing the amount of light that enters the posterior eye.*
lacrimal	lacrim/o-	tear	The **lacrimal** gland secretes tears that wash over the cornea and drain through the lacrimal ducts.
	-al	pertaining to	
ocular	ocul/o-	eye	**Ocular** is a word that *refers to the eye,* as in an ocular disease such as glaucoma.
	-ar	pertaining to	
ophthalmoscope	ophthalm/o-	eye	An **ophthalmoscope** is *an instrument used to examine the eye.*
	-scope	instrument used for examination	
photophobia	phot/o-	light	A patient with a corneal abrasion may be described as being **photophobic,** or having *a fear of pain-inducing exposure to light.*
	-phob/o-	fear of	
	-ia	pertaining to	
Disorders			
conjunctivitis	conjunctiv/o-	conjunctiva	Refers to *inflammation or infection of the conjunctiva; it is usually viral, bacterial, or allergenic in origin.*
	-itis	inflammation	
errors of refraction	*refringere*	From a Latin word meaning "to break up" (referring to light)	Refers to *distorted vision resulting from improper refraction of light as it enters the eye.* **Emmetropia (emmetros = well-proportioned/relaxed; -opia = condition of vision)** refers to *normal refractive condition of the eye.* Errors of refraction are described in the text.

Medical Terminology and Disorders   Disorders of the Senses: Eyes and Ears—cont'd

MEDICAL TERM	WORD PARTS	WORD PART MEANING OR DERIVATION	DESCRIPTION
Eye			
glaucoma	From the Greek word *glaukos*	Name given to any condition in which gray or green replaces the black color of the pupil	Also called the "silent thief of sight," glaucoma is the second most common cause of blindness in the United States. **Glaucoma** is *a group of eye conditions that cause damage to the optic nerve (CN II) and blindness*. The damage is due to increased intraocular pressure (IOP). There are four major types of glaucoma: open-angle glaucoma, angle-closure glaucoma, congenital glaucoma, and secondary glaucoma. Secondary glaucoma is due to drugs (corticosteroids), eye infections/trauma, or systemic diseases such as diabetes mellitus.
keratitis	kerat/o- -itis	cornea inflammation	*Refers to inflammation of the cornea.* **Keratitis** is most often caused by pathogens associated with the use of contact lenses. **Exposure keratitis** is caused by drying and ulceration of the cornea in response to incomplete closure of the eyelids (as occurs with **exophthalmos,** protrusion of the eyeball). **Photokeratitis** is due to excess UV radiation (snow blindness or welder's arc eye). Healing may cause scarring and necessitate a corneal transplant, or keratoplasty (-plasty = surgical repair of).
macular degeneration		From a Latin word *macula* meaning "spot"	Called **age-related macular degeneration (AMD)** and *results from damage to the macular cells of the retina with loss of vision in the center of the visual field (like a hole punched in the center of a picture).* **Dry AMD** is due is atrophy of the retina and loss of photoreceptors. **Wet AMD,** or **exudative AMD,** is due to neovascularization (new blood vessel growth), which causes blood or fluid to leak below the macula.
nystagmus		From a Latin word meaning "a nodding" or "drowsiness"	*Involuntary and rapid oscillating movements of the eyeball.* The movement may be side to side **(horizontal nystagmus),** up and down **(vertical nystagmus),** or rotary **(rotary or torsional nystagmus).**
retinopathy	retin/o- -pathy	retina disease	*Refers to permanent damage of the retina.* Retinopathy is often characterized by microvascular retinal changes and angiogenesis (formation of new blood vessels). The new blood vessels are fragile and leak fluid or blood into the eye; this causes retinal scarring and severe loss of vision or blindness. There are many causes of retinopathy, the most common being **diabetic retinopathy**.
strabismus		From a Greek word *strabismos* meaning "to squint"	Also called "crossed eyes." *A disorder in which two eyes do not align in the same direction and therefore do not focus on the same point.* There is **convergent strabismus,** whereby the eye(s) deviates medially, and **divergent strabismus,** whereby the eye(s) deviates laterally.
uveitis	uvea- -itis	From a Latin word meaning "grape" inflammation	*Inflammation of the uvea, the middle layer of the eye.* **Anterior uveitis** affects the front part of the eye, usually the iris, causing **iritis. Posterior uveitis** affects the choroid, the layer that supplies most of the blood to the retina. Posterior uveitis is most apt to cause loss of vision.
Ear			
myringotomy	myring/o- -otomy	eardrum incision into	A **myringotomy** is *an incision into the eardrum usually in an attempt to insert a plastic tube for the purpose of preventing the accumulation of fluid within the middle ear* as occurs in **otitis media.** Also called a *tympanoplasty* (tympan/o- = eardrum).
otoscope	ot/o- -scope	ear instrument for examination	An **otoscope** is *an instrument used to visualize the external auditory canal and the tympanic membrane (eardrum).*

Continued

Medical Terminology and Disorders   Disorders of the Senses: Eyes and Ears—cont'd

MEDICAL TERM	WORD PARTS	WORD PART MEANING OR DERIVATION	DESCRIPTION
Ear			
otosclerosis	ot/o-	ear	*Refers to an abnormal bone growth in the middle ear causing a gradual loss of hearing; causes bone conduction deafness.*
	-scler/o-	hard	
	-osis	condition of	
ototoxic	ot/o-	ear	Many drugs are considered to be ototoxic, harmful to the ear and causing a loss of hearing.
	-toxo-	poison	
	-ic	pertaining to	
presbycusis	presby/o-	old age	**Presbycusis** refers to *impaired hearing that develops with advancing age.*
	-acous/os	hearing condition	
Disorders			
Ménière's disease		Named after the French physician Ménière, who first described the disorder	*A disorder of the inner ear thought to be caused by a buildup of inner ear fluid (endolymph).* There are four main symptoms: hearing loss, a feeling of pressure in the ear, tinnitus or a roaring sound, and vertigo. The vertigo is most distressing, causing the person to experience a spinning sensation that, in turn, causes severe nausea, vomiting, and sweating.
kinetosis	kinesi/o-	From a Greek word *kinein,* meaning "to put in motion"	Also called **motion sickness** and **travel sickness** (car, plane, boat). Motion sickness occurs in response to excessive stimulation of the equilibrium receptors in the inner ear. The Greek word for *nausea* means "ship," a reference to seasickness.
	-osis	condition of	
otitis	ot/o-	ear	*A general term for inflammation or infection of the ear and* causes **otalgia** or **otodynia,** an earache. It is classified as otitis externa, otitis media, and otitis interna. **Otitis externa** is *an outer ear infection, most commonly "swimmer's ear."* **Otitis media** is *a middle ear infection with fluid or pus accumulation behind the tympanic membrane (eardrum).* The drum may burst, causing scarring of the tympanic membrane. Offending pathogens enter the middle ear from the pharynx (throat) via the eustachian tube. **Aerotitis media** is *inflammation of the middle ear caused by changes in atmospheric pressure, as in air travel.* **Otitis interna** *(inner ear inflammation/infection)* affects the sensory cells for both hearing and balance; vertigo is a common symptom.
	-itis	inflammation	

Get Ready for Exams!

Summary Outline

The sensory system allows us to experience the world through a variety of sensations: touch, pressure, pain, proprioception, temperature, taste, smell, vision, hearing, and equilibrium.

I. Receptors and Sensation
A. Receptor
  1. A receptor is a specialized area of a sensory neuron that detects a specific stimulus.
  2. The five types of receptors are chemoreceptors, pain receptors (nociceptors), thermoreceptors, mechanoreceptors, and photoreceptors.
B. Sensation
  1. A sensation is conscious or unconscious awareness of incoming sensory information.
  2. Perception is the conscious awareness of the sensation.
  3. There are four components of a sensation.
  4. Two characteristics of sensation are projection and adaptation.

II. General Senses
A. Pain
  1. Pain receptors (nociceptors) are free nerve endings.
  2. The stimuli for pain are tissue damage, lack of oxygen, and stretching or distortion of tissue.
B. Touch and pressure
  1. Receptors are mechanoreceptors that respond to forces that press, move, or deform tissue.
  2. The receptors for pressure are located in the skin, subcutaneous tissue, and deep tissue.
C. Temperature
  1. There are thermoreceptors for heat and cold.
  2. Thermoreceptors are found in free nerve endings and in other specialized sensory cells beneath the skin.
D. Proprioception
  1. Proprioceptors are located primarily in the muscles, tendons, and joints.
  2. Proprioceptors sense orientation or position.

III. Special Senses

A. Sense of smell: The nose
1. Olfactory receptors are chemoreceptors.
2. Sensory information travels along the olfactory nerve to the temporal lobe.
B. Sense of taste: The tongue
1. Taste buds contain chemoreceptors for taste.
2. There are four basic taste sensations: sweet, salty, sour, and bitter.
3. Sensory information travels along the facial, glossopharyngeal, and vagus nerves to the gustatory cortex in the parietal lobe.
C. Sense of sight: The eye
1. The visual accessory organs include the eyebrows, eyelids, eyelashes, lacrimal apparatus, and extrinsic eye muscles.
2. The eyeball has three layers: the sclera, choroid, and retina (contains the photoreceptors, rods, and cones).
3. The eyeball has two cavities. One is a posterior cavity filled with vitreous humor; the other is an anterior cavity filled with aqueous humor.
4. There are two sets of eye muscles: extrinsic and intrinsic eye muscles.
5. The extrinsic eye muscles move the eyeball.
6. The intrinsic eye muscles control the size of the pupil and shape of the lens for refraction.
7. Light must penetrate many structures to reach the retina.
8. Light stimulates the photoreceptors.
9. The electrical signal is carried to the occipital lobe via the optic nerve and visual pathway.
D. Sense of hearing: The ear
1. There are three parts of the ear: the external ear, middle ear, and inner ear.
2. The middle ear contains the ossicles.
3. The inner ear structure concerned with hearing is the cochlea. It contains the hearing receptors, or the organ of Corti (mechanoreceptors).
4. Hearing information is carried by the cochlear (CN VIII) to the temporal lobe.
5. Steps in hearing are summarized in Fig. 13.15.
E. Sense of balance: The ear
1. There are two types of equilibrium: static and dynamic.
2. The receptors are mechanoreceptors located in the vestibule (maculae) and semicircular canals (crista) of the inner ear.
3. The receptors in the vestibule are primarily responsible for static equilibrium.
4. The receptors for dynamic equilibrium are primarily responsible for dynamic equilibrium.
5. Balance information travels along the vestibular branch (CN VIII) to many areas of the brain, particularly the cerebellum.
6. Other parts of the body send signals to the brain that help with equilibrium: proprioceptors within muscles/joints and information from the eyes.

Review Your Knowledge

Matching: Senses
Directions: Match the following words with their descriptions. Some words may be used more than once.
a. sight
b. taste
c. smell
d. hearing
e. balance
1. ___ Involves rods and cones, the retina, and CN II
2. ___ Involves the organ of Corti and CN VIII
3. ___ Is the olfactory sense; uses chemoreceptors
4. ___ Uses mechanoreceptors; sensory information transmitted by the vestibular branch of CN VIII
5. ___ Gustatory sensation
6. ___ From photoreceptors to the occipital lobe
7. ___ From mechanoreceptors to the primary auditory cortex
8. ___ Involves the cristae and maculae from the vestibule and semicircular canals

Matching: Structures of the Eye
Directions: Match the following words with their descriptions. Some words may be used more than once.
a. choroid
b. vitreous humor
c. lens
d. cornea
e. iris
f. aqueous humor
g. conjunctiva
h. retina
1. ___ The layer of the eyeball that contains the photoreceptors
2. ___ The colored muscle portion of the eye that determines the size of the pupil
3. ___ The shape of this structure determined by the ciliary muscles; refracts light
4. ___ Layer of the eyeball that provides the blood supply for the retina
5. ___ Secreted by the ciliary body and drained by the canal of Schlemm
6. ___ Gel-like substance in the posterior cavity; maintains the shape of the eye and helps hold the retina in place
7. ___ Contains the radial and circular muscles; mydriasis and miosis
8. ___ The window of the eye; an avascular structure
9. ___ Layer that includes the macula lutea and fovea centralis
10. ___ Inner lining of the lids; "pink eye"

Matching: Structures of the Ear

Directions: Match the following words with their descriptions. Some words may be used more than once.

a. external ear

b. middle ear

c. inner ear

1. ___ Contains the malleus, incus, and stapes
2. ___ Connected to the pharynx by the eustachian tube
3. ___ Home of cerumen
4. ___ Location of the organ of Corti and CN VIII
5. ___ Cochlea, semicircular canals, and vestibule
6. ___ Endolymph and perilymph; mechanoreceptors
7. ___ Separated from the middle ear by the tympanic membrane
8. ___ Separated from the inner ear by the oval window
9. ___ Bone conduction deafness
10. ___ Nerve conduction deafness

Multiple Choice

1. The retina
   a. refracts light.
   b. contains rods and cones.
   c. covers the optic disc, the area of most acute vision.
   d. secretes vitreous humor.

2. What is the consequence of diminished blood flow to the choroid?
   a. Aqueous humor cannot be formed, and the intraocular pressure increases.
   b. Light cannot be refracted.
   c. The retina dies.
   d. The pupil constricts.

3. A drug or effect that is described as mydriatic
   a. decreases intraocular pressure.
   b. dilates the pupil.
   c. increases the secretion of aqueous humor.
   d. increases the numbers of cones.

4. Which of the following describes the inner ear?
   a. It contains the malleus, incus, and stapes.
   b. It connects with the pharynx by the eustachian tube.
   c. It is the location of the organ of Corti.
   d. It is concerned with bone conduction.

5. The organ of Corti
   a. is the receptor for hearing.
   b. refers to the ossicles within the middle ear.
   c. leans up against the tympanic membrane and "feels" its vibration.
   d. activates CN II.

6. Touch, pressure, pain, and temperature are
   a. mediated through mechanoreceptors.
   b. classified as general senses.
   c. interpreted in the precentral gyrus.
   d. senses that are interpreted in the occipital lobe.

7. Cranial nerves III, IV, and VI
   a. carry sensory information from the retina to the occipital lobe.
   b. carry sensory information from the organ of Corti to the primary auditory cortex.
   c. innervate the extrinsic eye muscles.
   d. are the motor nerves involved in the corneal reflex.

8. Which of the following is *not* a sense?
   a. Gustation
   b. Lacrimation
   c. Olfaction
   d. Proprioception

9. Which of the following best describes these structures: superior oblique, inferior oblique, superior rectus, inferior rectus, medial rectus, and lateral rectus?
   a. Cranial nerves that stimulate the extrinsic eye muscles
   b. Muscles that form the iris
   c. Middle ear structures
   d. Extrinsic eye muscles

10. Identify the sensation that matches the following descriptions: gustation, chemoreceptors, and CNs VII, IX, and X.
    a. Smell
    b. Lacrimation
    c. Taste
    d. Balance

11. Where are the receptors for static and dynamic equilibrium?
    a. Inner ear
    b. Cerebellum
    c. Ciliary body
    d. Cochlea

12. The vestibular apparatus refers to
    a. CN VIII and CN X.
    b. the vestibule and semicircular canals.
    c. the cochlea and organ of Corti.
    d. the retina and choroid.

13. Which of the following best describes this series of events: activation of nociceptors, transmission of the nerve impulse along the spinothalamic tract, and activation of the parietal lobe?
    a. Proprioception
    b. Anesthesia
    c. Pain
    d. Vision

14. The lens, suspensory ligaments, and ciliary muscles
    a. control the contractile activity of the extrinsic eye muscles.
    b. are concerned with refraction.
    c. are innervated by the optic nerve.
    d. move the eyeball medially.

15. Which of the following is *least* related to the eyelids?
    a. Levator palpebrae superioris
    b. CN III
    c. Ptosis, causing a "sleepy" appearance
    d. Optic nerve

Go Figure

1. Which of the following is correct according to Fig. 13.1 and Table 13.1?
   a. Sensory information travels from the occipital lobe to the photoreceptors.
   b. The photoreceptors are located within the occipital lobe of the brain.
   c. Fig. 13.1 identifies the four components of a sensation.
   d. All the receptors in Table 13.1 are identified in Fig. 13.1.

2. Which of the following is correct according to Fig. 13.3 and Table 13.1?
   a. The general senses include temperature, touch, smell, and proprioception.
   b. Nociceptors are stimulated when the temperature is extreme—too hot or too cold.
   c. Touch and pressure are the same sensations.
   d. The stimuli for thermoreceptors are changes in pressure or movement.

3. Which of the following is correct according to Fig. 13.5 and Table 13.1?
   a. Olfactory receptors are mechanoreceptors.
   b. Activation of chemoreceptors in the nasal mucosa elicits the sensation of smell in the olfactory cortex of the temporal lobe and the frontal lobe.
   c. The olfactory receptors are located in the olfactory cortex of the temporal and frontal lobes.
   d. Olfactory receptors are taste receptors

4. Which of the following is correct according to Fig. 13.6 and Table 13.2?
   a. The sense of taste is classified as a general sense.
   b. The receptors for the sense of taste are chemoreceptors.
   c. The tip of the tongue is responsible for differentiating among bitter, sour, salty, and sweet tastes.
   d. The gustatory sense (taste) is mediated by a nociceptor.

5. Which of the following is correct according to Fig. 13.7?
   a. The lacrimal gland is located medially and secretes aqueous humor.
   b. Tears are drained through openings in the canal of Schlemm.
   c. The lacrimal canals are located laterally and inferior to the lacrimal gland.
   d. The lacrimal puncta are part of the drainage system for tears.

6. Which of the following is correct according to Fig. 13.8?
   a. Vitreous humor fills the anterior cavity and gives shape to the cornea.
   b. Aqueous humor fills the posterior cavity and gently presses the retina against the choroid.
   c. The retina lies against the choroid in the posterior portion of the eyeball.
   d. The optic nerve receives sensory information from all structures within the eye, particularly the lens.

7. Which of the following is correct according to Fig. 13.8?
   a. Aqueous humor drains from the anterior cavity by way of the canal of Schlemm.
   b. Vitreous humor drains from the posterior cavity by way of the optic disc.
   c. The macula lutea and fovea centralis are called the "blind spot."
   d. All of the above are true.

8. Which of the following is correct according to Fig. 13.8?
   a. The retina, choroid, and sclera are layers of the posterior eyeball.
   b. Suspensory ligaments attach the lens to the cornea.
   c. The macula lutea and fovea centralis are intrinsic eye muscles.
   d. The iris is located posterior to the lens.

9. Which of the following is correct according to Fig. 13.9?
   a. The ciliary muscles are extrinsic eye muscles.
   b. The iris is composed of circular and radial muscles.
   c. The intrinsic eye muscles include the ciliary muscles and the superior and inferior oblique muscles.
   d. Mydriasis occurs in response to the constriction of the circular muscles of the iris.

10. According to Fig. 13.10, light
    a. enters the eye through the canal of Schlemm.
    b. is refracted by the choroid.
    c. must penetrate the cornea, lens, and "humors" before activating the retinal photoreceptors.
    d. is refracted by the retina so that it focuses on the lens.

11. Which of the following is correct according to Fig. 13.11?
    a. Refraction is accomplished by the contractile activity of the extrinsic eye muscles.
    b. Light is refracted so that it focuses on the retina.
    c. Refraction is accomplished by the contraction and relaxation of the iris.
    d. Ideally the lens focuses the light waves on the optic disc.

12. Which of the following is correct according to Fig. 13.12?
    a. The optic chiasm is located in the primary visual cortex.
    b. All fibers from the right eye cross at the optic chiasm and travel to the left side of the brain.
    c. All fibers from the left eye cross at the optic chiasm and travel to the right side of the brain.
    d. Some fibers from both the left and right eyes cross at the optic chiasm and travel to opposite sides of the brain.

13. Which of the following is correct according to Fig. 13.13?
    a. Bone conduction is an inner ear event.
    b. Nerve conduction is a middle ear event.
    c. The external ear is separated from the middle ear by the oval window.
    d. CN VIII receives input from receptors for both hearing and balance.

14. According to Fig. 13.14,
    a. The cochlear branch of CN VIII receives information from the semicircular canals and vestibule.
    b. The cristae are middle ear structures concerned with balance.
    c. The semicircular canals and vestibule house the organ of Corti.
    d. The cochlear branch of CN VIII carries information to the temporal lobe.

15. Which of the following is correct according to Fig. 13.15?
    a. Sound waves cause the tympanic membrane to vibrate.
    b. The vibrating tympanic membrane causes the middle ear ossicles to vibrate.
    c. The vibrating middle ear ossicles cause the oval window to move, thereby moving the endolymph.
    d. All of the above are true.

Endocrine System

http://evolve.elsevier.com/Herlihy

Objectives

1. List the functions of the endocrine system.
2. Discuss the role and function of hormones in the body, including the following:
   - Define *hormone*.
   - Explain the process by which hormones bind to the receptor sites of specific tissues (targets).
   - Explain the three mechanisms that control the secretion of hormones.
3. Discuss the pituitary gland, including the following:
   - Describe the relationship of the hypothalamus to the pituitary gland.
   - Describe the location, regulation, and hormones of the pituitary gland.
4. Identify the other major endocrine glands and their hormones, and explain the effects of hyposecretion and hypersecretion.

Key Terms

adenohypophysis (p. 264)
adrenal glands (p. 271)
biorhythms (p. 263)
catecholamines (p. 271)
endocrine glands (p. 260)
feedback control loops (p. 263)
hormone (p. 263)

hypothalamus (p. 264)
lock-and-key mechanism (p. 262)
neurohypophysis (p. 267)
organ-specific hormones (p. 277)
pancreas (p. 274)
parathyroid glands (p. 270)
pineal gland (p. 277)

receptor (p. 262)
second messenger (p. 262)
steroids (p. 262)
thymus gland (p. 277)
thyroid gland (p. 268)
tropic hormones (p. 267)

The nervous system and the endocrine system are the two chief communicating and coordinating systems in the body. They regulate almost all organ systems. Although the nervous and endocrine systems work together closely, they have several differences. The nervous system communicates through electrical signals called *nerve impulses*. Nerve impulses communicate information rapidly and generally achieve short-term effects. The endocrine system, in contrast, communicates through chemical signals called *hormones*. The endocrine system responds more slowly and generally exerts longer-lasting effects.

In general, the endocrine system and its hormones help regulate metabolic processes involving carbohydrates, proteins, and fats. Hormones also play an important role in growth and reproduction and help regulate water and electrolyte balance. When you become hungry, thirsty, hot, or cold, your body's response includes the secretion of hormones. Finally, hormones help your body meet the demands of infection, trauma, and stress. The study of the endocrine system is called *endocrinology*.

ENDOCRINE GLANDS

The endocrine system is composed of endocrine glands that are widely distributed throughout the body (Fig. 14.1). **Endocrine glands** secrete the chemical substances called *hormones*. Endocrine glands are ductless glands—that is, they secrete the hormones directly into the blood and not into ducts. For example, the pancreas secretes the hormone insulin into the blood, which then delivers the insulin to cells throughout the body. Many hormones are also secreted by organs, such as the stomach, kidney, and heart: these hormones will be described in later chapters. (Remember, an exocrine gland, such as the sweat gland, uses ducts or tiny tubes to carry its secretions to the surface of the body. Endocrine glands secrete hormones into the blood and not into ducts.)

CLASSIFICATION OF HORMONES

A hormone is a chemical messenger that influences or controls the activities of other tissues or organs. Chemically, hormones are classified as either proteins

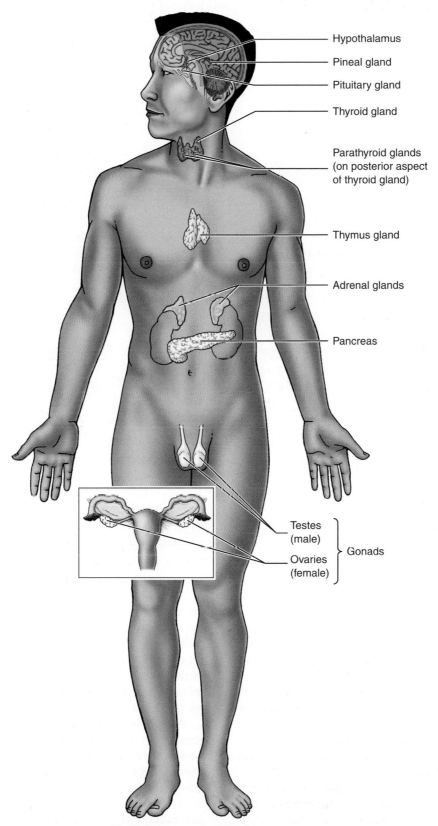

FIG. 14.1 Major endocrine glands of the body.

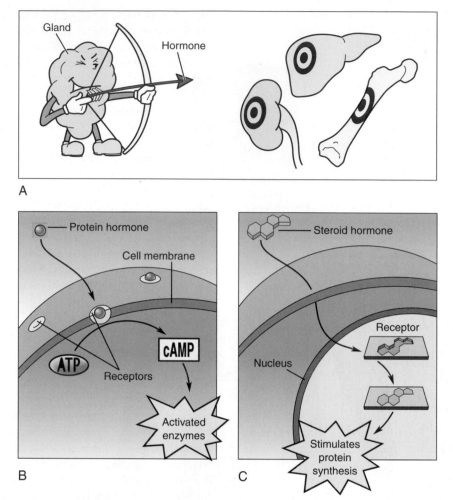

FIG. 14.2 What hormones do. (A) Hormones: aim at target tissues or target organs. (B) Protein hormones and membrane receptors. (C) Steroid hormones and intracellular receptors.

(and protein-related substances) or **steroids**. With the exception of secretions from the adrenal cortex and the sex glands, all hormones are protein or protein-related. The adrenal cortex and the sex glands secrete steroids.

TARGETS

Each hormone binds to a specific tissue, called its *target tissue* or *organ* (Fig. 14.2A). The target tissue may be located close to or at a distance from the endocrine gland. Some hormones, such as thyroid hormone and insulin, have many target tissues and therefore exert more widespread, or generalized, effects. Other hormones, such as parathyroid hormone (PTH), have fewer target tissues and therefore exert fewer effects.

HORMONE RECEPTORS

Hormones bind to the receptor sites of the cells of their target tissues. The two types of **receptors** are those located on the outer surface of the cell membrane (membrane receptors) and those located within the cell (intracellular receptors).

How do hormones recognize their target tissues? The hormone and its receptor can be compared with a **lock-and-key mechanism**. The key must fit the lock. The same is true for the hormone and receptor; a part of the hormone (key) "fits into" its receptor (lock) on the target. Unless the match is perfect, the hormone cannot lock into and stimulate the receptor. For example, the hormone insulin circulates throughout the body in the blood and is therefore delivered to every cell in the body. Insulin, however, can only stimulate the cells that have insulin receptors. Insulin does not affect cells that lack insulin receptors. The lock-and-key theory guarantees that a particular hormone affects only certain cells. The hormone-receptor relationship ensures specificity, meaning that there is a specific hormone for each receptor.

Protein hormones generally bind to receptor sites located on the cell membrane (see Fig. 14.2B). The interaction of the hormone with its receptor stimulates the production of a **second messenger** such as cyclic adenosine monophosphate (cAMP). The cAMP, in turn, helps activate the enzymes in the cell. For example, when epinephrine stimulates its receptors on the heart, cAMP is formed and then stimulates the heart itself.

The second type of receptor is located intracellularly (see Fig. 14.2C). Steroid hormones, which are lipid soluble, pass through the plasma membrane of the target

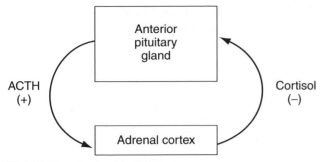

FIG. 14.3 **Negative feedback loop.**

cell and bind to receptors in the nucleus. The steroid–receptor complex then stimulates protein synthesis. The newly synthesized protein alters cellular function.

 Re-Think

1. What is the difference between an endocrine and exocrine gland?
2. Define *hormone*, and state how hormones are classified.
3. What is a target organ?
4. How does a hormone recognize its target cell?

CONTROL OF HORMONE SECRETION

Three mechanisms control the secretion of hormones: feedback control loops, biorhythms, and control by the central nervous system (CNS).

FEEDBACK LOOPS

Normal endocrine function depends on the normal plasma levels of hormones. Life-threatening complications develop when the glands hypersecrete or hyposecrete hormones. For example, if too much or too little steroid is secreted by the adrenal cortex, the person develops signs and symptoms that are potentially life threatening. So how does the adrenal cortex, a steroid-secreting gland, know when it has secreted enough steroid?

It "knows" through a negative **feedback control loop.** The pattern of adrenocorticotropic hormone (ACTH) and cortisol secretion is one example of a negative feedback loop (Fig. 14.3). ACTH, secreted by the anterior pituitary gland, stimulates its target organ (adrenal cortex) to secrete cortisol. As blood levels of cortisol increase, the cortisol in the blood chemically "tells" the anterior pituitary gland to slow further secretion of ACTH. The diminished ACTH, in turn, decreases the secretion of cortisol by the adrenal cortex.

What information was fed back to the anterior pituitary gland? It was the increasing level of cortisol in the blood. What was the response of the anterior pituitary gland? The gland decreased its secretion of ACTH. Because the cortisol diminished the secretion of the anterior pituitary gland, the response is referred to as *negative feedback control.* Why doesn't the adrenal cortex completely stop its secretion of cortisol? Over

time, the plasma level of cortisol declines as the hormone is degraded and eliminated from the body; the negative inhibition by cortisol is relieved, and ACTH is again secreted. (ACTH regulation is described more completely later in the chapter.)

Although negative feedback loops are the more common of the loops, there are also positive feedback loops. Unlike the inhibition of a negative feedback loop, a positive feedback loop causes an enhanced response, a self-amplification cycle in which a change is the stimulus for an even greater change in the same direction. For example, during early labor, the head of the baby stretches the cervix, the neck of the uterus. The stretch causes nerve impulses to travel from the cervix to the brain, which in turn causes the secretion of a hormone called *oxytocin.* The oxytocin is carried by the blood to the uterus, where it stimulates the contraction of the uterus. In response to uterine contraction, the cervix is stretched further by the baby's head, causing the release of additional oxytocin. This positive feedback cycle continues until the baby is born. Positive feedback loops are often designed to produce a rapid response.

BIORHYTHMS

Blood levels of most hormones are also controlled by **biorhythms.** A biorhythm is a rhythmic alteration in a hormone's rate of secretion. Some **hormones,** such as cortisol, are secreted in a circadian rhythm. A circadian rhythm (*circa-* means "around"; *-dian* means "day") is a 24-hour rhythm; its pattern repeats every 24 hours. Because of its circadian rhythm, cortisol secretion is highest in the morning hours (peak at 8 AM) and lowest in the evening hours (lowest at midnight). The female reproductive hormones represent another biorhythm. They are secreted in a monthly pattern—hence, the monthly menstrual cycle.

Unfortunately, biorhythms can be disturbed by travel and alterations in sleep patterns. For example, jet lag and the symptoms of fatigue experienced by persons who work the night shift are related to alterations of biorhythms. More recently, alterations in biorhythms have also been linked to disturbances in cholesterol metabolism and diseases such as cancer. The problem has become so acute that some hospitals have developed staffing schedules based on biorhythms.

Sometimes drugs are administered on a schedule that mimics normal biorhythms. For example, steroids are administered in the morning, when natural steroid levels are highest. Coordinating with the natural rhythms increases the effectiveness of the drug and causes fewer side effects. The effect of biorhythms on drug effects is so important that a branch of pharmacology addresses this issue: chronopharmacology. The time of drug administration may have a profound effect on its activity.

CONTROL BY THE CENTRAL NERVOUS SYSTEM

The CNS helps control the secretion of hormones in two ways: activation of the hypothalamus and stimulation of the sympathetic nervous system. Think about this. The CNS exerts a powerful influence over the endocrine system. Because the CNS is also the center for our emotional lives, it is not surprising that our emotions, in turn, affect the endocrine system.

For example, when we are stressed out, the CNS causes several of the endocrine glands to secrete stress hormones, thereby alerting every cell in the body to the threat. Many women have experienced the effect of stress on the menstrual cycle. Stress can cause the menstrual period to occur early or late; it may even cause the cycle to skip a month. These effects illustrate the power of emotions and the CNS on our body. In fact, the functions of the nervous system and the endocrine system are so closely related that the word *psychoneuroendocrinology* is used.

 Re-Think

1. Explain the difference between negative and positive feedback control.
2. Explain why the menstrual cycle is called a biorhythm.

 Sum It Up!

The endocrine system is composed of endocrine glands widely distributed throughout the body. The endocrine glands secrete hormones. Hormones are classified as either protein (protein-like) or steroids. They exert widespread metabolic effects throughout the body and affect every organ system. Hormones stimulate target tissues by binding to cell receptors. The receptors are located either on the cell membrane or within the cell. Three control mechanisms regulate the secretion of hormones: negative and positive feedback loops, biorhythms, and CNS activity.

PITUITARY GLAND AND THE HYPOTHALAMUS

The pituitary gland, also called the *hypophysis* (hye-POF-is-sis), is a pea-sized gland located in a depression of the sphenoid bone. It is attached to the undersurface of the **hypothalamus** by a short stalk called the *infundibulum*. The pituitary contains two main parts: the anterior pituitary gland and posterior pituitary gland. The major hormones and their target glands are shown in Fig. 14.4A.

The secretions of both the anterior and posterior lobes of the pituitary gland are dependent upon the hypothalamus, although in different ways. The secretion of the anterior pituitary gland is controlled by the hypothalamic secretion of hormones called *releasing hormones* and *release-inhibiting hormones*—they either stimulate or inhibit the secretion of anterior pituitary hormones. For example, prolactin-releasing hormone, secreted by the hypothalamus, stimulates the pituitary gland to secrete prolactin. Prolactin-inhibiting hormone (PIH), secreted by the hypothalamus, inhibits the secretion of prolactin by the anterior pituitary gland.

How do the hypothalamic hormones reach the anterior pituitary gland? The hypothalamus secretes its hormones into a network of capillaries (tiny blood vessels) that connect the hypothalamus with the anterior pituitary gland (see Fig. 14.4B). These connecting capillaries are called the *hypothalamic–hypophyseal portal system*. Thus, hormones secreted by the hypothalamus flow through the portal capillaries to the anterior pituitary.

 Do You Know...

Why the Pituitary Gland Is "Uppity" but Not Snotty?

The pituitary gland is also known as the *master gland*, and a pretty important gland it is! When first discovered, however, the pituitary gland was relegated to the lowly role of mucus secretion (pituita is the Greek word for "mucus"). The gland was credited with secreting mucus as a cooling agent. After cooling the body, mucus was then eliminated through the nose. Obviously, this is not true. Mucus is secreted by the mucous membrane that lines the nasal passages and does not act as a coolant. Mucus merely does the nasal housework—it traps the dust and gets blown out of your nose. The pituitary gland, on the other hand, has more important things to do. It secretes many hormones and controls much of the endocrine function of the body. Unfortunately, this master gland is stuck with the name pituitary (mucus-making). Its other name, hypophysis, isn't much more flattering; it means "undergrowth" (referring to its location under the brain). Mucus and undergrowth—humbling for a master gland!

ANTERIOR PITUITARY GLAND

The anterior pituitary gland is composed of glandular epithelial tissue and is also called the **adenohypophysis** (ad-eh-no-hye-POF-i-sis). The anterior pituitary gland secretes six major hormones (Table 14.1; Fig. 14.4A). These hormones control other glands and affect many organ systems. In fact, the anterior pituitary affects so many other glands that it is often called the *master gland*.

The hormones of the anterior pituitary include thyroid-stimulating hormone (TSH), ACTH, growth hormone (GH), the gonadotropins, and prolactin (PRL). Here's an easy way to remember these hormones.

PRO	Prolactin
ATHletes	ACTH
Got	Gonadotropins (FSH, LH)
To	TSH
GROW	Growth hormone

GROWTH HORMONE

Growth hormone (GH) is also called *somatotropin* or *somatotropic hormone*. Its primary effects are on the growth of bones, cartilage, and skeletal muscles, thereby determining a person's size and height. GH also exerts powerful metabolic effects. It causes amino acids to be built into proteins and fats to be broken down and used for energy. It also stimulates the conversion of protein to glucose (gluconeogenesis), especially during periods of fasting between meals. GH thus causes blood glucose levels to rise. GH also affects electrolyte balance: it stimulates the kidneys to reabsorb sodium (Na^+), potassium (K^+), and chloride (Cl^-) and the digestive

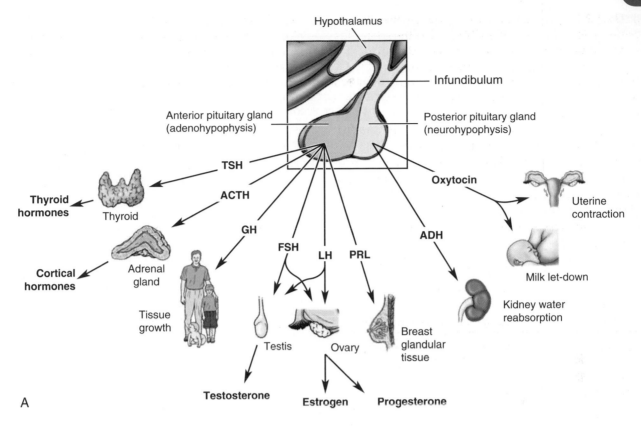

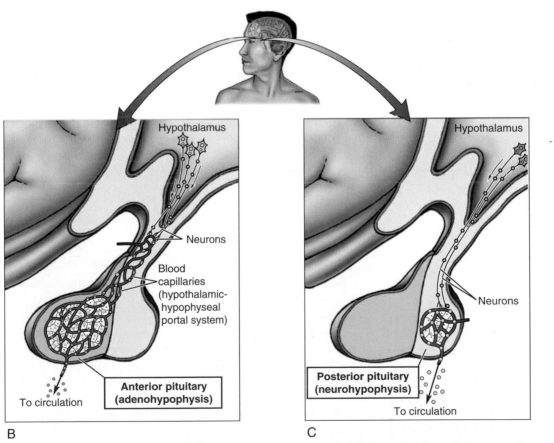

FIG. 14.4 Pituitary gland. (A) Hormones and target organs of the anterior and posterior pituitary glands. (B) Relationship of the hypothalamus to the anterior pituitary gland. (C) Relationship of the hypothalamus to the posterior pituitary gland.

Table 14.1   Hormones and Their Functions

HORMONE	FUNCTION
Anterior Pituitary Gland	
Growth hormone (GH)	Stimulates the growth of all tissues and organs, especially bone, cartilage, and skeletal muscle; stimulates the transport of amino acids into cells and the synthesis of glucose during periods of fasting
Prolactin	Stimulates the breast to develop; maintains milk production after birth; also called lactogenic hormone
Thyroid-stimulating hormone (TSH)	Stimulates the thyroid gland to produce thyroid hormones (T_3 and T_4)
Adrenocorticotropic hormone (ACTH)	Stimulates the adrenal cortex to secrete steroids, especially cortisol
Gonadotropic hormones	
Follicle-stimulating hormone (FSH)	Stimulates the development of ova and sperm
Luteinizing hormone (LH)	Causes ovulation in women; stimulates secretion of progesterone in women and testosterone in men
Posterior Pituitary Gland	
Antidiuretic hormone (ADH)	Stimulates water reabsorption by the kidneys; also constricts blood vessels
Oxytocin	Contracts uterine muscle during labor; releases milk from the mammary glands during breast-feeding (milk let-down reflex)
Hormones of the Thyroid and Parathyroid Glands	
Thyroid hormones (T_3, T_4)	Triiodothyronine (T_3) and tetraiodothyronine (T_4, or thyroxine) secreted by the thyroid gland; control metabolic rate and regulate physical and neurologic growth and development
Calcitonin	Secreted by the thyroid gland; regulates calcium and phosphate (decreases plasma levels of calcium and phosphate)
Parathyroid hormone (PTH)	Secreted by the parathyroid glands; regulates calcium and phosphate (increases plasma calcium; exerts a phosphaturic effect)
Hormones of the Adrenal Gland	
Catecholamines	Secreted by the adrenal medulla
Epinephrine	Stimulate the "fight-or-flight" response; epinephrine increases blood glucose
Norepinephrine	
Steroids	Secreted by the adrenal cortex.
Cortisol	Glucocorticoid that helps regulate glucose, fat, and protein metabolism; is part of the stress response. Cortisol increases blood glucose.
Aldosterone	Mineralocorticoid that causes the kidneys to reabsorb sodium and water and excrete potassium; helps regulate extracellular fluids and electrolytes (especially Na^+ and K^+).
Sex hormones	The androgens (especially testosterone) help develop the secondary sex characteristics in the female and male.
Hormones of the Pancreas	
Insulin	Secreted by beta cells of the islets of Langerhans; helps regulate the metabolism of carbohydrates, proteins, and fats; lowers blood glucose levels
Glucagon	Secreted by the alpha cells of the islets of Langerhans; increases blood glucose levels
Other Hormones	
Estrogens and progesterone	Secreted by the ovaries; stimulate the development of the ova (eggs) and development of secondary sex characteristics in the female. Promote conditions necessary for pregnancy.
Testosterone	Secreted primarily by the testes; chief male androgen; stimulates development of sperm and secondary sex characteristics in the male
Thymosins	Stimulates maturation of the T lymphocytes; secreted by the thymus gland
Melatonin	Secreted by the pineal gland; helps set the biorhythms and participates in the sleep–wake cycle

tract to absorb dietary calcium. These electrolytes then become available to growing tissue. In addition to the direct effects of GH on tissue growth, it also stimulates growth indirectly. GH stimulates the liver to produce growth stimulants called *insulin-like growth factors* (or somatomedins). GH is secreted during periods of exercise, sleep, and hypoglycemia.

As its name implies, GH exerts a profound effect on growth. A person who hypersecretes GH as a child develops gigantism and will grow very tall, often achieving a height of 8 or 9 feet. If hypersecretion of GH occurs in an adult after the epiphyseal discs of the long bones have sealed, only the bones of the jaw (called "lantern jaw"), eyebrow ridges, nose, hands, and feet enlarge. This condition is called *acromegaly*. GH deficiency in childhood causes the opposite effect, a pituitary dwarfism. With this condition, body proportions are normal, but the person's height is very short.

PROLACTIN

Prolactin (PRL) is also called *lactogenic hormone*. As its name suggests (*pro-* means "for"; *-lact-* means "milk"), PRL stimulates the growth of the mammary glands and the production of milk after childbirth. As long as the lactating mother continues to breast-feed, PRL levels remain high, and milk is produced. The role of PRL in males is not fully understood but is known to increase the secretion of testosterone.

TROPIC HORMONES

The remaining hormones of the anterior pituitary gland are **tropic hormones,** which are aimed at and control other glands. They include the following:

- **Thyrotropin, or thyroid-stimulating hormone (TSH).** The target gland for TSH is the thyroid gland, stimulating it to secrete two thyroid hormones.
- **Adrenocorticotropic hormone (ACTH).** The target gland for ACTH is the adrenal cortex, stimulating it to secrete steroids.
- **Gonadotropic hormones.** The target glands for the gonadotropic hormones are the gonads, or sex glands (ovaries and testes). The two gonadotropins are follicle-stimulating hormone (FSH) and luteinizing hormone (LH). FSH stimulates the development of ova (eggs) in the female and sperm in the male. LH causes ovulation in the female and causes the secretion of sex hormones in both the male and the female. LH in the male is also called interstitial cell–stimulating hormone (ICSH) because it stimulates the interstitial cells in the testes to synthesize and secrete testosterone. (These hormones are described further in Chapter 26.)

POSTERIOR PITUITARY GLAND

The posterior pituitary gland is also controlled by the hypothalamus, but not through the secretion of releasing hormones. The posterior pituitary gland is an extension of the hypothalamus (see Fig. 14.4C). It is composed of nervous tissue and is therefore called the neurohypophysis (noo-roh-hye-POF-i-sis). The two hormones of the posterior pituitary gland are produced in the hypothalamus and transported to the gland, where they are stored until needed. The two hormones are antidiuretic hormone (ADH) and oxytocin.

ANTIDIURETIC HORMONE

Antidiuretic hormone (ADH) is released from the posterior pituitary gland in an attempt to conserve water. The primary target organ for ADH is the kidney. ADH causes the kidney to reabsorb water from the urine and return it to the blood. By so doing, the amount of urine that the kidney excretes decreases—hence, the term *antidiuretic hormone* (*anti-* means "against"; *diuresis* means "urine flow").

What are the signals for the release of ADH? ADH is released in response to a concentrated blood (increased osmolarity) and decreased blood volume; both occur in dehydration. The hypothalamic cells that sense the increasing osmolarity of the blood are called *osmoreceptors*. Other triggers for the release of ADH are stress, trauma, and drugs such as morphine. Alcohol, in contrast, inhibits ADH secretion—hence, the excessive urination that accompanies beer drinking!

In the absence of ADH, a profound diuresis occurs, and the person may excrete up to 25 L/day of dilute urine. This ADH deficiency disease is called *diabetes insipidus* and should not be confused with the more common *diabetes mellitus*, which is an insulin deficiency. (The effect of ADH on the kidneys is described in Chapter 24.)

ADH also causes the blood vessels to constrict, thereby elevating blood pressure. Because of this blood pressure–elevating effect, ADH is also called *vasopressin* (vay-so-PREHS-in). (A vasopressor agent is one that elevates blood pressure.)

OXYTOCIN

The second posterior pituitary hormone is oxytocin. The target organs of oxytocin (ahk-see-TOH-sin) in the female are the uterus and the mammary glands (breasts). Oxytocin release occurs in response to neuroendocrine reflexes, that is, in response to signals from the nervous system. Oxytocin stimulates the muscles of the uterus to contract and plays a role in labor and the delivery of a baby. The word *oxytocin* literally means "swift birth," and an oxytocic drug is one that causes uterine contractions and hastens delivery. You have probably heard of the use of IV "pit" (or Pitocin, the trade name for oxytocin) to initiate labor.

Oxytocin also plays a role in breast-feeding. When the baby suckles at the breast, oxytocin is released and stimulates contraction of the smooth muscles around the mammary ducts within the breasts, thereby releasing breast milk. The release of milk in response to suckling is called the *milk let-down reflex* (discussed further in Chapter 26). The role of oxytocin in the male is not fully understood; it is thought to help move the semen along the male reproductive tract. Oxytocin has recently been dubbed the bonding or relationship hormone; it seems that a high blood level of oxytocin generates feelings of goodwill and an urge to be cooperative, protective, and friendly. It makes sense that breast-feeding and the release of oxytocin facilitate bonding between Mom and Baby.

? Re-Think

1. Why is the pituitary gland sometimes called the master gland? Why do some call the hypothalamus the master gland?
2. What "happens" in the hypothalamic–hypophyseal portal system?
3. List the six hormones secreted by the anterior pituitary gland and two hormones secreted by the posterior pituitary gland.
4. Describe the influence of the hypothalamus on both the anterior and posterior pituitary hormonal secretion.

◎ Sum It Up!

The pituitary gland is called the master gland because it controls many other endocrine glands. The anterior pituitary gland (adenohypophysis) is controlled by hypothalamic hormones, called *releasing hormones* and *release-inhibiting hormones*. These hormones are secreted by the hypothalamus into the hypothalamic–hypophyseal portal system. The anterior pituitary gland secretes six major hormones: growth hormone, ACTH, TSH, prolactin, and gonadotropins (FSH and LH). The posterior pituitary gland is an extension of the hypothalamus and is called the *neurohypophysis*. The posterior pituitary gland secretes two hormones, ADH and oxytocin ADH conserves water by the action on the kidneys. Oxytocin participates in labor and in breast-feeding through the milk let-down reflex.

THYROID GLAND

The **thyroid gland** is located in the anterior neck; it is situated anterior to the trachea (Fig. 14.5A) and is easily palpated (i.e., you can feel thyroid nodules or enlargement). The thyroid gland is butterfly shaped and has two large lobes connected by a band of tissue called the *isthmus* (ISS-muss). The thyroid gland contains two types of cells: the follicular cells, located within the thyroid follicle, and the parafollicular cells, located between the follicles. Each type of cell secretes a particular hormone (see Table 14.1).

THYROID FOLLICLE

The thyroid gland is composed of many secretory units called *follicles*. The cavity in each follicle is filled with a clear, viscous substance called *colloid*. Follicular cells secrete two thyroid hormones: triiodothyronine (try-eye-oh-doh-THY-roh-neen) (T_3) and tetraiodothyronine (tet-rah-eye-oh-doh-THY-roh-neen) (T_4, or thyroxine). The term *thyroid hormones* refers to T_3 and T_4 collectively.

WHAT THYROID HORMONES (T_3 AND T_4) DO

The thyroid hormones T_3 and T_4 have similar functions, although T_3 is more potent. Thyroid hormones regulate all phases of metabolism; they increase the release of energy from carbohydrates and fatty acids, increase protein synthesis, and determine the

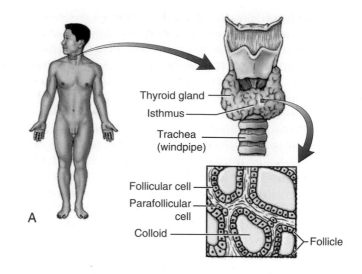

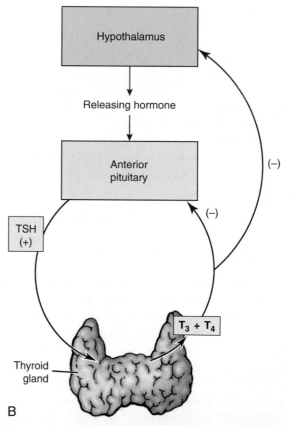

FIG. 14.5 Thyroid gland. (A) Location; the follicular cells (thyroid follicle) and parafollicular cells. (B) Negative feedback control of the secretion of T_3 and T_4.

number of calories required to "keep it running" at rest. The "keep it running" at rest is called the *basal metabolic rate* or BMR. Thyroid hormones: think metabolic rate!

In addition, thyroid hormones are essential for the normal maturation of the nervous system and for normal growth and development; they also play a permissive role in that they are necessary for the proper functioning of all other hormones. Perhaps the best way to describe the effects of thyroid hormones is to observe the effects of thyroid hormone deficiency (hypothyroidism) and excess (hyperthyroidism).

Hypothyroidism in an adult results in a sloweddown metabolic state characterized by a slow heart rate, sluggish peristalsis resulting in constipation, a low body temperature, low energy, loss of hair, and weight gain. If an infant is born with no thyroid gland, a condition called *cretinism* develops. An infant with cretinism fails to develop both physically and mentally. The child will be short and stocky, with abnormal skeletal development and signs of severe developmental delay.

An excess of thyroid hormones produces hyperthyroidism, a speeded-up metabolic state that is characterized by an increase in heart rate, an increase in peristalsis resulting in diarrhea, elevation in body temperature, hyperactivity, weight loss, and wide emotional swings. The elevation in body temperature reflects the heat-producing or calorigenic effects of thyroid hormones. In fact, in a severe hyperthyroid state, body temperature can elevate into lethal ranges.

 Do You Know...

About Graves' Disease and the "Eye-Pad" Thing?

Graves' disease is a hyperthyroid state characterized by bulging eyes, a condition called *exophthalmia*. The eyes bulge forward because the fat pads behind the eyeball enlarge and push the eyeballs forward in the eye socket. Why do the eyepads enlarge? Because of the hormonal changes associated with Graves' disease. Why is exophthalmia of concern? In addition to the cosmetic issue, there is the possibility of corneal ulceration and loss of vision. The eyelids are unable to cover and lubricate the corneas of the bulged eyeballs. Consequently, the corneas dry out, ulcerate, and impair vision.

REGULATION OF SECRETION

The regulation of thyroid gland activity is illustrated in Fig. 14.5B. The hypothalamus secretes a hypothalamic releasing hormone, which stimulates the anterior pituitary to secrete TSH. TSH stimulates the thyroid gland to secrete T_3 and T_4. When the plasma levels of the thyroid hormones increase sufficiently, negative feedback inhibition prevents further secretion of TSH.

THE NEED FOR IODINE

SYNTHESIS OF THYROID HORMONE

The synthesis of T_3 and T_4 requires iodine salts called *iodides*. The iodides come from dietary sources; they are absorbed into the blood and are then actively pumped into the follicular cells of the thyroid gland, where they are used in the synthesis of the thyroid hormones. Tetraiodothyronine, or thyroxine, contains four (*tetra-*) iodine atoms and therefore is called T_4. Triiodothyronine (*tri-*) contains three iodine atoms and is called T_3.

IODINE DEFICIENCY

Why does an iodine-deficient diet cause the thyroid gland to enlarge? In an iodine-deficient state, the amount of T_3 and T_4 production decreases because iodine is necessary for the synthesis of the thyroid

hormones. With insufficient iodine, thyroid hormones cannot be made in quantities great enough to shut off the secretion of TSH through negative feedback control. Persistent stimulation of the thyroid gland by TSH causes the thyroid gland to enlarge; an enlarged thyroid gland is called a *goiter* (GOYH-ter).

 Do You Know...

What a Goiter Is Doing on the Ceiling of the Sistine Chapel?

Like many artists of the Renaissance period, Michelangelo had a fascination with goiters (from the Latin *guttur*, meaning "throat"). One of his paintings, called the "Separation of Light from Darkness," shows the Creator with a very obvious nodular goiter. It is no accident that the artist equates the appearance of the goiter with the first day of creation. Why? Michelangelo was very familiar with goiters, having grown up in the iodine-poor region of Italy (before the days of iodized salt). Michelangelo was obsessed with anatomy, having spent many hours dissecting corpses and sketching innards. He shared the view of his contemporaries that goiters were a sign of beauty and privilege, so of course he gifted God a huge goiter. Other artists not only painted gnarly goiters, but they also illustrated rather hefty body types, thereby connecting the goiter with the weight gain of hypothyroidism.

Some medical historians offer a different "take" on Michelangelo's divine goiter. It has been suggested by some that Michelangelo himself had a goiter and actually painted God in his own goitrous image. This view is certainly consistent with Michelangelo's lofty opinion of himself. It has also been suggested that the "self-portrait" theory represents his petulant response to the demand of Pope Julius that he paint the ceiling, a task that Michelangelo did not enjoy.

Clinical assessment of thyroid function makes use of the iodine-pumping activity of the gland. For example, if a patient drinks radioactive iodine (^{131}I), the thyroid gland pumps the radioactive iodine from the blood into the gland. The rate of iodine uptake by the thyroid gland can be determined by a gamma ray scanner placed over the thyroid gland. Increased iodine uptake is observed in hyperthyroid and iodine-deficient patients, whereas a decrease in iodine uptake is noted with hypothyroid patients. Larger therapeutic doses of ^{131}I can be used to destroy thyroid tissue in the hyperthyroid state.

 Re-Think

1. Name the two thyroid hormones.
2. Name the term that describes the general effects of thyroid hormones.
3. Why does a hypothyroid person have an elevated plasma TSH level?
4. Why does an iodine-deficient diet cause goiter formation?

CALCITONIN

The parafollicular cells of the thyroid gland secrete a hormone called *calcitonin*. Although calcitonin is secreted by the thyroid gland, it is not called "thyroid hormone" as are T_3 and T_4. The effects of calcitonin are very different from those of T_3 and T_4. Calcitonin helps regulate blood levels of calcium and phosphate. Calcitonin is secreted in response to elevated blood levels of calcium and stimulates osteoblastic (bone-making) activity in the bones, thereby moving calcium from the blood into the bone. Calcitonin also increases the excretion of calcium and phosphate in the urine. In general, calcitonin acts as an antagonist to parathyroid hormone.

PARATHYROID GLANDS

Four tiny parathyroid glands lie along the posterior surface of the thyroid gland (Fig. 14.6). The **parathyroid glands** secrete PTH. The stimulus for the release of PTH is a low blood level of calcium. PTH has three target organs: bone, digestive tract (intestine), and kidneys. The overall effect of PTH is to increase blood calcium levels, which it does in three ways:

1. PTH increases the release of calcium from bone tissue, called *resorption*. (Do not confuse the word *resorption* with *reabsorption*.) It does so by stimulating osteoclastic (bone breakdown) activity. In response, calcium moves from the bone to the blood.
2. PTH stimulates the kidneys to reabsorb calcium from the urine. At the same time, PTH causes the kidneys to excrete phosphate. The excretion of phosphate by the kidneys is called its *phosphaturic* (foss-foh-TOOR-ik) *effect*. The urinary excretion of phosphate is important because of the inverse relationship of phosphate and calcium in the blood. The inverse relationship means that as phosphate levels decrease, calcium levels increase; when phosphate levels increase, calcium levels decrease. Thus, to raise blood calcium levels, it is necessary to lower blood phosphate levels.
3. Working with vitamin D, PTH increases the absorption of dietary calcium by the digestive tract (intestine). Thus, a vitamin D deficiency can decrease the dietary absorption of calcium. Remember from Chapter 7 that a daily but brief exposure to sunlight increases the production of vitamin D by the skin.
4. Blood calcium levels control the secretion of both calcitonin and PTH through negative feedback control. High blood calcium levels stimulate secretion of calcitonin, whereas low blood calcium levels inhibit secretion of calcitonin and stimulate secretion of PTH.

PTH DEFICIENCY AND HYPOCALCEMIC TETANY

What is the hand in Fig. 14.7 doing? The hand and wrist muscles are contracted and cannot relax, thereby producing a carpal spasm. What causes the carpal spasm? Calcium normally stabilizes nerve and muscle membranes. With insufficient PTH, blood calcium declines, causing hypocalcemia. Consequently, the nerve and muscle membranes become unstable and continuously fire electrical signals, causing the muscles to remain contracted. Sustained skeletal muscle contraction is referred to as *tetany* (TET-ah-nee). Hypocalcemic tetany not only contorts the wrist; more seriously, it causes sustained contractions of

the muscles of the larynx (laryngospasm) and the breathing muscles. Inability of these muscles to relax causes asphyxiation and death. Hypocalcemia is life threatening!

 Do You Know...

About "Bones, Stones, Moans, and Groans"?

Occasionally, a person develops a hypersecreting parathyroid gland tumor. The excess PTH stimulates osteoclastic activity in the bones, thereby moving calcium from the bones to the blood and causing hypercalcemia. Bone pain results from persistent osteoclastic activity (bones and groans). Hypercalcemia causes excess calcium to be filtered into the urine, causing hypercalciuria (hye-per-kal-see-YOOR-ee-ah); the excess calcium in the urine precipitates out as kidney stones (bones, stones, and groans). Hypercalcemia also depresses the nervous, cardiac, and gastrointestinal systems causing a variety of symptoms, including depression (moans), fatigue, bradycardia, anorexia, and constipation. The Groan Zone, indeed!

 Re-Think

1. What is the most important effect of PTH?
2. List the target organs of PTH.
3. Why does a deficiency of PTH cause hypocalcemia and tetany?

 Do You Know...

Why Mr. Graves's Face Is a-Twitching?

Mr. Graves just had a thyroidectomy. As part of his postsurgical care, his nurse periodically tapped the area over the facial nerve. "He is twitching," observed his nurse and immediately reported this observation as a positive Chvostek's sign. Hyperirritability of the facial nerve occurs when the blood levels of calcium decrease. Sometimes the parathyroid glands, which are embedded in the thyroid gland, are mistakenly removed or injured during thyroid surgery. If the parathyroid glands are removed, blood calcium levels decrease because there is no PTH. The nerves become so irritable that they fire continuously, causing continuous muscle contraction (tetany). Unless treated with intravenous calcium, the person may develop a fatal hypocalcemic tetany.

 Sum It Up!

The thyroid gland and parathyroid glands are located in the anterior neck region. The follicular cells of the thyroid gland secrete two iodine-containing hormones: T_3 and T_4. These hormones regulate the body's metabolic rate, affecting the metabolism of carbohydrates, proteins, and fats. The basal metabolic rate (BMR) is the metabolic rate of the body at rest; it refers to the number of calories needed to maintain life in the resting state. Excess secretion of T_3 and T_4, called *hyperthyroidism*, increases the body's metabolic rate. Hypothyroidism causes a hypometabolic state. The thyroid gland also secretes calcitonin, which is concerned with calcium and phosphate regulation. The parathyroid glands secrete PTH, which increases blood calcium levels through its effect on three target organs: bone, kidneys, and digestive tract. PTH also exerts a phosphaturic effect.

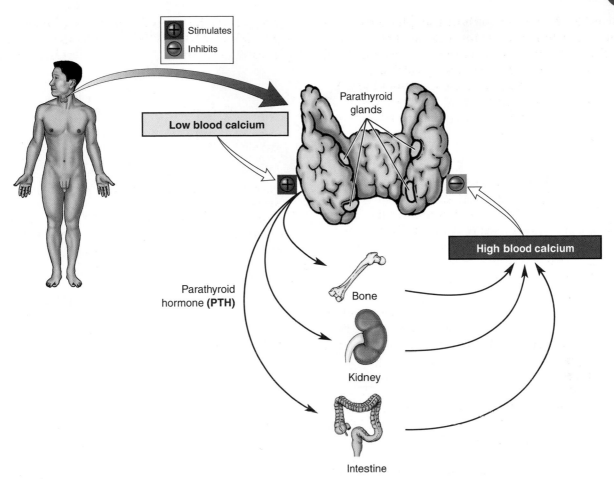

FIG. 14.6 **Parathyroid glands.** Parathyroid hormone (PTH) and three target organs (bone, kidneys, and intestine).

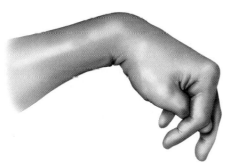

FIG. 14.7 **Carpal spasm.**

ADRENAL GLANDS

The two small glands located above the kidneys are called **adrenal glands** (*ad* means "near"; *renal* means "kidney"; Fig. 14.8A). An adrenal gland consists of two regions: an inner medulla and an outer cortex. The medulla and the cortex secrete different hormones (see Table 14.1). Although the adrenal gland secretes two different types of hormones from two distinct regions, there is some interaction between the medulla and cortex, especially in the hormonal response to stress.

ADRENAL MEDULLA

The adrenal medulla is the inner region of the adrenal gland and is considered an extension of the sympathetic nervous system. Remember from Chapter 12 that the sympathetic nervous system is called the "fight-or-flight" system. Chromaffin cells in the adrenal medulla secrete two hormones: epinephrine (85%) and norepinephrine (15%).

Epinephrine (adrenaline) and norepinephrine, classified as **catecholamines** (kat-eh-KOHL-ah-meens), are secreted in emergency or stress situations. You may have heard the expression, "I can feel the adrenaline flowing." It is another way of saying, "I'm ready to meet the challenge." The catecholamines, like the sympathetic nervous system, help the body respond to stress by causing the following effects:

- Elevating blood pressure
- Increasing heart rate
- Converting glycogen to glucose in the liver, thereby making more glucose available to the cells
- Increasing metabolic rate of most cells, thereby providing more energy
- Causing bronchodilation (opening up of the breathing passages) to increase the flow of air into the lungs

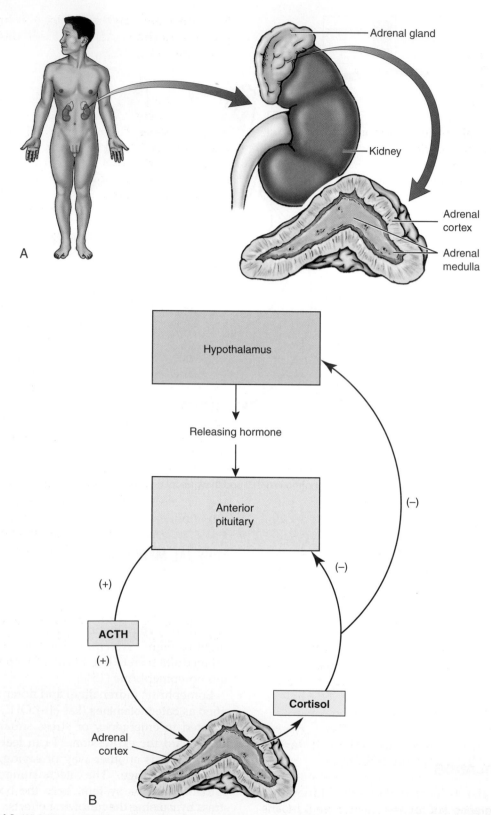

FIG. 14.8 (A) Adrenal glands: adrenal medulla and adrenal cortex. (B) Negative feedback control of the secretion of cortisol.

- Changing blood flow patterns, causing dilation of the blood vessels to the heart and muscles and constriction of the blood vessels to the digestive tract

Some medullary cells extend into the outer cortical layer. When stress activates the sympathetic fight-or-flight response, the medullary cells stimulate the cortex to secrete steroids (also stress hormones).

ADRENAL CORTEX

The adrenal cortex, the outer region of the adrenal gland (see Fig. 14.8A), secretes hormones called *steroids*. Steroids are lipid-soluble hormones made from cholesterol. The adrenal cortex secretes three steroids: glucocorticoids, mineralocorticoids, and sex hormones. Adrenal cortical hormones are essential for life. If the adrenal cortex is removed or its function is lost, death will occur unless steroids are administered. An easy way to remember the functions of the adrenal cortical steroids is that they regulate sugar, salt, and sex.

Glucocorticoids	Sugar
Mineralocorticoids	Salt
Sex hormones	Sex

GLUCOCORTICOIDS

As their name implies, the glucocorticoids affect carbohydrates. They convert amino acids into glucose by gluconeogenesis, thereby maintaining blood glucose levels between meals. This action ensures a steady supply of glucose for the brain and other cells. Glucocorticoids also affect protein and fat metabolism, burning both substances as fuel to increase energy production.

The chief glucocorticoid is cortisol. Cortisol is a hormone that is secreted in greater amounts during times of stress. *Stress* refers to physiological stress such as disease, physical injury, hemorrhage, infection, pregnancy, extreme temperature, and emotional stress, such as anger and worry. In fact, it is thought that the abdominal fat associated with heart disease is deposited in response to stress-induced chronic secretion of cortisol. Yet another reason to relax!

Control of Cortisol Secretion

The secretion of cortisol involves the hypothalamus, anterior pituitary gland, and adrenal gland (see Fig. 14.8B). The hypothalamus secretes a releasing hormone, which then stimulates the anterior pituitary gland to secrete ACTH. ACTH, in turn, stimulates the adrenal cortex to secrete cortisol. Through negative feedback control, the cortisol inhibits the further secretion of ACTH and additional cortisol.

MINERALOCORTICOIDS

The chief mineralocorticoid is aldosterone (al-DOS-ter-own). Aldosterone is often called the salt-retaining (NaCl) hormone. The primary target organ of aldosterone is the kidney where it acts to reabsorb sodium and water and eliminate potassium. Through its action on the kidney aldosterone plays an important role in the regulation of blood volume, blood pressure, and the concentration of electrolytes. In the absence of aldosterone, the body loses Na^+ and water, and both blood volume and blood pressure decline. (Aldosterone is described further in Chapter 24.).

SEX HORMONES

The sex hormones—secreted in small amounts—include the female hormones, primarily estrogens, and male hormones, called *androgens* (primarily testosterone). The sex hormones of the ovaries usually mask the effects of the adrenal sex hormones. In females, the masculinizing effects of the adrenal androgens, such as increased body hair, may become evident after menopause, when levels of estrogen and progesterone from the ovaries decrease.

NEGATIVE FEEDBACK...AGAIN

Yet, another reason to understand negative feedback control and ACTH/cortisol! Consider this situation. A patient is given prednisone (cortisol-like) as a drug for the treatment of arthritis. As blood cortisol levels rise, the secretion of ACTH by the anterior pituitary gland is inhibited by negative feedback. In the absence of ACTH, the adrenal gland becomes "lazy" and stops its production of cortisol. As long as the person continues to take the prednisone, blood cortisol levels remain high. If, however, the person suddenly discontinues the drug, the lazy adrenal gland no longer produces cortisol in response to ACTH, and the person may develop a lethal acute adrenal cortical insufficiency. (Remember: Steroids are essential for life.) Because of lazy adrenal cortical response, steroid drugs are never discontinued abruptly; dosage is tapered off over an extended period. This gradual reduction in drug dose gives the lazy adrenal gland time to recover and regain its ability to respond to ACTH.

 Do You Know...

Why Ms. Cushing Has a Moon Face, Buffalo Hump, and Facial Hair While Mr. Addison Is Bronzed?

The Ms. and Mr. both have steroid issues. Ms. Cushing has been taking prednisone (cortisol) for an arthritic condition. Chronically elevated blood levels of steroids cause a condition called *Cushing's syndrome*. It is characterized by truncal obesity, moon face, buffalo hump, and virilization. Long-term exposure to elevated cortisol affects the mobilization and metabolism of fat. Excess fat accumulates in the cheeks (moon face), between the shoulders (buffalo hump), and on the trunk (truncal obesity). The masculinized appearance (virilization) is due to the androgenic activity of the steroid, providing the distressed Ms. Cushing her facial hair, deeper voice, and acne. Mr. Addison, on the other hand, has too little steroid and hypersecretes ACTH, thus begging his adrenal cortex to "kick in." His excess ACTH, however, is derived from pro-opiomelanocortin (POMC); the pigmentation associated with the POMC causes the bronzed appearance. Too much steroid—Cushing's syndrome. Too little steroid—Addison's disease.

Re-Think

1. List the two catecholamines secreted by the adrenal medulla.
2. List the three groups of steroids secreted by the adrenal cortex.
3. Explain the following: A person has been taking prednisone for 1 year. She suddenly stops taking the drug and develops a life-threatening acute adrenal cortical insufficiency.

 Sum It Up!

The adrenal glands are composed of the medulla and the cortex; both secrete stress hormones. The adrenal medulla is an extension of the sympathetic nervous system ("fight or flight") and secretes two catecholamines called *epinephrine* (adrenaline) and *norepinephrine*. The adrenal cortex secretes three steroids: the glucocorticoids (cortisol), the mineralocorticoids (aldosterone), and the sex hormones. The adrenal cortex is controlled by a hypothalamic-releasing hormone and ACTH from the anterior pituitary gland. The functions of the adrenal cortex are concerned with the regulation of sugar, salt, and sex.

PANCREAS

The **pancreas** (PAN-kree-ass) is a long, slender organ that lies transversely across the upper abdomen, extending from the curve of the duodenum to the spleen (see Fig. 14.1). The pancreas functions as both an exocrine gland and an endocrine gland. (Its exocrine function is concerned with the digestion of food and is discussed in Chapter 23.)

The pancreas secretes at least five hormones; we are concerned primarily with two hormones: insulin and glucagon. Consult Ms. PIG in Fig. 14.9; she will help remind you that the *p*ancreas secretes *i*nsulin and *g*lucagon (**P**ancreas, **I**nsulin, **G**lucagon). The hormone-secreting cells of the pancreas are called the *islets of Langerhans*. The islets of Langerhans have several types of cells: the alpha cells, which secrete glucagon, and the beta cells, which secrete insulin. Both insulin and glucagon help regulate the metabolism of carbohydrates, proteins, and fats. We are particularly interested in the regulation of blood glucose.

INSULIN

SECRETION AND EFFECTS

Fig. 14.9 illustrates the relationship of the blood glucose level to the pancreatic hormones. Insulin is released in response to increased blood levels of glucose, as occurs after a meal. The secretion of insulin decreases as blood levels of glucose decrease. Insulin has many target tissues and therefore exerts widespread effects:

- Insulin helps transport glucose into most cells. Without insulin, glucose remains outside the cells, thereby depriving the cell of its fuel. (The liver and brain require glucose for their metabolic needs but do not require insulin for the transport of glucose across the cell membrane.) Insulin is the only hormone that lowers blood glucose!
- Insulin helps control carbohydrate, protein, and fat metabolism in the cell. Insulin stimulates the breakdown of glucose (glycolysis) for energy and stimulates the liver and skeletal muscles to store excess glucose as glycogen (glycogenesis). Insulin also increases the transport of amino acids into cells and then stimulates the synthesis of protein from the amino acids. Finally, insulin promotes the making of fats from fatty acids.
- Diabetes mellitus is often defined as a lack of insulin. However, some diabetics with adult-onset, or type 2, diabetes mellitus have excess insulin (hyperinsulinemia) and are still hyperglycemic. What's that about? Under normal conditions, insulin binds to the insulin receptors on the cell membrane. What if:
  1. The insulin receptors are damaged? The damaged receptors cannot respond to the insulin, and the person becomes hyperglycemic. The hyperglycemia then triggers the release of additional insulin and the person becomes hyperinsulinemic.
  2. There are a diminished number of receptors? The number of insulin receptors on the membrane can increase or decrease. Obesity and lack of exercise can cause the number of insulin receptors to decrease. This means that obese people can secrete plenty of insulin, but their cells cannot respond to that insulin. The good news is that weight loss and exercise increase the number of insulin receptors, thereby improving the insulin response and relieving the symptoms of diabetes.
  3. Excess fat (adipose) tissue secretes hormones that oppose the effects of insulin? Some cytokines antagonize insulin, causing a state of insulin resistance.

A strong link obviously exists among insulin resistance, obesity, and diabetes. A new term, *metabolic syndrome*, addresses this issue.

 Do You Know...

Why Some Diabetic Persons Require an Injection of Insulin, Whereas Others Can Take a Pill?

Some diabetic persons require insulin injections, and others control their diabetes with a pill. The difference is that the pancreas of a person with severe diabetes produces no insulin, so this person must receive insulin injections. Such people have insulin-dependent diabetes. In contrast, the pancreas of a person with another form of diabetes may still be able to produce some insulin. This person may not require insulin injections and may benefit from noninsulin oral medication. Some diabetic pills work by stimulating the person's pancreas to produce more insulin. Others work by suppressing the hepatic (liver) synthesis of glucose. A person with diabetes who does not require insulin injections is considered to have non–insulin-dependent diabetes.

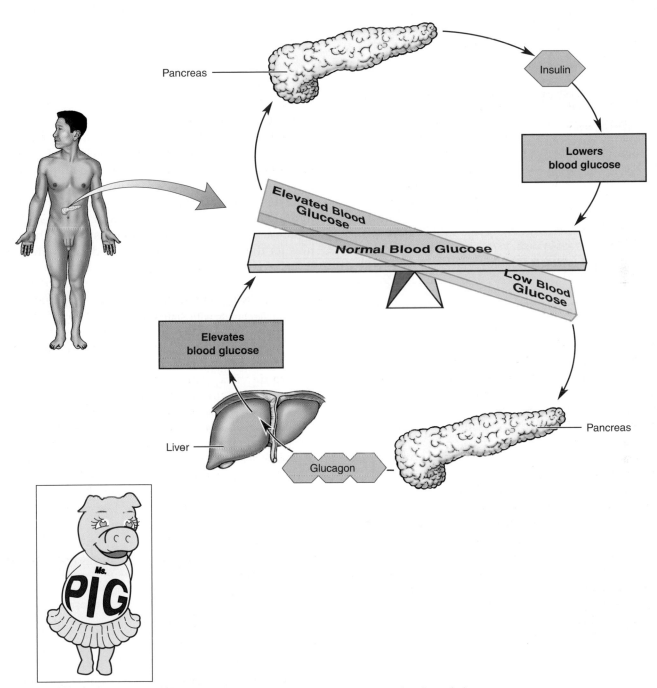

Pancreas

Insulin

Lowers blood glucose

Elevated Blood Glucose

Normal Blood Glucose

Low Blood Glucose

Elevates blood glucose

Liver

Glucagon

Pancreas

Ms. PIG

FIG. 14.9 Pancreatic regulation of blood glucose: insulin and glucagon.

Diabetes Mellitus: "A Melting Down of the Flesh and Limbs into Urine"

Because insulin plays such an important role in the metabolism of all types of foods (carbohydrates, proteins, and fats), a deficiency of insulin causes severe metabolic disturbances. Insulin deficiency or insulin ineffectiveness is called *diabetes mellitus* (dye-ah-BEE-teez mell-EYE-tus). Before insulin therapy was discovered, diabetes mellitus was described as a "melting down of the flesh and the limbs into urine." This description attests to the devastating effects of untreated type I (juvenile-onset) diabetes mellitus. The child took 1 year literally to "melt away." Read on to understand the physiological effects of insulin deficiency; note specifically the three "polys" of diabetes mellitus: polyuria, polydipsia, and polyphagia.

- **Hyperglycemia.** Excess glucose in the blood is called *hyperglycemia.* This condition is caused by two factors. The first is the inability of glucose to enter the cells, where it can be burned for energy. Failure to move the glucose into the cells causes it to accumulate in the blood. The second is the making of additional glucose. In the absence of insulin, the body makes glucose from protein (gluconeogenesis). The excess glucose cannot be used by the cells and therefore accumulates in the blood. In essence, the diabetic body converts its protein to glucose that it cannot burn as fuel and then eliminates it in the urine. The body is "starving in the midst of plenty" (of glucose).
- **Glucosuria or glycosuria.** Glucose in the urine is called *glucosuria* or *glycosuria.* The hyperglycemia causes excess glucose to be eliminated in the urine.
- **Polyuria.** Excretion of a large volume of urine is called *polyuria.* Whenever the kidneys excrete a lot of glucose, they must also excrete a lot of water. Glucosuria therefore causes polyuria.
- **Polydipsia.** Excessive thirst is called *polydipsia.* Polyuria causes an excessive loss of body water, thereby stimulating the thirst mechanism in an attempt to replace the water lost in the urine.
- **Polyphagia.** *Polyphagia* refers to excessive eating. Despite plenty of glucose in the blood, the cells cannot use it; instead, the diabetic eats excessive amounts of food to fuel the cells. Despite the polyphagia, the diabetic person continues to lose weight.
- **Acidosis.** An excess of H^+ in the blood causes acidosis. Because the cells cannot burn glucose as fuel, they burn fatty acids instead. The rapid, incomplete breakdown of fatty acids produces strong acids (H^+) called *ketoacids.* This process causes a condition called *diabetic ketoacidosis.*

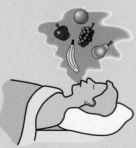

- **Fruity odor to the breath.** The rapid, incomplete breakdown of fatty acids causes the formation of acetone, a ketone body. Acetone smells fruity and makes the patient's breath smell like rotten apples. A fruity odor is a sign of ketoacidosis. Treatment of diabetic ketoacidosis requires the prompt administration of insulin and the correction of the fluid and electrolyte disturbances.

Who Dawn Is and What Her Phenomenon Is?

Dawn refers to the early morning hours, as in sunrise. Diabetics are often hyperglycemic in the early morning hours (at dawn), despite insulin therapy and the lack of food intake during the night. Why? Throughout the night, the person secretes GH. GH stimulates gluconeogenesis and increases blood glucose; this accounts for the early morning hyperglycemia. An adjustment in the timing and type of insulin therapy generally corrects the dawn phenomenon.

GLUCAGON

Glucagon, a second pancreatic hormone, is secreted by the alpha cells of the islets of Langerhans. Its primary action is to increase blood glucose levels (see Fig. 14.9). Glucagon raises the blood glucose level in two ways: by stimulating the conversion of glycogen to glucose in the liver and by stimulating the conversion of proteins into glucose (gluconeogenesis). Both these processes ensure a supply of glucose for the busy cells. The stimulus for the release of glucagon is a decrease in blood levels of glucose.

How One Rebounds with Somogyi?

A diabetic person takes insulin to lower his or her blood glucose level. If too much insulin is taken, the blood glucose level becomes too low (hypoglycemia). The hypoglycemia, in turn, stimulates the secretion of glucose-elevating hormones such as glucagon, cortisol, growth hormone, and epinephrine; this causes hyperglycemia. The hyperglycemia requires additional insulin to lower blood glucose levels. The additional insulin again causes hypoglycemia; thus a vicious cycle of hypoglycemia and hyperglycemia occurs. The Somogyi effect is a rebound phenomenon in which hypoglycemia is followed by hyperglycemia as a result of a hormonal overreaction to the low blood sugar level.

1. What are the two pancreatic hormones?
2. What is the stimulus for the secretion of each pancreatic hormone?
3. What is the only hormone that lowers blood glucose?

A number of hormones, particularly those secreted by the pancreas, regulate blood glucose levels. The pancreas secretes two hormones that affect blood glucose: insulin and glucagon. Insulin works in two ways to decrease blood glucose levels: (1) it increases the transport of glucose from the blood into the cells, and (2) it stimulates the cells to burn glucose as fuel. Diabetes mellitus develops when the pancreas fails to secrete insulin or the receptors on the target tissues fail to respond to insulin. Glucagon antagonizes the effects of insulin by increasing blood glucose levels. Insulin is the only hormone that decreases blood glucose levels.

GONADS

The gonads are the sex glands and refer to the ovaries in the female and to the testes in the male. The gonads not only produce ova (eggs) and sperm but also secrete hormones. The gonads are therefore glands. The ovaries secrete two female sex hormones: estrogen and progesterone. A female appears female (i.e., size, hair distribution, and fat distribution) primarily because of estrogen. The testes secrete testosterone; a male appears male primarily because of testosterone. (Reproductive anatomy and physiology are discussed in Chapter 26 .)

THYMUS GLAND

The **thymus gland** lies in the thoracic cavity behind the sternum. The thymus gland secretes hormones called *thymosins,* which play a role in the immune system (described in Chapter 21).

PINEAL GLAND

The **pineal (PIN-ee-al) gland** is a cone-shaped gland located close to the thalamus in the brain. It has been called the body's "biological clock," controlling many of its biorhythms. The pineal gland secretes a hormone called *melatonin,* which affects the reproductive cycle by influencing the secretion of hypothalamic-releasing hormones. In general, melatonin plays an important role in sexual maturation.

Melatonin is also thought to play a role in the sleep–wake cycle. The amount of melatonin secreted is related to the amount of daylight. Melatonin secretion is lowest during daylight hours and highest at night. As melatonin levels increase, the person becomes sleepy. Melatonin is therefore said to have a tranquilizing effect. Persons who work night shifts and sleep during the day have a reversed cycle of melatonin production. The reversal of the melatonin cycle is related to the fatigue experienced by night shift workers. Elevated melatonin levels have also been implicated in a type of depression called *seasonal affective disorder* (SAD). This condition occurs most commonly in parts of the world where daylight hours are shorter during the winter season.

OTHER HORMONES

ORGAN-SPECIFIC HORMONES

The glands identified in Fig. 14.1 make up the endocrine system, but numerous hormone-secreting cells are scattered throughout the body. These hormones usually control the activities of a particular organ. For example, hormone-secreting cells in the digestive tract secrete cholecystokinin and gastrin, which help regulate digestion. The kidneys secrete erythropoietin, which helps regulate red blood cell production. The liver secretes a number of hormones, including insulin-like growth factor (IGF-1). IGF-1 mediates the action of growth hormone. (**Organ-specific hormones** are described in later chapters.)

PROSTAGLANDINS

The prostaglandins (pross-tah-GLAN-dins) are hormones derived from a fatty acid called *arachidonic* (ah-RAK-i-don-ik) *acid.* The prostaglandins are produced by many tissues and generally act locally, near their site of secretion. The prostaglandins play an important role in the regulation of smooth muscle contraction and the inflammatory response. Prostaglandins are also thought to increase the sensitivity of nerve endings to pain. Drugs such as aspirin and ibuprofen block the synthesis of prostaglandins and are therefore useful in relieving pain and inflammation.

ADIPOSE TISSUE HORMONES

Excess adipose tissue acts as a gland—a very nasty gland—that secretes hormones called *cytokines.* First, a word about excess fat; there is bad fat and worse fat. How so? There's the bad fat that collects around the thighs. There's also a worse fat that collects around the abdominal area. The abdominal fat associated with excess visceral fat (surrounding the organs).

The cost is high with regard to heart disease, diabetes mellitus, cancer, and joint disease. Read on!

Heart and Blood Vessels

Most believe that obesity is a risk for heart disease merely because excess weight overburdens the heart. Although this is true, excess adipose tissue, through its cytokines, affects the heart and blood vessels in other ways. For example, adipose tissue contains many narrow blood vessels; in fact, miles of additional blood vessels may be required to carry blood throughout the excess fat. The additional narrowed blood vessels increase blood pressure and strain the heart. Adipose tissue secretes several cytokines that cause the blood vessels to become even narrower. The cytokines also stimulate the immune system, causing inflammation—an important risk factor for heart disease. In fact, inflammation plays a larger role in heart attacks than the narrowing of the coronary (heart) arteries by cholesterol. The cytokines also stimulate blood clotting. Blood clots, in turn, impair blood flow to the heart and brain, thereby predisposing the obese person to heart attack and stroke.

Diabetes Mellitus

Adipose tissue secretes several cytokines that adversely affect glucose metabolism and predispose the person to type 2 diabetes mellitus. First, the cytokines oppose the action of insulin, thereby decreasing the transport of glucose into the cells. Second, the cytokines stimulate the liver to make excess glucose. Both these actions increase blood glucose levels, causing hyperglycemia, a hallmark of diabetes mellitus. In short, cytokines make the obese person resistant to insulin.

Cancer

Fat cells secrete estrogen, a hormone that has been linked to several types of cancer, especially breast cancer.

Joint Disease

The added body weight puts additional stress on joints such as the knees. The joints simply cannot support the extra weight. An apology to cytokines is in order. Many cytokines cause undesirable effects, as noted previously, but most cytokines exert important and beneficial physiological effects (see Chapter 21).

? **Re-Think**

1. List the hormones secreted by the gonads and pineal gland.
2. What is meant by *organ-specific hormones*? List two examples.
3. Why is adipose tissue considered a "nasty gland"?
4. Where are prostaglandins produced? List two functions of the prostaglandins.

 Sum It Up!

The gonads are glands that include the ovaries in the female and the testes in the male. The ovaries secrete estrogens and progesterone; the testes secrete testosterone. Other endocrine glands include the thymus, liver, and pineal gland. The thymus gland plays an important role in the immune response. The pineal gland is thought to be the body's "biological clock," affecting reproduction, biorhythms, and the sleep–wake cycle. Other hormone-secreting cells are scattered throughout the body. Prostaglandins are secreted by many cells throughout the body and generally act locally. They are chemical mediators of pain and inflammation. Excess adipose tissue functions as a "nasty" endocrine gland that contributes to the development of heart disease, diabetes mellitus , cancer, and joint disease.

As You Age

1. In general, age-related endocrine changes include an alteration in the secretion of hormones, circulating levels of hormones, metabolism of hormones, and biological activity of hormones.
2. Although most glands decrease their levels of secretion, normal aging does not lead to deficiency states. For example, although adrenal cortical secretion of cortisol decreases, negative feedback mechanisms maintain normal plasma levels of the hormones, thereby preserving water and electrolyte homeostasis.
3. Changes in the thyroid gland cause a decrease in the secretion of thyroid hormones, thereby decreasing the metabolic rate.
4. Decreased secretion of growth hormone causes a decrease in muscle mass and an increase in storage of fat.
5. A diminishment of circadian control of hormone secretion occurs.

 Medical Terminology and Disorders   Disorders of the Endocrine System

MEDICAL TERM	WORD PARTS	WORD PART MEANING OR DERIVATION	DESCRIPTION
Words			
adrenal	ad-	near	The **adrenal** glands sit atop the kidneys.
	-ren/o-	kidney	
	-al	pertaining to	
adenohypophyseal	aden/o-	gland	The **adenohypophysis** is *the anterior pituitary gland that is located under the hypothalamus.* The **neurohypophysis** (neur/o = nerve) is *the posterior pituitary gland; it is a downward extension of the hypothalamus.*
	-hypophysis-	From a Greek word meaning "to grow under"	
	-al	pertaining to	
adrenocorticotropic	adren/o-	adrenal gland	**Adrenocorticotropic hormone (ACTH)** stimulates the adrenal cortex to secrete steroids.
	-cortic/o-	cortex	
	-troph/o-	nourishment, development	
	-ic	pertaining to	
androgen	andr/o-	male	An **androgen,** such as testosterone, *stimulates the development of male or virilizing characteristics.*
	-gen	origin or production	
endocrine	endo-	within	**Endocrine** glands secrete hormones "within the body"; they are transported around the body by the blood.
	-crin/o-	to secrete	

MEDICAL TERM	WORD PARTS	WORD PART MEANING OR DERIVATION	DESCRIPTION
gonadotropic	gonad/o-	gonad	**Gonadotropic** hormones (FSH and LH) target the gonads, the ovaries, and the testes.
	-troph/o-	nourishment or development	
	-ic	pertaining to	
glycemia.	-glyc/o-	glucose	**Glycemia** refers to the presence of glucose in the blood. **Normoglycemia** refers to the normal amount of glucose in the blood. **Hyperglycemia** is *an increase in the amount of glucose in the blood.* **Hypoglycemia** is a decrease in the amount of glucose in the blood.
	-emia	condition of the blood	

Disorders

Adrenal Gland Disorders

adrenal cortical insufficiency and excess			Excess cortisol or cortisol-like drugs will produce a cluster of symptoms called **Cushing's syndrome.** The syndrome is an expression of altered carbohydrate, protein, and fat metabolism. It also reflects a mineralocorticoid-induced blood volume expansion. Adrenal cortical deficiencies are classified as acute (described in the text) and chronic. Chronic adrenal insufficiency is called *Addison's disease*; the life-threatening symptoms are primarily related to Na⁺ and blood volume depletion
pheochromocytoma	pheochromocyt/o-	catecholamine-secreting cell	**Pheochromocytoma** is *a benign tumor of the adrenal medulla that hypersecretes the catecholamines epinephrine and norepinephrine.*
	-oma	tumor	

Pituitary Gland Disorders

somatotropic hormone imbalances	somat/o-	body	*Hypersecretion of somatotropic hormone (growth hormone [GH]). The conditions are described in the text.*
	-troph/o-	nourishment, development	
	-ic	condition of	
diabetes insipidus	dia-	through	*A condition caused by a lack of ADH secretion* **(central diabetes insipidus)** *or by the lack of the response of the kidney to ADH* **(nephrogenic diabetes insipidus).** Further described in the text.
	-betes	From a Greek word *bainein,* meaning "to go or pass"	
	insipidus	Reference to the word *insipid,* meaning "tasteless"	
syndrome of inappropriate ADH (antidiuretic hormone) secretion	anti-	against	Abbreviated as **SIADH. SIADH** is caused by excess ADH secretion resulting in excess water reabsorption by the kidney, expansion of blood volume, and decreased plasma sodium.
	-diuretic	to increase the flow of urine	

Pancreatic Disorders

diabetes mellitus	dia-	through	*A deficiency or ineffectiveness of insulin.* There are several types of diabetes mellitus (DM), which is epidemic in the United States: **Type 1 DM,** also called **juvenile-onset diabetes,** usually develops in children and must be treated with insulin. **Type 2 DM** is called **adult-onset diabetes.** The typical adult-onset diabetic is older, obese, and sedentary. **Gestational diabetes mellitus** refers to the appearance of diabetic symptoms only during pregnancy. The symptoms usually subside when the baby is delivered. Unfortunately, in the United States, type 2 diabetes is appearing in children. The development of **MODY** (**m**aturity-**o**nset **d**iabetes in **y**outh) is related to lifestyle (diet, exercise, obesity). Further described in text.
	-betes	From the Latin word *bainein,* meaning "to go or pass"	
	mellitus	honey or sweet	

Continued

Medical Terminology and Disorders   Disorders of the Endocrine System—cont'd

MEDICAL TERM	WORD PARTS	WORD PART MEANING OR DERIVATION	DESCRIPTION
Parathyroid Gland Disorders			
hyperparathyroidism	hyper-	above or excessive	*Refers to an excess secretion of parathyroid hormone (PTH) causing bone resorption and elevation of plasma calcium (hypercalcemia).*
	-parathyroid/o-	parathyroid	
	-ism	condition of	
hypoparathyroidism	hypo-	below or deficient	*Refers to the diminished secretion of parathyroid hormone (PTH) causing low plasma levels of calcium (hypocalcemia) and tetany. Further described in the text.*
	-parathyroid/o-	parathyroid	
	-ism	condition of	
Thyroid Gland Disorders			
goiter	goiter	From a Latin word meaning "struma" (throat enlargement)	*An enlargement of the thyroid gland, which may or may not be functioning normally.* A **toxic nodular goiter** contains nodules that excrete excess T_3 and T_4, thereby causing a hyperthyroid state. A **nontoxic goiter,** such as a goiter induced by an iodine-deficient diet, does not secrete excess T_3 and T_4. The person is most often euthyroid or experiences mild hypothyroidism.
hyperthyroidism	hyper-	above or excessive	Also called an "overactive thyroid"; **hyperthyroidism** is due to excess synthesis of thyroid hormones (T_3, T_4) by the thyroid gland. **Graves' disease** is the most common type and is described in the text. **Thyrotoxicosis,** which presents as severe hyperthyroidism, is due to an increase in the release of stored T_3 and T_4 from the thyroid gland. **Thyroid storm,** or **thyrotoxic crisis,** is an extreme and life-threatening manifestation of **thyrotoxicosis:** clinical presentation includes extreme elevation in body temperature and cardiac stimulation (tachycardia) progressing to heart failure.
	-thyroid/o-	thyroid	
	-ism	condition of	
hypothyroidism	hypo-	below or deficient	Also called a "sluggish thyroid" and **myxedema** in the adult (described in the text). **Myxedema coma** is *an extreme and life-threatening form of hypothyroidism.* **Cretinism** is *neonatal hypothyroidism;* insufficient treatment with thyroid hormones results in severe physical and mental developmental abnormalities.
	-thyroid/o-	thyroid	
	-ism	condition of	

Get Ready for Exams!

Summary Outline

The endocrine system and the nervous system are the two major communicating and coordinating systems in the body. The endocrine system communicates through chemical signals called *hormones.*

I. Hormones
  A. Classification of hormones
   1. Hormones are secreted by endocrine glands directly into the blood.
   2. Hormones are classified as proteins (protein-related substances) and steroids.

  B. Hormone receptors
   1. Hormones are aimed at receptors of target organs.
   2. Receptors are located on the outer surface of the membrane or inside the cell.
   3. Hormone secretion is controlled by three mechanisms: feedback control, biorhythms, and control by the central nervous system.

II. Pituitary Gland
  A. Hypothalamic–hypophyseal portal system
   1. The portal system is a system of capillaries that connects the hypothalamus and the anterior pituitary.

2. The portal system transports releasing hormones from the hypothalamus to the anterior pituitary gland.

B. Hormones of the anterior pituitary gland

1. Growth hormone stimulates growth and maintains blood glucose levels during periods of fasting.
2. Prolactin (lactogenic hormone) stimulates milk production by the breasts.
3. Tropic hormones stimulate other glands to secrete hormones. These include thyroid-stimulating hormone (TSH), adrenocorticotropic hormone (ACTH), and the gonadotropins (FSH, LH).
4. Thyroid-stimulating hormone stimulates the thyroid gland.
5. Adrenocorticotropic hormone (ACTH) stimulates the adrenal cortex.
6. The gonadotropic hormones (FSH and LH) stimulate the gonads (ovaries and testes).

C. Hormones of the posterior pituitary gland

1. Antidiuretic hormone (ADH) stimulates the kidney to reabsorb water.
2. Oxytocin stimulates the uterine muscle to contract for labor and stimulates the breast to release milk during suckling (milk let-down reflex).

III. Other Endocrine Glands

A. Thyroid gland

1. The follicular cells synthesize triiodothyronine (T_3) and tetraiodothyronine, or thyroxine (T_4). T_3 and T_4 regulate metabolic rate.
2. The parafollicular cells secrete calcitonin. Calcitonin lowers blood calcium level.

B. Parathyroid glands

1. The parathyroid glands secrete parathyroid hormone (PTH).
2. PTH stimulates the bones, kidneys, and intestines to increase blood calcium levels.

C. Adrenal gland

1. The adrenal medulla secretes the catecholamines epinephrine and norepinephrine and causes the "fight-or-flight" response.
2. The adrenal cortex secretes the steroids: glucocorticoids, mineralocorticoids, and sex hormones.

D. Pancreas

1. The pancreas secretes insulin and glucagon.
2. Insulin lowers blood glucose levels, whereas glucagon increases blood glucose levels.

E. Gonads

1. The ovaries are stimulated by the gonadotropins and secrete estrogens and progesterone.
2. The testes are stimulated by the gonadotropins and secrete testosterone.

F. The thymus gland plays an important role in the immune response.

G. The pineal gland houses the "biological clock" and secretes melatonin.

H. Other hormones include organ-specific hormones (cholecystokinin), prostaglandins, and hormones of adipose tissue.

Review Your Knowledge

Matching: Glands

Directions: Match the following words with their descriptions. Some words may be used more than once.

a. pancreas
b. adrenal cortex
c. anterior pituitary gland
d. adrenal medulla
e. thyroid gland
f. parathyroid glands
g. posterior pituitary gland
h. hypothalamus

1. ___ Contains the beta cells of the islets of Langerhans
2. ___ Secrete glucocorticoids, mineralocorticoids, and androgens
3. ___ Its hormonal secretion is controlled by ACTH
4. ___ Secretes iodine-containing hormones
5. ___ Secretes releasing hormones
6. ___ Secretes ACTH, TSH, prolactin, growth hormone, and the gonadotropins
7. ___ Its hormone moves calcium from the bone to the blood
8. ___ Secretes both insulin and glucagon
9. ___ Part of the "fight-or-flight" system; secretes catecholamines
10. ___ The neurohypophysis; secretes ADH and oxytocin

Matching: Hormones

Directions: Match the following words with their descriptions in the right column. Some words may be used more than once.

a. aldosterone
b. insulin
c. prolactin
d. growth hormone
e. parathyroid hormone
f. epinephrine
g. T_3 and T_4
h. oxytocin
i. ACTH
j. ADH

1. ___ Stimulates osteoclastic activity to increase blood calcium
2. ___ Regulates metabolic rate
3. ___ Lowers blood glucose
4. ___ Cortisol is released in response to this hormone.
5. ___ Stimulates the breast to produce milk
6. ___ Catecholamine that participates in the "fight-or-flight" response
7. ___ The neurohypophyseal hormone that controls water balance
8. ___ Prednisone (cortisol) shuts down the secretion of this adenohypophyseal hormone
9. ___ Also called somatotropic hormone
10. ___ The mineralocorticoid that is called the salt-retaining hormone

Multiple Choice

1. Which of the following is true about cortisol?
   a. It is a catecholamine.
   b. It is secreted by the adrenal cortex in response to ACTH.
   c. It stimulates the secretion of ACTH.
   d. It is secreted by the adrenal medulla in response to sympathetic nerve stimulation.

2. Aldosterone is
   a. a mineralocorticoid secreted by the adrenal cortex.
   b. the primary regulator of blood glucose.
   c. an adenohypophyseal hormone that stimulates the adrenal cortex to secrete cortisol.
   d. a neurohypophyseal hormone that causes the kidneys to reabsorb water.

3. The pancreas
   a. secretes steroids that are concerned with sugar, salt, and sex.
   b. is controlled by a hormone secreted by the anterior pituitary gland.
   c. secretes both insulin and glucagon.
   d. secretes hormones that only lower blood glucose levels.

4. Which of the following best describes the function of insulin?
   a. Regulates blood volume
   b. Stimulates cells to make glucose (gluconeogenesis)
   c. Causes ketone body formation and acidosis
   d. Lowers blood glucose

5. As plasma levels of calcium decrease,
   a. insulin is secreted.
   b. the parathyroid glands secrete calcitonin.
   c. the kidneys excrete calcium and phosphate.
   d. PTH is secreted, thereby stimulating osteoclastic activity.

6. Which of the following is true of TSH?
   a. Secreted by the thyroid gland
   b. Is an iodine-containing thyroid hormone
   c. Secreted in response to declining plasma levels of calcium
   d. Stimulates the thyroid gland to secrete T_3 and T_4

7. Hypocalcemic tetany is
   a. a consequence of a deficiency of PTH.
   b. caused by calcitonin deficiency.
   c. a consequence of osteoclastic activity.
   d. of concern because it causes osteoporosis.

8. Which of the following is true of glucagon, epinephrine, growth hormone, and cortisol?
   a. All are secreted by the anterior pituitary gland.
   b. All are secreted in response to hypocalcemia.
   c. All raise blood glucose.
   d. All are steroids.

9. Hyperglycemia, polyuria, polydipsia, polyphagia, and ketoacidosis are characteristic of a deficiency in
   a. cortisol.
   b. insulin.
   c. catecholamines.
   d. neurohypophyseal hormones.

10. Which of the following is *not* a steroid?
    a. Adrenal cortical hormones
    b. ACTH
    c. Estrogen
    d. Androgens

11. Which gland is most related to the following: BMR, iodine pump, T_3/T_4?
    a. Anterior pituitary
    b. Thyroid
    c. Parathyroid
    d. Neurohypophysis

12. Which of the following is *not* part of the thyroid–pituitary feedback control loop?
    a. TSH
    b. T_3, T_4
    c. Thyroxine
    d. PTH

13. Which of the following most accurately describes the hypothalamic–hypophyseal portal system?
    a. The band of connective tissue connecting the anterior and posterior lobes of the pituitary gland
    b. The capillary network that connects the hypothalamus with the adenohypophysis
    c. The large nerve that connects the hypothalamus with the neurohypophysis
    d. The tubes that provide a constant flow of cerebrospinal fluid for storage within the portal capillaries

14. Which of the following is the target of the hypothalamic-releasing hormones?
    a. Neurohypophysis
    b. Beta cells of the islets of Langerhans
    c. Anterior pituitary gland
    d. Adrenal cortex

15. Which of the following is *not* true of antidiuretic hormone (ADH)?
    a. Secreted by the neurohypophysis
    b. Also called *vasopressin*
    c. Stimulates the kidney, causing water reabsorption
    d. Is the salt-retaining hormone

Go Figure

1. Which of the following is correct according to Fig. 14.1?
   a. All endocrine glands are located in the abdominal cavity.
   b. No endocrine glands are located in the pelvic cavity.
   c. The pituitary gland is located within the thoracic cavity.
   d. The thyroid and parathyroid glands are located in the neck.

2. Which of the following is correct according to Fig. 14.2?
   a. All hormone receptors are located on the outer cell membrane.
   b. Steroid receptors are generally located on the outer surface of the cell membrane.
   c. Hormones that bind to receptors on the outer surface of the cell membrane may activate a second chemical messenger, such as cAMP.
   d. All hormone receptors are located intracellularly.

3. According to Fig. 14.4 which of the following is *not* true?
   a. The adenohypophysis secretes TSH, growth hormone, prolactin, the gonadotropins, and ACTH.
   b. The posterior pituitary gland secretes ADH and oxytocin.
   c. The hypothalamic–hypophyseal portal system allows the anterior and posterior pituitary glands to "swap" hormones.
   d. Hypothalamic-releasing hormones control the secretion of the adenohypophysis.

4. Which of the following is correct according to Fig. 14.5?
   a. T_3 and T_4 are adenohypophyseal hormones.
   b. TSH stimulates the parathyroid glands.
   c. T_3 and T_4 stimulate the thyroid gland to secrete thyroxine.
   d. The secretion of TSH is inhibited by increased plasma levels of T_3 and T_4.

5. Which of the following is correct according to Fig. 14.5?
   a. The thyroid gland partially surrounds the trachea, a respiratory structure.
   b. The thyroid gland is a mediastinal structure.
   c. The parafollicular cells form a cavity filled with colloid.
   d. T_3 and T_4 stimulate the follicular cells to secrete TSH.

6. Which of the following is correct according to Figs. 14.6?
   a. PTH increases plasma calcium levels through its effects on bone, kidneys, and intestine.
   b. The stimulus for the release of PTH is hypercalcemia.
   c. PTH moves calcium from the blood into the bone.
   d. As plasma levels of calcium increase, PTH levels increase.

7. Which of the following is correct according to Fig. 14.8?
   a. ACTH stimulates the secretion of catecholamines.
   b. Cortisol stimulates the adenohypophyseal secretion of ACTH.
   c. ACTH is a hypothalamic-releasing hormone.
   d. ACTH secretion decreases as plasma levels of cortisol increase.

8. Which of the following is correct according to Fig. 14.8?
   a. Cortisol is secreted by the inner adrenal medulla.
   b. The anterior pituitary gland is the target gland of ACTH.
   c. The adenohypophysis is the target gland of a hypothalamic releasing hormone.
   d. The adrenal cortex is the target gland of cortisol.

9. Which of the following is correct according to Fig. 14.9?
   a. The pancreas secretes insulin and glucagon in response to hyperglycemia.
   b. Insulin is secreted in response to an increase in the blood glucose level.
   c. Glucagon lowers the blood glucose level.
   d. Glucagon is secreted in response to hyperglycemia.

Objectives

1. Describe three functions of blood.
2. Describe the composition of blood, including the following:
   - Describe the three types of blood cells: erythrocytes, leukocytes, and thrombocytes.
   - Explain the formation of blood cells.
3. Explain the composition, characteristics, and functions of red and white blood cells and platelets, including the breakdown of red blood cells and the formation of bilirubin.
4. Identify the steps of hemostasis.
5. Describe the four blood types.
6. Describe the Rh factor.

Key Terms

albumin (p. 285)
anemia (p. 286)
basophils (p. 293)
bilirubin (p. 290)
clotting cascade (p. 295)
coagulation (p. 294)
cyanosis (p. 289)
eosinophils (p. 293)
erythrocytes (p. 285)
erythropoietin (p. 290)

fibrin (p. 294)
hematocrit (p. 285)
hemoglobin (p. 288)
hemolysis (p. 298)
hemopoiesis (p. 286)
hemostasis (p. 294)
jaundice (p. 290)
leukocytes (p. 285)
lymphocytes (p. 286)
monocytes (p. 286)

neutrophils (p. 292)
plasma (p. 285)
platelets (p. 285)
red blood cells (p. 285)
reticulocytes (p. 287)
serum (p. 285)
thrombocytes (p. 285)
white blood cells (p. 285)

Long before modern medicine, blood was viewed as the part of the body that possessed a mysterious life force. Blood was literally referred to as the *river of life*. This belief arose from the observation that severe bleeding episodes often ended in death, suggesting that the life force flowed out of the body with the blood. Blood was also credited with determining personality traits and emotions. For example, feuding groups often attributed the cause of the troubled relationship to bad blood. Anger was said to cause the blood to boil, whereas fear could generate blood-curdling screams. Blood could also become bad or impure through ethical and moral transgressions, a view often reflected in the causes of such diseases as syphilis and AIDS. The qualities of blood seemed so magical that a sharing of a few drops of blood could make one's friend a blood brother. Although we no longer speak of blood in such terms, we do recognize that an adequate blood supply is essential for life. We are still fascinated by blood and have a fancy word for its study: hematology. (*Hemat-* is the root word meaning "blood.")

Blood flows through a closed system of blood vessels. The force that pushes the blood through the vessels is the pumping action of the heart (see Chapter 16).

WHAT BLOOD DOES

Blood performs three general functions: transport, regulation, and protection.

- Blood transports many substances around the body. For example, blood delivers oxygen (O_2) and nutrients to every cell in the body. Blood also picks up waste material from the cells and delivers the waste to organs that eliminate it from the body. Nutrients, ions, hormones, and many other substances use blood as the vehicle for movement throughout the body.

- Blood participates in the regulation of fluid and electrolyte balance, acid–base balance, and body temperature.
- Blood helps protect the body from infection. Blood also contains clotting factors, which help protect the body from excessive blood loss.

COMPOSITION OF BLOOD

CHARACTERISTICS

Blood is a type of connective tissue that contains blood cells dispersed within a liquid intercellular matrix. The color of blood varies from a bright red to a darker blue-red. The difference in color is caused by the amount of O_2 in the blood; well-oxygenated blood is bright red, whereas O_2-poor blood is blue-red. The amount of blood varies, depending on body size, gender, and age. The average adult has 4 to 6 L of blood.

 Do You Know...

Why George Washington's 9 Pints of Blood Went Down the Drain?

You probably remember George Washington for chopping down the cherry tree, for his penchant for truth, and for being the first president—but here is something you probably didn't know about George's medical history. George had been quite ill with a long winter cold, pneumonia, and throat infection. Despite many home remedies and much attention, the infection lingered and worsened. Enter the "quacks"! Immediately before his death, George was bled of 9 pints of blood in an attempt to rid his body of disease. This commonly used procedure was called *bloodletting*.

The practice of bloodletting had been around since before the days of Hippocrates (circa 350 BC). Bloodletting grew out of the belief that health was the result of a balance of the four body humors (fluids): blood, phlegm, black bile, and yellow bile. Disease was therefore attributed to an imbalance of the humors. By draining George's blood, the bloodletter hoped to balance George's unbalanced humors. (Not funny!) The fact that George died immediately after being drained of 9 pints is not surprising. At a time when he needed all the help he could get from his blood, he was literally drained and probably plunged into a state of low-volume circulatory shock. Although the practice of bloodletting, as described in this case, has been discredited, the practice of bloodletting hasn't completely died out. It has, however, been cleaned up and refined. "Therapeutic phlebotomy," or the removal of blood for therapeutic purposes, is routinely performed in the treatment of polycythemia vera and hemochromatosis, conditions characterized by excess red blood cells, iron, and blood volume. And our little leech on p. 297 is a natural-born phlebotomist when it comes to maintaining blood flow in edematous tissues.

We retain a friendly reminder of our former bloodletting ways in the barbershop pole. Barbers and surgeons were the early bloodletters, and the pole advertised their trade. The barbershop pole is striped red and white. Red represents blood, white represents the tourniquet, and the pole itself represents the stick that the patient squeezed to dilate the veins for easy puncturing. Fortunately, today's barbers go for your hair and not your jugular.

Other characteristics of blood include pH (normal, 7.35 to 7.45) and viscosity. Blood *viscosity* (vis-KOS-i-tee) refers to the thickness of the blood and affects the ease with which blood flows through the blood vessels. Viscosity is best demonstrated by comparing the flow of water and molasses. If water and molasses are poured out of a bottle, the molasses flows more slowly. Molasses is said to be more viscous, or thicker, than water. Blood is normally three to five times more viscous than water.

BLOOD HAS TWO PARTS

Blood is composed of two parts: the plasma and the formed elements (blood cells and cell fragments). The **plasma** is a pale-yellow fluid composed mostly of water; it also contains proteins, ions, nutrients, gases, and waste. The plasma proteins consist of **albumin** (al-BYOO-min), clotting factors, antibodies, and complement proteins. In general, the plasma proteins help regulate fluid volume, protect the body from pathogens, and prevent excessive blood loss in the event of injury. **Serum** is the plasma minus the clotting proteins.

The blood cells and cell fragments include the following:

- **Red blood cells** (RBCs) are also called **erythrocytes** (eh-RITH-roh-sytes) (from *erythro*, meaning "red"). RBCs are primarily involved in the transport of O_2 to all body tissues.
- **White blood cells** (WBCs) are also called **leukocytes** (LOO-koh-sytes) (from *leuko*, meaning "white"). WBCs protect the body from infection.
- **Platelets** (PLAYT-lets) are also called **thrombocytes** (THROM-boh-sytes). Platelets protect the body from bleeding.

The two parts of blood can be observed in a test tube. If a sample of blood is collected in a tube and spun in a centrifuge, two phases appear; the heavier blood cells appear at the bottom of the tube, whereas the lighter plasma accumulates at the top.

The separation of blood into two phases forms the basis of a blood test called the *hematocrit* (Hct) or *packed cell volume* (Fig. 15.1). The **hematocrit** (hee-MAT-oh-krit) is the percentage of blood cells in a sample of blood. A sample of blood is normally composed of 45% blood cells and 55% plasma. The blood cell component is composed mainly of RBCs. A small layer of cells between the plasma and the RBCs is called the *buffy coat* and consists of WBCs and platelets. Because the buffy coat is so thin, any change in the Hct is generally interpreted as a change in the numbers of RBCs. For example, a person with a low Hct is considered to be anemic, with a lower than normal number of RBCs. A word of caution! Because the Hct is expressed as a percentage (%), any change in blood volume affects the Hct. For example, a dehydrated patient has a diminished blood volume. Thus, the ratio of RBCs to blood volume increases. The elevated Hct therefore represents not an

BLOOD SAMPLE

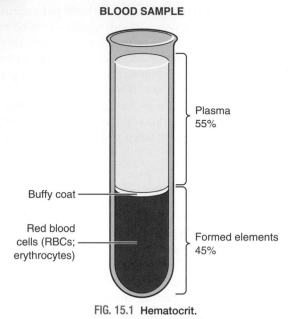

FIG. 15.1 **Hematocrit.**

increase in RBCs but a decrease in blood volume. Conversely, an expanded blood volume, as occurs in heart failure, decreases the Hct. The lowered Hct represents not a decrease in RBCs but an increase in blood volume. In essence, the RBCs have been diluted by the excess water in the blood. An expanded blood volume causes a "dilutional anemia."

 Re-Think

1. List the two parts of blood.
2. List the three types and functions of blood cells.
3. Describe the effect of anemia (a deficiency of RBCs) on the hematocrit.
4. Describe the effects of dehydration or overhydration on the hematocrit.

ORIGIN OF BLOOD CELLS

The process of blood cell formation is called **hemopoiesis** (hee-moh-POY-ess-iss). The three types of blood cells (RBCs, WBCs, and platelets) are made in hemopoietic tissue. The two types of hemopoietic tissue in the adult are the red bone marrow and the lymphatic tissue.

Blood formation in the red bone marrow is called *myeloid hemopoiesis.* (Myeloid comes from the Greek word meaning "bone marrow.") Blood formation in the lymphatic tissue (described in Chapter 21) is called *lymphoid hemopoiesis.* Red bone marrow is found primarily in the ends of long bones, such as the femur, and in flat and irregular bones, such as the sternum, cranial bones, vertebrae, and bones of the pelvis.

HEMOPOIESIS AND RED BONE MARROW

How does the red bone marrow produce three different types of blood cells? They are produced in the red bone marrow from the same cell, called a *stem cell.* Under

the influence of specific growth factors, the stem cell differentiates into a RBC, a WBC, or a platelet. Note the stem cell in Fig. 15.2. In line 1, the stem cell differentiates into the RBC (erythrocyte). In lines 2, 3, and 4, the stem cells form five different types of WBCs (leukocytes). The **lymphocytes** and **monocytes** originate in the bone marrow; some of the lymphocytes then mature and reproduce in the lymphatic tissue. In line 5, the stem cell differentiates into a *megakaryocyte* (meg-ah-KAIR-ee-oh-syte), a large blood cell that breaks up into tiny cell fragments called *platelets* or *thrombocytes.*

BONE MARROW WOES: TOO LITTLE, TOO MUCH

BONE MARROW DEPRESSION

Cheer up! Even bone marrow gets depressed. Under certain conditions, the bone marrow cannot produce enough blood cells. Bone marrow depression is called *myelosuppression.* What happens if the bone marrow is depressed? Depressed bone marrow leads to a severe deficiency of RBCs, causing a serious form of **anemia** called *aplastic anemia.* Myelosuppression can also cause a deficiency of WBCs (leukocytes) called *leukopenia* (loo-koh-PEE-nee-ah). The leukopenic person is more prone to infection and may die from a common cold. Depressed bone marrow may also produce inadequate numbers of platelets, or thrombocytes. This condition is called *thrombocytopenia* (throm-boh-sye-toh-PEE-nee-ah). The thrombocytopenic person is at risk for abnormal bouts of bleeding or hemorrhage. Why the concern for bone marrow depression? Because many drugs, especially cytotoxic cancer drugs, radiation, and a variety of diseases depress the bone marrow. Clinically, this is a huge problem. As a point of interest, Madame Curie, co-discoverer of the radioactive elements radium and polonium, died of a radiation-induced aplastic anemia. Seems that she routinely carried the radioactive elements in the pockets of her lab coat—obviously, years before radiation safety became an issue.

BONE MARROW OVERACTIVITY

Then, there is the hyperactive bone marrow known as *polycythemia vera,* or the overactivity and excess production of blood cells. The excess thickened blood (increased viscosity) burdens the heart, overwhelms the clotting system, and produces a beet-red, ruddy face (caused by the increase in RBC production). To help this condition, the patient may be given a drug that depresses the bone marrow or undergo therapeutic phlebotomy (fleh-BOHT-oh-mee) to remove excess blood.

 Re-Think

1. Where does most hemopoiesis occur?
2. What is the difference between myeloid and lymphoid hemopoiesis?
3. What are three consequences of myelosuppression? Of bone marrow overactivity?

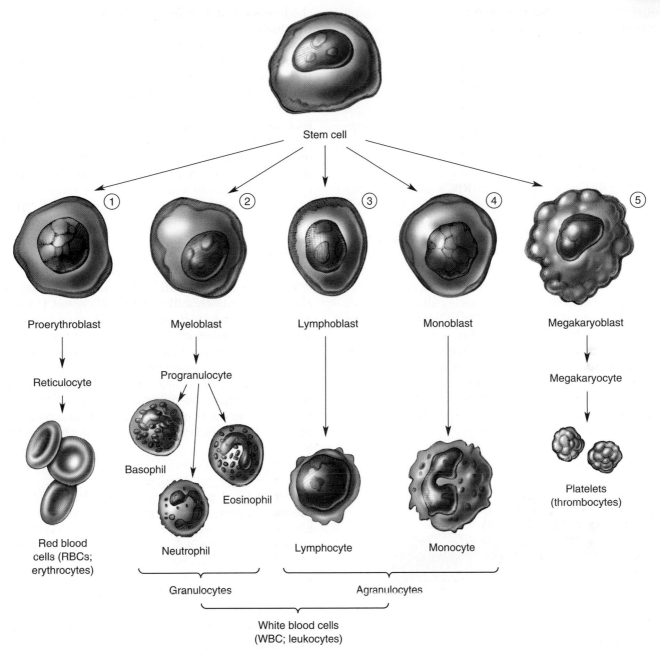

FIG. 15.2 Differentiation of a stem cell into RBCs, WBCs, and platelets.

Sum It Up!

Blood is composed of plasma and blood cells. The RBCs (erythrocytes) carry O₂; the WBCs (leukocytes) protect against infection, and the platelets (thrombocytes) prevent bleeding. The hematocrit is a measure of the ratio of the blood cells to blood volume. Myelosuppression and polycythemia vera are two examples of altered bone marrow activity.

BLOOD CELLS

RED BLOOD CELLS

The RBCs are the most numerous of the blood cells. Between 4.5 and 6.0 million RBCs are in 1 µl (microliter) of blood. The rate of production by the red bone marrow is several million RBCs per second. The production of RBCs is called *erythropoiesis* (eh-rith-roh-poy-EE-sis). RBCs are primarily concerned with the transport of O₂ and carbon dioxide.

The stem cell within the red bone marrow differentiates into a proerythroblast and eventually into a mature erythrocyte (RBC) (Fig. 15.2, column 1). Note the **reticulocyte** (reh-TIK-yoo-loh-syte), the immature RBC. Reticulocytes can develop into mature RBCs within 48 hours of release into the blood. The number of reticulocytes in blood is normally very small (0.5% to 1.5%). Why measure the reticulocyte count? A high reticulocyte count may indicate blood loss or an iron-deficient state. Why? A loss of blood stimulates the bone marrow to make more RBCs. The more severe the blood loss, the greater the bone marrow activity, and the higher the number of reticulocytes prematurely added to the circulation. The reticulocytes simply don't have time to mature in the bone marrow. Conversely, a low reticulocyte count might indicate that the patient's bone marrow is unable to make RBCs, as in myelosuppression. Hence, changes in the reticulocyte count can provide valuable diagnostic clues.

SHAPE AND CONTENTS

What do RBCs look like? First, RBCs are large. They are so large that they are unable to wiggle through the blood vessels wall. The RBCs stay in the blood vessels and do not roam around the tissue spaces, as do the WBCs. Second, RBCs are flexible disc-shaped cells that have a thick outer rim and a thin center (Fig. 15.3). Because the RBC can bend, it can squeeze its way through tiny blood vessels called *capillaries*. This flexibility allows the RBC to deliver O_2 to every cell in the body. The RBC's ability to bend is important. If the RBC were not able to bend, it would not fit through the tiny blood vessels, and tissue cells would be deprived of O_2 and die. Decreased oxygenation and cell death occur in a condition known as *sickle cell disease*. Instead of bending, the RBCs assume a

sickle or C shape and block blood flow through the tiny blood vessels.

RBC size and shape matter! While reading the results of a blood smear, you may come across the terms *anisocytosis* and *poikilocytosis*, which pertain to shape. Anisocytosis (ahn-ISS-oh-syte-OH-sis) refers to unequal-sized RBCs, whereas poikilocytosis (poy-KEE-loh-syte-OH-sis) refers to irregularly shaped RBCs. Both are found in anemia and other blood disorders. Is the RBC smaller than normal or *microcytic*, as in iron deficiency anemia, or larger than normal or *macrocytic*, as in vitamin B_{12} deficiency anemia? What about its color? Is the RBC *hypochromic* (pale), *normochromic* (normal in color), or *hyperchromic* (deeper red)? These are all commonly used terms to describe RBCs.

The content of the RBC is also unique. The RBC normally loses almost all its organelles as it matures. Having no mitochondria, the RBC is not powered aerobically; rather, it produces adenosine triphosphate (ATP) anaerobically. Think about it; the RBC does not metabolically use up the O_2 that it is transporting throughout the body. Also, the RBC, lacking a nucleus and DNA, cannot replicate; the "old" RBC is removed from the blood and replaced by a new RBC made in the bone marrow. We now know what the RBC does not contain, so what does it contain? Read on.

HEMOGLOBIN

RBCs are filled with a large protein molecule called **hemoglobin** (Fig. 15.4). Hemoglobin (hee-moh-GLOH-bin) consists of two parts: globin (protein) and heme, an iron-containing substance. Hemoglobin contains

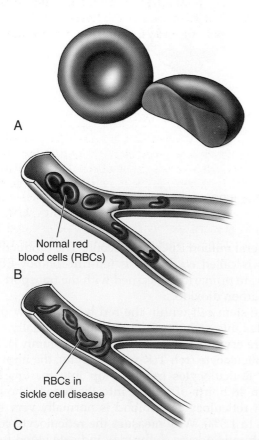

FIG. 15.3 (A) The RBCs are large and doughnut shaped. (B) The RBCs must bend to fit through the blood vessel. (C) Sickled RBCs blocking the flow of blood through the blood vessel.

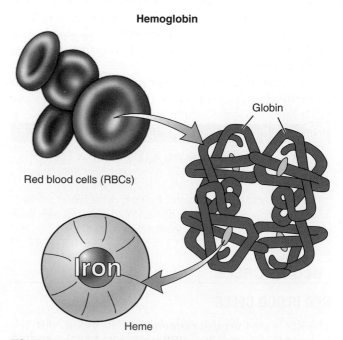

FIG. 15.4 RBCs filled with hemoglobin. Hemoglobin is formed by globin chains and iron-containing heme.

four globin chains, with each globin having a heme group. The hemoglobin molecule is responsible for RBC function.

What is so important about heme? As the RBCs circulate through the blood vessels in the lungs, O_2 attaches loosely to the iron atom in the heme. The oxygenated hemoglobin is referred to as *oxyhemoglobin* (OX-ee-HEEM-oh-globe-in). Then, as the blood flows to the various tissues in the body, the O_2 detaches from the hemoglobin. The unloaded O_2 diffuses from the blood to the cells, where it is used during cellular metabolism.

The globin portion of hemoglobin also plays a role in gas transport. Globin transports some of the carbon dioxide (CO_2) from its site of production in the metabolizing cells to the lungs, where it is excreted. The CO_2-hemoglobin complex is called *carbaminohemoglobin* (kahr-bam-ih-no-hee-moh-GLOH-bin). To repeat: Hemoglobin carries both O_2 and CO_2 but at different sites.

WHY BLOOD CHANGES ITS COLOR

The color of blood changes from bright red to blue-red. When hemoglobin is oxygenated, blood appears bright red. When hemoglobin is unoxygenated, blood assumes a darker blue-red color. Thus, blood coming from the lungs is well oxygenated and appears red. Blood leaving the tissues has given up its O_2 and appears blue-red. When a person is deprived of O_2, the blood is a blue-red color, causing the skin to look blue, or cyanotic. **Cyanosis** is a sign of hypoxemia, a deficiency of O_2 in the blood. Cyanosis is always cause for concern and should prompt a search for the underlying cause of the hypoxemia. Sometimes a person who has been exposed to cold temperature appears cyanotic. What is going on here? The cold causes the cutaneous blood vessels to constrict, slowing blood flow and providing additional time for O_2 to diffuse from the blood into the tissues. Less oxyhemoglobin…bluish!

But wait! Why can a person appear cherry red and be hypoxemic at the same time? It's a carbon monoxide (CO) thing. Blood is bright red when the hemoglobin is saturated with O_2. CO, like O_2, binds to the iron and also makes the blood appear bright cherry red. When CO occupies the iron site, however, no O_2 can be carried by the hemoglobin. Therefore, the person with CO poisoning can be both cherry red and hypoxemic. CO poisoning is deadly and very common. By the way, 20% of the hemoglobin of a cigarette smoker is unavailable for O_2 transport because of the presence of CO in the smoke.

WHAT IS ESSENTIAL FOR HEMOGLOBIN PRODUCTION?

What does the body need to make adequate amounts of hemoglobin? In addition to correct genetic coding for protein synthesis, and healthy bone marrow, the body requires certain raw materials. Some of the essential precursors include iron, vitamin B_{12}, and folic acid. A deficiency of any of the raw materials results in a specific type of anemia. Recall that the heme, the O_2-carrying component of hemoglobin, contains iron. A diet deficient in iron can result in inadequate hemoglobin synthesis and a condition called *iron deficiency anemia*. Young women are more prone to iron deficiency anemia than young men, as might be expected. Women not only are more apt to get caught up in rigorous and unhealthy dieting, but they also tend to lose more iron because of the blood loss associated with menstruation and fetal demands during pregnancy. Persons with a low income also have a higher incidence of iron deficiency anemia because iron-rich foods such as meat are expensive. Another group of persons at risk for iron deficiency anemia is those who have had gastrectomy and other gastric bypass surgeries. The surgical loss of acid-secreting cells impairs iron absorption. And for you forensic sleuths? The iron in hemoglobin can combine with a chemical called *luminal*, causing a blue glow (chemiluminescence). Thus, when luminal is sprayed at a crime scene, trace amounts of blood glow, despite the heroic cleansing and bleaching efforts of the perp.

A deficiency of raw materials, such as folic acid and vitamin B_{12}, can cause other specific anemias, described in the Medical Terminology and Disorders table (p. 303). It is critical to determine the type of anemia so as to provide the appropriate treatment.

 Do You Know...

Why There Is a Needle in This Hip Bone?

Because the red bone marrow is the site of blood cell production, certain abnormalities of blood cells can be detected through a bone marrow biopsy. In this procedure, a needle is inserted into the red bone marrow, usually at the iliac crest (hip bone). A sample of bone marrow is withdrawn, or aspirated, and then studied microscopically. The analysis includes the numbers and types of blood cells and the specific developmental characteristics of each cell type.

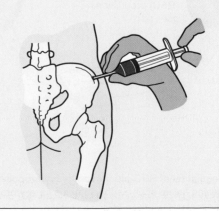

REGULATION OF RBC PRODUCTION

New RBCs are constantly added to the circulation, and old, worn-out RBCs are constantly removed from the circulation. Fig. 15.5 indicates that the RBC count is maintained through negative feedback control between the amount of O_2 in the blood and a hormone called *erythropoietin*. When the O_2 in the body tissues decreases, the kidneys sense the need for additional O_2 and secrete a hormone called **erythropoietin** (eh-RITH-roh-POY-eh-tin). The erythropoietin (EPO) stimulates the bone marrow to produce additional RBCs. The increase in the number of RBCs causes an increase in the amount of O_2 transported to the tissues. As tissue O_2 increases, the stimulus for EPO release diminishes, and the bone marrow slows its rate of RBC production.

Three clinical thoughts about EPO follow:

- Note what happens in a person who is chronically hypoxemic, such as a person with emphysema (a chronic lung disorder). The low O_2 in the blood stimulates the secretion of excess EPO, causing additional RBC production. Thus, a person with emphysema often has polycythemia (excess RBCs) secondary to chronic lung disease. Similarly, a person who moves to a high-altitude location experiences a mild hypoxemia, which, in turn, stimulates EPO secretion and a rise in the RBC count. Both the emphysema-induced and altitude-induced polycythemias are called *secondary polycythemias*, meaning that the polycythemia is secondary to the condition that is causing the excess secretion of EPO.
- Athletes sometimes use EPO as a drug. The drug increases RBC production, thereby increasing the amount of O_2 delivered to exercising muscle and enhancing athletic performance. The administration of EPO under this condition is a form of blood doping and is illegal.
- Patients with declining kidney function do not produce enough EPO and therefore become anemic. This type of anemia is called *anemia of chronic renal (kidney) failure.*

? Re-Think

1. What is a reticulocyte? What diagnostic information may be gained by knowing the reticulocyte count?
2. Differentiate between oxyhemoglobin and carbaminohemoglobin.
3. What role does iron play in the hemoglobin molecule?
4. How does EPO regulate the numbers of RBCs in the blood?

REMOVAL AND BREAKDOWN OF RED BLOOD CELLS

How does the body know when an RBC needs to be removed from the circulation? The life span of an RBC is about 120 days. Because the mature RBC has no nucleus, it cannot reproduce and must be replaced as it wears out. The signal for RBC removal? With time, as it performs its job, the RBC eventually gets misshapen, ragged around the edges, and fragile; the poor thing looks worn out! The ragged RBC membrane is detected by the macrophages that line the spleen and liver. The macrophages, or "big eaters," remove the RBCs from the circulation and phagocytose them.

RECYCLE!

As the old, worn-out RBC is dismantled, its components are recycled or excreted. The hemoglobin is broken down into globin and heme (Fig. 15.6). The globin is broken down into various amino acids that are later used in the synthesis of other proteins.

The heme is further broken down into iron and bile pigments. The iron is stored in the liver until it is needed by the bone marrow for the synthesis of new hemoglobin. The liver removes bile pigments, especially bilirubin, from the blood and excretes them into the bile. Bile eventually flows into the intestines and is excreted from the body in the feces. What if RBC breakdown is excessive, as in hemolysis? The excess **bilirubin** in the blood, called *hyperbilirubinemia*, is deposited in the skin, causing it to appear yellow or jaundiced. Because the **jaundice** is caused by hemolysis, it is called *hemolytic jaundice*. Bilirubin metabolism and jaundice are further described in the Ramp It Up!: Bilirubin and Jaundice box (pp. 301-302).

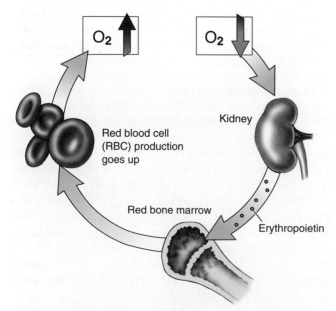

FIG. 15.5 Regulation of RBC production by erythropoietin. Note decreasing levels of O_2 as the stimulus for erythropoietin secretion.

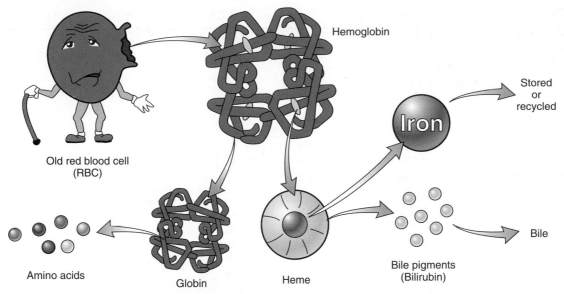

Hemoglobin

Old red blood cell
(RBC)

Iron

Stored
or
recycled

Amino acids

Globin

Heme

Bile pigments
(Bilirubin)

Bile

FIG. 15.6 Breakdown of old RBCs. Note the recycling of amino acids and iron and the excretion of bilirubin in the bile.

 Do You Know...

Who This Little Yellow Bird Called Icterus Is?

The term *icterus* is a Greek word for "little yellow bird." Icterus is the same as jaundice. The ancient Greeks thought that a jaundiced person could be cured by gazing at the yellow bird. We now know that bird watching is not the cure. Jaundice is caused by an elevation of bilirubin in the blood (hyperbilirubinemia). The hyperbilirubinemia can be caused by excessive blood cell destruction (hemolysis) or the reduction in the elimination of bilirubin from the blood (via the liver and bile). When jaundice is present, it is essential to determine the cause of the hyperbilirubinemia. The cure? Treat the underlying cause of the jaundice.

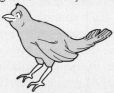

 Do You Know...

About Bilirubin, Kernicterus, and Sulfa Drugs?

Normally, bilirubin is transported by the plasma proteins, especially albumin, in the blood. In pharmacology terms, bilirubin is said to be tightly bound to albumin. As long as the bilirubin is bound to the albumin, it is not free to leave the blood and stain the tissues yellow. Enter the sulfa drugs. If an infant (younger than 2 months old) is given a sulfa drug to treat an infection, the drug binds to the albumin and displaces or frees the bilirubin. The free bilirubin enters the tissues, staining them yellow. Because the blood–brain barrier of the infant is not fully developed, the bilirubin can enter the central nervous system (CNS), causing brain damage (kernicterus). The same thing happens when a pregnant woman is given a sulfa drug. The drug crosses the placental barrier, enters the fetal blood, and causes an excess of free bilirubin. Thus, the administration of sulfa drugs to an infant or to a pregnant or nursing mother is contraindicated.

WHITE BLOOD CELLS

WBCs, or leukocytes, are large round cells that contain nuclei. WBCs lack hemoglobin and are less numerous than RBCs. WBCs function primarily to protect the body by destroying pathogens and removing dead tissue and other cellular debris by phagocytosis. When an infection is present in the body, the numbers of WBCs generally increase. This increase in the number of WBCs is called *leukocytosis* (loo-koh-syte-OH-sis). A few infections cause leukopenia, a decrease in the numbers of WBCs. Leukocytes vary widely with respect to life span: granulocytes may live only a few hours, whereas some lymphocytes may live for years.

Normally, 1 µl of blood contains 5000 to 10,000 WBCs (Table 15.1). This number is somewhat misleading because the WBCs spend less than 12 hours in the

 Sum It Up!

RBCs are filled with hemoglobin; the heme (iron) portion carries O_2 as oxyhemoglobin, and the globin portion carries CO_2 as carbaminohemoglobin. Normal RBCs are formed only in the presence of adequate raw materials, normal genetic information that directs hemoglobin synthesis, and healthy bone marrow. RBC production is regulated by erythropoietin, which in turn responds to tissue levels of O_2. Hemoglobin is degraded into globin, iron, and bilirubin. The iron and amino acids (globin) are recycled, and the bilirubin is excreted in the bile.

Re-Think

1. Explain why excess hemolysis causes jaundice.
2. When an RBC is dismantled what is the fate of the globin? Heme? Bilirubin?

Table 15.1   Types and Functions of Blood Cells

CELL TYPE	NORMAL RANGE	PRIMARY FUNCTION
Red blood cells (RBCs)	Men: 4.5–6.0 million/μL Women: 4.2–5.4 million/μL	Transport oxygen and carbon dioxide
Hemoglobin (Hgb)	Men: 13.5–17.5 g/100 mL Women: 12–16 g/100 mL	
Hematocrit (Hct)	Men: 40%–50% Women: 37%–47%	
Reticulocytes	0.5%–1.5%	
White blood cells (WBCs)*	5000–10,000/μL	Protect the body from infection
Platelets (thrombocytes)	150,000–450,000/μL	Help control blood loss from injured blood vessels

μL, Microliter.
*See Table 15.2 for the WBC differential count.

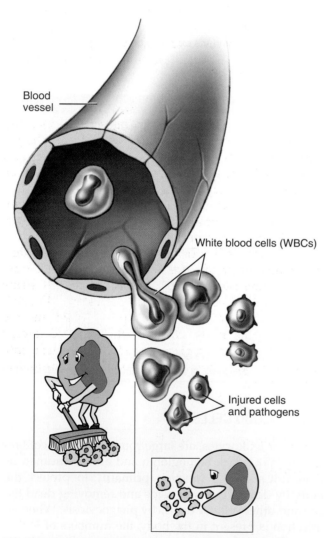

Blood vessel

White blood cells (WBCs)

Injured cells and pathogens

FIG. 15.7 White blood cells are involved in phagocytosis. Note the WBCs leaving the blood in search of injured cells in the tissues.

blood; they leave the blood vessels and migrate to connective tissue or to the site of an infection or inflammation, where they work and live out their lives (Fig. 15.7). Thus, the number of WBCs distributed throughout the body is much larger than what is suggested by the WBC count in the blood.

Table 15.2   White Blood Cells (WBCs) Differential Count*

TYPE OF WBC	PERCENTAGE OF TOTAL WBC COUNT	FUNCTION OF CELL
Granulocytes		
Neutrophils	55–70	Phagocytosis
Eosinophils	1–3	Inflammatory responses, parasitic infection, allergies
Basophils	0–1	Inflammatory responses, release of heparin
Agranulocytes		
Lymphocytes	25–38	Immunity
Monocytes	3–8	Phagocytosis

*A differential WBC count indicates the percentage of each type of WBC.

TYPES OF WHITE BLOOD CELLS

WBC production is called *leukopoiesis* (loo-koh-poy-EE-sis) (see Fig. 15.2). Each of the five types of WBCs has a different name, appearance, and function (Table 15.2). How do we tell the difference? WBCs are classified according to granules in their cytoplasm. WBCs that contain granules are called *granulocytes*. Other WBCs do not have granules in their cytoplasm and are called *agranulocytes*. Granulocytes are produced in the red bone marrow and are further classified according to their staining characteristics.

GRANULOCYTES

The three types of granulocytes are neutrophils, basophils, and eosinophils. The **neutrophil** (NOO-troh-fil) is the most common granulocyte. Neutrophils (which are pale or stain lavender) account for 55% to 70% of the total WBC population and usually remain in the blood for about 10 to 12 hours. The neutrophil's most important role is phagocytosis and the release of antimicrobial chemicals. These cells quickly move to the site of infection, where they phagocytose pathogens and remove tissue debris. The battle between the neutrophils and pathogens at the site of infection creates pus, a collection of dead neutrophils, parts of cells, and fluid.

Sometimes, the body can wall off the collection of pus from the surrounding tissue, forming an abscess. Abscess formation is one way that the body can prevent the spread of infection. The neutrophil plays such an important role in the defense of the body that a deficiency of neutrophils (neutropenia or granulocytopenia) is considered life threatening. Be sure that you understand these WBC terms: *leukopenia, granulocytopenia,* and *neutropenia.*

Because it plays such an important role in protecting the body from infection, the neutrophil is often the center of attention clinically. Depending on its age, appearance, and its actions at the moment, the neutrophil has many nicknames. The neutrophil is a round cell that contains a nucleus that can have many shapes and different sizes. Because of the many-shaped (polymorphic) nucleus, neutrophils are called *polymorphs,* or *polymorphonuclear leukocytes* (PMNs). Sometimes, they are simply called *polys.*

The nucleus of the mature neutrophil appears segmented when viewed under a microscope. Mature neutrophils are therefore called *segs.* The nucleus of the immature neutrophil looks like a thick curved band—hence the name *band cells.* Because the band resembles the shape of a staff, the band cells are also called *staff cells.* Neutrophils are also called *stab cells.*

Do You Know
What Is a "Shift to the Left"?

This is a clinical phrase illustrating the response of the WBCs to a pathogen. As the body tries to mount an attack against a pathogen, it needs more neutrophils. The production of the neutrophils may be so rapid that the time for cells to mature is inadequate. A greater proportion of the neutrophils is therefore immature and appears banded. When immature neutrophils (bands) become prominent in the differential WBC count (lab test), the condition is termed a *shift to the left.* The term is derived from early studies that used tabular headings to report the numbers of each cell type. The cell types were listed across the top of the printout, starting with bands on the left and the more mature neutrophils on the right. Thus, a shift to the left indicates an infection.

The second type of granulocytic WBCs, called **basophils** (BAY-so-fils), is normally present in small numbers. Basophils make up less than 1% of the WBCs and absorb a dark blue stain. The basophil plays a role in the inflammatory response, primarily through its release of histamine. The basophil also releases heparin, an anticoagulant. Because basophils are found in abundance in areas with large amounts of blood, such as the lungs and liver, the release of heparin is thought to reduce the formation of tiny blood clots and facilitates the movement of WBCs throughout the injured tissue.

The third type of granulocytic WBC is the **eosinophil** (ee-oh-SIN-oh-fil). The prefix eos- means rosy and refers to the staining characteristic of the eosinophil. Eosinophils are present in small numbers, constituting only 1% to 3% of the WBCs. They are involved in the inflammatory response, secreting chemicals that weaken and destroy large parasites (tapeworm, hookworm), engage in phagocytosis, and become elevated in persons with allergies.

AGRANULOCYTES

The two types of agranulocytes are lymphocytes and monocytes. The lymphocytes are produced in the red bone marrow; some migrate to and then mature and reproduce in the lymphatic tissue (lymph nodes, liver, spleen, lymphatic nodules). Lymphocytes constitute 25% to 38% of the WBCs and perform an important role in the body's immune response. Monocytes are the second type of agranulocyte.

Monocytes leave the blood for tissues, where they differentiate into large cells called *macrophages.* Macrophages are very efficient phagocytes; as the name indicates, the macrophages are "big eaters." In addition to phagocytosis, the macrophage plays another important role. It also chops up the engulfed foreign particle and pushes a piece of the foreign particle onto its surface; this process is called *antigen presentation* (Chapter 21).

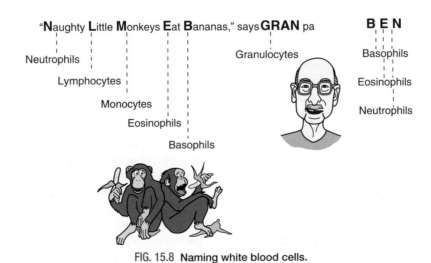

FIG. 15.8 **Naming white blood cells.**

GOOD NEWS, BAD NEWS

The bad news is that clinically, you must know the names and classifications (granulocytes, agranulocytes) of the WBCs. The good news is that you can use the monkey business in Fig. 15.8. "Naughty Little Monkeys Eat Bananas," says **GRAN**pa **BEN**. "Naughty Little Monkeys Eat Bananas" identifies the type of WBCs—**n**eutrophils, **l**ymphocytes, **m**onocytes, **e**osinophils, and **b**asophils. **GRAN**pa **BEN** indicates that the granulocytes are **b**asophils, **e**osinophils, and **n**eutrophils.

 Re-Think

1. Classify the neutrophil, and identify its primary function.
2. List the two agranulocytes.
3. What is the origin of the macrophage?
4. What are two functions of the macrophage?

PLATELETS

Platelets are tiny cell fragments of the larger megakaryocytes. Normally, each microliter of blood contains between 150,000 and 450,000 platelets or thrombocytes. They are produced in the red bone marrow (see Fig. 15.2) and have a life span of 5 to 9 days. The production of the platelet is called *thrombopoiesis* (THROM-boh-poy-EE-sis).

Platelets prevent blood loss. (Platelet function is more fully described later in the "Hemostasis" section.) Failure of the bone marrow to replace platelets at an adequate rate results in a deficiency of platelets called *thrombocytopenia*, which is characterized by petechiae—little pinpoint hemorrhages under the skin—and potentially lethal bleeding episodes.

BLOOD COUNTS

A complete blood count (CBC) is a laboratory test that provides information about the composition of the blood. A CBC provides the normal range of the numbers of RBCs, WBCs, and platelets. In addition to the numbers of blood cells, the CBC provides information specific to each cell type. Relative to the RBC, the CBC indicates the normal hemoglobin content of the RBC, the normal Hct, and the percentage of the reticulocytes (the immature RBCs). With regard to information concerning the WBCs, a CBC indicates the percentage of each type of WBC (the differential WBC count).

DIFFERENTIAL COUNT

A differential WBC count indicates the percentage of each type of WBC (see Table 15.2). The differential count provides valuable diagnostic information because it indicates which specific WBC is involved. For example, one infection may cause an elevation primarily in the numbers of neutrophils, but a different infection may cause an elevation in the monocytes.

 Sum It Up!

The WBCs (leukocytes) protect the body by destroying pathogens and removing dead tissue and other cellular debris by phagocytosis. The five types of WBCs are granulocytes (neutrophils, basophils, and eosinophils) and agranulocytes (lymphocytes and monocytes).

HEMOSTASIS: PREVENTION OF BLOOD LOSS

Injury to a blood vessel causes bleeding. Bleeding usually stops spontaneously when the injury is minor. What causes the bleeding to stop? The process that stops bleeding is called **hemostasis**, which literally means that the blood (*hemo*) stands still (*stasis*). Hemostasis involves three events: blood vessel spasm, the formation of a platelet plug, and blood clotting (Fig. 15.9). (Do not confuse the words *hemostasis* and *homeostasis*.)

BLOOD VESSEL SPASM

When a blood vessel is injured, the smooth muscle in the blood vessel wall responds by contracting in a process called *vascular spasm*. (*Vascular* refers to blood vessels.) Vascular spasm causes the diameter of the blood vessel to decrease, thereby decreasing the amount of blood that flows through the vessel. In the smallest vessels, vascular spasm stops the bleeding completely. In the larger vessels, vascular spasm alone may slow bleeding but is generally insufficient to stop bleeding.

FORMATION OF A PLATELET PLUG

When a blood vessel is torn, the inner lining of the vessel activates the platelets. The platelets become sticky and adhere to the inner lining of the injured vessel and to each other. By sticking together, they form a platelet plug, which diminishes bleeding at the injured site. Over several minutes, the plug will be invaded by activated blood-clotting factors and will eventually evolve into a stable, strong blood clot. In addition to forming a plug, the platelets also release chemicals that further stimulate vascular spasm and help activate the blood-clotting factors. Thus, the platelets participate in all three phases of hemostasis.

BLOOD COAGULATION

Vascular spasm and a platelet plug alone are not sufficient to prevent the bleeding caused by a large tear in a blood vessel. With a more serious injury to the vessel wall, bleeding stops only if a blood clot forms. Blood clotting, or **coagulation**, is the third step in the process of hemostasis. A blood clot is formed by a series of chemical reactions that result in the formation of a netlike structure. The net, or framework, of the clot is composed of protein fibers called **fibrin**. As

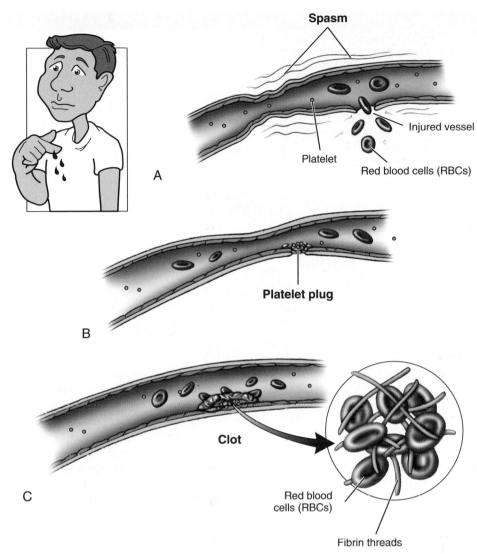

Spasm

Injured vessel

Platelet

Red blood cells (RBCs)

A

Platelet plug

B

Clot

Red blood
cells (RBCs)

Fibrin threads

C

FIG. 15.9 **Steps in hemostasis. (A) Blood vessel spasm. (B) Formation of the platelet plug. (C) Blood clotting (coagulation).**

blood flows through the fibrin net, large particles in the blood, such as RBCs and platelets, become trapped within it. The fibrin net and the trapped elements are called a *blood clot*. The blood clot seals off the opening in the injured blood vessel and stops the bleeding.

FORMATION OF THE BLOOD CLOT

How does the clot form? The clot is the result of a series of reactions in which a number of clotting factors are activated. The series of reactions in which one clotting factor activates another clotting factor is called the **clotting cascade**.

Follow the three stages of blood coagulation identified in Fig. 15.10.

- Stage I. Injury to the blood vessel wall activates various clotting factors. These clotting factors normally circulate in the blood in their inactive form. When activated, the clotting factors produce prothrombin activator (PTA).
- Stage II. In the presence of calcium, platelet chemicals, and PTA, prothrombin is activated to form thrombin.

- Stage III. Thrombin activates fibrinogen. Activated fibrinogen forms the fibrin fibers, or fibrin net. The net traps other blood cells and particles to form the clot. Other factors then stabilize and strengthen the clot.

CLOT RETRACTION

What happens to the clot after it forms? It becomes smaller as water is squeezed out. This process is called *clot retraction*. As the clot retracts, the edges of the injured blood vessels are also pulled together. This pulling together slows bleeding and sets the stage for repair of the blood vessel.

CLOT BUSTING: FIBRINOLYSIS

Are you stuck with the clot forever? No! After the clot accomplishes its task, it is dissolved by a process called *fibrinolysis* (fye-brin-OL-is-sis) (Fig. 15.11). A substance called *plasmin* gradually dissolves the clot. Plasmin is formed from its inactive form, plasminogen (plaz-MIN-o-jen), which normally circulates within the blood. Tissue plasminogen activator (TPA), formed by injured tissue, activates plasminogen.

Do You Know...

What Queen Victoria, the "Royal Disease," and Factor VIII Have in Common?

Hemophilia A is a bleeding disorder caused by the deficiency of a clotting factor called *factor VIII*, or the hemophilic factor. Hemophilia was common in the royal families of Europe; hence, it was called the "royal disease." Why was hemophilia so prevalent in the royal families? Hemophilia is genetically transmitted. Because of the tendency of the royals to intermarry (e.g., cousin marrying cousin), the gene carrying hemophilia was kept in the family and expressed frequently in the royal offspring. Queen Victoria of England carried the gene for hemophilia. Victoria, being both reproductively prolific and politically astute, placed a descendant on every major throne in Europe. As each descendant married and intermarried, the incidence of hemophilia increased. (See the Medical Terminology and Disorders table at the end of the chapter for other forms of hemophilia.)

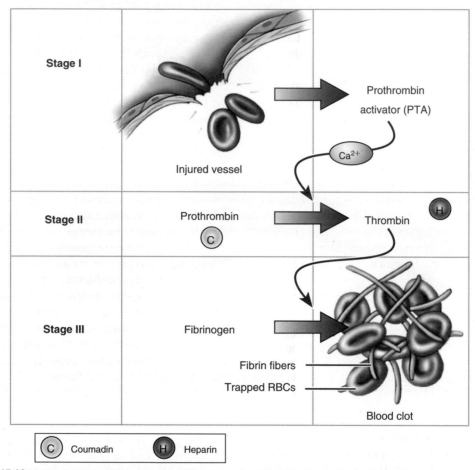

FIG. 15.10 Three stages of blood clotting. The sites of Coumadin *(C)* and heparin *(H)* activity are indicated.

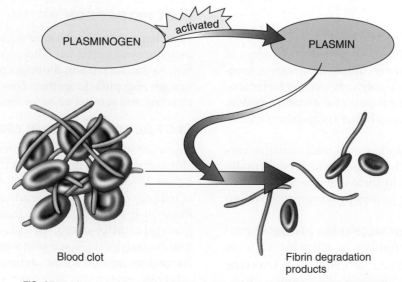

FIG. 15.11 Fibrinolysis, also called "clot busting"; activation of plasminogen.

PREVENTION OF EXCESSIVE CLOT FORMATION

Natural Mechanisms

- Although the body must be able to stop bleeding, it is equally essential for it to prevent excessive clot formation. Several natural mechanisms prevent clot formation. Three of the most important mechanisms are a smooth inner lining (endothelium) of the blood vessels, the secretion of heparin (an anticoagulant), and exercise

- The inner lining (endothelium) of the blood vessels is smooth and shiny and allows blood to flow easily along its surface. If the surface of the endothelium becomes roughened or lined with cholesterol plaques, however, coagulation factors are activated, and blood clots are apt to form.

- Heparin is an anticoagulant secreted by mast cells. Mast cells are related to basophils and are concentrated in and around the liver and lungs, sites where the blood is stagnant and therefore apt to clot easily.

- Exercise helps prevent the development of blood clots in two ways. First, exercise decreases platelet stickiness and platelet activation of the clotting cascade. Secondly, the massaging effect of contracting leg muscles prevents the stagnation of blood in the deep veins of the legs where blood clots tend to form. The improved blood flow, in turn, prevents the accumulation of activated clotting factors such as thrombin.

 Do You Know...

Why This Toe Needs This Leech?

This toe was accidentally severed from its owner. In reattaching the toe to the foot, the surgeon recognized that the toe graft would be successful only if the blood supply to the toe was good. Frequently, after surgery of this type, blood clots and edema (swelling) develop at the graft site, resulting in a decrease in blood flow. Leeches, or bloodsuckers, may be applied to the site of the graft. As the hungry leech attaches to the skin to feed, it drains the excess fluid (edema) and injects a potent anticoagulant. The anticoagulant prevents blood clotting at the graft site, thereby maintaining a good blood flow and improving the chances for successful grafting. Enter the celebrities. The rich and famous have discovered that leeches "take away the years." Attach a hungry leech to some puffy whatever, and—presto—the swelling subsides. Leeches are making it big and bringing in big bucks!

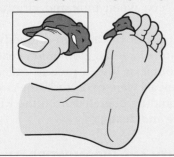

Use of Medications That Prevent Excessive Clot Formations

At times, the administration of drugs that interfere with hemostasis may be necessary. Antiplatelet drugs and anticoagulants are two groups of drugs used for this purpose. A third group of drugs called *fibrinolytic agents* dissolves clots that have already formed.

The blood clot is called a *thrombus*; the process of blood clot formation is called *thrombosis*. The problem? A piece of the thrombus can break off, forming a traveling blood clot called an *embolus*. The embolus may lodge in the smaller blood vessels of other organs, blocking the flow of blood to the organ and resulting in organ damage, such as a pulmonary infarct (necrosis), heart attack, or brain attack (stroke). A common killer disorder, called *deep vein thrombosis* (DVT), is particularly lethal. A clot in the deep veins of the legs gives rise to an embolus. The embolus travels to the blood vessels of the lungs, where it blocks blood flow and often causes sudden death.

Thrombosis may be prevented by the administration of two types of anticoagulants: heparin and warfarin (Coumadin). Heparin, designated "H" in Fig. 15.10, acts as an antithrombin agent. Another anticoagulant, Coumadin (warfarin), also prevents clot formation. Like heparin, Coumadin interferes with the clotting scheme but does so at a different step. Coumadin, designated "C" in Fig. 15.10, decreases the hepatic (liver) utilization of vitamin K in the synthesis of prothrombin, causing hypoprothrombinemia (hye-poh-pro-THROM-ben-EE-mee-ah), a diminished amount of prothrombin in the blood. Less prothrombin means less thrombin, and less thrombin means that blood clotting is diminished.

Another category of drugs, called *clot busters* or *fibrinolytic agents*, dissolves potentially lethal clots. As shown in Fig. 15.11, plasminogen activators dissolve clots. The clot busters, such as TPA, have revolutionized the treatment of myocardial infarction (heart attacks caused by blood clots in the blood vessels of the heart) and brain attacks (blood clots in the blood vessels of the brain).

 Do You Know...

About Harry Clotter, His Spinach Salad, and His PT?

Harry was diagnosed with deep vein thrombosis (DVT) after a 15-hour nonstop flight on his broomstick. After a 3-day stay in the hospital with heparin therapy, he was discharged on Coumadin (warfarin) and directed not to eat spinach. Why no spinach? The drug Coumadin works by blocking the utilization of vitamin K in the hepatic synthesis of prothrombin. Because spinach contains a lot of vitamin K, it reduces the effectiveness of Coumadin, thereby reversing its anticoagulant effects. So leave the spinach to Popeye, Harry. Harry was also advised to lose the stick and walk.

Harry was also directed to have his prothrombin (PT) time measured regularly. The PT is a blood test that measures the time it takes for a sample of blood to clot. Coumadin blocks the synthesis of prothrombin, so it induces hypoprothrombinemia and prolongs the PT. Because Coumadin can prolong the PT, the person is at risk for bleeding. Conversely, too little Coumadin provides inadequate anticoagulation, predisposing the person to clot formation; hence, the need for regular monitoring. PT values are reported as international normalized ratio (INR) units in an attempt to standardize laboratory test results. Harry's physician would most likely aim for an INR between 2 and 3.

Sum It Up!

The process that stops bleeding after injury is called *hemostasis*. Hemostasis involves three events: blood vessel spasm, the formation of a platelet plug, and blood clotting (coagulation). Clotting occurs when a series of clotting factors are activated (coagulation cascade) producing thrombin; thrombin causes the conversion of fibrinogen into a fibrin clot. Blood clots are eventually dissolved by plasmin. It is also important to prevent excessive clot formation. This is achieved through natural anticoagulant activity (smooth endothelium, heparin secretion by mast cells, and exercise). Medications are frequently used to prevent excessive clotting: antiplatelet drugs (aspirin), anticoagulants (heparin and coumadin), and fibrinolytic or clot-busting drugs.

Do You Know...

About Miss Muffet, Her Curds, Whey, and Blood Clot?

As you know, little Miss Muffet sat on her tuffet eating her curds and whey—that is, her soured milk. (The lumps in soured milk are called *curds*, and the watery part is called *whey*. So much for Muffet's diet.) What does this have to do with blood? *Thrombosis* (blood clotting) is from a Greek word meaning "to curdle," as in the curdling of milk. *Serum* is from a Latin word that refers to whey or the watery residue left after milk has curdled. Miss Muffet didn't really have a blood clot, but her diet inspired blood-clotting vocabulary. Her tuffet and arachnophobic personality are another story!

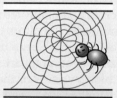

? Re-Think

1. Use the following words to explain the steps in coagulation: fibrinogen, thrombin, fibrin, PTA, and prothrombin.
2. Why might excessive doses of aspirin, heparin, Coumadin, and TPA cause bleeding?
3. Provide two reasons that exercise helps prevent the development of potentially lethal blood clots.

BLOOD TYPES

The history of medicine has recorded attempted blood transfusions since its earliest days. Although some were successful, others were medical disasters. The earliest physicians recognized that a severely wounded person was in need of blood. They did not realize, however, that blood from one person cannot always be mixed with blood from another. These physicians unknowingly demonstrated by disaster the presence of different blood types.

ANTIGENS AND BLOOD TYPES

Blood is classified according to specific antigens on the surface of the RBC. An antigen is a substance that the body recognizes as foreign. As a foreign substance, an antigen stimulates an antigen–antibody response. This response is designed to attack and destroy the antigen.

The ABO grouping contains four blood types: A, B, AB, and O. The letters A and B refer to the antigen on the RBC membrane. Table 15.3 shows what it means to be type A, B, AB, or O.

- A person with type A blood has the A antigen on the RBC.
- A person with type B blood has a B antigen on the RBC.
- A person with type AB blood has both A and B antigens on the RBC.
- A person with type O blood has neither A nor B antigen on the RBC.

Remember that the antigen is located on the RBC membrane.

ANTIBODIES AND BLOOD TYPE

In addition to the antigens on the RBC membranes, specific antibodies are found in the plasma of each blood type (see Table 15.3).

- A person with type A blood has anti-B antibodies in the plasma.
- A person with type B blood has anti-A antibodies in the plasma.
- A person with type AB blood has neither anti-A nor anti-B antibodies in the plasma.
- The person with type O blood has both anti-A and anti-B antibodies in the plasma.

ANTIGEN–ANTIBODY INTERACTION

Table 15.3 indicates that type A blood contains the A antigen and anti-B antibodies. What would happen if a person had the A antigen on his or her RBCs and anti-A antibodies in his plasma? The A antigen and the anti-A antibody would cause a clumping reaction much like the curdling seen when milk and vinegar are mixed together.

This clumping of the antigen–antibody interaction is called *agglutination*. Agglutination reactions cause the RBCs to burst or lyse, a process called **hemolysis**. If rapid hemolysis were to occur in the circulation, hemoglobin would be liberated from the RBCs, causing kidney failure and death.

COMPATIBILITY AND INCOMPATIBILITY OF BLOOD TYPES

The curdling, or agglutination, reaction has important implications for blood transfusions. Some blood

Table 15.3 ABO Blood Groups

BLOOD TYPE*	ANTIGEN (RBC MEMBRANE)	ANTIBODY (PLASMA)	CAN RECEIVE BLOOD FROM	CAN DONATE BLOOD TO
A (40%)	A antigen	Anti-B antibodies	A, O	A, AB
B (10%)	B antigen	Anti-A antibodies	B, O	B, AB
AB† (4%)	A antigen / B antigen	No antibodies	A, B, AB, O	AB
O‡ (46%)	No antigen	Both anti-A and anti-B antibodies	O	O, A, B, AB

*Number in parentheses indicates the percentage of the population with this blood type.
†Type AB, universal recipient.
‡Type O, universal donor.

types mix without undergoing agglutination reactions; they are said to be *compatible blood groups*. Other blood groups agglutinate, causing severe hemolysis. These blood groups are incompatible. To avoid giving a person incompatible blood, donor blood is first typed and cross-matched.

What do blood typing and cross-matching mean? First, the blood type (A, B, AB, or O) is determined. Then, a sample of donor blood (blood from the person who is donating it) is mixed (cross-matched) with a sample of recipient blood (blood from the person who is to receive the donated blood). Any evidence of agglutination indicates that the donor blood is incompatible with the recipient's blood.

Suppose a recipient of a blood transfusion has type A blood. She or he then can be given type A blood and type O blood (see Table 15.3). No antigen–antibody reaction (agglutination) would occur because type A donor blood has the A antigen and the recipient has only anti-B antibodies (plasma). The type O donor blood does not cause agglutination because that person's RBC has neither the A nor the B antigen. Type A and type O blood are therefore compatible with type A blood.

Note what happens, however, if the type A recipient receives type B blood (see Table 15.3). Type B donor blood has the B antigen on each RBC surface. The plasma antibodies of the recipient are anti-B antibodies. The B antigen and the anti-B antibodies cause agglutination; thus, type B blood is incompatible with

type A blood. What happens if the type A recipient is given type AB blood? In this case, the RBC contains both A and B antigens. The plasma of the recipient contains anti-B antibodies. When types A and AB are mixed, an agglutination reaction then occurs; these blood groups are incompatible. The administration of incompatible blood groups forms the basis of hemolytic blood transfusion reactions. The presence or absence of antibodies dictates the compatibility/incompatibility characteristics of the four blood groups (see Table 15.3).

Note in Table 15.3 that type O blood can be given to people in all four blood groups. Type O blood is therefore called the *universal donor*. For this reason, blood banks stock a large supply of type O blood. Note also that someone with type AB blood can receive all four types of blood; this person is called a *universal recipient*. Table 15.3 also indicates the prevalence of the four blood types. Type A blood occurs in 40% of the population, 10% of the population has type B, 4% has type AB, and 46% has type O. Thus, type O is the most common and type AB is the least common. (What blood type are you?)

? Re-Think

1. Why can't a person with type O blood safely receive a transfusion of type AB blood?
2. Why can't you change a person's blood type from type A to type O by giving him or her several transfusions of type O blood?

Rh CLASSIFICATION SYSTEM

Blood is also classified according to the Rh factor. The Rh factor is an antigen located on the membrane of the RBC. The Rh factor was named for the rhesus monkey, in which it was first detected. If an RBC contains the Rh factor, the blood is said to be Rh-positive (+). If the RBC lacks the Rh factor, it is said to be Rh-negative (−). Thus, A+ blood refers to type A (A antigen) blood that also has the Rh factor, whereas A− blood is type A blood that does not have the Rh factor. Approximately 85% of the population is Rh positive (+).

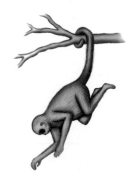

Plasma does not naturally carry anti-Rh antibodies. In two conditions, however, the plasma of an Rh-negative (−) person can develop anti-Rh antibodies.

The first condition involves the accidental administration of Rh-positive (+) blood to an Rh-negative (−) person. If Rh-positive (+) blood from a donor is administered to an Rh-negative (−) person (the recipient), the Rh antigen of the donor stimulates the recipient to produce anti-Rh antibodies. The recipient is now said to be sensitized. If the Rh-negative (−) person is later given a second transfusion of Rh-positive (+) blood, the anti-Rh antibodies in the plasma of the recipient will attack the Rh antigen of the Rh-positive (+) donor blood, causing agglutination and hemolysis.

The Rh factor may cause a serious problem in a second condition, that of an Rh-negative (−) pregnant mother who is carrying an Rh-positive (+) fetus (Fig. 15.12). During this first pregnancy, the fetus grows to term and is delivered uneventfully. During late pregnancy or childbirth, however, some of the fetus's Rh-positive (+) blood crosses the placenta and enters the mother's blood. The Rh antigen stimulates the mother's immune system to produce anti-Rh antibodies. In other words, the mother has become sensitized during her first pregnancy. If the mother becomes pregnant for a second time with an Rh-positive (+) fetus, the anti-Rh antibodies move from the mother's circulation into the fetus's circulation. These anti-Rh antibodies attack the fetus's RBCs, causing agglutination and hemolysis. In response, the fetus becomes jaundiced and anemic as the RBCs undergo hemolysis.

This hemolytic condition is called *erythroblastosis fetalis*. The hemolysis causes a rapid rise in plasma levels of bilirubin. The hyperbilirubinemia (increased bilirubin in the blood), in turn, causes severe jaundice and a condition called *kernicterus*. Kernicterus (kehr-NIK-tehr-ahs), caused by the staining of a part of the brain with bilirubin, is characterized by impaired mental development. The great tragedy is that kernicterus is preventable. Every woman should know her blood type and recognize the need for early prenatal care!

Erythroblastosis fetalis can be prevented by the administration of the drug RhoGAM. RhoGAM is administered to the Rh-negative mother during pregnancy and within 72 hours after delivery. RhoGAM surrounds, or coats, the fetus's Rh-positive (+) antigens, thereby preventing them from stimulating the development of anti-Rh antibodies by the mother.

Other antigens in the maternal and fetal blood are capable of inducing hemolysis, hyperbilirubinemia, and jaundice. Consequently, a newer and more inclusive term than *erythroblastosis fetalis* is *hemolytic disease of the newborn* (HDN). HDN includes all antigen–antibody reactions, including the Rh factor, that cause hemolysis and jaundice.

Visit any newborn nursery, and you will see a little yellow baby "sunbathing" in an isolette. What's that about? It has been known for years that ultraviolet radiation (sunlight) hastens the disappearance of jaundice. Phototherapy provides ultraviolet radiation, which helps break down the bilirubin deposited in the skin so that it can be eliminated from the body.

 Sum It Up!

Blood is classified according to the antigens on the surface of the RBC. The ABO grouping contains four blood types: A (A antigens), B (B antigens), AB (A and B antigens), and O (neither A nor B antigens). An antigen–antibody reaction, called *agglutination*, occurs when blood is mismatched. Type AB blood is the universal recipient blood. Type O blood is the universal donor blood. The Rh factor is another type of antigen on the RBC. Rh-positive blood has the Rh factor on the RBC, whereas Rh-negative blood does not contain the Rh factor.

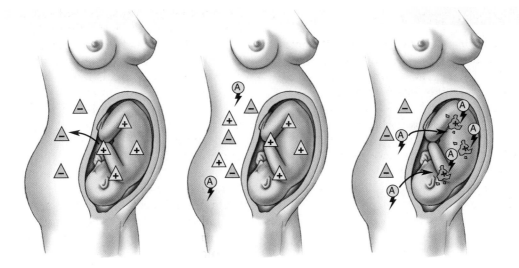

 Rh– Red blood cell (RBC) of mother

 Rh+ RBC of fetus with Rh antigen on surface

 Anti–Rh antibody made against Rh+ RBC

 Hemolysis of Rh+ RBC

FIG. 15.12 Rh-negative (–) mother, Rh-positive (+) fetus.

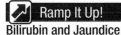 **Ramp It Up!**

Bilirubin and Jaundice

The story of bilirubin, how it is formed and excreted, has important clinical significance—namely, that of understanding the development of jaundice.

Normal Bilirubin Metabolism. Panel 1. (see figure on next page) Bilirubin comes from red blood cells (RBCs). When RBCs are broken down, the hemoglobin releases bilirubin into the blood. The bilirubin attaches to a plasma protein and is transported to the liver. At this stage, the bilirubin is called *protein-bound bilirubin* or *unconjugated bilirubin*. The liver changes the bilirubin by removing the plasma protein and attaching glucuronic acid to the bilirubin by the process of conjugation. The bilirubin is now called *conjugated bilirubin*. The liver then excretes the conjugated bilirubin into the bile; the bile flows through a series of bile ducts into the intestines of the digestive tract. Bilirubin and its breakdown products form the basis of many diagnostic tests.

Hyperbilirubinemia and Jaundice. Normally, the production and elimination of bilirubin is balanced so that the plasma level of bilirubin remains constant and low. With hemolytic, hepatocellular, or hepatobiliary dysfunction, however, the plasma concentration of bilirubin may increase. As the plasma level of bilirubin increases, the person develops hyperbilirubinemia, excess bilirubin in the blood. The bilirubin leaves the blood and stains the skin and mucous membranes a yellow color, called *jaundice.* The intensity of the jaundice reflects the plasma levels of bilirubin; the higher the bilirubin, the deeper the jaundice. The jaundice is most evident in the skin, sclerae (whites of the eyes), and mucous membranes of the mouth. Hyperbilirubinemia and jaundice occur for three reasons: prehepatic, hepatic, and posthepatic dysfunctions (*hepatic* refers to the liver).

Prehepatic Dysfunction. Panel 2. Excess bilirubin (hyperbilirubinemia) is produced whenever RBCs are broken down too rapidly (hemolysis). The excess bilirubin overwhelms the liver, meaning that the liver cannot clear the excess bilirubin from the blood. The hyperbilirubinemia causes jaundice. Because the jaundice is due to hemolysis and because the dysfunction occurs before the hepatic events, it is called *prehepatic* and *hemolytic jaundice*. For instance, normal neonates frequently have a mild hyperbilirubinemia and jaundice, called *normal physiologic jaundice*, as they attempt to get rid of excess RBCs. The jaundice is usually not severe and resolves without therapy. Some neonates, however, experience a blood incompatibility that causes severe hemolysis, hyperbilirubinemia, and intense jaundice. This is of concern and must be treated because severe hyperbilirubinemia in the neonate poses the risk of brain damage as the bilirubin stains and damages brain tissue; this complication is referred to as *kernicterus*.

Hepatic Dysfunction. Panel 3. The liver damaged by conditions such as hepatitis and cirrhosis creates two bilirubin-related problems. First, some of the hepatic cells are damaged and therefore are unable to conjugate bilirubin. Therefore, the blood levels of unconjugated bilirubin increase. Second, some of the undamaged hepatic cells are able to conjugate bilirubin. However, the inflamed hepatic tissues obstruct the flow of bile through the tiny bile canals and trap it within the liver. The conjugated bilirubin is then absorbed into the blood. Thus, hepatic dysfunction may be characterized by an elevation of both the unconjugated and conjugated bilirubin. The resulting hyperbilirubinemia causes jaundice and is called *hepatocellular jaundice*.

Continued

Bilirubin and Jaundice

Bilirubin and Jaundice

Panel 1
Normal Bilirubin Metabolism

RBCs

Bilirubin + plasma protein
(unconjugated bilirubin)

(Blood vessel)

Bile
(conjugated bilirubin)

Bilirubin

Intestines

Panel 2
Prehepatic Dysfunction (Hemolytic Jaundice)

RBCs

↑ unconjugated bilirubin

Bile

Bilirubin

Intestines

Panel 3
Hepatic Dysfunction

RBCs

↑ unconjugated bilirubin
↑ conjugated bilirubin

"Sick" liver

Bile

Bilirubin

Intestines

Panel 4
Posthepatic Dysfunction (Obstructive Jaundice)

RBCs

↑ conjugated bilirubin

Gallstone

No bilirubin

Intestines

Posthepatic Dysfunction. Panel 4. The liver is undamaged and is able to conjugate bilirubin and excrete it into the bile and larger bile ducts (biliary tree). However, obstruction to the flow of bile within the biliary tree causes a backup of bile into the liver. The "obstructed" bile contains conjugated bilirubin, which is then absorbed into the blood, causing hyperbilirubinemia and jaundice. Because the jaundice is due to the obstruction, as often occurs with inflammation, gallstones, and tumors, it is called *obstructive jaundice*. Because the dysfunction occurs after the liver has conjugated the bilirubin, it is called *posthepatic dysfunction.*

Diagnostic Tests for Jaundice. The serum bilirubin test helps diagnose jaundice and differentiate between the causes of jaundice. The serum bilirubin blood test measures two types of bilirubin: the amount of unconjugated bilirubin (recorded as the indirect reading) and the amount of conjugated bilirubin (recorded as the

direct reading). The total serum bilirubin is determined by adding the values of the indirect and direct readings. The total serum bilirubin is the amount of bilirubin the blood and is an indication of the intensity of the jaundice. It does not identify the cause of the jaundice. The cause of the jaundice is indicated by the indirect and direct readings. The indirect reading measures the amount of unconjugated bilirubin in the blood and, if elevated, is indicative of hemolytic jaundice or prehepatic dysfunction (see panel 2). The direct reading measures the amount of conjugated bilirubin in the blood and, if elevated, is indicative of obstructive jaundice or posthepatic dysfunction (see panel 4). Hepatocellular dysfunction, reflecting damage of some liver cells and intrahepatic swelling, can elevate both the indirect and direct readings. Hence, the serum bilirubin test indicates both the intensity of the jaundice and the specific causes of the jaundice.

As You Age

1. The volume and composition of blood remain constant with age, so most laboratory values remain normal. Alterations in laboratory values for blood usually indicate alterations in other organ systems. For example, the fasting blood glucose level increases with aging. This alteration is not the result of changes in the blood, however. Rather, it is the result of age-related changes associated with insulin. The same is true regarding serum lipid levels. Serum lipid levels increase 25% to 50% after the age of 55, but the increase is caused by an altered metabolism and not by changes in the blood and blood-forming organs.

2. The amount of red bone marrow decreases with age. The total number of blood cells remains normal, but older persons take longer to form new blood cells and hence recover more slowly from bleeding episodes.

3. An age-related decline occurs in white blood cell (WBC) activity. Although WBC activity still increases in response to infection, it does so more slowly.

Medical Terminology and Disorders   Disorders of the Blood

MEDICAL TERM	WORD PARTS	WORD PART MEANING OR DERIVATION	DESCRIPTION
Words			
ecchymosis	ecchy-	From the Greek word *eccym*, meaning "to pour out"	An **ecchymosis** is *a formation of escaped blood in the tissues from a blood vessel that has ruptured (commonly called a* bruise).
	-osis	condition or increase	
hematocrit	hemat/o-	blood	The **hematocrit** is *the ratio of the blood cells to the volume of the blood sample.*
	-crit	to separate	
normochromic	norm/o-	normal	**Normochromic** red blood cells (RBCs) contain a normal amount of hemoglobin; therefore, the color is normal. A hypochromic cell is pale, whereas a hyperchromic cell appears a deeper red.
	-chrom/o-	color	
	-ic	pertaining to	
myelodysplasia	myel/o-	bone marrow	Refers to *a group of disorders in which the bone marrow fails to produce blood cells, causing a reduction in RBCs, white blood cells (WBCs), and platelets.*
	-dys-	faulty	
	-plasia	formation	
petechiae		From an Italian word meaning "flea-bite," a reference to the appearance of petechiae	**Petechiae** are *tiny purple or red spots resulting from bleeding under the skin's surface.*
purpura		From a Latin word meaning "purple garment"	**Purpura** are *red or purple splotches under the skin or mucous membrane and are due to bleeding.*
Disorders			
anemia	an-	without	**Anemia** is *a deficiency of RBCs or hemoglobin, diagnostically indicated by a low hematocrit.* The reduction in RBCs leads to varying degrees of hypoxemia, the basis for most of the signs and symptoms. The etiological classification is based on the causes of anemia. Some of the anemias are described in the text. The macrocytic and normochromic anemias include folic acid deficiency anemia and pernicious anemia. Pernicious anemia is due to poor absorption of vitamin B_{12}, which in turn is due to the absence of adequate intrinsic factor normally secreted by the parietal cells in the stomach.
	-emia	condition of the blood	
hemolytic disorders	hem/o-	blood	**Hemolytic** refers to *the breakdown of RBCs, which leak their contents (hemoglobin, bilirubin, K^+) into the plasma.* There are many causes of hemolysis: infections, especially streptococcus and staphylococcus; antibody-inducing drugs; diseases such as sickle cell anemia (hemolytic crisis); the administration of incompatible blood; and hemolytic disease of the newborn (HDN).
	-lysis-	breakdown	
	-ic	pertaining to	

Continued

📖 Medical Terminology and Disorders   Disorders of the Blood—cont'd

MEDICAL TERM	WORD PARTS	WORD PART MEANING OR DERIVATION	DESCRIPTION
hemostatic disorders	hem/o-	blood	**Hemostatic** refers *to disorders that impair the ability of the blood to clot*. Disorders can be inherited or acquired (which is more common). **Thrombocytopenia,** *a reduction in platelets,* presents as spontaneous bleeding, such as hematuria, and prolonged bleeding from minor injuries. **Heparin-induced thrombocytopenia and thrombosis syndrome (HITTS),** also known as **white clot syndrome,** is of particular concern because of the frequent use of heparin as an anticoagulant. Heparin induces an immune response that causes platelet aggregation. **Hemophilia** refers to a group of bleeding disorders characterized by delayed coagulation and caused by a deficiency of a coagulation factor. **Hemophilia A,** the most common type, is due to a Factor VIII deficiency. Factor IX deficiency is called **hemophilia B** or **Christmas disease,** named for Stephan Christmas, the first patient diagnosed with factor IX deficiency. The chief symptom is bleeding, often into joints **(hemarthrosis).** Hemophilia (phil/o- = love) literally means "love of bleeding"; in this instance, love should be understood as a tendency to bleed. **Von Willebrand's disease** is the most common hereditary coagulation defect. It is a deficiency of von Willebrand factor, a protein that is necessary for platelet stickiness. **Disseminated intravascular coagulation (DIC),** despite its reference to coagulation, is characterized by excessive bleeding. An underlying condition stimulates accelerated clotting, depleting blood clotting factors and platelets and causing profuse hemorrhage.
	-stasis	stop or stand	
	-ic	pertaining to	
leukemias	leuk/o-	white	Also called *cancer of the blood,* **leukemia** is a hematological malignant condition in which there are excessive, immature ("blasts"), and abnormally functioning leukocytes. There are several classification systems. There are acute and chronic leukemias. There are also lymphocytic and myelocytic leukemias. The **lymphoblastic** or **lymphocytic leukemias** are caused by abnormal changes in bone marrow cells that give rise to B lymphocytes. The **myeloid** or **myelocytic leukemias** are caused by abnormal changes in bone marrow cells that give rise to RBCs, platelets, and some WBCs. Because the bone marrow becomes infiltrated with immature and abnormal leukocytes, hemopoiesis (blood formation) is severely impaired. The patient becomes anemic, thrombocytopenic, and neutropenic.
	-emia	blood condition	
hemorrhage	hem/o-	blood	**Hemorrhage** refers to *active bleeding*. The patient becomes symptomatic with a loss of 15% to 30% of the total blood volume. **Hemorrhage** is classified in stages depending on the amount of blood loss. Hemorrhage may be internal, as in the loss of blood from a ruptured aneurysm, or external as in bleeding from a laceration on the arm. With severe hemorrhage the patient can "bleed out" or "bleed to death." This is known in medical terminology as **exsanguinations** (*ex* = out of) and (*sanguis* = blood).
	-rrhage	to burst forth	
septicemia	sept-	rotten	Also called *blood poisoning* and refers to *the presence of harmful substances in the blood, such as pathogens and toxins*. Septicemia can cause a life-threatening septic shock.
	-emia	blood condition	

Get Ready for Exams!

Summary Outline

Blood has three main functions: it delivers oxygen to all cells; it helps regulate body functions, such as body temperature; and it protects the body from infection and bleeding.

I. **Blood Functions**
   A. Transport (O_2, CO_2, nutrients)
   B. Regulation (fluid/electrolyte, acid–base, temperature)
   C. Protection (infection, blood loss)

II. **Composition and Characteristics of Blood**
   A. Blood is composed of plasma and blood cells.
   B. The blood cells originate in the bone marrow and lymphoid tissue.
   C. Hemopoiesis: erythropoiesis, leukopoiesis, and thrombopoiesis

III. **Blood Cells**
   A. Red blood cells (RBCs) or erythrocytes
      1. RBCs are filled with hemoglobin.
      2. Oxyhemoglobin transports oxygen, and carbaminohemoglobin transports carbon dioxide.
      3. RBC production is regulated by erythropoietin (senses oxygen).
   B. White blood cells (WBCs)
      1. WBCs are classified as granulocytes and agranulocytes.
      2. The granulocytes are neutrophils, basophils, and eosinophils.
      3. The nongranulocytes are the lymphocytes and monocytes.
   C. Platelets
      1. Platelets are thrombocytes.
      2. Platelets are involved in hemostasis.

IV. **Hemostasis**
   A. Stages of hemostasis
      1. The three stages of hemostasis are blood vessel spasm, formation of a platelet plug, and blood coagulation.
      2. The three stages of blood coagulation are summarized in Fig. 15.10.
   B. Dissolving clots and preventing clot formation
      1. Eventually, the clot dissolves by a process called *fibrinolysis;* clot dissolution is achieved primarily by plasmin.
      2. Natural anticoagulant mechanisms include a smooth endothelial lining and heparin.

V. **Blood Types**
   A. ABO blood types
      1. There are four types of blood: A, B, AB, and O.
      2. The A and B antigens are on the membrane of the RBC.
      3. Blood plasma contains anti-A and anti-B antibodies.
      4. Blood antigen and antibodies are summarized in Table 15.3.
   B. Rh factor
      1. An Rh-positive person has the Rh antigen on the RBC membrane; an Rh-positive person does not have anti-Rh antibodies in the plasma.
      2. The Rh factor must be considered when blood is transfused; an Rh-negative person cannot receive Rh-positive blood.
      3. An Rh-negative mother carrying an Rh-positive baby may give birth to a baby with hemolytic disease of the newborn (HDN).

Review Your Knowledge

Matching: Blood Cells
Directions: Match the following words with their descriptions. Some words may be used more than once.
   a. platelets
   b. white blood cells
   c. red blood cells
   1. ___ Contains the antigens A and B
   2. ___ Requires erythropoietin for production
   3. ___ The reticulocyte is an immature cell of this type
   4. ___ Includes the neutrophil, eosinophil, and basophil
   5. ___ A deficiency causes petechiae and bleeding
   6. ___ Stickiness and plug both describe the functional role of this cell type
   7. ___ Primarily concerned with infection
   8. ___ Measured as the hematocrit
   9. ___ Classified as granulocytes and agranulocytes
   10. ___ Primarily concerned with the delivery of oxygen

Matching: Blood Clots
Directions: Match the following words with their descriptions. Some words may be used more than once.
   a. embolus
   b. plasmin
   c. heparin
   d. warfarin (Coumadin)
   e. thrombus
   1. ___ A blood clot in the leg
   2. ___ Drug that interferes with the hepatic utilization of vitamin K in the synthesis of prothrombin
   3. ___ A traveling or moving blood clot
   4. ___ Enzyme that dissolves clots
   5. ___ An anticoagulant that works by removing thrombin (antithrombin activity)

Matching: Blood Types
Directions: Match the following blood types with their descriptions. Some may be used more than once.
   a. A
   b. B
   c. AB
   d. O
   1. ___ The blood cells that contain neither the A antigen nor the B antigen
   2. ___ The universal donor
   3. ___ This blood type can receive type B and type A blood

4. ___ This blood type contains only anti-B antibodies

5. ___ This blood type contains both anti-A and anti-B antibodies

Multiple Choice

1. The erythrocyte
   a. is phagocytic.
   b. contains hemoglobin and transports oxygen.
   c. initiates blood coagulation.
   d. produces antibodies that are involved in the immune response.

2. The neutrophil
   a. is a T lymphocyte.
   b. is a granulocytic phagocyte.
   c. secretes antibodies.
   d. activates plasmin.

3. Thrombin
   a. activates fibrinogen.
   b. is responsible for the formation of the platelet plug.
   c. is inactivated by vitamin K.
   d. is inactivated by prothrombin.

4. What statement is true regarding the administration of type A+ blood to a type O– recipient?
   a. The blood types are compatible; no hemolytic reaction is expected.
   b. Persons with O– blood are allergic to type A+ blood.
   c. The administration of type A+ blood to a type O– recipient causes hemolysis.
   d. Persons with type O– blood can safely receive type A+ blood.

5. Erythropoietin
   a. is synthesized by the bone marrow.
   b. stimulates the bone marrow to make neutrophils.
   c. is released by the kidney in response to hypoxemia.
   d. is located within the RBC, where it binds loosely with O_2.

6. Which of the following is most likely to cause jaundice?
   a. Anemia
   b. A deficiency of erythropoietin
   c. A deficiency of intrinsic factor
   d. Hemolysis

7. Which of the following is a true statement?
   a. The reticulocyte is an immature thrombocyte.
   b. The neutrophil is a phagocytic granulocyte.
   c. The neutrophil, basophil, and eosinophil are fragments of the megakaryocyte.
   d. A deficiency of reticulocytes causes hypoprothrombinemia.

8. Hypoprothrombinemia and a prolonged prothrombin time is
   a. associated with bleeding.
   b. symptomatic of pernicious anemia.
   c. a consequence of heparin therapy.
   d. a consequence of thrombocytopenia.

9. Characteristics of hyperbilirubinemia include which of the following?
   a. Can be caused by hemolysis
   b. Causes jaundice
   c. Can cause kernicterus
   d. All of the above

10. Activation of plasminogen
    a. stimulates phagocytosis.
    b. activates the clotting cascade.
    c. dissolves blood clots.
    d. stimulates erythropoiesis.

11. Which of the following is most descriptive of neutrophils, lymphocytes, and monocytes?
    a. Granulocytes
    b. Thrombocytes
    c. Leukocytes
    d. Megakaryocytes

12. Clinically, a hematocrit is used to assess which of the following?
    a. The rate at which thrombin causes blood to clot
    b. The phagocytic activity of WBCs
    c. The percentage of RBCs in a sample of blood
    d. The number reticulocytes in a sample of blood

13. Which of the following is true of the words *hemostasis, hemolytic,* and *hematuria*?
    a. All refer to diseases of the blood.
    b. All refer to conditions that cause red blood cell destruction and jaundice.
    c. All refer to conditions that are caused by the failure of the red bone marrow to make RBCs.
    d. All refer to blood.

14. Which of the following is true of the words *neutropenia, thrombocytopenia,* and *granulocytopenia*?
    a. All refer to states of deficiency.
    b. All refer to leukocyte function.
    c. All refer to types of anemia.
    d. All refer to causes of leukocytosis.

15. Which of the following is *least* related to heme?
    a. Oxygen
    b. Phagocytosis
    c. RBC
    d. Iron

Go Figure

1. According to Fig. 15.1, a hematocrit reveals the
   a. composition of the buffy coat.
   b. composition of plasma.
   c. numbers and types of leukocytes.
   d. percentage of RBCs in a sample of blood.

2. Which of the following is correct according to Fig. 15.2?
   a. The reticulocyte is an immature thrombocyte.
   b. Neutrophils, basophils, and eosinophils are granulocytic and leukocytic.
   c. The megakaryocyte matures into an agranulocytic leukocyte.
   d. The mature erythrocyte is filled with granules and multiple nuclei.

3. Which of the following is correct according to Fig. 15.2?
   a. The stem cell is also called the *reticulocyte.*
   b. Platelets give rise to megakaryocytes.
   c. Lymphocytes and monocytes are granulocytes.
   d. Stem cells can differentiate into RBCs, WBCs, and platelets.

4. Which of the following is correct according to Fig. 15.4?
   a. Heme is a chain of amino acids.
   b. The globin chains are located within the RBCs; the heme is located on the outer surface of the RBC.

c. Heme is an iron-containing molecule.

d. RBCs are tucked within the four globin chains.

5. Which of the following is correct according to Fig. 15.5?

a. Erythropoiesis is stimulated by low levels of CO_2 in the blood.

b. The secretion of erythropoietin increases as blood levels of O_2 decrease.

c. Erythropoietin is secreted by the liver and stimulates the kidney to produce RBCs.

d. Erythropoietin is secreted by the bone marrow in response to decreased blood levels of O_2.

6. Which of the following is *not* correct according to Fig. 15.6?

a. Heme contains iron.

b. Bilirubin is one of the degradation products of heme.

c. Iron generated by the degradation of heme can be stored or recycled.

d. Only the globin part of hemoglobin can produce bilirubin.

7. Which of the following is correct according to Fig. 15.6?

a. Rapid hemolysis generates excess bilirubin.

b. Bilirubin is a degradation product of the globin chains.

c. Bilirubin is used to synthesize globin.

d. When heme is degraded, the iron is excreted into the bile for elimination in the stools.

8. Which of the following is correct according to Fig. 15.7?

a. Injured cells and pathogens diffuse into the blood vessels, where they are phagocytosed by the WBCs.

b. Hemoglobin-filled leukocytes squeeze out of the blood vessels in to carry O_2 to the injured cells.

c. Bilirubin-filled platelets plug small holes in the blood vessel wall.

d. Leukocytes squeeze through the blood vessel wall to phagocytose injured cells and pathogens.

9. According to Fig. 15.8, GRANpa BEN

a. is a reference to all RBCs.

b. refers to the granulocytes: basophils, eosinophils, and neutrophils.

c. refers to the agranulocytes: monocytes and lymphocytes.

d. refers to all blood cells produced by the red bone marrow.

10. Which of the following is correct according to Fig. 15.9?

a. Hemostasis is another name for trauma-induced hemorrhage.

b. Blood vessel spasm, platelet activation, and blood coagulation all play a role in hemostasis.

c. Fibrin threads are the most important component of the platelet plug.

d. *Hemostasis* and *homeostasis* mean the same thing.

11. Which of the following is correct according to Fig. 15.10?

a. Thrombin enhances the conversion of fibrinogen to fibrin strands.

b. Prothrombin activator is a consequence of blood vessel injury.

c. Coumadin interferes with the synthesis of prothrombin.

d. All of the above are true.

12. Which of the following is correct according to Fig. 15.10?

a. Thrombin enhances the synthesis of prothrombin.

b. Coumadin exerts an antithrombin effect.

c. Both Coumadin and heparin exert an anticoagulant effect by decreasing the hepatic utilization of vitamin K in the synthesis of prothrombin.

d. Heparin exerts an antithrombin effect, thereby delaying blood clotting.

13. Which of the following is correct according to Fig. 15.11?

a. Fibrin degradation products form blood clots in the presence of plasmin.

b. Plasmin works exclusively on platelets.

c. Plasmin dissolves clots.

d. Tissue plasminogen activators are drugs that enhance blood coagulation.

14. Which of the following is correct according to Fig. 15.12?

a. Anti-Rh antibodies are produced by the fetus.

b. The mother is initially Rh+ and becomes Rh− as anti-Rh antibodies accumulate.

c. The fetus is initially Rh+ and becomes Rh− as the disorder progresses.

d. The mother is Rh−, and the fetus is Rh+.

Anatomy of the Heart

Objectives

1. Describe the location of the heart.
2. Name the three layers and the covering of the heart.
3. Explain the function of the heart as two separate pumps.
4. Identify the four chambers and great vessels of the heart.
5. Explain the functions of the four heart valves.

6. Describe the physiological basis of the heart sounds.
7. Describe blood flow through the heart.
8. List the vessels that supply blood to the heart.
9. Identify the major components of the heart's conduction system.

Key Terms

aortic valve (p. 314)
atrioventricular valves (p. 313)
atrial conducting fibers (p. 318)
atrium (p. 312)
automaticity (p. 319)
AV node (p. 318)
bicuspid valve (p. 314)
cardiology (p. 308)
chordae tendineae (p. 313)
conduction system (p. 315)

coronary arteries (p. 315)
electrocardiogram (ECG) (p. 319)
endocardium (p. 310)
epicardium (p. 310)
great vessels (p. 313)
heart (p. 308)
His-Purkinje system (p. 319)
interatrial septum (p. 312)
interventricular septum (p. 312)
mitral valve (p. 314)

myocardium (p. 310)
pacemaker (p. 318)
pericardium (p. 310)
precordium (p. 309)
Purkinje fibers (p. 318)
rhythmicity (p. 319)
SA node (p. 318)
semilunar valves (p. 313)
tricuspid valve (p. 314)
ventricles (p. 312)

Throughout history, many functions have been attributed to the heart. Some philosophers have called it "the seat of the soul." The ancient Egyptians, for example, weighed the heart after a person's death because they believed that the weight of the heart equaled the weight of the soul. The heart has also been described as the seat of wisdom and understanding; accordingly, it thinks and makes plans. More often than not, however, history has portrayed the heart as the seat of the emotions. An overly compassionate person is described as soft-hearted, a generous person has a heart of gold, and a grief-stricken person is broken-hearted. The heart too gives one a sense of identity. Ask a person to point to herself... she will point to her heart and not to her brain. The word *courage* implies all of this and more. *Courage* is derived from a French word meaning "heart" and has long been used as a metaphor for inner strength; it is a word that fully embraces heart knowledge and heart power. Enter the world of the physiologist...the heart is defined as an adaptable, hard-working, and efficient pump...no feeling, thinking, or pining away.

The word root *cardi/o* refers to the heart. The study of the heart, especially with regard to diagnosis and treatment of disorders of the heart, is called cardiology.

FUNCTION, LOCATION, AND SIZE OF THE HEART

The heart is a hollow muscular organ. Its primary function is to pump and force blood through the blood vessels of the body, providing every cell in the body with vital nutrients and oxygen. The heart pumps an average of 72 times each minute for your entire lifetime. If you live until you are 75 years old, your heart will beat in excess of 3 billion times. Puts the Energizer Bunny to shame!

The adult heart is about the size of a closed fist and weighs less than 1 pound. The heart sits in the thoracic cavity within the lower mediastinum, between the two lungs and behind the sternum (Fig. 16.1). Two-thirds of the heart is located to the left of the midline of the sternum, and one-third is located

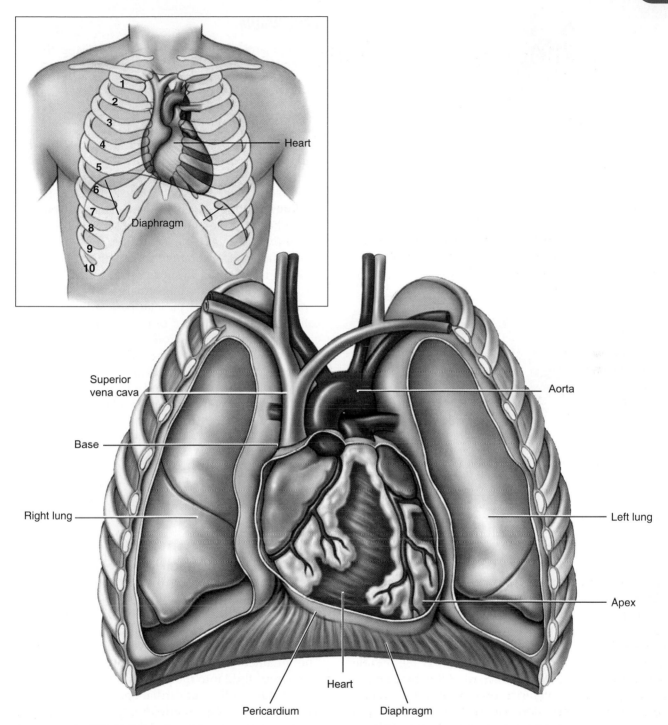

FIG. 16.1 Location of the heart. Note the location with regard to rib numbers, lungs, and diaphragm.

to the right. The upper flat portion of the heart, called the *base,* is located at the level of the second rib. The lower, more pointed end of the heart is the apex; it is located at the level of the fifth intercostal space. The **precordium** refers to the area of the anterior chest wall overlying the heart and great vessels. You need to know the precise location of the heart because you will be asked to evaluate different heart sounds, accurately position electrodes for an electrocardiogram, and provide life-saving cardiopulmonary resuscitation (CPR).

LAYERS AND COVERING OF THE HEART

The heart is made up of three layers of tissue: endocardium, myocardium, and epicardium (Fig. 16.2).

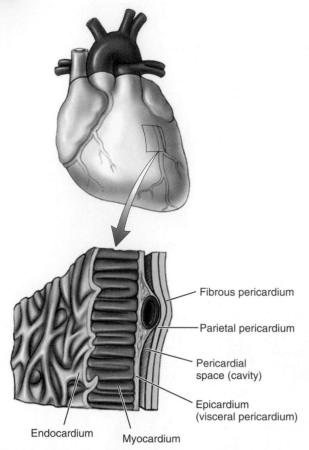

FIG. 16.2 Layers of the heart, pericardium, and pericardial space.

ENDOCARDIUM

The **endocardium** (en-doh-KAR-dee-um) is the heart's innermost layer. The endocardium also lines the valves and is continuous with the blood vessels that enter and leave the heart. The smooth and shiny surface allows blood to flow over it easily.

MYOCARDIUM

The **myocardium** (my-oh-KAR-dee-um) is the middle layer of the heart and is the thickest of the three layers. The myocardium is composed of cardiac muscle that contracts and pumps blood through the blood vessels. Myocardial fibers are striated and interconnected in a way that encourages the rapid spread of the electrical signal over the myocardium and a well-coordinated and forceful muscle contraction. (Review muscle contraction in Chapter 9, especially the "sliding" of actin and myosin.)

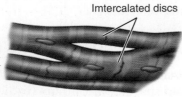

Cardiac muscle

EPICARDIUM

The **epicardium** (ep-i-KAR-dee-um) is the thin outermost layer of the heart. The epicardium also helps form the pericardium.

PERICARDIUM

The heart is supported by a slinglike structure called the **pericardium**. The pericardium attaches the heart to surrounding structures, such as the diaphragm and the large blood vessels that attach to the heart. The pericardium has three layers. The innermost layer (closest to the heart) is the epicardium, also called the *visceral pericardium*. The visceral pericardium folds back and becomes the *parietal pericardium*. The parietal pericardium attaches to the outer fibrous pericardium that anchors the heart to its surrounding structures. Between the visceral pericardium and parietal pericardium is a space called the *pericardial space*, or *pericardial cavity*. The pericardial membranes are serous membranes that secrete a small amount of slippery serous fluid (10 to 30 mL) into the pericardial space. The pericardial fluid lubricates the surfaces of the membranes and allows them to slide past one another with little friction or rubbing.

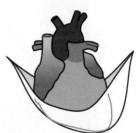

At times, the pericardial membranes become inflamed; this condition is called *pericarditis* and is characterized by pain and a sound called a *friction rub*. The friction rub is similar to the sound of scratchy sandpaper and is best heard when the stethoscope is placed over the left sternal border, near the apex of the heart. The inflamed pericardial membranes also secrete excess serous fluid into the pericardial space. This collection of fluid in the pericardial space (called *pericardial effusion*) may compress the heart externally, making it difficult for the heart to relax and fill with blood. Consequently, the heart is unable to pump a sufficient amount of blood to the body. This life-threatening condition is called *cardiac tamponade* (TAM-pon-ade). Cardiac tamponade may be treated by inserting a long needle into the pericardial space and aspirating (sucking out) the serous fluid through the needle.

❓ Re-Think

1. Locate the heart with specific references to the sternum and ribs.
2. List the three layers of the heart. Identify the pumping layer.
3. What is the function of the pericardium?

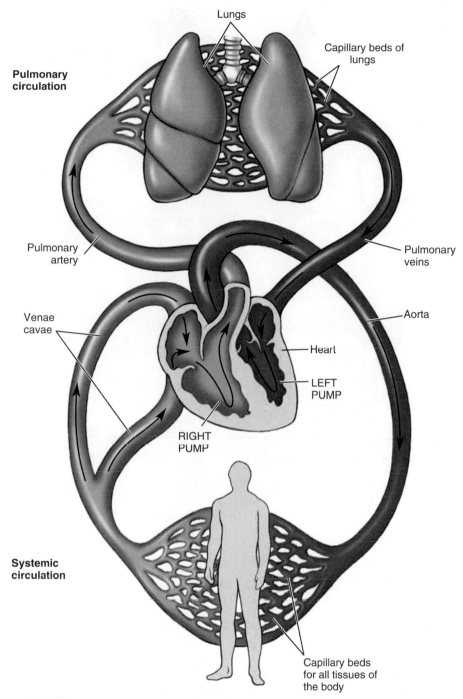

FIG. 16.3 Double pump and two circulations: pulmonary and systemic circulations.

A DOUBLE PUMP AND TWO CIRCULATIONS

The myocardium enables the heart to pump blood. The heart is a double pump that beats as one. The pumps are the right heart and the left heart (Fig. 16.3). The right heart receives unoxygenated blood from the superior and inferior venae cavae, large veins that collect blood from all parts of the body. The right heart, which is colored blue because it contains unoxygenated blood, pumps blood to the lungs, where the blood is oxygenated.

The path that the blood follows from the right side of the heart to and through the lungs and back to the left side of the heart is called the *pulmonary circulation*. The function of the pulmonary circulation is to pump blood through the lungs to pick up oxygen and get rid of carbon dioxide. Oxygen diffuses from the lungs into the blood for delivery to the tissues, whereas carbon dioxide diffuses from the blood into the lungs for excretion.

The left heart receives the oxygenated blood from the lungs and pumps it to all the organs of the body. The left heart is colored red because it contains oxygenated

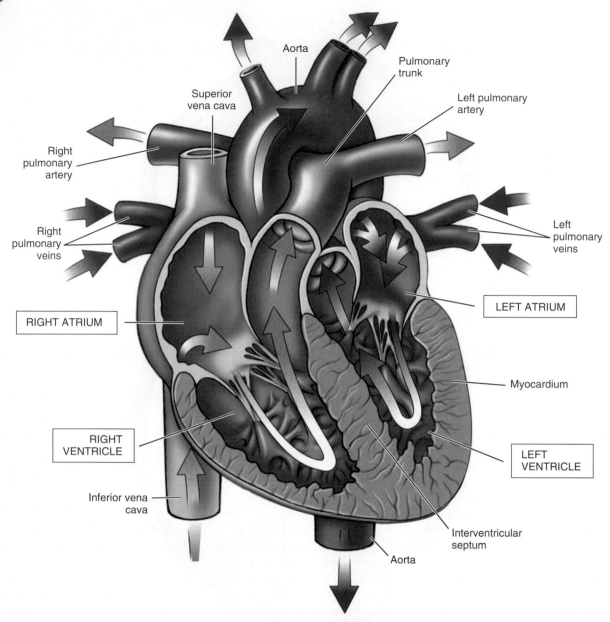

FIG. 16.4 **Chambers of the heart and the great vessels. The *arrows* indicate the blood flow through the heart.**

blood. The path that the blood follows from the left heart to all the organs of the body and back to the right heart is called the *systemic circulation*. The systemic circulation is the larger of the two circulations.

Re-Think

1. What is the right pump (heart)? Left pump (heart)?
2. Why are the two circulations color-coded red and blue?
3. What is the difference between the pulmonary and systemic circulations?

THE HEART'S CHAMBERS AND GREAT VESSELS

The heart has four chambers: two atria and two ventricles (Fig. 16.4). The atria (sing., **atrium**) are the upper chambers and receive the blood into the heart. The

ventricles (VEN-tri-kuls) are the lower chambers and pump blood out of the heart. The right and left hearts are separated from one another by two septa (sing., septum). The **interatrial septum** separates the two atria; the **interventricular septum** separates the two ventricles. Note the color coding. All structures that carry unoxygenated blood (right heart) are colored blue. All structures (left heart) that carry oxygenated blood are colored red.

RIGHT ATRIUM

The right atrium is a thin-walled cavity that receives unoxygenated blood from the superior and inferior venae cavae. The superior vena cava collects blood from the head and upper body region, whereas the inferior vena cava receives blood from the lower part of the body.

RIGHT VENTRICLE

The right ventricle receives unoxygenated blood from the right atrium. The primary function of the right ventricle is to pump blood through the pulmonary arteries to the lungs.

LEFT ATRIUM

The left atrium is a thin-walled cavity that receives oxygenated blood from the lungs through four pulmonary veins.

LEFT VENTRICLE

The left ventricle receives oxygenated blood from the left atrium. The primary function of the left ventricle is to pump blood into the systemic circulation. Blood leaves the left ventricle through the aorta, the largest artery of the body. Note the thickness of the myocardial layer of the ventricles as compared with the thinner atrial muscle. The thick muscle is needed to create enough force to pump blood out of the heart. Note also that the left ventricular myocardium is thicker than the right ventricular myocardium. This difference is the result of the greater amount of force required to pump blood into the systemic circulation (aorta).

As noted, the thickness of the myocardium reflects the amount of work performed by the myocardium. If a ventricle is forced to overwork, it will eventually enlarge—a condition called *ventricular hypertrophy*. For example, a chronically hypertensive (high blood pressure) person generally develops left ventricular hypertrophy. Why? The high blood pressure in the aorta makes it more difficult for the left ventricle to pump blood into the aorta. The left ventricle works harder and therefore enlarges, or hypertrophies. If the blood pressure is not lowered, the left ventricle will eventually weaken and fail as a pump. For the same reason, a person with pulmonary artery hypertension develops right ventricular hypertrophy and right heart failure.

GREAT VESSELS OF THE HEART

The large blood vessels attached to the heart are called the **great vessels**. They include the superior and inferior venae cavae, pulmonary trunk, four pulmonary veins, and the aorta.

 Sum It Up!

The heart, a hollow muscular organ that pumps blood, is located within the mediastinum of the thoracic cavity. The heart has three layers: endocardium, myocardium, and epicardium. It is supported and anchored by a slinglike pericardium. The heart is a double pump; the right heart pumps blood to the pulmonary circulation, and the left heart pumps blood to the systemic circulation. The heart has four chambers: two atria and two ventricles. The upper atria are receiving chambers, and the lower ventricles are pumping chambers. The great blood vessels carry blood to and from the heart.

HEART VALVES

The heart has four valves (Fig. 16.5). The purpose of the heart valves is to keep the blood flowing in a forward direction. The valves lie at the entrance and exit of the ventricles. Two of the valves are called **atrioventricular valves** (AV valves), which are located between the atria and the ventricles. Blood flows from the atria through the AV valves into the ventricles. AV valves, which look like basketball nets, are entrance valves because they allow blood to enter the ventricles.

The other two valves are classified as **semilunar valves**, so-named because the cusps of the valves resemble a half-moon (*semi-* means "half," *lunar* means "moon"). The semilunar valves control the outflow of blood from the right and left ventricles and are therefore exit valves.

ATRIOVENTRICULAR VALVES

The AV valves are located between the atria and the ventricles on each side of the heart. The AV valves have cusps or leaflets (see Fig. 16.5). When the ventricles are relaxed, the cusps hang loosely within the ventricles; in this position, the valves are open and permit the flow of blood from the atria into the ventricles.

What closes the AV valves? Pressure! When the ventricles contract, the heart muscle compresses or squeezes the blood in the ventricles. The blood then gets behind and pushes the cusps upward toward the atria, into a closed position. The closed AV valves prevent the backward flow of blood from the ventricles to the atria.

Why are the cusps not pushed completely through the openings, into the atria, as the pressures within the ventricles increase during muscle contraction? The cusps are attached to the ventricular wall by tough fibrous bands of tissue called **chordae tendineae** (KOR-day ten-din-EE-ay). The chordae tendineae, in turn, are attached to papillary muscles in the ventricular walls. As blood pushes the cusps into a closed position, the papillary muscles contract, pulling on the chordae tendineae. The stretched chordae tendineae hold on to the cusps and prevent them from "blowing" through into the atria, like a storm-blown, inside-out umbrella.

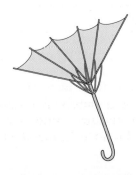

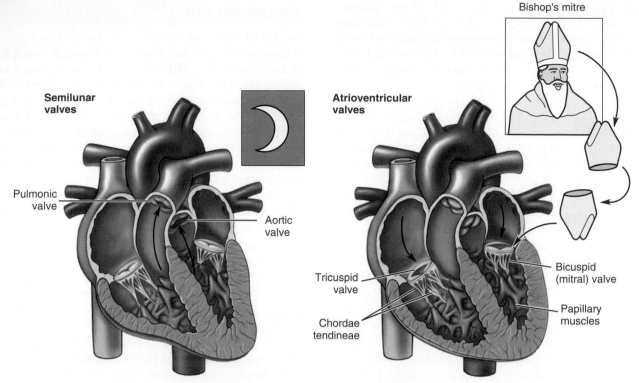

FIG. 16.5 Valves of the heart: semilunar valves and atrioventricular valves.

The right AV valve is located between the right atrium and the right ventricle. The right AV valve is called the **tricuspid valve** because it has three cusps. When the tricuspid valve is open, blood flows from the right atrium into the right ventricle. When the right ventricle contracts, however, the tricuspid valve closes and prevents blood from flowing back into the right atrium. The valve ensures a forward flow of blood.

The left AV valve is located between the left atrium and the left ventricle. The left AV valve is called the **bicuspid valve** because it has two cusps. It is also known as the **mitral valve** because it resembles a bishop's mitre—a hat with two cusps or flaps. When the mitral valve is open, blood flows from the left atrium into the left ventricle. When the left ventricle contracts, the mitral valve closes and prevents the flow of blood from the left ventricle back into the left atrium.

SEMILUNAR VALVES

The two semilunar valves (exit valves) are the pulmonic and aortic semilunar valves (see Fig. 16.5).

PULMONIC VALVE

The pulmonic semilunar valve is also called the *right semilunar valve*. It is located between the right ventricle and the pulmonary trunk. When the right ventricle relaxes, the valve is in a closed position. When the right ventricle contracts, thus increasing intraventricular pressure, blood from the ventricle forces the pulmonic valve open. Blood then flows into the pulmonary

trunk, the large vessel that carries the blood from the right ventricle to the right and left pulmonary arteries and lungs. When the right ventricle relaxes, the pulmonic valve snaps closed and prevents any blood from returning to the right ventricle from the pulmonary trunk.

AORTIC VALVE

The aortic semilunar valve or the left semilunar valve is located between the left ventricle and the aorta. When the left ventricle relaxes, the valve is in a closed position. When the left ventricle contracts, thus increasing intraventricular pressure, blood from the ventricles forces the **aortic valve** open and flows into the aorta. When the left ventricle relaxes, the aortic valve snaps closed and prevents any backflow of blood from the aorta into the ventricle.

How and why do the semilunar valves close? Pressure! The semilunar valves close when the pressure in the pulmonary trunk and the aorta becomes greater than the pressure in the relaxed ventricles. The blood in these large blood vessels gets behind the cusps of the valves, snapping them closed. The closed semilunar valves prevent the backward flow of blood from the pulmonary trunk and aorta into the ventricles. To repeat: Valves open and close in response to the changing pressures within the heart chambers.

Valves are sometimes defective; they can become narrow or incompetent. Narrowing of the valve is called *stenosis*. A stenotic valve makes it difficult for a heart chamber to force blood through the stenosed valve, thereby increasing the work of the pumping chamber. Thus, aortic valve stenosis increases the work of the left ventricle, causing left ventricular hypertrophy and failure. What happens when a heart valve becomes leaky? A leaky, or incompetent, valve allows blood to regurgitate or leak back into the chamber from which it has just been pumped. For example, an incompetent aortic valve allows blood that has been pumped into the aorta to leak back into the left ventricle. The left ventricle must then pump the same blood again. Over time, stenotic and leaky valves damage the heart.

 Re-Think

1. List and locate the atrioventricular valves.
2. List and locate the semilunar valves.
3. Explain the reason for the following: When the ventricles contract, the AV valves close and the semilunar valves open.
4. Explain the reason for the following: When the ventricles relax, the AV valves open, and the semilunar valves close.

HEART SOUNDS

The heart sounds ("lubb-dupp, lubb-dupp") are made by the vibrations caused by the closure of the valves. When valves become faulty, the heart sounds change. Abnormal heart sounds are called *murmurs*.

The heart sounds can be heard through a stethoscope placed over the chest wall. The first heart sound (the "lubb") is called S_1. S_1 is caused by the closure of the AV valves at the beginning of ventricular contraction; it is best heard over the apex of the heart. The second heart sound (the "dupp") is called S_2. S_2 is caused by the closure of the semilunar valves at the beginning of ventricular relaxation. S_2 can be heard best at the base of the heart. Listening to S_1 and S_2 is like the sound made by drumming two fingers on a table. Sometimes extra sounds (called S_3 and S_4) can be heard; they are due to vibrations caused by the rapid flow of blood into the ventricles. When both S_3 and S_4 occur, a "gallop rhythm" is heard, which sounds like a galloping horse.

 Sum It Up!

The purpose of the heart valves is to keep blood flowing forward. There are four heart valves. The two atrioventricular valves are the tricuspid (right heart) and the bicuspid or mitral valves (left heart). The two semilunar valves are the pulmonic (right heart) and aortic (left heart) semilunar valves. The heart sounds ("lubb-dupp") are caused by the closure of the valves. S_1 (lupp) is caused by the closure of the AV valves at the beginning of ventricular contraction. S_2 (dupp) is caused by closure of the semilunar valves at the beginning of ventricular relaxation.

PATHWAY OF BLOOD FLOW THROUGH THE HEART

The arrows in Fig. 16.4 indicate the pathway of blood as it flows through the heart. Unoxygenated blood enters the right atrium from the superior and inferior venae cavae. The blood flows through the tricuspid valve into the right ventricle. From the right ventricle, the blood flows through the pulmonic valve into the pulmonary trunk. The pulmonary trunk branches into the right and left pulmonary arteries. The right and left pulmonary arteries carry unoxygenated blood to the right and left lungs for gas exchange. The blood releases carbon dioxide as waste and picks up a fresh supply of oxygen. Note the blue color coding of the right heart structures.

The oxygenated blood flows through four pulmonary veins from the lungs into the left atrium. From the left atrium, the blood flows through the bicuspid, or mitral, valve into the left ventricle. Left ventricular contraction forces blood through the aortic valve into the aorta for distribution to the systemic circulation. The pathway of blood flow through the heart and pulmonary circulation is summarized in Fig. 16.6.

 Re-Think

1. What is the cause of "lubb" (S_1) and "dupp" (S_2)?
2. Describe the path of the flow of blood through the right heart. Describe the path of the flow of blood through the left heart.

BLOOD SUPPLY TO THE MYOCARDIUM

Although blood constantly flows through the chambers of the heart, this blood does not nourish the myocardium. The blood supply that nourishes and oxygenates the myocardium is provided by the coronary arteries (Fig. 16.7). The arteries supplying the myocardium are called **coronary arteries** because they resemble a crown encircling the heart. The coronary arteries arise from the base of the ascending aorta, just distal to the aortic semilunar valve.

The two main coronary arteries are the left and right coronary arteries. The right coronary artery nourishes the right side of the heart, especially the right ventricle. It also supplies blood to the parts of the electrical **conduction system**, including the sinoatrial (SA) node and the atrioventricular (AV) node. These nodes are important in establishing the normal heart rate and rhythm and will be described more fully later in the chapter. The left coronary artery branches into the left anterior descending (LAD) artery and the circumflex artery. These arteries carry blood to the left side of the heart, especially the left ventricular wall and interventricular septum. Small branches of the right and left coronary

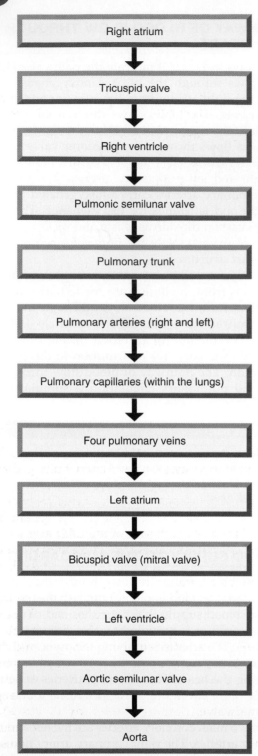

FIG. 16.6 **Blood flow through the heart and pulmonary circulation.**

arteries fuse, forming interconnections, called *anastomoses*, that help maintain an adequate blood supply to the myocardium, despite pressure fluctuations within the heart. The coronary veins collect the blood that nourishes the myocardium. The coronary veins carry the blood to the coronary sinus, which empties the blood into the right atrium.

Coronary blood flow has three important characteristics:

- Coronary blood flow can increase. The heart must have a constant supply of oxygenated blood. Under resting conditions, the heart muscle removes almost all the oxygen from the blood flowing through the coronary arteries. Thus, if the heart needs more oxygen, coronary arteries dilate, and blood flow increases. With exertion, coronary blood flow can increase up to nine times in the normal heart. However, coronary arteries that have severe fatty plaque buildup are usually maximally dilated at rest. With exertion, coronary blood flow cannot increase, and the myocardium experiences oxygen deprivation. Thus, patients with coronary artery disease will often experience pain (angina) with exertion.

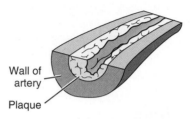

Wall of artery

Plaque

- Coronary blood flow is greatest during myocardial relaxation. Why? Because contraction of the myocardium externally compresses or squeezes the coronary arteries, thereby cutting off blood flow. When the heart muscle relaxes, the coronary arteries open, thereby restoring blood flow. When the relaxation phase is shortened, as in a "racing heart," coronary blood flow decreases, and the myocardial cells may experience signs of oxygen deprivation, causing chest pain (angina).
- Coronary arteries can form anastomoses, or multiple connections between the arteries. An anastomosis allows blood to flow around an artery that is blocked. Additional collateral blood vessels develop in response to chronic diminished coronary blood flow, as often occurs with aging and chronic coronary artery disease. For this reason, older persons often experience less myocardial damage from a heart attack than younger persons.

? Re-Think

1. What is the purpose of coronary blood flow?
2. Name the two coronary arteries. Name the two branches of the left coronary artery.
3. Why is coronary blood flow highest when the myocardium is relaxed?

ISCHEMIA AND INFARCTION

If coronary blood flow diminishes, the myocardium experiences oxygen deprivation (ischemia) and soon informs its owner of the situation. For example, a coronary artery may become partially occluded by fatty

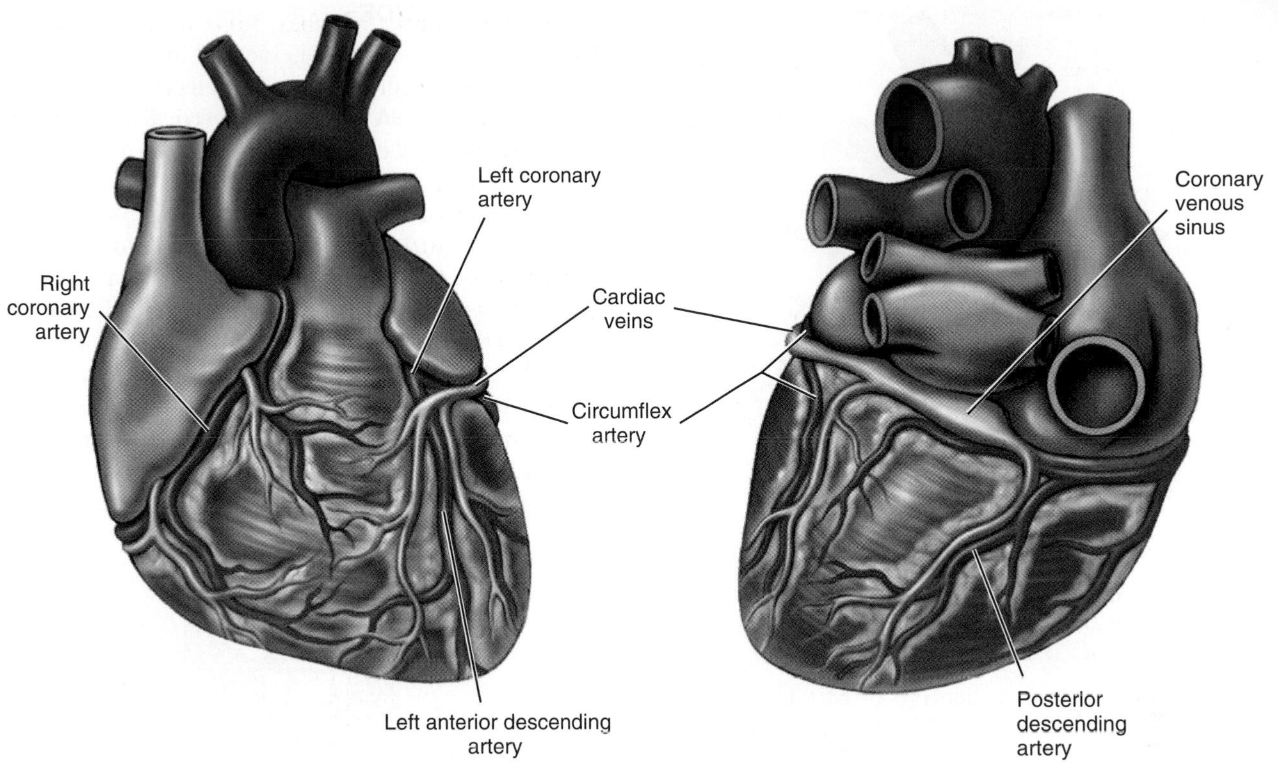

FIG. 16.7 **Blood supply to the heart: coronary blood vessels.**

plaque or blood vessel spasm, thereby diminishing coronary blood flow. The person experiences chest pain that often radiates to the left shoulder and down the left arm into the fingers (referred pain). "Pain at the pump"? Think angina. Angina is often relieved by rest and the administration of drugs such as nitroglycerin and beta-adrenergic blockers that decrease the work of the heart.

Do You Know...

About Balloons and CABGs as Treatment for Coronary Artery Disease?

Angina is usually caused by the accumulation of fatty plaque within the coronary arteries. Coronary artery occlusion is often treated with balloon therapy. A deflated balloon is inserted into the coronary artery. It is then inflated against the fatty plaque, flattening the plaque against the arterial wall and restoring coronary blood flow. A stent is then inserted to maintain the opening of the coronary vessel. A stent is a hollow, wire mesh cylinder that looks like a tiny Slinky. Improved cardiac blood flow improves myocardial oxygenation, reduces chest pain, and prevents myocardial damage. A patient may not be a suitable candidate for balloon angioplasty and stent; instead, he or she may require a CABG (pronounced like the vegetable, cabbage). CABG refers to a *coronary artery bypass graft*, whereby the surgeon bypasses the obstructions in the coronary vessels with donor blood vessels.

Sometimes, the coronary artery occlusion worsens when a platelet-containing fatty plaque ruptures and completely blocks coronary blood flow. The oxygen-deprived myocardial cells die, causing a myocardial

infarction (MI), or heart attack. A man having a heart attack often experiences nausea and vomiting, diaphoresis (profuse sweating), and severe crushing chest pain. With a fist clenched over his heart, he may complain that the pain feels as though an elephant is sitting on his chest. Occlusion of the LAD artery is particularly devastating because it oxygenates so much of left ventricle. For this reason, occlusion of the LAD is called the *widow maker*.

Older people and women who experience an MI may present a very different clinical picture. For example, many do not experience crushing chest pain and diaphoresis. They often complain of fatigue and digestive symptoms, such as heartburn and upset stomach. Depending on the severity and location of the infarction, the person may recover uneventfully or experience a lethal electrical disturbance (dysrhythmia), cardiogenic shock, or heart failure. Time to treatment is crucial! Cardiologists have a saying: "Time is muscle." The faster the intervention, the less myocardial damage is sustained.

CARDIAC ENZYMES AND LEAKY CELLS

The dead myocardial cells leak enzymes into the blood, causing plasma elevations of cardiac enzymes such as creatine phosphokinase (CPK), aspartate aminotransferase (AST), and lactic dehydrogenase (LDH). A regulator myocardial protein, called *troponin*, also leaks out of the necrotic myocardium into the blood. Thus, plasma elevations of CPK, AST,

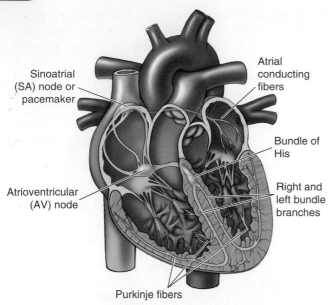

Sinoatrial (SA) node or pacemaker

Atrial conducting fibers

Bundle of His

Atrioventricular (AV) node

Right and left bundle branches

Purkinje fibers

FIG. 16.8 Conduction system of the heart.

LDH, and troponin are indicative of MI. The leaked enzymes thus provide a valuable diagnostic tool for heart attacks.

◎ Sum It Up!

Blood flows from the right atrium to the right ventricle, where it is pumped to the lungs for oxygenation (pulmonary circulation). Oxygenated blood returns to the left atrium and then to the left ventricle where it is pumped into the aorta and systemic circulation. The myocardium (pump) is nourished by the left and right coronary arteries. Coronary blood flow must be maintained if the heart is to function normally. Coronary blood flow is greatest during ventricular relaxation. Occlusion of the coronary arteries is a major cause of disability and death.

CARDIAC CONDUCTION SYSTEM

How does the heart know when to contract (pump) and when to relax? The heart's conduction system initiates an electrical signal and then moves that signal along a special pathway through the heart. The cardiac conduction system not only provides the stimulus (cardiac impulse) for muscle contraction but also coordinates the pumping activity of the atria and ventricles. First, both atria must contract, forcing blood into the relaxed ventricles. Then, the ventricles contract, forcing blood out of the heart. The cardiac conduction system gets it going and keeps it organized!

PARTS OF THE CARDIAC CONDUCTION SYSTEM

The conduction system is located within the walls and septum of the heart. The conduction system consists of the following structures: the sinoatrial node, the atrial conducting fibers, the atrioventricular node, and the His-Purkinje system (Fig. 16.8).

SINOATRIAL NODE

The sinoatrial (SA) node is located in the upper posterior wall of the right atrium. An electrical signal originates within the **SA node**. The electrical signal is called the *action potential* or the *cardiac impulse*. In this chapter, we use the term *cardiac impulse*.

The SA node fires a cardiac impulse 60 to 100 times per minute (average, 72 times/min). Because the firing of the SA node sets the rate at which the heart beats, or contracts and relaxes, the SA node is called the **pacemaker** of the heart. The heart rate is set by this pacemaker, just as the speed of a race is set by the pace car. If the electrical signal originates outside of the SA node, it is referred to as *ectopic*.

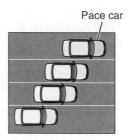

Pace car

ATRIAL CONDUCTING FIBERS

The cardiac impulse spreads from the SA node through both atria along the **atrial conducting fibers**. The signal also spreads to the AV node.

ATRIOVENTRICULAR NODE

The atrioventricular (AV) node is located in the floor of the right atrium, near the interatrial septum. The purpose of the **AV node** is twofold: (1) it acts as a path for the cardiac impulse to travel from the atrial conducting fibers into the ventricular bundle of His, and (2) the AV node slows the cardiac impulse as it moves through the AV node into the bundle of His.

The slowing of the cardiac impulse by the AV node is important because it delays ventricular activation and allows the relaxed ventricle time to fill with blood during atrial contraction.

NOTE: Do not confuse the AV node with the AV valve.

HIS-PURKINJE SYSTEM

The cardiac impulse next enters the bundle of His, specialized conduction tissue located in the interventricular septum. The bundle of His divides into two branches: the right and left bundle branches. These branches send out numerous long fibers called **Purkinje fibers**. Purkinje (pur-KIN-jee) fibers are distributed throughout the ventricular myocardium. Purkinje fibers conduct the cardiac impulse very rapidly throughout the ventricles, thereby ensuring a coordinated contraction of both ventricles.

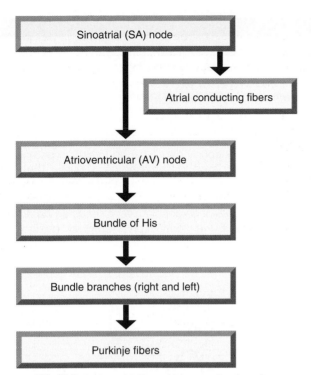

FIG. 16.9 Pathway followed by a cardiac impulse.

The pathway followed by the cardiac impulse in the **His-Purkinje system** is summarized in Fig. 16.9. Be sure you can trace the path of the cardiac impulse from its origin, the SA node, to its destination, the Purkinje fibers.

AUTOMATICITY AND RHYTHMICITY

Your heart has automaticity and rhythmicity. **Automaticity** refers to the ability of cardiac pacemaker cells to generate their own electrical signal with no help from extrinsic nerves coming from the central nervous system. The signal arises automatically (see the Ramp It Up!: Pacemaker Cells box). Because cardiac tissue fires a cardiac impulse regularly, the heart is said to have **rhythmicity**. Feel the rhythmicity of your heart rate at the radial (wrist) pulse.

NORMAL, SLOW, AND SLOWER

Not all pacemaker cells fire at the same rate. The SA node is *the* pacemaker of the heart; it sets the heart rate between 60 and 100 beats/min. There are many other pacemaker cells within the heart, but they fire at a slower rate. For example, when the SA node fails to function as a pacemaker, the AV takes over and fires at a slower rate of 40 to 60 beats/min. Sometimes the ventricles assume the pacemaker role and fire at a much slower rate of 30 to 40 beats/min. Impaired pacemaker activity is common and often requires the insertion of an artificial pacemaker.

At times, the rhythm of the heart is disturbed; the heart is then said to be dysrhythmic (meaning "difficulty with rhythm"). Some dysrhythmias are relatively harmless; others are life threatening and demand immediate attention. For example, ventricular fibrillation is a life-threatening dysrhythmia because it causes the ventricular myocardium to fibrillate. A fibrillating muscle merely quivers and is unable to contract and pump blood. Dysrhythmias that are caused by excess electrical activity are called *tachydysrhythmias*, whereas dysrhythmias characterized by diminished electrical activity are called *bradydysrhythmias*.

> **? Re-Think**
>
> 1. Trace the electrical signal (cardiac impulse) from its origin to the ventricles.
> 2. Why is it important that the AV node slows the conduction of the cardiac impulse from the atria to the ventricles?
> 3. What happens if the AV nodal rate exceeds the rate of the SA node?

ELECTROCARDIOGRAM

The cardiac impulse that stimulates muscle contraction is an electrical signal. The entire electrical activity of the heart is measured by placing electrodes on the surface of the chest and attaching the electrodes to a recording device. The record of these electrical signals is called an **electrocardiogram (ECG)** (Fig. 16.10).

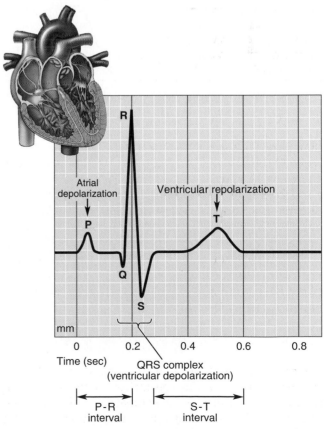

FIG. 16.10 Electrocardiogram (ECG).

↗ Ramp It Up!

Pacemaker Cells

Before answering the question, "What is a pacemaker cell?," let's review the terms used to describe an action potential. Resting membrane potential (RMP) refers to the electrical charge across the membrane of a resting cell. The RMP is negative; that is, the inside of the resting cell is negative. When the cell is stimulated, it depolarizes to threshold potential. If threshold potential is not reached, the signal decays, and the cell returns to its RMP. If, however, threshold potential is reached, the cell proceeds to depolarize fully to +20 mV. At the end of depolarization (+20mV), the cell repolarizes, meaning that it returns to its negative RMP. The cell remains at RMP until it is stimulated again. This last sentence is key: the cell remains in its RMP until it is stimulated again (see Chapter 10 for a more complete description of the action potential).

Panel A shows the action potential of the SA node (pacemaker) cell. The SA node does not have a stable RMP; the cell momentarily rests at −60 mV. The membrane immediately and spontaneously depolarizes to its threshold potential (−40 mV) and fires an action potential. The important term is *spontaneous depolarization*. The slope of the spontaneous depolarization is called the *pacemaker potential*. Repolarization resets the action potential to −60 mV. The spontaneous depolarization immediately begins again, thereby firing a second action potential. Note that a pacemaker cell is not stimulated to fire an action potential—it fires "on its own"—and it fires rhythmically.

Panel A: SA node action potential

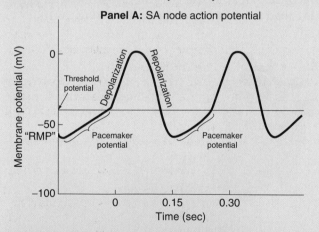

Can the rate of spontaneous depolarization change?

Yes. The faster the rate of spontaneous depolarization, the faster the heart rate. The slower the rate of spontaneous depolarization, the slower the heart rate. Several factors affect the rate of spontaneous depolarization. First, autonomic nerve stimulation affects the rate of spontaneous depolarization. Sympathetic nerve stimulation increases the rate of spontaneous depolarization, thereby increasing heart rate. Excessive sympathetic stimulation can cause tachycardia and tachydysrhythmias. Parasympathetic or vagal stimulation slows the rate of spontaneous depolarization, thereby slowing heart rate. Intense vagal discharge, in fact, can cause bradycardia and heart block, and even cardiac standstill. Hormones and drugs also affect the rates of depolarization.

Panel B shows a comparison of the action potential of the SA and AV nodes. Note that both the SA and AV nodes can both spontaneously depolarize to threshold potential. Thus, both cells have pacemaker capabilities. The SA node, however, is *the* pacemaker. Why? The SA node spontaneously depolarizes at a faster rate than the AV node. Once the SA node depolarizes, it sends an electrical signal throughout the conduction system of the heart, including the AV node. Consequently, all cells, including the AV node, must repolarize and thus reset to the RMP. Why isn't the AV node the pacemaker? The SA depolarizes at a faster rate.

Panel B: SA and AV node action potentials

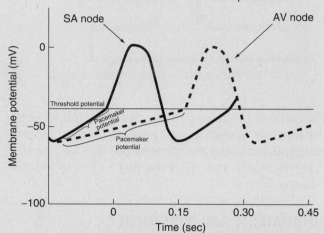

Can the AV node ever become the pacemaker?

Yes. If the rate of SA node activity slows too much or if the rate of the AV node increases too much, the AV node can assume the role of pacemaker activity. This is called *nodal rhythm*. For example, a diseased SA node, such as in sick sinus syndrome or scarring of the conduction pathway, can seriously depress SA node activity, thereby allowing the AV to take over as pacemaker. Typically, the slower nodal rhythm generates a heart rate of 40 to 50 beats/min.

There are even pacemaker cells in the conduction tissue of the ventricles. These ventricular pacemaker cells spontaneously depolarize very slowly and therefore rarely function as the pacemaker. However, in complete heart block, a condition in which no electrical signal crosses the AV node into the His-Purkinje system, the ventricular pacemaker cells take over as the pacemaker, typically generating a heart rate of 30 to 40 beats/min. This excessively slow heart rate decreases cardiac output and requires the implantation of an artificial pacemaker. An artificial pacemaker "drives" the ventricles at a higher rate, thereby increasing cardiac output.

The components of the ECG include a P wave, a QRS complex, and a T wave. The P wave reflects the electrical activity associated with atrial depolarization. The QRS complex reflects the electrical activity associated with ventricular depolarization. Depolarization precedes and triggers contraction of the heart muscle. The T wave reflects the electrical activity associated with ventricular repolarization. (See Chapter 10 for a review of polarization, depolarization, and repolarization.)

In addition to identifying areas of depolarization and repolarization, the P, QRS, and T deflections (waves) of the ECG provide other useful information. For example, the P-R interval represents the time it takes for the cardiac impulse to travel from the atria (P wave) to the ventricles (QRS complex). Other measurements include the width of the QRS complex and the length of the S-T interval. Normal sinus rhythm (NSR) means that the ECG appears normal and that the impulse originates in the SA node.

Note that the ECG is recorded on special graph paper that allows electrical events to be timed. The clinician can determine whether the electrical signals are moving too fast or too slow or generating an irregular pattern.

◎ Sum It Up!

Heart muscle contracts in response to an electrical signal called the *cardiac impulse*, which spreads throughout the heart, coordinating cardiac muscle contraction. The cardiac impulse normally arises within the SA node and spreads throughout both atria over specialized conduction tissue. The cardiac impulse then enters the AV node, where it is momentarily delayed before entering the His-Purkinje system in the ventricles. Cardiac conduction tissue displays automaticity and rhythmicity. The electrical events are recorded as the electrocardiogram (ECG).

Note: The As You Age box and the Medical Terminology and Disorders table appear in Chapter 17.

Get Ready for Exams!

Summary Outline

The heart is a four-chambered pump that delivers blood to the pulmonic and systemic circulations.

I. Function, Location, and Size of the Heart
  A. The heart (size of a fist) is located in the lower mediastinum, toward the left side of the sternum.
  B. It is located between the second rib and fifth intercostal space.
  C. The heart pumps blood throughout the body, delivering oxygen and nutrients and picking up waste.

II. The Heart's Layers and Covering
  A. The heart has three layers: endocardium, myocardium, and epicardium.
  B. The heart is supported by a slinglike pericardium.
  C. Two layers of the pericardium form the pericardial space (contains serous fluid).

III. A Double Pump and Two Circulations
  A. The right heart pumps blood to the lungs for oxygenation (called the pulmonary circulation).
  B. The left heart pumps blood throughout the rest of the body (called the systemic circulation).

IV. The Heart's Chambers and Great Vessels
  A. The heart has four chambers: two atria and two ventricles.
  B. The atria receive the blood and the ventricles pump the blood to the pulmonary and systemic circulations.

V. Heart Valves
  A. The purpose of heart valves is to keep blood flowing in a forward direction.
  B. Two atrioventricular (AV) valves are the tricuspid valve (right heart) and the bicuspid (mitral) valve (left heart).
  C. The two semilunar valves are the pulmonic valve (right heart) and the aortic valve (left heart).

VI. Heart Sounds
  A. The heart sounds ("lubb-dupp") are made by the vibrations caused by closure of the valves.
  B. The "lubb" (S_1) is caused by the closure of the AV valves at the beginning of ventricular contraction. The "dupp" (S_2) is caused by the closure of the semilunar valves at the beginning of ventricular relaxation.

VII. Pathway: Blood Flow Through the Heart
  A. The right heart receives blood from the venae cavae and pumps it to the lungs for oxygenation. The left heart receives oxygenated blood from the lungs and pumps it to the systemic circulation.
  B. Blood flow through the heart is summarized in the flowchart in Fig. 16.6.
  C. Shunts alter the path of blood flow through the heart.

VIII. Blood Supply to the Myocardium
  A. The left and right coronary arteries supply the myocardium with oxygen and nutrients. The left coronary artery branches into the left anterior descending (LAD) artery and the circumflex artery.
  B. The coronary veins drain the unoxygenated blood and empty it into the coronary sinus, which empties into the right atrium.

IX. Cardiac Conduction System
  A. The SA node generates an electrical signal (cardiac impulse) that moves throughout the heart in a coordinated way. The electrical signal causes the myocardium to contract.
  B. The pathway followed by the cardiac impulse is summarized in Fig. 16.9.
  C. Cardiac muscle displays automaticity and rhythmicity.
  D. The SA node is the pacemaker of the heart. Pacemaker cells throughout the heart fire at different rates: normal, slow, and slower.
  E. The electrical activity of cardiac muscle is recorded as an electrocardiogram.

Review Your Knowledge

Matching: Structures of the Heart

Directions: Match the following words with their descriptions. Some words may be used more than once.

a. left ventricle
b. coronary arteries
c. right atrium
d. left atrium
e. right ventricle
f. myocardium
g. pericardium
h. precordium

1. _g_ Slinglike structure that supports the heart
2. _b_ Delivers oxygenated blood to the myocardium
3. _f_ Layer of the heart that contains actin and myosin; arranged in sarcomeres
4. _c_ Chamber that receives unoxygenated blood from the venae cavae
5. _D_ Chamber that receives oxygenated blood from the four pulmonary veins
6. _a_ Chamber that pumps blood into the aorta
7. _a_ Chamber that has the thickest myocardium
8. _e_ Chamber that pumps blood into the pulmonary artery
9. _d_ The left ventricle receives oxygenated blood from this chamber
10. _h_ Refers to the area of the chest that overlies the heart

Matching: Valves

Directions: Match the following words with their descriptions. Some words may be used more than once.

a. aortic
b. tricuspid
c. bicuspid
d. pulmonic

1. _d_ The semilunar valve through which blood exits the right ventricle
2. _d_ The exit valve for the right ventricle
3. _b_ The atrioventricular valve that "sees" unoxygenated blood
4. _c_ The valve that is also called the mitral valve
5. _a_ The semilunar valve through which blood exits the left ventricle
6. _c_ The AV valve that "sees" oxygenated blood
7. _c_ The AV valve located between the left atrium and left ventricle
8. _d_ If "leaky," this valve allows blood to flow backward from the pulmonary trunk
9. _d_ This valve is located in the right heart and does not have chordae tendineae
10. _c_ This valve is located in the left heart and has chordae tendineae

Multiple Choice

1. Which of the following is *not* true of the heart?
   a. The heart is located within the mediastinum.
   b. The apex is located to the left of the sternal midline at the level of the fifth intercostal space.
   c. The base of the heart is located at the level of the second rib.
   d. The precordium is composed of cardiac muscle.

2. Which of the following is descriptive of the myocardium?
   a. Composed of contractile proteins called actin and myosin
   b. Thicker in the ventricles than the atria
   c. Thicker in the left ventricle than the right ventricle
   d. All of the above

3. Which of the following is the function of a valve?
   a. Regulates the direction of the flow of blood through the heart
   b. Regulates the amount of oxygen bound to hemoglobin
   c. Regulates heart rate
   d. Directs the progression of the cardiac impulse from the SA node throughout the His-Purkinje system

4. Which of the following is true regarding the structures of the electrical conduction system?
   a. The AV node is the pacemaker.
   b. In normal sinus rhythm, the electrical signal arises within the SA node.
   c. The His-Purkinje system spreads the electrical signal from the right atrium to the left atrium.
   d. The purpose of the AV node is to increase the speed at which the cardiac impulse moves from the atria to the ventricles.

5. Which of the following is true of the aortic valve?
   a. "Sees" oxygenated blood
   b. Causes right ventricular hypertrophy if the valve is stenotic
   c. Allows blood to flow from the ventricle into the pulmonary trunk
   d. Classified as an AV valve

6. Which of the following pacemaker cells of the heart normally determines heart rate?
   a. Atrial conducting fibers
   b. SA node
   c. Ventricular myocardial cells
   d. AV node

7. The coronary arteries
   a. exit the aorta at a point immediately distal to the aortic semilunar valve.
   b. fill the right atrium with blood with each myocardial contraction.
   c. connect the right and left atria.
   d. deliver most O_2 and nutrients to the myocardium while the myocardium is contracted.

8. Which of the following blood flow statements is true?
   a. Blood is pumped by the right atrium through the mitral valve into the right ventricle.
   b. Blood is pumped by the right ventricle into the pulmonary trunk toward the lungs.
   c. Blood is pumped by the left ventricle through the mitral valve into the aorta.
   d. Blood flows from the pulmonary capillaries → pulmonary arteries → left atrium.

9. Which of the following carries oxygenated blood?
   a. Right ventricle
   b. Both AV valves
   c. Both semilunar valves
   d. Pulmonary veins

10. The chordae tendineae are necessary for the proper functioning of the
    a. SA node.
    b. pericardium.
    c. pulmonic semilunar valve.
    d. mitral valve.

11. Which of the following groups is most related to the pumping function of the heart?
    a. Semilunar, atrioventricular
    b. Bicuspid, tricuspid
    c. Aorta, venae cavae
    d. Actin, myosin

12. The His-Purkinje system
    a. is responsible for the P wave on the ECG.
    b. transmits the action potential from the AV node to the SA node.
    c. is the ventricular electrical conduction system.
    d. transmits the action potential from the ventricular myocardial cells to the AV node.

13. Which of the following is a consequence of the QRS complex?
    a. Opening of the AV valves
    b. Ventricular myocardial contraction
    c. Closure of the semilunar valves
    d. Ventricular myocardial relaxation

14. Which of the following electrical events is most descriptive of a pacemaker cell?
    a. Spontaneous depolarization
    b. Myocardial ischemia
    c. Actin, myosin
    d. Contraction, relaxation

15. Which of the following is *least* characteristic of normal sinus rhythm?
    a. The action potential arises within the SA node.
    b. The QRS complex and the T wave are ventricular electrical events.
    c. The origin of the action potential is described as being ectopic.
    d. Each P wave is followed by a QRS complex.

16. Myocardium, cardiomyopathy, and electrocardiogram all refer to
    a. contraction and relaxation of the heart.
    b. diseases of the heart.
    c. diagnostic tests of the heart.
    d. the heart.

Go Figure

1. Which of the following is correct according to Fig. 16.1?
    a. The apex (tip) of the heart is at the level of the 10th intercostal space.
    b. The apex of the heart is located to the left of the midsternal line.
    c. The heart is located within the left pleural cavity
    d. The base of the heart is located at the level of the fifth intercostal space.

2. Which of the following is correct according to Fig. 16.2?
    a. The endocardium forms the inner layer of the pericardium.
    b. The myocardium and endocardium form the pericardial space (cavity).

c. The endocardium forms the "sling" that supports the heart.
    d. The epicardium and parietal pericardium form the pericardial space (cavity).

3. Which of the following is correct according to Fig. 16.3?
    a. The left heart pumps blood to the lungs for oxygenation.
    b. The right heart pumps blood into the systemic circulation.
    c. The systemic circulation delivers unoxygenated blood to the lungs for oxygenation.
    d. The right heart is color-coded blue and delivers blood to the lungs for oxygenation.

4. Which of the following is correct according to Fig. 16.4?
    a. Pulmonary veins are color-coded red, meaning that they carry oxygenated blood.
    b. All arteries carry oxygenated blood.
    c. The venae cavae carry blood to the left side of the heart.
    d. The left side of the heart carries unoxygenated blood.

5. Which of the following is correct according to Fig. 16.5?
    a. All AV valves are located in the right heart.
    b. All semilunar valves are located in the left heart.
    c. Both AV valves contain cusps and are attached to papillary muscles of the ventricular wall by chordae tendineae.
    d. Both semilunar valves attach to the papillary muscles of the ventricular walls by chordae tendineae

6. Which of the following is correct according to Fig. 16.5?
    a. The bicuspid valve has three leaflets and "sees" unoxygenated blood.
    b. The tricuspid valve is also called the mitral valve.
    c. The bicuspid and tricuspid valves are semilunar valves.
    d. Blood exits the ventricles by the pulmonic and aortic semilunar valves.

7. According to Fig. 16.6, a correct sequence for the flow of blood is
    a. right atrium → mitral valve → right ventricle → pulmonic semilunar valve.
    b. mitral valve → left ventricle → left atrium → pulmonary veins.
    c. pulmonary veins → pulmonic semilunar valve→ left atrium → bicuspid valve.
    d. pulmonary arteries → pulmonary capillaries → pulmonary veins → left atrium.

8. Which of the following is correct according to Fig. 16.7?
    a. The left anterior descending (LAD) artery and the circumflex artery are branches of the left coronary artery.
    b. Only the oxygen-carrying blood vessels are displayed in this figure.
    c. The cardiac veins and the coronary sinus supply oxygenated blood to the left ventricular myocardium.
    d. The right and left coronary arteries pump blood from the left ventricle through the aortic valve into the aorta.

9. Which of the following is correct according to Fig. 16.8?
    a. The sinoatrial node is located within the interatrial septum and is the pacemaker of the heart.
    b. The AV node is located on the cusps of the AV valves.

c. Fast-conducting Purkinje fibers are located within the ventricles.

d. The electrical signal normally arises within the AV node.

10. According to Fig. 16.8, the proper sequence of the cardiac impulse is

a. SA node → AV node → bundle of His → Purkinje fibers.

b. AV node → atrial conducting fibers → mitral valve → papillary muscles.

c. Sinoatrial node → venae cavae → AV node → tricuspid valve.

d. Purkinje fibers → bundle of His → AV node → atrial conducting fibers.

11. Which of the following is correct according to Fig. 16.10?

a. The P and T waves are atrial events.

b. The QRS complex indicates the time it takes for the electrical signal to travel from the SA node to the AV node.

c. The P-R interval indicates the time it takes for the electrical signal to travel from the right atrium to the left atrium.

d. The P-R interval indicates the time it takes for the electrical signal to travel from the atria to the ventricles.

Function of the Heart

Objectives

1. Define the cardiac cycle with respect to systole and diastole.
2. Describe the autonomic innervation of the heart, including sympathetic and parasympathetic innervation.
3. Define cardiac output, including the following:
   - Describe the effect of Starling's law of the heart on cardiac output.
   - Describe the inotropic effect on cardiac output.
   - Explain how changes in heart rate and/or stroke volume change cardiac output.
4. Define specific clinical vocabulary used to describe cardiac function, including the following:
   - Define preload (end-diastolic volume), and explain how it affects cardiac output.
   - Define afterload, and identify the major factor that determines afterload.
   - Define chronotropic, inotropic, and dromotropic effects.
5. Define heart failure, and differentiate between right-sided and left-sided heart failure.

Key Terms

afterload (p. 331)
cardiac cycle (p. 325)
cardiac output (p. 328)
cardiac reserve (p. 330)
chronotropic effect (p. 332)
diastole (p. 325)
dromotropic effect (p. 332)

ejection fraction (p. 331)
end-diastolic volume (EDV) (p. 330)
heart failure (p. 327)
inotropic effect (p. 329)
preload (p. 331)
pulmonary edema (PE) (p. 333)
Starling's law of the heart (p. 329)

stroke volume (p. 329)
sympathomimetic (p. 328)
systole (p. 325)
vagolytic (p. 328)
vagomimetic (p. 328)
venous return (p. 328)

The heart functions as a pump that supplies blood to every cell in the body. The heart is a hard worker; on a daily basis the human heart accomplishes the work equivalent to lifting a ton of weight from the ground to the top of a five-story building. The heart is also an adaptable pump. For example, the heart alters its pumping activity to meet the demands of day-to-day physiological functions such as eating, exercise, and responding to changes in environmental temperature; it also adapts to disease. How does the heart know when to beat faster or slower, or weaker or stronger? The coordinated and adaptable heart is the focus of the first part of this chapter, "The Coordinated and Adaptable Pump." The second part of this chapter, "Heart Talk," defines terminology that is commonly used in clinical situations. The third part, "The Failing Heart: When the Heart Can't Pump," describes the failing heart.

THE COORDINATED AND ADAPTABLE PUMP

CARDIAC CYCLE

The **cardiac cycle** is the sequence of events that occurs during one heartbeat. A cardiac cycle is a coordinated contraction and relaxation of the chambers of the heart. Contraction of the heart muscle (myocardium) is called **systole** (SIS-toh-lee). Contraction of the heart muscle during systole pumps blood out of a chamber. Relaxation of the myocardium is called **diastole** (dye-ASS-toh-lee). Blood fills a chamber during diastole.

Atrial and ventricular muscle activity is closely coordinated. For example, during atrial systole, the ventricles are in diastole. In this way, when the atria contract, they pump blood into the relaxed ventricles.

The cardiac cycle has three stages (Fig. 17.1):
- *Atrial systole.* The atria contract (systole) and pump blood into the ventricles. During atrial systole, the atrioventricular (AV) valves are open, and the ventricles are relaxed.
- *Ventricular systole.* At the end of atrial systole, the ventricles contract; this is called ventricular systole. As ventricular contractions begin, blood is forced against the AV valves, causing them to snap shut. The blood pushes the semilunar valves open, allowing blood to flow into the pulmonary trunk and aorta.

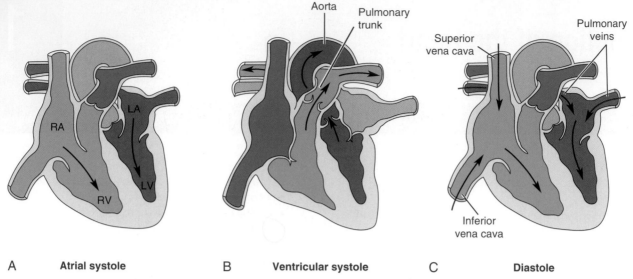

FIG. 17.1 Stages of the cardiac cycle. (A) Atrial systole. (B) Ventricular systole. (C) Diastole.

• *Diastole.* For a brief period during the cardiac cycle, both the atria and the ventricles are in diastole. As the chambers relax, blood flows into the atria. Because the AV valves are open at this time, much of this blood also flows passively into the ventricles. The period of diastole therefore is a period of filling (of blood); atrial systole follows. The cycle then repeats itself.

How long does the cardiac cycle last? With a heart rate (HR) of 70 beats/min, the duration of the cardiac cycle is 0.8 second. All chambers rest for 0.4 second. As HR increases, the duration of the cardiac cycle shortens. With a dramatic increase in HR, the period of rest (diastole) may shorten so much that cardiac function diminishes. An episode of tachycardia may thus be accompanied by chest pain. Why? First, because of a decreased filling time, the amount of blood that enters the ventricles decreases so that less blood is pumped. Second, because coronary blood flow to the myocardium occurs during diastole, the diminished period of diastole decreases coronary blood flow. Decreased coronary blood flow, in turn, results in poor oxygenation of the myocardium and pain.

NOTE: The valves of the heart open and close in response to pressure changes. Think of the valves during the three stages of the cardiac cycle. Are they open or closed?

? Re-Think

1. Define *systole* and *diastole.*
2. Why is it important that the atria and ventricles do not contract at the same time?
3. Why is coronary blood flow greatest during ventricular diastole?
4. Why does extreme tachycardia cause chest pain?

⊚ Sum It Up!

The cardiac cycle is the coordinated sequence of events that occurs during one heartbeat. The cardiac cycle has three stages: atrial systole, ventricular systole, and ventricular diastole. Cardiac muscle contraction is called *systole*; cardiac muscle relaxation is called *diastole*. The duration of the cardiac cycle (resting heart) is 0.8 second; duration changes with a change in heart rate. When heart rate increases the duration of the cardiac cycle decreases; the phase of the cardiac cycle that shortens most is diastole (the resting phase).

AUTONOMIC CONTROL OF THE HEART

The autonomic nervous system (ANS) plays an important role in coordinating and adapting cardiac function.

WHY THE AUTONOMIC NERVOUS SYSTEM?

In the previous chapter, we learned that specialized cardiac tissue displays automaticity and rhythmicity. The electrical signal, the cardiac impulse, arises within the sinoatrial (SA) node and then spreads throughout the heart, causing the heart muscle to contract. If the heart is capable of initiating its own cardiac impulse, why are the autonomic nerves needed? Although the ANS does not cause the cardiac impulse, it can affect the rate at which the cardiac impulse is fired and the speed at which it travels throughout the heart. The ANS can also make the heart muscle contract more forcefully; thus, the ANS can change the pumping activity of the heart. For example, if a person suddenly sprints down the street, his or her heart autonomically or automatically responds to the increased need for more oxygenated blood; it beats faster and stronger.

AUTONOMIC WIRING

As described in Chapter 12, the ANS has two branches: the sympathetic and parasympathetic branches.

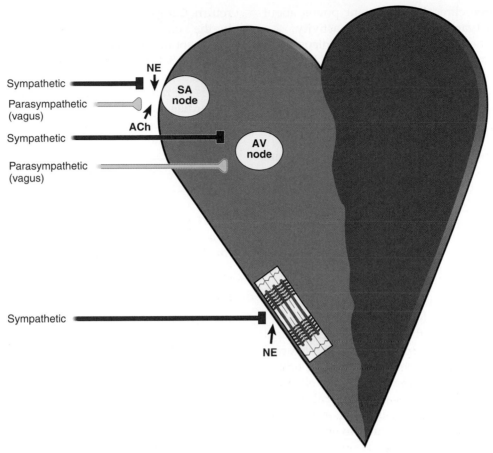

FIG. 17.2 Autonomic innervation of the heart. Sympathetics: adrenergic fibers are red and secrete NE. Parasympathetics: cholinergic fibers are green and secrete ACh.

Refer to Fig. 17.2 and note the autonomic wiring of the heart. Sympathetic nerves supply the SA node, AV node, and ventricular myocardium (the sarcomere represents heart muscle). Parasympathetic nerves, also called the *vagus nerve*, innervate the SA node and the AV node; there is no parasympathetic or vagal innervation of the ventricular myocardium.

AUTONOMIC FIRING

What happens when the ANS fires?

Sympathetic Stimulation
- Increases SA node activity, thus increasing heart rate
- Increases the speed at which the cardiac impulse travels from the SA node throughout the AV node and His-Purkinje system
- Increases the force of myocardial contraction

There are four clinically important points regarding excess sympathetic activity on the heart and blood vessels:

- Excess sympathetic activity produces the "fight-or-flight" response. You will often observe these symptoms (racing and pounding heart) in people who are very anxious, such as during panic attacks. The symptoms are frightening, and the person is convinced of an impending heart attack. Many trips to the emergency room (ER) are panic related.

- Excess sympathetic activity plays a key role in some disease states. For example, most of the signs and symptoms of circulatory shock are caused by excess sympathetic firing. Similarly, the progressive deterioration of patients with **heart failure** is in large measure caused by persistent sympathetic nerve stimulation. Some of the drugs used to treat heart failure are aimed at minimizing the sympathetic effects.
- Excess sympathetic activity often causes tachydysrhythmias ("fast" rhythm disorders).
- You will be giving drugs that resemble or block the effects of sympathetic activity. For example, epinephrine (Adrenalin) and dopamine increase HR and myocardial contractile force. You will also be giving drugs that block the sympathetic effects, including beta- and alpha-adrenergic blockers.

Parasympathetic (Vagus Nerve) Stimulation
- Decreases SA node activity, thereby decreasing heart rate
- Decreases the speed at which the cardiac impulse travels from the SA node to and through the AV node into the His-Purkinje system
- Exerts no effect on the strength of myocardial contraction because there are no parasympathetic (vagal) fibers innervating the ventricular myocardium

There are three clinically important points about parasympathetic (vagal) nervous system activity:

- In the resting heart, vagal tone is more intense than sympathetic activity. For example, the SA node would like to fire at a rate of 90 beats/min. However, the "braking" or inhibiting effect of the vagus nerve slows SA node firing to a rate of 72 beats/min, the normal resting heart rate. If the vagus nerve were interrupted, the HR would increase to 90 beats/min.
- Certain conditions (heart attack) and drugs (digoxin) can cause excess vagal discharge. Excess vagal discharge causes bradycardia (bray-dee-KAR-dee-ah) (<60 beats/min) and increases the tendency of the heart to develop life-threatening electrical rhythm disturbances. Excess vagal discharge also slows the conduction of the cardiac impulse through the heart, causing heart block (a condition in which the signal has difficulty traveling from the atria to the ventricles). The abnormally slow rhythms are called *bradydysrhythmias* (bray-dee-diss-RITH-mee-ahs).
- You will be giving drugs that alter the effects of vagal activity. For example, digoxin decreases the HR and slows the speed at which the cardiac impulse travels from the atria to the ventricle. Because the effects of digoxin "mimic" vagal stimulation, it is called a **vagomimetic** (vag-oh-mihm-EHT-ik) drug. A drug may also produce effects that are similar to an inhibition of vagal discharge. For example, atropine is used to relieve bradycardia because it blocks the effects of vagal stimulation and increases heart rate. Because of its blocking effects on the vagus nerve, atropine is called a **vagolytic** (vag-oh-LIT-ik) drug.

 Do You Know...

Why a Patient May "Brady-Down"?

Most persons respond to stress with excess sympathetic activity; for most persons, stress is **sympathomimetic**. Sometimes, however, a patient responds to fear or anxiety with an intense discharge of the parasympathetic (vagus) nerves. Vagal discharge to the heart causes a dangerous bradycardia and decline in cardiac output and blood pressure. The patient is said to "brady-down." The administration of a vagolytic drug, such as atropine, relieves the vagal effects and restores the heart rate to normal.

Re-Think

1. If the electrical signal (cardiac impulse) arises within the SA node spontaneously, why is the heart innervated by the ANS?
2. Describe a sympathomimetic effect on heart rate and force of myocardial contraction.
3. Describe a vagomimetic effect on heart rate.

CARDIAC OUTPUT AND VENOUS RETURN

To understand how the heart alters its pumping activity, you must understand cardiac output and venous

return. **Cardiac output** is the amount of blood pumped by the ventricle in 1 minute. The normal cardiac output is about 5 L/min. Because the total blood volume is about 5 L (5000 mL), the entire blood volume is pumped through the heart every minute. **Venous return** is the rate of blood flow back to the heart. Its effect on cardiac output is described later.

Two factors determine cardiac output: HR and stroke volume.

> **Cardiac Output = Heart Rate × Stroke Volume**

Heart Rate

The HR is the number of times the heart beats each minute. The HR is caused by the rhythmic firing of the SA node, the pacemaker of the heart. The normal adult resting HR is between 60 and 100 beats/min, with an average of 72 beats/min. Resting heart rates differ for many reasons, including size, gender, and age.

- *Size.* Size affects heart rate; generally, the larger the size, the slower the rate. Our feathered and furry friends dramatically illustrate this point. The HR of a hummingbird, for example, is more than 200 beats/min, whereas that of a grizzly bear is only about 30 beats/min. Why do heart rates differ? The small hummingbird has a very high metabolism and therefore requires a large amount of oxygen. The metabolism of a grizzly is much slower, requiring less oxygen. Similarly, a tiny baby has a faster HR than a larger adult.
- *Gender.* Women have slightly faster heart rates than men.
- *Age.* Generally, the younger the person, the faster the rate. The normal adult heart rate, for example, is 70 to 80 beats/min, whereas a normal child's HR is around 100 beats/min. An infant's HR is about 120 beats/min, and fetal heart rates are about 140 beats/min.

In addition to the variation in HR according to size, age, and gender, a person's HR can change for a variety of other reasons, such as exercise, stimulation of the autonomic nerves, hormonal influence, pathology, and various medications.

- *Exercise.* Exercise increases HR. Check your pulse as you exercise and note the increase; also note the decrease in pulse when you rest. At rest, the HR may be 65 beats/min but may increase to well over 100 beats/min with exercise.
- *Stimulation of the autonomic nerves.* Firing of the sympathetic nerve stimulates the SA node, causing an increase in HR. Stimulation of the parasympathetic (vagus) nerve slows the rate.
- *Hormonal influence.* Several hormones affect heart rate. For example, epinephrine and norepinephrine (adrenal gland hormones) and thyroid hormone increase HR.
- *Pathology.* Many disease states affect HR. For example, a sick SA node may fire too slowly, thereby

slowing the heart too much. Vagal discharge following a heart attack (myocardial infarction) slows the rate, predisposing the heart to lethal rhythm disorders. A high fever, hyperthyroidism, and persistent sympathetic activity can increase heart rate, overworking the heart and causing it to fail.

- *Medications.* Many drugs affect heart rate; some are administered for the purpose of changing heart rate. Digoxin and beta-adrenergic blockers slow heart rate, whereas beta-adrenergic agonists, such as epinephrine and dopamine, increase heart rate. Heavy coffee drinkers often experience palpitations (the heart feels "jumpy," as if it has extra beats) because of the stimulatory effect of caffeine on the heart. Because some drugs can profoundly alter HR, it must be monitored when these drugs are used. For example, digoxin should not be administered if the HR is less than 60 beats/min.

Stroke Volume

Stroke volume is the second factor affecting cardiac output. **Stroke volume** is the amount of blood pumped by the ventricle per beat. An average resting stroke volume is 60 to 80 mL/beat (about 2 ounces). At rest, the ventricles pump out only about 67% of the blood in the ventricles. Therefore, if the ventricles can be made to contract more forcefully, a greater percentage of the blood can be pumped per beat. In other words, a greater force of contraction can increase stroke volume. Like HR, stroke volume can change thereby affecting cardiac output.

> ### ? Re-Think
>
> 1. Define *cardiac output* and *venous return.*
> 2. What two factors determine cardiac output?

How to Change Stroke Volume

The stroke volume can be altered in two ways: through Starling's law of the heart and through an inotropic effect.

Starling's Law of the Heart. The relationship of myocardial stretch to myocardial contractile force is referred to as **Starling's law of the heart**. The greater the stretch of the myocardium, the stronger the force of contraction. For example, an increase in the amount of blood entering the ventricle, the venous return, causes the ventricle to stretch (Fig. 17.3). Stretch increases the force of contraction, which in turn increases stroke volume. Conversely, a decrease in the amount of blood entering the ventricles causes less stretch. As a result, the force of contraction decreases, thereby decreasing stroke volume (see the Ramp It Up!: Starling's Law of the Heart and Inotropism box on p. 330).

What is the purpose of Starling's law of the heart? It allows the heart to pump out the same amount of blood it receives. In other words, Starling's law allows the heart to match cardiac output with venous return on a beat-to-beat basis.

Inotropic Effect. A second way to increase stroke volume is by strengthening the force of myocardial contraction without stretching the myocardial fibers. This is called a positive **inotropic** (in-o-TROH-pik) **effect.** Stimulation of the heart muscle by sympathetic nerves causes a positive inotropic effect. Certain hormones and drugs, such as epinephrine, also cause this effect. Digoxin is the most famous of the positive inotropic drugs. Some medications cause a negative inotropic effect. A negative inotropic effect is a decrease in the force of contraction, resulting in a weaker myocardial contraction. A negative inotropic effect is most often

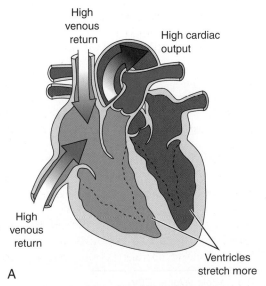

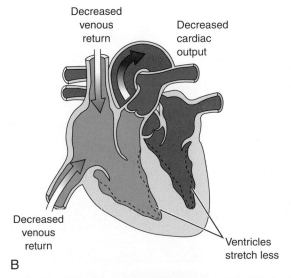

FIG. 17.3 Starling's law of the heart, matching venous return with cardiac output. (A) A large venous return. (B) A smaller venous return.

associated with the failing heart (see the Ramp It Up!: Starling's Law of the Heart and Inotropism box below).

Do You Know...
About Atrial Kick?

About 70% of blood flows passively from the atria into the ventricles. Atrial contraction (systole) accounts for the remaining 30%; it is called the *atrial kick*. With atrial fibrillation the contribution from atrial kick is missing, and cardiac output declines. Atrial kick—it's a good thing!

CHANGING CARDIAC OUTPUT

Because cardiac output is determined by HR and stroke volume, cardiac output can be altered by changing either or both. The healthy heart can increase cardiac output four to five times the resting cardiac output; an Olympic athlete can do even better! The capacity to increase cardiac output above the resting cardiac output is called the **cardiac reserve**. A person with a diseased heart may have little cardiac reserve and therefore becomes easily fatigued with mild exercise.

Ramp It Up!
Starling's Law of the Heart and Inotropism

Cardiac output is determined by HR and stroke volume (CO = HR × SV). By changing either or both, the heart adapts to changing body needs. There are two mechanisms whereby stroke volume and, therefore, cardiac output can be altered: Starling's law of the heart and inotropism.

Starling's law of the heart refers to the relationship of myocardial stretch to myocardial contractile force. It is based on the mechanical properties of muscle contraction (described in Chapter 9 ...the sliding filament mechanism of muscle contraction). Recall that the force of skeletal muscle contraction is proportional to the number of cross-bridges formed when actin and myosin interact. The greater the number of cross-bridges, the greater is the force of muscle contraction. The important point is this: the length of the cardiac muscle continues to change as blood flows into the ventricles during diastole. The accumulation of blood stretches the muscle, realigns the actin and myosin, changes the numbers of cross-bridges, and therefore increases contractile force. Refer to the curve in Panel A and note the following:

1. *The labeling of the horizontal and vertical lines.* The horizontal line is the myocardial stretch or **end-diastolic volume (EDV)**. It is determined by the amount of blood in the ventricle at the end of diastole and indicates how much the ventricular muscle has been stretched. The vertical line represents myocardial contractile force or stroke volume.
2. *What happens when EDV changes?* Note the EDV and stroke volume at point A. When EDV increases, stroke volume increases. This is indicated by moving from point A to point B. When EDV decreases, stroke volume

decreases. This is indicated by moving from point B back to point A. The relationship of EDV to SV is Starling's law of the heart. The curve is referred to as the *ventricular function curve.* This mechanism allows the stroke volume (and cardiac output) to match venous return on a beat-to-beat basis. In other words, when more blood returns to the heart, more blood is pumped out of the heart. When less is returned, less is pumped.

Inotropic Effects. An inotropic effect refers to a change in myocardial contractile force achieved without stretching the muscle fibers as occurs in Starling's law of the heart. Inotropic effects can be positive or negative. Refer to panel B and note the following:

1. Locate point A on the curve labeled "normal." Note the EDV and SV.
2. Draw a vertical line from point A to point B on the upper curve labeled "(+) inotropic effect." What is this saying? A positive inotropic effect is an increase in the myocardial contractile force (SV) achieved without stretching the myocardium. A (+) inotropic effect can be elicited by sympathetic nerve stimulation and by certain drugs, such as dopamine and digoxin. These drugs are called (+) inotropic agents.
3. Draw a vertical line from point A to point C on the lower curve labeled "(–) inotropic effect." What is this saying? A negative inotropic effect is a decrease in the force of myocardial contractile force achieved independently of myocardial stretch. A (–) inotropic effect describes the failing heart. Unfortunately, some drugs elicit a (–) inotropic effect.

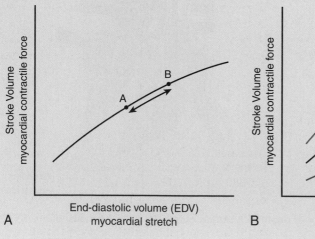

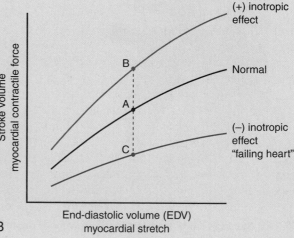

? Re-Think

1. Explain how Starling's law of the heart changes the force of myocardial contraction.
2. Explain how an inotropic effect changes the force of myocardial contraction.
3. How does the heart match cardiac output and venous return?
4. Explain why cardiac output can remain unchanged even if heart rate changes.

◎ Sum It Up!

Cardiac output is determined by multiplying heart rate and stroke volume. The heart rate is the number of times the heart beats each minute. The normal adult resting heart rate is between 60 and 100 beats/min (average, 72 beats/min). Heart rates differ for three main reasons: size, gender, and age. A person's heart rate may also change in response to exercise, stimulation of the ANS, hormonal influence, pathology, and various medications. Stroke volume is the amount of blood ejected by the ventricle in one beat. Stroke volume can be altered through Starling's law of the heart or an inotropic effect. Cardiac output can increase or decrease in response to changing HR and/or stroke volume. The heart is able to match cardiac output and venous return on a beat-to-beat basis.

The following major sections, "Heart Talk" and "The Failing Heart: When the Heart Can't Pump," are clinically focused and may be omitted in nonmedical courses.

HEART TALK

HEART TALK: CLINICAL TERMS

Clinically, cardiac function is described using special vocabulary.

END-DIASTOLIC VOLUME

The EDV refers to the amount of blood in the ventricle at the end of its resting phase (diastole). The EDV determines how much the ventricle is stretched and is the basis of Starling's law of the heart.

PRELOAD

The **preload** is the amount of blood in the ventricles at the end of diastole; it is the same as the EDV. Note in Fig. 17.4 that the filling of the right heart by the funnel illustrates preload. An increased preload stretches the ventricles, causing a stronger force of contraction. The stronger contraction increases stroke volume and cardiac output. Drugs can also affect preload. For example, a drug may dilate the veins, causing blood to pool in the veins, thereby decreasing venous return, preload, stroke volume, and cardiac output. Another drug may constrict the veins; this increases blood flow to the ventricles, thereby increasing venous return, preload, stroke volume, and cardiac output.

? Re-Think

1. Explain why a decrease in venous return decreases cardiac output.
2. Explain why venous return, EDV, preload, and the Starling effect "make" the same point.

EJECTION FRACTION

When the ventricle contracts, it pumps about 67% of its volume (EDV); therefore, some blood remains in the ventricle. The percentage of the EDV that is pumped is called the **ejection fraction**. The ejection fraction is an indication of cardiac health. For example, a healthy heart can increase its ejection fraction to 90% with exercise. A weakened failing heart is characterized by a decrease in ejection fraction, perhaps as low as 30%.

AFTERLOAD

Afterload refers to resistance or opposition to the flow of blood. Note in Fig. 17.4 that the pinched aorta represents an increased afterload, demanding that the left ventricle work harder to overcome the resistance. The pinched aorta can represent a number of clinical conditions such as aortic valve stenosis and systemic hypertension. If the person develops high blood pressure, afterload increases and the ventricle must work harder to pump blood into the aorta. Like any other muscle that overworks, the left ventricular myocardium enlarges or hypertrophies. The enlarged left ventricle will eventually fail as a pump.

What about afterload and the right ventricle? Its afterload is determined by the pressure within the pulmonary trunk and pulmonary arteries. If pulmonary artery pressure rises (increased afterload), the right ventricle must work harder to pump blood and therefore hypertrophies. Right ventricular hypertrophy frequently occurs in response to chronic lung diseases such as emphysema and asthma. The elevation in pulmonary artery pressure and right ventricular hypertrophy is called *cor pulmonale* (kohr pul-mah-NAL-ee). Cor pulmonale often causes the right ventricle to fail as a pump.

Afterload can be altered by drugs. For example, a drug that relaxes and dilates the blood vessels in the peripheral circulation can lower blood pressure and therefore decrease the afterload. The reduction in afterload reduces the work of the heart. Conversely, a drug that constricts blood vessels in the periphery increases afterload, thereby increasing the workload of the heart.

INOTROPIC EFFECT

An inotropic effect is a change in myocardial contraction that is not caused by stretch of the myocardial fibers. A positive inotropic effect is an increase in contractile force, whereas a negative inotropic effect is a decrease in contractile force. Sympathetic nerve stimulation and hormones such as epinephrine and norepinephrine cause a positive inotropic effect.

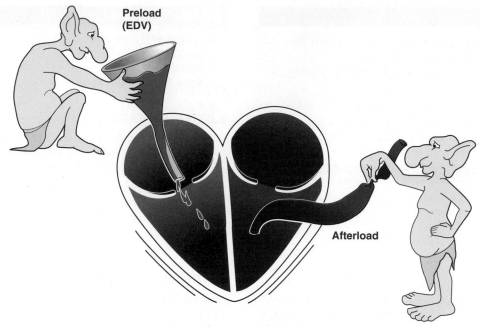

Preload (EDV)

Afterload

FIG. 17.4 **Preload and afterload.**

CHRONOTROPIC EFFECT

A **chronotropic** (KRON-oh-TROH-pik) **effect** is a change in heart rate. Anything that increases HR causes a positive chronotropic effect, whereas anything that decreases HR causes a negative chronotropic effect. Sympathetic nerve stimulation causes a positive chronotropic effect, whereas vagal (parasympathetic) stimulation causes a negative chronotropic effect.

DROMOTROPIC EFFECT

A **dromotropic** (DROM-oh-TROH-pik) **effect** is a change in the speed at which the cardiac impulse travels from the SA node through the AV node and the His-Purkinje system. If the speed of the cardiac impulse increases, it is called a *positive dromotropic effect*; a decrease in the speed causes a negative dromotropic effect. Sympathetic nerve stimulation causes a positive dromotropic effect, whereas vagal (parasympathetic) stimulation causes a negative dromotropic effect. The negative dromotropic effect may be so pronounced that the person develops a heart block.

HEART TALK: RECEPTOR LANGUAGE

Heart talk often involves the autonomic receptors of the heart and their responses to autonomic stimulation and to drugs. (Refer to the Chapter 12 discussion of receptors in the heart and blood vessels.)

BETA₁-ADRENERGIC RECEPTOR ACTIVATION

The sympathetic nerves innervate the SA node, AV node, His-Purkinje system, and ventricular myocardium. The neurotransmitter for the adrenergic neuron is norepinephrine. The cardiac adrenergic receptors for norepinephrine are called *beta₁-adrenergic receptors*. Activation of the beta₁ receptors causes a positive chronotropic effect, a positive dromotropic effect, and a positive inotropic effect. The increase in HR and stroke volume increases cardiac output. A drug that activates beta₁-adrenergic receptors is called a *beta₁-adrenergic agonist*. Examples include dopamine and epinephrine. Note that beta₁-adrenergic receptor activation is the same as a sympathomimetic effect.

BETA₁-ADRENERGIC RECEPTOR BLOCKADE

Blockade of the beta₁-adrenergic receptors prevents cardiac beta₁-adrenergic receptor activation. People taking beta₁-adrenergic blockers, such as propranolol, will not increase their HR when their sympathetic nerves fire as in exercise or stress. If a person is tachycardic (HR >100 beats/min) from excessive sympathetic nervous stimulation, a beta₁-adrenergic blocker can decrease the HR and the force of myocardial contraction; this results in a decrease in cardiac output and blood pressure.

? Re-Think

1. Define *ejection fraction*. Why can activation of the sympathetic nerves increase the ejection fraction?
2. Why is systemic hypertension referred to as an increase in afterload?
3. Describe the effects of a sympathomimetic drug using the words *chronotropic, inotropic,* and *dromotropic effects.*
4. What is the effect of a beta₁-adrenergic agonist on heart rate, stroke volume, and cardiac output?
5. What is the name of the neurotransmitter that activates a beta₁-adrenergic receptor?

MUSCARINIC (CHOLINERGIC) RECEPTOR ACTIVATION

The parasympathetic (vagus) nerves supply the SA and the AV nodes. The neurotransmitter for the cholinergic neuron is acetylcholine (ACh). The cardiac cholinergic receptors for ACh are called *muscarinic receptors*. Activation of the muscarinic receptors causes a negative chronotropic effect and a negative dromotropic effect. There is no effect on myocardial contractile force because there is no parasympathetic innervation to the ventricular myocardium. The administration of a cholinergic (muscarinic) agonist drug causes a negative chronotropic effect and a negative dromotropic effect. Note that muscarinic receptor activation is the same as a parasympathomimetic or vagomimetic effect.

MUSCARINIC (CHOLINERGIC) RECEPTOR BLOCKADE

The muscarinic receptors can also be blocked. Muscarinic-blocking drugs act by blocking the effects of ACh at the muscarinic receptors. Muscarinic blockade relieves the inhibiting effects of ACh at the receptors, thereby increasing HR and increasing the speed of the cardiac impulse from the atria to the ventricles. Atropine is an example of a muscarinic blocker that is often used to relieve bradycardia and heart block (slowing of the cardiac impulse through the heart).

Note the duplication in terminology (your worst terminology nightmare!). The muscarinic receptors are activated by ACh. Because ACh is secreted by a cholinergic fiber, a muscarinic agonist is also called a *cholinergic agonist*. A muscarinic blocker is also called an *antimuscarinic agent*, a *cholinergic blocker*, or an *anticholinergic agent*. Unfortunately, this terminology is used frequently in pharmacology, so you need to start building your autonomic vocabulary now.

 Re-Think

1. Why is a muscarinic agonist called a vagomimetic drug?
2. What is the effect of a vagomimetic drug, such as atropine, on heart rate?
3. What is the name of the neurotransmitter that activates the muscarinic receptors?

⊚ **Sum It Up!**

Cardiac function is often described using special vocabulary, such as EDV, preload, ejection fraction, and afterload. Inotropic, chronotropic, and dromotropic effects describe changes in cardiac contractile force, heart rate, and conduction velocity through the heart. Cardiac function is also described in receptor terminology, specifically the beta$_1$-adrenergic and muscarinic receptors.

THE FAILING HEART: WHEN THE HEART CAN'T PUMP

The heart functions as a double pump. The right ventricle pumps blood to the lungs for oxygenation, and the left ventricle pumps blood into the aorta for distribution to the systemic circulation. What happens when either or both pumps fail?

🦉 **Do You Know...**

Why BNP Is Used in the Assessment of Heart Failure?

Brain natriuretic peptide (BNP) is secreted by the walls of the ventricles in response to stretch. The failing heart is characterized by pooling of blood in the ventricular chambers and stretching of the myocardial fibers, thereby increasing the secretion of BNP. An elevation in BNP is thus suggestive of ventricular dilation and heart failure.

LEFT HEART FAILURE

When the left ventricle fails to pump blood into the aorta, two things happen: blood backs up in the lungs, and the heart is unable to pump a sufficient amount of blood to the systemic circulation.

BACKWARD FAILURE

What happens when the blood backs up (Fig. 17.5)? The blood backs up into the structures "behind" the left ventricle—namely, the left atrium, pulmonary veins, and, most important, the pulmonary capillaries. The pooled blood increases the pressure within the pulmonary capillaries and forces fluid into the lungs. The presence of fluid in the lungs impairs oxygenation of blood. The accumulation of fluid within the lungs is called **pulmonary edema (PE)**. The signs and symptoms of PE are exertional dyspnea (difficulty breathing upon exertion), cyanosis (bluish appearance), blood-tinged (pink and frothy) sputum and cough, orthopnea (or-THOP-nee-ah) (inability to breathe while lying down), tachycardia, and restlessness. Because these symptoms are largely caused by the backup of blood behind the failed ventricle, the condition is called *backward failure*. Note that the signs and symptoms of left-sided heart failure are predominantly respiratory!

 Do You Know...

About Two- and Three-Pillow Dyspnea?

A patient with heart failure may develop pulmonary edema and dyspnea. There is a simple way to determine the severity of the dyspnea: ask the patient how many pillows he uses at night. A patient with no pulmonary edema can lie flat and use a single pillow. As fluid collects in the alveoli (lungs), a patient must sit up to breathe (orthopnea). Thus, he tends to use two or three pillows, depending on the severity of the edema and dyspnea—hence the name *two-* or *three-pillow dyspnea*.

FORWARD FAILURE

There is also a "forward" component to left heart failure. For example, if the damaged left ventricle cannot pump enough blood to the systemic circulation, all the organs of the body receive inadequate oxygen. The decreased cardiac output causes additional systemic signs and symptoms to develop. For example, the kidneys filter less water for excretion as urine.

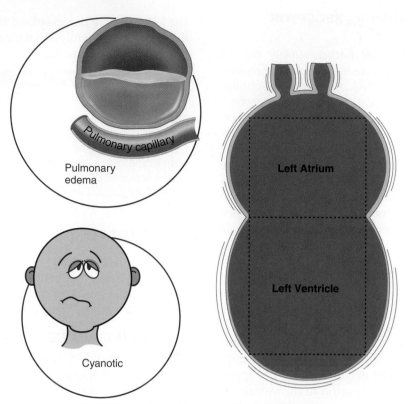

FIG. 17.5 Left-sided heart failure: backward failure.

The kidneys also reabsorb excess salt and water, causing an increase in blood volume and edema formation. The decrease in cardiac output also stimulates the sympathetic nervous system. Sympathetic activity stimulates the heart and blood vessels in a way that temporarily improves cardiac output. Over time, however, the improvement diminishes, and additional signs of heart failure develop. The heart begins to show the wear and tear of continuous and excessive sympathetic activity.

What usually causes the left heart to fail? Two common causes are myocardial infarction (MI) and chronic hypertension (increased blood pressure). If a person suffers an acute MI, a part of the left ventricular myocardium may be destroyed. The damaged myocardium is unable to contract and fails as a pump. More commonly, the left heart fails in response to chronic hypertension. Increased blood pressure overworks the heart, eventually causing the left ventricle to enlarge (left ventricular hypertrophy) and then fail.

> **?** **Re-Think**
>
> 1. Why does left-sided heart failure cause pulmonary edema?
> 2. Differentiate between forward and backward heart failure.
> 3. Explain why a positive inotropic drug, such as digoxin, relieves backward and forward heart failure.

RIGHT HEART FAILURE

When the right ventricle fails (Fig. 17.6), blood backs up into the veins that return blood to the right heart. Blood backs up into the superior vena cava, thereby slowing venous drainage from the head via the jugular veins. The congestion of the jugular veins causes jugular vein distention (JVD), which is visible as the veins in the neck pulsate. Blood also backs up into the veins that drain the liver, spleen, and digestive organs, causing hepatomegaly (enlarged liver), splenomegaly (enlarged spleen), and digestive symptoms. Right-sided failure is also characterized by ankle, or pedal, edema; ankle edema can be so severe that the skin remains indented when you depress an area of skin with your thumb. This "indentation" response is called *pitting edema.*

The right heart most often fails as a consequence of left-sided failure; when one side of the heart fails, the other side will eventually fail. Another common cause is chronic lung disease, such as emphysema. The diseased lungs make it difficult for the right ventricle to pump blood into the pulmonary circulation. The overworked right ventricle becomes enlarged (right ventricular hypertrophy) and eventually fails.

> **?** **Re-Think**
>
> 1. Why does right-sided heart failure cause JVD, hepatomegaly, and pedal edema rather than pulmonary edema?
> 2. Translate the following into lay terminology: A patient with an ejection fraction of 35% was given a drug (digoxin) that exerted positive inotropic, negative dromotropic, and negative chronotropic effects.

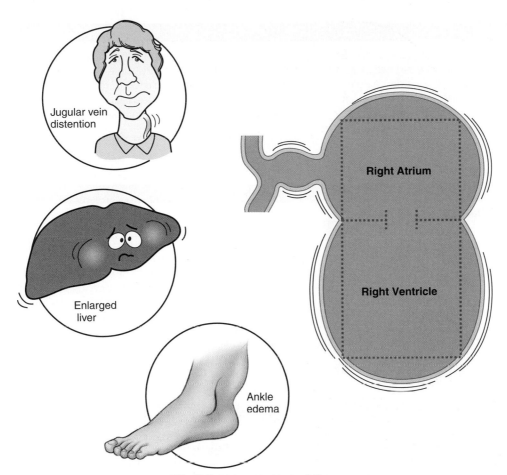

FIG. 17.6 Right-sided heart failure.

 Do You Know...

Why CVP Is Elevated in Heart Failure?

Central venous pressure (CVP) is considered a direct measurement of the pressure in the right atrium and superior vena cava (the large vein that empties blood into the right atrium). The CVP reading is obtained by threading a catheter through the subclavian vein into the superior vena cava. When the heart fails, blood backs up in the vena cava, thereby elevating venous pressure. Thus, an elevated CVP is indicative of a failing heart.

Let's see if you can follow the rationale for the treatment in the following case studies.

- *Case 1.* A patient in left-sided heart failure and pulmonary edema is given a positive inotropic drug, a potent diuretic, oxygen, and morphine. The rationale for this is that the failing heart muscle contracts weakly. A positive inotropic drug such as digoxin or dopamine strengthens myocardial contraction. The increased force of contraction results in an increased cardiac output, decreased pooling of blood in the pulmonary capillaries (decreases pulmonary edema), and increased blood flow to the kidney, which results in greater excretion of urine. A potent diuretic, such as furosemide (Lasix), blocks the absorption of sodium and water by the kidney, thereby ridding the body of excess water and decreasing the edema.

The oxygen and morphine improve oxygenation and relieve the anxiety caused by poor oxygenation.

- *Case 2.* An older patient with symptoms of right-sided failure and a fast HR is given a beta$_1$-adrenergic blocker. The rationale for this is that heart failure is characterized by excess sympathetic nerve stimulation. Long-term sympathetic stimulation damages the heart, causing the heart to fail eventually. The administration of a beta$_1$-adrenergic receptor blocker diminishes the response to sympathetic activity and protects the heart from further damage.

- *Case 3.* An older patient has mild right-sided failure and is given an angiotensin-converting enzyme (ACE) inhibitor. An ACE inhibitor decreases afterload, acts like a diuretic, and decreases the secretion of aldosterone from the adrenal cortex. The decreased afterload decreases the workload of the heart. The diuretic effect excretes water and relieves the edema. The decrease in the secretion of aldosterone has two effects: it causes diuresis, and it prevents myocardial damage. (Chronic secretion of aldosterone causes structural damage, called *remodeling*, to the heart muscle.)

Clearly, the healthy heart is a magnificent, adaptable pump. Pump failure adversely affects the functioning of every organ system and is a common cause of disability and death.

Sum It Up!

The heart functions as a double pump. Either or both pumps can fail. When the left heart fails, fluid backs up into the lungs, causing pulmonary edema (backward failure). The failing left heart is also unable to pump sufficient blood to the organs of the body; the result is poor tissue oxygenation (forward failure). Right-sided failure causes JVD, ankle edema, and congestion of the abdominal organs. The treatment of heart failure is aimed at strengthening of myocardial contractile force, removing excess water, decreasing the work of the heart, and protecting the heart from excess sympathetic nerve activity.

 Do You Know...

What's with the Octopus and the Takotsubo?

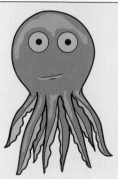

Most persons intuitively believe that one can die of a broken heart, the death of a loved one most often being cited as its cause. Until recently, however, the broken heart was not recognized as an official diagnosis of cardiac dysfunction or grief-related death. Today the diagnosis of a broken heart is very real and now has several fancy names...transient apical ballooning, stress cardiomyopathy, and takotsubo (TACK-ott-sue-boh) cardiomyopathy. The signs and symptoms of the broken heart resemble those of a heart attack, especially the chest pain and dyspnea. One of the diagnostic challenges is to differentiate the signs of the broken heart from those of a heart attack.

What's going on with the broken heart? Although the underlying cause isn't known, one theory proposes that extreme stress causes an intense sympathetic nervous system discharge and exposure of the heart to a large amount of catecholamines (epinephrine and norepinephrine). The catecholamines, in turn, cause coronary artery spasm, a diminishment of oxygen to the myocardial cells, and myocardial cell dysfunction. The coronary artery spasm induces structural changes in the left ventricular (LV) wall. In response to ischemic conditions, the lower part of the LV, called the *apex*, contracts ineffectively and "balloons"—hence the name *apical ballooning*, the hallmark structural defect of this cardiomyopathy. The upper part of the LV narrows and also contracts less in a dysfunctional way.

So, what's with the octopus and the takotsubo? The shape of the left ventricle of the broken heart resembles the shape of the fishing pot used to catch an octopus. The Japanese word for "fishing pot" is *tsubo,* and the word for "octopus" is *tako*...hence the word *takotsubo.* Takotsubo cardiomyopathy...an apt description for a grief-stricken heart.

Good news for the broken heart...in most persons the cardiomyopathy resolves in 2 to 3 weeks with no permanent damage. Obviously, the symptoms of the cardiac distress must be treated and the stressful events leading up to the cardiac event addressed...not an easy thing!

 As You Age

1. Contrary to popular opinion, no significant age-related decline occurs in resting cardiac output. When cardiac output declines, it is a result of age-related disease processes such as arteriosclerosis.
2. An age-related decline occurs in exercise cardiac output. The heart cannot respond as quickly or as forcefully to the increased workload of the exercised heart. Exertion, sudden movements, and changes in position may cause a decrease in cardiac output, resulting in dizziness, loss of balance, and falls.
3. Several structural changes in the heart contribute to the impaired response to exercise: heart muscle loses elasticity and becomes more rigid, heart valves become thicker and more rigid, the number of pacemaker cells decreases, and the aging heart cells have a decreased ability to use oxygen.
4. An age-related increase occurs in blood pressure, which increases the work the heart must do to pump blood into the systemic circulation.

Medical Terminology and Disorders   Disorders of the Heart

MEDICAL TERM	WORD PARTS	WORD PART MEANING OR DERIVATION	DESCRIPTION
Words			
bradycardia	brady-	abnormally slow	**Bradycardia** is *an abnormally slow heart rate (<60 beats/min).*
	-cardi/o-	heart	
	-ia	condition of	
cardiogram	cardi/o-	heart	A **cardiogram** is *a recording of the electrical events of the heart.*
	-gram	record	
ectopic	ec-	out of	An **ectopic** beat is one that originates outside the SA node. Examples include premature atrial and ventricular beats.
	-top/o-	place	
	-ic	condition of	
pericardium	peri-	around	The **pericardium** is *a slinglike membrane that surrounds the heart.*
	-cardi/o-	heart	
	-ium	tissue or structure	
tachycardia	tachy-	fast	**Tachycardia** is *an abnormally fast heart rate (>120 beats/min).*
	-cardi/o-	heart	
	-ia	condition of	
Disorders			
angina pectoris	angina	From the Greek word *ankhone,* meaning "to strangle"	**Angina pectoris**, also called *chest pain,* signals a diminished coronary blood flow to the heart. There are three forms of angina pectoris: 1. **Chronic stable angina (or exertional angina)** is triggered by physical activity and/or emotional excitement. The decreased coronary flow is due to changes associated with fatty plaque buildup (atherosclerosis). 2. **Variant angina (Prinzmetal's angina, vasospastic angina)** is caused by diminished blood flow resulting from spasm of the coronary arteries. 3. **Unstable angina** is a medical emergency; the diminished blood flow is due to severe coronary artery disease and complicated by vasospasm, rupture of the plaques, and formation of thrombi.
	pectoris	From the Latin word *pectus,* meaning "chest"	
coronary artery disease and atherosclerosis	coronary	Related to the veins and arteries	Also referred to as **CAD**, or **coronary heart disease** (CHD). Coronary blood flow is reduced because of a progressive narrowing of the coronary blood vessels that deprives the myocardium of O_2 and nutrients. Diminished coronary blood flow is most often caused by **atherosclerosis**, an inflammation-induced accumulation of fatty plaques on the inner lining of the coronary blood vessels. With time the fatty plaques reduce the elasticity of the arteries, causing them to thicken and harden *(sclerosis);* the plaque reduces coronary blood flow and can eventually rupture, causing thrombotic occlusion of the coronary artery. Untreated, atherosclerosis commonly progresses to myocardial infarction. A **myocardial infarction (MI)**, or "**heart attack**," refers to *the death or necrosis* (**infarction**) *of the heart muscle* (**myocardium**) *caused by insufficient oxygenated blood.*
	athero/o-	From the Greek word *ather/o,* meaning "oatmeal" or "gruel"	
	-scler/o-	harden	
	-osis	condition of	
carditis	cardi/o-	heart	**Carditis** is *inflammation of the heart;* this includes the following conditions: endocarditis, myocarditis, and pericarditis. **Endocarditis** is *an inflammation of the endocardium, the inner lining of the heart and valves.* It is most often caused by bacterial infection; bacteria enter the blood from any infected part of the body, particularly infected gums and dental procedures. **Myocarditis** is *an inflammation of the heart muscle and is most often associated with viral infection.* **Pericarditis** is *an inflammation of the outer lining of the heart (pericardium).* **Pericarditis** may be accompanied by the accumulation of serous or purulent exudates in the pericardial space, which, in turn, may cause **cardiac tamponade** *(external compression of the heart)* and heart failure.
	-itis	inflammation	

Continued

Medical Terminology and Disorders   Disorders of the Heart—cont'd

MEDICAL TERM	WORD PARTS	WORD PART MEANING OR DERIVATION	DESCRIPTION
cardiomegaly	cardi/o-	heart	**Cardiomegaly,** *an enlarged heart,* is not a disease, but a consequence of an underlying disorder. There are two types of cardiomegaly:
	-megal/o-	large	
	-y	condition of	1. **Dilative cardiomegaly** develops when the heart weakens and becomes dilated by the increased blood volume, as in heart failure.
			2. **Hypertrophic cardiomegaly** refers to the hypertrophy (growth in size) of the myocardium in response to an increased workload.
cardiomyopathy	cardi/o-	heart	**Cardiomyopathy** is a *disease of the heart muscle that results in weak and insufficient pumping activity.* In its earliest stage, cardiomyopathy is often asymptomatic, but it gradually progresses to cardiomegaly and heart failure. There are four types:
	-my/o-	muscle	
	-path	disease of	
	-y	condition of	1. In **dilated cardiomyopathy,** the cardiac chambers dilate.
			2. In **hypertrophic cardiomyopathy,** the myocardium thickens or hypertrophies.
			3. In **ischemic cardiomyopathy,** the myocardium thins and weakens because of a poor blood supply.
			4. In **restrictive cardiomyopathy,** the thickened myocardium prevents ventricular filling.
congenital heart defects	con-	together or with	*Heart and defects of the great vessels that are present from birth* are called **congenital heart defects.** The term includes structural defects, such as septal defects, valvular disorders, absence or incomplete development of cardiac structures, and disturbances in cardiac rhythm. Congenital heart defects are also classified as **cyanotic** or **acyanotic,** depending upon the degree of O_2 saturation. Examples of congenital heart defects are septal defects, patent ductus arteriosus, tetralogy of Fallot, transposition of the great vessels, tricuspid atresia, and coarctation of the aorta. Septal defects create **shunts** (left-to-right, right-to-left) because of the pressure differences within the chambers. A **ventriculoseptal** defect (**VSD**) is the most common congenital heart defect.
	-gen/o-	origin	
	-al	pertaining to	
dysrhythmia	dys-	faulty	*Any disturbance in normal cardiac rhythm* is referred to a **dysrhythmia.** Dysrhythmias are classified in several ways. According to rate: normal sinus rhythm, bradycardia, and tachycardia. According to mechanism: automaticity, reentry, junctional, and fibrillation. According to origin: atrial, junctional, ventricular, heart blocks, and arrhythmias that cause sudden death. **Bradydysrhythmias** (brady- = slow) are *rhythm disturbances that are characterized by excessively slow activity.* Slow electrical conduction through the heart causes varying degrees of heart block (first, second, complete). **Tachydysrhythmias** (tachy- = fast) are *rhythm disturbances that are characterized by excessive electrical activity.* Fast rhythm disorders include tachycardia, flutter, and fibrillation. These dysrhythmias may be atrial, ventricular, or both. Generally the ventricular rhythm disorders are more acute, demanding prompt attention.
	-rhythm/o-	rhythm	
	-ia	condition of	
heart failure			**Described in the text.**
valvular disorders	valvul/o-	valve	Some examples of **valvular disorders** include semilunar and AV valves, which are incompletely formed, too narrow, or incompetent. Tricuspid atresia is an example of an incompletely formed valve. **Valvular stenosis** (i.e., mitral valve stenosis) is a narrowing of a valve restricting the flow of blood. An **incompetent valve** is a leaky valve; it does not do its job, which is to prevent backflow of blood.
	-ar	pertaining to	

Get Ready for Exams!

Summary Outline

The heart pumps blood through the blood vessels, supplying the cells of the body with oxygen and nutrients and carrying away the waste products of metabolism. The heart functions in a coordinated and adaptable manner to perform its tasks.

I. **The Coordinated and Adaptable Pump**
   A. Cardiac cycle
      1. The cardiac cycle is a sequence of events that occurs during one heartbeat.
      2. The events of the cardiac cycle include atrial and ventricular systole (contraction) and diastole (relaxation).
   B. Heart: autonomic control
      1. The autonomic nervous system (ANS) allows the heart to respond to changing body needs.
      2. Stimulation of the sympathetic nerves increases heart rate (SA node), conduction velocity (AV node), and contractile force (myocardium).
      3. Stimulation of the parasympathetic nerves (vagus) decreases heart rate and conduction velocity.
   C. Cardiac output (CO) and venous return
      1. CO is the amount of blood pumped by the ventricle in 1 minute.
      2. CO is determined by heart rate (HR) and stroke volume (SV).
      3. Many factors can change HR and/or SV.
      4. Venous return is the rate of blood flow back to the heart.
   D. How stroke volume can be changed
      1. SV can be changed by Starling's law of the heart (stretch).
      2. SV can be changed by an inotropic effect (nonstretch).

II. **Heart Talk**
   A. Heart talk: clinical terms
      1. Includes the definition and description of commonly used clinical terms such as preload, afterload, ejection fraction, inotropic effect, chronotropic effect, and dromotropic effect
   B. Heart talk: receptor terminology
      1. Includes the definitions of beta$_1$-adrenergic receptor activation, beta$_1$-adrenergic receptor blockade, muscarinic receptor activation, and muscarinic receptor blockade

III. **The Failing Heart: When the Heart Can't Pump**
   A. Left heart failure
      1. The left heart can fail, producing symptoms caused by a backup of blood into the pulmonic circulation (pulmonary edema); referred to as backward failure.
      2. The failing left heart is unable to pump enough blood to the systemic circulation, producing symptoms related to poor tissue oxygenation; referred to as forward failure.
   B. Right heart failure
      1. Blood backs up behind the failed right ventricle, causing jugular vein distention, hepatomegaly, splenomegaly, digestive problems, and ankle edema.

Review Your Knowledge

Matching: Cardiac Function Terms
Directions: Match the following words with their descriptions. Some words may be used more than once.

a. inotropic effect
b. cardiac output
c. stroke volume
d. diastole
e. systole
f. Starling's law of the heart

1. _b_ 5000 mL/min
2. _c_ 70 mL/beat
3. _b_ Stroke volume times heart rate
4. _e_ Phase of the cardiac cycle that refers to myocardial contraction
5. _d_ Phase of the cardiac cycle during which the ventricles fill with blood
6. _d_ Phase of the cardiac cycle that refers to myocardial relaxation
7. _f_ Change in myocardial contraction that is caused by stretching of the heart muscle
8. _a_ Change in myocardial contraction that is not caused by stretching of the heart muscle
9. _c_ Amount of blood pumped by the ventricle in one beat
10. _b_ Amount of blood pumped by the ventricle in 1 minute

Matching: Loads and Effects
Directions: Match the following words with their descriptions. Some words may be used more than once.

a. afterload
b. preload
c. ejection fraction
d. dromotropic effect
e. chronotropic effect

1. _b_ Amount of blood in the ventricle at the end of its resting phase
2. _c_ Percentage of the end-diastolic volume (EDV) pumped by the ventricle
3. _a_ Arteriolar constriction and hypertension cause this to increase
4. _b_ Forms the basis of Starling's law of the heart
5. _e_ The effect of a drug that changes heart rate
6. _d_ Digoxin slows the speed of the cardiac impulse through the conduction system, thereby potentially causing a heart block
7. _b_ Same as end-diastolic volume (EDV)
8. _c_ May decline from 67% to 30% in the failing heart

Multiple Choice

1. Which of the following statements is correct about cardiac output?
   a. Cardiac output is determined by the heart rate and pulse.
   b. Stimulation of the sympathetic nerves decreases cardiac output.
   c. Cardiac index is the same as cardiac output.
   d. Cardiac output is determined by heart rate and stroke volume.

2. Which statement is true of ventricular diastole?
   a. Blood is ejected from the ventricles.
   b. The semilunar valves are open.
   c. The atrioventricular valves are closed.
   d. Blood fills the ventricles.

3. Which of the following statements is true of ventricular systole?
   a. Blood fills the ventricles.
   b. The atrioventricular valves remain open throughout ventricular systole.
   c. The semilunar valves remain closed throughout ventricular systole.
   d. Blood is ejected from the ventricles.

4. Which of the following most accurately describes the vagus nerve?
   a. Sympathetic, NE, activates muscarinic receptors, increases heart rate.
   b. Parasympathetic, ACh, activates beta-adrenergic receptors, slows heart rate.
   c. Parasympathetic, ACh, activates muscarinic receptors, slows heart rate.
   d. ACh, activates muscarinic receptors, increases heart rate

5. Which of the following is most related to bradycardia?
   a. <60 beats/min
   b. "fight or flight"
   c. (+) chronotropic effect
   d. $Beta_1$-adrenergic receptor activation

6. An increased venous return stretches the ventricular myocardium, thereby increasing stroke volume and cardiac output. Which of the following best describes this effect?
   a. Cardiac reserve
   b. Cardiac cycle
   c. (-) inotropic effect
   d. Starling's law of the heart

7. Which of the following is defined as a change of the force of myocardial contraction that is not due to the stretching of the ventricular myocardial fibers?
   a. Cardiac cycle
   b. Cardiac reserve
   c. Starling's law of the heart
   d. Inotropic effect

8. An increase in preload is most apt to
   a. decrease cardiac output due to vagal stimulation.
   b. increase cardiac output because of Starling's law of the heart.
   c. decrease stroke volume.
   d. decrease the ejection fraction.

9. A positive inotropic agent is most apt to
   a. increase cardiac output.
   b. decrease heart rate.
   c. decrease stroke volume.
   d. decrease venous return.

10. What is the response to left ventricular systole?
    a. Closure of the aortic semilunar valve
    b. Ejection of a bolus of blood into the aorta
    c. Opening of the mitral valve
    d. Decreased left intraventricular pressure

11. Which of the following combinations is a cardiac response to vagal nerve stimulation?
    a. Decreased heart rate, prolonged P-R interval, (–) chronotropic effect
    b. (+) inotropic effect, decreased cardiac output, tachycardia
    c. Increased stroke volume, increased heart rate, increased cardiac output
    d. (-) inotropic effect, (–) chronotropic effect, tachycardia

12. Which of the following is the result of a (+) inotropic effect?
    a. Increased heart rate
    b. Increased stroke volume
    c. Decreased cardiac output
    d. Decreased ejection fraction

13. Which of the following is *least* true of the stroke volume?
    a. Refers to the amount of the blood ejected from the ventricle in one heart beat
    b. Is expressed as mL/min
    c. Is affected by the force of myocardial contraction
    d. Is one of the determinants of cardiac output

14. A change in end-diastolic volume (EDV) causes a change in which of the following?
    a. Stroke volume
    b. Cardiac output
    c. Force of myocardial contraction
    d. All of the above

15. Which of the following refers to the amount of blood in the ventricles at the end of ventricular relaxation?
    a. Afterload
    b. Ejection fraction
    c. Stroke volume
    d. Preload

16. Which of the following refers to the resistance or opposition to the flow of blood from the heart?
    a. Afterload
    b. End-diastolic volume (EDV)
    c. Preload
    d. Ejection fraction

Go Figure

1. Which of the following is true according to Fig. 17.1?
   a. The semilunar valves are open during atrial systole.
   b. The AV valves are closed during ventricular systole.
   c. Blood is pumped out of the atria during ventricular systole.
   d. The AV valves remain closed during atrial systole.

2. According to Fig. 17.1, during ventricular systole
   a. blood flows passively from the atria into the ventricles.
   b. blood is pumped into the pulmonary arteries and the aorta.
   c. blood is pumped by the atria into the ventricles.
   d. all valves are open.

3. Which of the following is true according to Fig. 17.2?
   a. The neurotransmitter for the vagus nerve is norepinephrine.
   b. The vagus nerve is a sympathetic nerve.
   c. The ventricular myocardium is innervated only by sympathetic nerves.
   d. The SA node is subject only to vagal effects.

4. According to Fig. 17.2, the postganglionic parasympathetic fiber
   a. secretes NE.
   b. secretes a transmitter that binds to a beta$_1$-adrenergic receptor.
   c. is cholinergic.
   d. is adrenergic.

5. Which of the following is true according to Fig. 17.2?
   a. Sympathetic firing affects the force of myocardial contraction.
   b. The AV node can be stimulated only by ACh.
   c. The SA node contains receptors that respond only to ACh.
   d. The fibers that are color-coded red are cholinergic.

6. Which of the following is true according to Fig. 17.3?
   a. An increase in venous return stretches the ventricular myocardium, thereby decreasing cardiac output.
   b. An increase in venous return increases cardiac output because of Starling's law of the heart.
   c. A decrease in venous return has no effect on cardiac output.
   d. A decrease in venous return increases cardiac output because of Starling's law of the heart.

7. Which of the following is true according to Fig. 17.4?
   a. Increased venous return increases preload.
   b. Increased venous return decreases EDV.
   c. Increased EDV increases afterload.
   d. Dilation of the aorta and peripheral blood vessels increases afterload.

8. Which of the following is true according to Fig. 17.5?
   a. When the left heart fails, the patient appears cyanotic because he is in pain.
   b. The cyanosis and pulmonary edema are most likely caused by pulmonic valve stenosis.
   c. When the left heart fails, blood backs up in the pulmonary capillaries, causing fluid accumulation in the lungs and hypoxemia.
   d. The earliest symptoms of acute left-sided failure are pedal (ankle) edema and abdominal bloating.

9. Which of the following is true according to Fig. 17.6?
   a. Right-sided heart failure usually develops in response to an occlusion of the left anterior descending (LAD) artery.
   b. The right ventricle can't pump blood efficiently, so fluid accumulates in the lungs.
   c. The consequences of right-sided heart failure are ankle edema, jugular vein distension (JVD), and enlarged liver.
   d. Right-sided failure is usually due to aortic valve stenosis.

Objectives

1. Describe the pulmonary and systemic circulations.
2. Describe the structure and function of arteries, capillaries, and veins, including the following:
   - List the three layers of tissue found in arteries and veins.
   - Explain the functions of conductance, resistance, exchange, and capacitance vessels.
3. List the major arteries of the systemic circulation that are branches of the ascending aorta, aortic arch, and descending aorta.
4. List the major veins of the systemic circulation.
5. Describe the following special circulations: blood supply to the head and brain, hepatic circulation, and fetal circulation.
6. Explain pulse and its use as an assessment tool.

Key Terms

aorta (p. 346)
arteries (p. 343)
arterioles (p. 343)
capacitance vessels (p. 346)
capillaries (p. 343)
circle of Willis (p. 351)
conductance vessels (p. 345)
ductus arteriosus (p. 356)

ductus venosus (p. 354)
exchange vessels (p. 345)
fetal circulation (p. 353)
foramen ovale (p. 356)
hepatic portal system (p. 353)
pulmonary circulation (p. 342)
pulse (p. 356)
resistance vessels (p. 345)

special circulations (p. 351)
systemic circulation (p. 343)
umbilical arteries (p. 354)
umbilical vein (p. 354)
veins (p. 343)
venae cavae (p. 349)
venules (p. 343)

The circulatory system consists of the heart and blood vessels. The historical description of the heart and blood vessels is intriguing. The ancients knew that the heart played an important role in pumping blood through the body, but no one described the intricate role of the blood vessels. The ancient Greeks thought that blood moved throughout the body like an ocean tide. Blood was seen as washing out from the heart through a series of blood vessels and then ebbing back to it through those same blood vessels, with impurities removed from the blood as it washed through the lungs. Not until the 17th century did the English physician William Harvey, described as a crackpot by his fellow scientists, identify the system of blood vessels and thus provide the first accurate description of the circulation.

CIRCLES, CIRCUITS, AND CIRCULATIONS

The blood vessels are a series of connected hollow tubes that begin and end in the heart. The blood vessels form a path through the body, much like the system of highways and roads that enables us to travel from place to place. Note the path of the delivery truck in Fig. 18.1. Leaving the bakery, the truck travels on a major highway and exits onto a smaller road. The truck then arrives at a grocery store, where it makes a delivery. The empty truck returns to the bakery through a number of connecting roads. Note the circle, or circuit, from bakery to grocery store to bakery.

The heart and blood vessels also form a circuit. The heart pumps blood into the large artery. The blood flows through a series of blood vessels back to the heart. Moving from heart to blood vessels to heart, the blood forms a circuit, or circulation. This arrangement ensures a continuous one-way movement of blood. As Chapter 16 explained, the two main circulations are the pulmonary circulation and the systemic circulation.

The **pulmonary circulation** carries blood from the right ventricle of the heart to the lungs and back to the left atrium of the heart (see Fig. 16.3). The pulmonary circulation transports unoxygenated blood to the lungs, where oxygen is loaded and carbon dioxide is unloaded. Oxygenated blood then returns to the left side of the heart to be pumped into the systemic circulation.

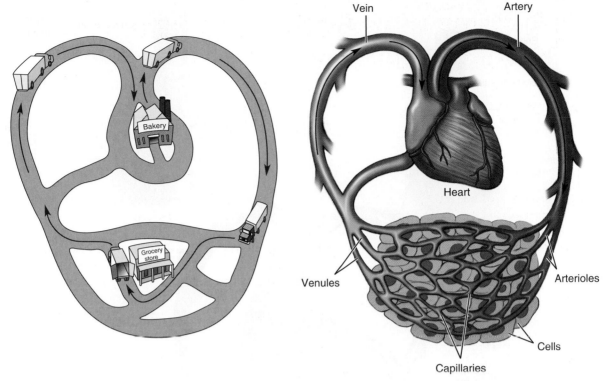

FIG. 18.1 **A circuit or route: the circulatory system.**

The **systemic circulation** is the larger circulation; it provides the blood supply to the rest of the body. The systemic circulation carries oxygen and other nutrients to the cells and picks up carbon dioxide and other waste.

BLOOD VESSELS

NAMING THE BLOOD VESSELS

Note the different types of blood vessels (Fig. 18.2), their relationship to the heart, and the color-coding. The blood vessels are the body's highways; they are anatomically classified as arteries, capillaries, and veins (Table 18.1).

ARTERIES

Arteries are blood vessels that carry blood away from the heart. The large arteries repeatedly branch into smaller and smaller arteries as they are distributed throughout the entire body. As they branch, the arteries become much more numerous but smaller in diameter. The smallest arteries are called **arterioles** (ar-TEER-ee-ohls). Most of the arteries are color-coded red because they carry oxygenated blood.

CAPILLARIES

Blood flows from the arterioles into the capillaries. The **capillaries** (KAP-i-lair-ees) are the smallest and most numerous of all the blood vessels. They connect the arterioles with the venules. Because the body has so many of them, a capillary is close to every cell in the body. This arrangement provides every cell with a continuous supply of oxygen and other nutrients. The capillaries are colored from red to purple to blue. Why? At the capillary level, the blood gives up its oxygen to the tissues; the unoxygenated blood leaving the tissues is therefore bluish.

VEINS

Blood flows from the capillaries into the veins. **Veins** are blood vessels that carry blood back to the heart. The smallest veins are called **venules** (VEN-yools). The small venules converge to form fewer but larger veins. The largest veins empty the blood into the right atrium of the heart. Most of the veins are color-coded blue because they carry unoxygenated blood.

 Re-Think

1. Differentiate between the pulmonary and systemic circulations.
2. Define *artery*. Why are most arteries color-coded red?
3. Define *vein*. Why are most veins color-coded blue?
4. Why does the color-coding for capillaries change from red to purple to blue?

BLOOD VESSEL WALLS: THE LAYERED LOOK

With the exception of the capillaries, the blood vessels are composed of three layers (or tunics) of tissue (see Fig. 18.2): tunica intima, tunica media, and tunica adventitia.

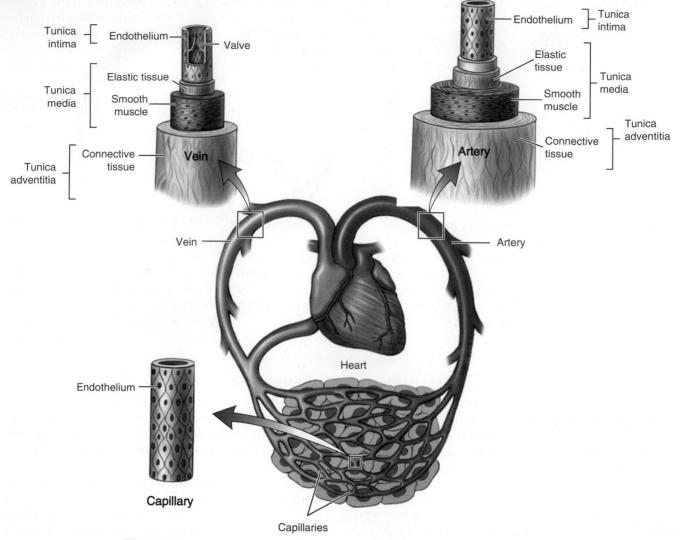

FIG. 18.2 Blood vessel wall layers: the tunica intima, tunica media, and tunica adventitia.

Table 18.1	Structure and Function of Blood Vessels	
VESSEL	**STRUCTURE**	**FUNCTION**
Artery	Thick wall with three layers: tunica intima (endothelial lining), tunica media (elastic tissue and smooth muscle), and tunica adventitia (connective tissue)	Called *conductance vessels* because they carry blood from the heart to the arterioles
Arteriole	Small artery but with three layers, mostly smooth muscle	Called *resistance vessels* because the contraction and relaxation of the muscle changes vessel diameter, which alters resistance to blood flow
Capillary	Layer of endothelium on a basement membrane	Called *exchange vessels* because nutrients, gases, and wastes exchange between the blood and interstitial fluid
Vein (venules)	Thin wall with less smooth muscle and elastic tissue than an artery or arteriole Three layers (intima, media, and adventitia), but thinner and less elastic than an artery; contain valves	Venules and veins collect and return blood from the tissues to the heart. They are called *capacitance vessels* because they hold or store blood.

1. *Tunica intima.* The tunica (TOO-nik-kah) intima is the innermost layer, an endothelium. The endothelial lining forms a slick, shiny surface continuous with the endocardium, the inner lining of the heart. Blood flows easily and smoothly along this surface.
2. *Tunica media.* The tunica media is the middle layer. It is the thickest layer and is composed primarily of elastic tissue and smooth muscle; the thickness and composition vary according to the function of the blood vessel. The large arteries, for example, contain considerable elastic tissue so that they can stretch in response to the pumping of blood by the heart. The smallest of the arteries, the arterioles, are composed primarily of smooth muscle. The muscle allows the arterioles to contract and relax, thereby changing the diameter of the arteriole.
3. *Tunica adventitia.* The outer layer is called the *tunica adventitia* (ad-ven-TEESH-ah). Composed of tough connective tissue, its main function is to support and protect blood vessels.

BLOOD VESSELS: WHAT THEY DO

Note how the structure of the blood vessels changes from artery to capillary to vein (see Fig. 18.2 and Table 18.1). As always, the structure is related to its function. The following is a functional classification of blood vessels.

ARTERIES

The walls of the large arteries are thick, tough, and elastic because they must withstand the high pressure of the blood pumped from the ventricles. Because the primary function of the large arteries is to conduct blood from the heart to the arterioles, the large arteries are called **conductance vessels**.

ARTERIOLES

The arterioles are the smallest of the arteries. They are composed primarily of smooth muscle and spend most of their time contracting and relaxing. By changing their diameter, the arterioles affect resistance to the flow of blood. A narrow (constricted) vessel offers an increased resistance to blood flow; a wider (dilated) vessel offers less resistance. Because of their effect on resistance, the arterioles are called **resistance vessels**.

CAPILLARIES

The capillaries have the thinnest walls of any of the blood vessels. The capillary wall is made up of a single layer of endothelium lying on a delicate basement membrane. The thin capillary wall enables water and dissolved substances, including oxygen, to move across the capillary wall from the blood into the tissue spaces, where they become available for use by

the cells. The capillary also allows waste from the metabolizing cell to diffuse from the tissue spaces into the capillaries for transport by the blood to the organs of excretion. The capillaries are called **exchange vessels** because they allow for an exchange of nutrients and waste.

> ### ? Re-Think
>
> 1. Why are the layers of the arteries thicker than those of the capillaries?
> 2. Explain the color coding of arteries, capillaries, and veins.

VEINS AND VENULES

As the capillaries begin to converge to form venules, the structure of the wall changes again. The venule wall is slightly thicker than the capillary wall. As the venules converge to form larger veins, the walls become even thicker. The tunica media of the vein, however, is much thinner than the tunica media of the artery. This difference is appropriate because pressure in the veins is much less than the pressure in the arterial blood vessels.

In addition to thinner walls, the veins differ in another way; most veins contain one-way valves. These valves direct the flow of blood toward the heart. The valves are most numerous in the veins of the lower extremities, where they prevent backflow, helping move blood up and away from the ankles toward the heart.

While the valves facilitate the movement of venous blood toward the heart, the veins sometimes need some "outside" help. This is particularly true of the veins of the lower extremities. The problem? Although blood pressure is very high in the arterial circulation, it decreases to almost 0 mm Hg in the veins. The pressure in the veins is so low, in fact, that it alone cannot return blood from the veins back to the heart. The "outside" help is the skeletal muscle pump. As Fig. 18.3 shows, the large veins in the leg are surrounded by skeletal muscles. When the skeletal muscles are

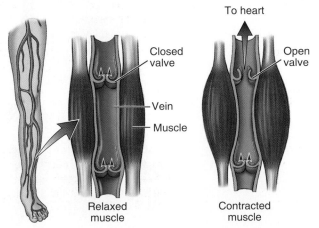

FIG. 18.3 Skeletal muscle pump. Note lumen of veins and positions of valves with muscle relaxation and contraction.

relaxed and blood flow slows, the valves close. As the skeletal muscles contract, they squeeze the large veins, thereby opening the valves and forcing blood toward the heart. This mechanism is called the *skeletal muscle pump*. The pump explains the beneficial effects of exercise for your patients. Exercise improves venous return of blood to the heart and prevents stagnation of blood and thrombosis (blood clot formation).

In addition to carrying blood back to the heart, the veins play another role. The veins store blood. In fact, about 70% of the total blood volume is found on the venous side of the circulation. Because the veins store blood, they are called **capacitance vessels**. (*Capacitance* refers to storage.) When this stored blood is needed, the veins constrict (venoconstriction) and move blood to the heart for circulation.

 Re-Think

1. Why are the layers of the arteries thicker than those of the capillaries?
2. Why are the arterioles called resistance vessels?
3. Why are the capillaries called exchange vessels?
4. Why are the large arteries and veins not suitable for exchange?
5. Why do the veins, but not the arteries, contain valves?

 Sum It Up!

The blood vessels are a series of connected hollow tubes that form a circuit. There are two circulations: the pulmonary circulation and the systemic circulation. The three types of blood vessels are arteries (conductance), capillaries (exchange), and veins (capacitance). The arterioles are tiny arteries called *resistance vessels*. Because the blood pressure within the veins is so low, "outside" help in the form of the skeletal muscle pump assists in the return of the blood to the heart. There are three layers of most blood vessel walls: tunica intima, tunica media, and tunica adventitia. The composition of the layers differs depending on the function of the blood vessel.

MAJOR ARTERIES OF THE SYSTEMIC CIRCULATION

The major arteries of the systemic circulation include the aorta and the arteries arising from the aorta.

AORTA

The **aorta** (ay-OR-tah) is the mother of all arteries; its average diameter is that of a garden hose. The aorta originates in the heart's left ventricle (Fig. 18.4),

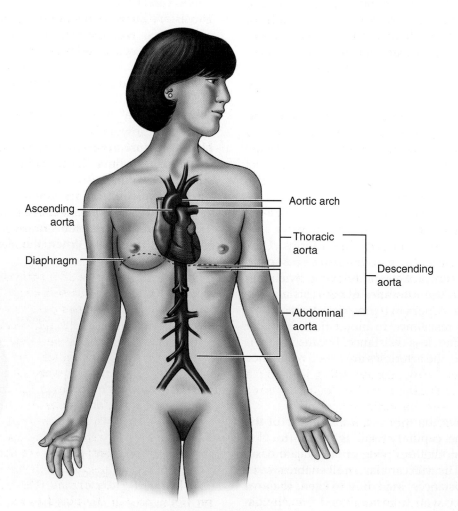

FIG. 18.4 **Naming the parts of the aorta.**

extends upward from the left ventricle, curves in an archlike fashion, and then descends through the thoracic and abdominopelvic cavities. The aorta ends in the pelvic cavity, where it splits into two common iliac arteries.

The aorta is divided into segments, each named according to two systems. One system is the path that the aorta follows as it courses through the body. In this system, the aorta is divided into the ascending aorta, the arch of the aorta, and the descending aorta. In the second naming system, the aorta is named according to its location within the body cavities. Thus, we have the thoracic aorta and the abdominal aorta.

 Re-Think

1. Where does the aorta begin and end?
2. List five words that describe parts of the aorta.
3. Why is the aorta considered the mother of all arteries?

BRANCHES OF THE AORTA

All systemic arteries are direct or indirect branches of the aorta. In other words, the arteries arise directly from the aorta, or they arise from vessels that are themselves branches of the aorta. For example, the coronary arteries arise directly from the ascending aorta. The brachial artery in the right arm, however, arises from the axillary artery. The axillary artery has its origin in the subclavian artery, an extension of the brachiocephalic artery, which arises from the arch of the aorta. The brachial artery therefore arises indirectly from the aorta.

The systemic arteries are described in the order in which they arise from the aorta. Refer to Fig. 18.5 as you read the text to identify the arteries and the structures that they supply.

BRANCHES OF THE ASCENDING AORTA

The ascending aorta arises from the left ventricle of the heart. It begins at the aortic semilunar valve and extends upward to the aortic arch. The right and left coronary arteries branch from the ascending aorta at a point that is immediately distal to the aortic semilunar valve. The coronary arteries are distributed throughout the heart and supply oxygenated blood to the myocardium.

BRANCHES OF THE AORTIC ARCH

The aortic arch extends from the ascending aorta to the beginning of the descending aorta. The following three large arteries arise from the aortic arch:

• The brachiocephalic artery is a large artery on the right side of the body. Refer to Fig. 18.5 for the names of the arteries that extend from, or branch off, the brachiocephalic artery. These arteries supply the right side of the head and neck and the arm and hand regions. (There is no left brachiocephalic artery.)

• The left common carotid artery extends upward from the highest part of the aortic arch and supplies the left side of the head and neck. Note that the left common carotid artery arises directly from the aorta, whereas the right common carotid artery arises from the brachiocephalic artery. (The common carotid arteries are described later in the section entitled Special Circulations.)

• The left and right subclavian arteries supply blood to the shoulders and upper arms. The right subclavian artery is an extension of the brachiocephalic artery while the left subclavian artery arises from the aortic arch. The subclavian arteries give rise to the vertebral arteries (→brain) and also extend toward the shoulder as the axillary arteries; they then enter the arm as the brachial arteries. At the elbow the brachial artery divides into the ulnar and radial arteries, which supply the forearm. The distal radial artery, in particular, comes close to the surface at the wrist and is the site where the radial pulse can be assessed. Extensions of the ulnar and radial arteries form arteries that supply the hand.

BRANCHES OF THE DESCENDING AORTA (THORACIC AORTA)

The thoracic aorta is the upper portion of the descending aorta. It extends from the aortic arch to the diaphragm. Intercostal arteries arise from the aorta and supply the intercostal muscles between the ribs. Other small arteries supply the organs in the thorax.

BRANCHES OF THE DESCENDING AORTA (ABDOMINAL AORTA)

The abdominal aorta extends from the thoracic aorta to the lower abdomen. Branches of the abdominal aorta include the following:

• The celiac (SEE-lee-ack) trunk is a short artery that further divides into three smaller arteries: the gastric artery supplies the stomach, the splenic artery supplies the spleen, and the hepatic artery supplies the liver.

• Two mesenteric (MEZ-en-tair-ik) arteries are the superior and inferior segments. The superior mesenteric artery supplies blood to most of the small intestine and part of the large intestine. The other part of the large intestine receives its blood supply from the inferior mesenteric artery.

• Two renal arteries supply blood to the right and left kidneys. Other branches of the abdominal aorta include the gonadal arteries and the lumbar arteries.

The distal abdominal aorta splits into the right and left common iliac arteries. The common iliac arteries divide into the internal and external iliac arteries. The internal iliac artery supplies the pelvic organs and external reproductive organs. The external iliac artery provides most of the blood to the lower extremities. The external iliac artery extends into the thigh as the

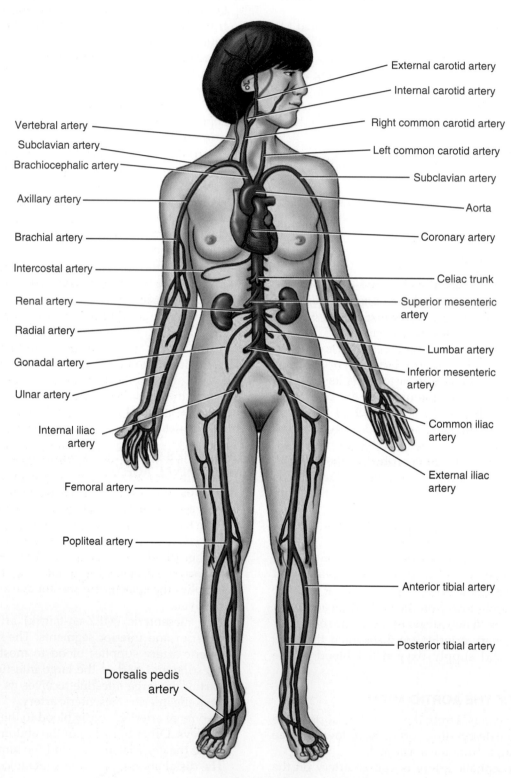

Vertebral artery

Subclavian artery

Brachiocephalic artery

Axillary artery

Brachial artery

Intercostal artery

Renal artery

Radial artery

Gonadal artery

Ulnar artery

Internal iliac artery

Femoral artery

Popliteal artery

Dorsalis pedis artery

External carotid artery

Internal carotid artery

Right common carotid artery

Left common carotid artery

Subclavian artery

Aorta

Coronary artery

Celiac trunk

Superior mesenteric artery

Lumbar artery

Inferior mesenteric artery

Common iliac artery

External iliac artery

Anterior tibial artery

Posterior tibial artery

FIG. 18.5 Major arteries.

femoral artery, becoming the popliteal artery, and then the anterior and posterior tibial arteries. The anterior tibial artery continues into the foot as the dorsalis pedis artery. Palpation of the dorsalis pedis pulse is used to assess blood flow in the foot.

 Re-Think

1. Identify the origin of the right and left common carotid arteries.
2. Identify the origin of the right and left subclavian arteries.
3. List five arteries that emerge directly from the aorta.
4. List in sequence the arteries arising from the aorta extending to the hand
5. List in sequence the arteries arising from the aorta extending to the foot.

MAJOR VEINS OF THE SYSTEMIC CIRCULATION

If you look at the back of your hand, you can see several veins but no arteries. Why? The arteries are usually located in deep and well-protected areas. Many of the veins, however, are located more superficially and can be seen. These are called *superficial veins*. Deep veins are located more deeply and usually run parallel to the arteries. With few exceptions, the names of the deep veins are the same as the names of the companion arteries. For example, the femoral artery is accompanied by the femoral vein. In Figs. 18.5 and 18.6, note the similarity in the names of many of the arteries and veins. Good news! If you learn the names of the arteries, you'll also know most of the names of the veins.

VENAE CAVAE

The veins carry blood from all parts of the body to the venae cavae for delivery to the heart. The **venae cavae** are the main veins. They are divided into the superior vena cava (SVC) and the inferior vena cava (IVC). Veins draining blood from the head, shoulders, and upper extremities empty into the SVC. Veins draining the lower part of the body empty into the IVC. The SVC and IVC empty into the right atrium.

 Do You Know...

Why Your Veins May Hum?

About 20% of the cardiac output flows to the brain and must therefore be returned to the right side of the heart. The large flow of blood through the jugular veins causes the walls of the veins to vibrate; the vibration can be heard as a venous hum in the upper chest near the clavicle (collarbone). The condition is benign but may be confused with a heart murmur. How do we differentiate between a heart murmur and venous hum? The venous hum disappears when the patient is placed in a supine position or if the clinician presses on the jugular vein. A true heart murmur is not affected by a change of position or compression of the jugular vein.

VEINS THAT EMPTY INTO THE SUPERIOR VENA CAVA

The SVC receives blood from the head, shoulder, and upper extremities. Veins may drain directly or indirectly into the SVC. For example, the brachiocephalic veins empty directly into the SVC. The axillary vein, however, drains into the subclavian vein, which drains into the brachiocephalic vein, which in turn drains into the SVC. Refer to Fig. 18.6 to help trace the flow of venous blood from a distal site to the vena cava, as follows:

- The cephalic vein is a superficial vein that drains the lateral arm region and carries blood to the axillary vein toward the SVC.
- The basilic vein is a superficial vein that drains the medial arm region. The cephalic and basilic veins receive unoxygenated blood from the ulnar and radial veins in the forearm. They are joined by the median cubital vein (anterior aspect of the elbow). Blood samples are often drawn from the median cubital vein.
- The axillary vein receives blood from the blood vessels in the arm and delivers it to the subclavian vein. The subclavian vein receives blood from the axillary vein and from the jugular veins and delivers it to the brachiocephalic vein (→ superior vena cava).
- The jugular veins drain blood from the head and drain into the subclavian veins. The external jugular veins drain blood from the face, scalp, and neck. The internal jugular veins drain blood from the brain. The internal jugular vein, in fact, is the main vein that drains the brain. Because the jugular veins are so close to the heart (right atrium), the pressure in the jugular veins reflects the pressure of blood in the right side of the heart. A person in right-sided heart failure has a higher-than-normal pressure in the right heart. This is observed clinically as pulsating jugular veins and is referred to as *jugular vein distention* (JVD). As a clinician, you will be observing, measuring, and recording JVD.
- The azygos vein is a single vein that drains the thorax and empties directly into the SVC.

 Do You Know...

What the Subclavian Stole?

"Thou shalt not steal." Good advice! It even applies to blood, with a condition called *subclavian steal syndrome*. This is how the heist goes down. A person develops an occlusion in the subclavian artery proximal to the origin of the vertebral artery. (Remember, the vertebral artery supplies blood to the posterior brain, and the subclavian artery supplies blood to the shoulder and arm.) When the affected arm is exercised, the subclavian artery is unable to supply enough blood. Blood pressure in the exercising shoulder and arm decreases, causing a retrograde (backward) flow of blood from the vertebral artery to the subclavian artery. The subclavian artery robs the posterior brain of blood, causing neurological symptoms such as impaired vision, dizziness, and syncope (fainting).

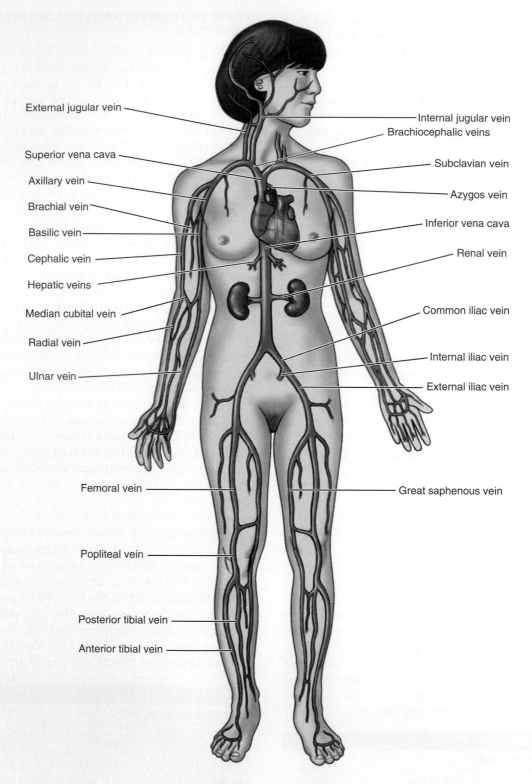

External jugular vein

Superior vena cava

Axillary vein

Brachial vein

Basilic vein

Cephalic vein

Hepatic veins

Median cubital vein

Radial vein

Ulnar vein

Femoral vein

Popliteal vein

Posterior tibial vein

Anterior tibial vein

Internal jugular vein

Brachiocephalic veins

Subclavian vein

Azygos vein

Inferior vena cava

Renal vein

Common iliac vein

Internal iliac vein

External iliac vein

Great saphenous vein

FIG. 18.6 **Major veins.**

VEINS THAT EMPTY INTO THE INFERIOR VENA CAVA

The IVC returns blood to the heart from all regions of the body below the diaphragm. Follow the venous drainage from the leg to the right atrium in Fig. 18.6.

- The tibial veins drain the calf and foot regions. The posterior tibial vein drains into the popliteal vein (behind the knee) and then the femoral vein (in the thigh). The femoral vein enters the pelvis as the external iliac vein; it joins with the internal iliac vein and continues as the common iliac vein. The common iliac vein continues as the IVC.
- The great saphenous (SAF-en-us) veins are the longest veins in the body. They begin in the foot, ascend along the medial side, and merge with the femoral vein to become the external iliac vein. These veins

receive drainage from the superficial veins of the leg and thigh region. The great saphenous veins also connect with the deep veins of the leg and thigh. Thus, blood can return from the lower extremities to the heart by several routes. The great saphenous veins are sometimes "borrowed" by cardiac surgeons. Portions of a vein are surgically removed and transplanted into the heart to bypass clogged coronary arteries.

- The renal veins drain the right and left kidneys, emptying blood directly into the IVC.
- The hepatic veins drain the liver, emptying blood directly into the upper IVC. Because the hepatic veins are so close to the heart, congestion of the right heart often causes congestion in the hepatic veins and liver.

Do You Know...
What Varicose Veins Look Like?

Varicose veins are distended and twisted veins, usually involving the superficial veins in the legs. Varicosities can develop in other veins. Hemorrhoids, for example, are varicose veins that affect the veins in the anal region. Persons who are alcoholic often develop varicose veins at the base of the esophagus—esophageal varices. Esophageal varices are apt to rupture, causing a massive life-threatening hemorrhage.

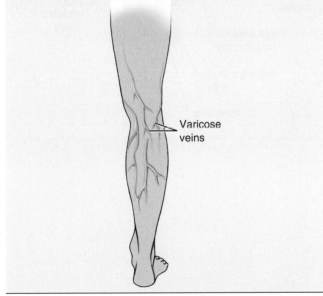
Varicose veins

Re-Think

1. Functionally, in what way does the venae cavae resemble the aorta?
2. List five veins that empty directly into the venae cavae.
3. List the sequence of veins as you trace a drop of blood from the left hand to the right atrium.
4. List the sequence of veins as you trace a drop of blood from the foot to the right atrium.

Sum It Up!

The arrangement and names of the major arteries and veins are summarized in Figs. 18.5 and 18.6. All systemic arteries are direct or indirect branches of the aorta, the main artery that arises from the left ventricle. The aorta is classified as the ascending aorta, arch of the aorta, and descending aorta. The descending aorta is described as the thoracic aorta and the abdominal aorta. Most veins throughout the body drain directly or indirectly into the superior and inferior venae cavae and then into the right atrium of the heart.

SPECIAL CIRCULATIONS

Most organs receive oxygen-rich blood from a single large artery, whereas oxygen-poor blood is drained by large veins. Several organs have circulations that are arranged differently. These special circulations include the blood supply to the head and brain, the blood supply to the liver, and the arrangement of the blood vessels in the unborn child (fetal circulation).

BLOOD SUPPLY TO THE HEAD AND BRAIN

The brain requires a continuous supply of blood; even a few minutes without oxygen alters the level of consciousness and causes brain damage. To ensure a rich supply of blood, the head is supplied by two pairs of arteries: carotid arteries and vertebral arteries (Fig. 18.7A).

ARTERIES OF THE HEAD AND NECK

The right common carotid artery, arising from the brachiocephalic artery, and the left common carotid artery, arising directly from the aortic arch (see Fig. 18.7B), ascend in the anterolateral neck. At about the level of the mandible, the common carotid arteries split to form the external and internal carotid arteries. The external carotid arteries supply the superficial areas of the neck, face, and scalp. The internal carotid arteries extend to the anterior part of the brain. Once inside the cranium, the internal carotid arteries divide, sending numerous branches to various parts of the brain. The internal carotid arteries supply most of the blood to the brain.

Vertebral arteries pass upward in the posterolateral neck from the subclavian arteries toward the brain. As the vertebral arteries extend up into the cranium, they join to form a single basilar artery (see Fig. 18.7B). Numerous branches from the basilar artery supply areas of the brain around the brain stem and cerebellum. Other branches of the basilar artery connect with branches of the internal carotid arteries forming a circle of arteries at the base of the brain. This circular arrangement of arteries is called the circle of Willis (see Fig. 18.7B). Arising from the circle of Willis are many arteries that penetrate the brain and maintain its rich supply of blood.

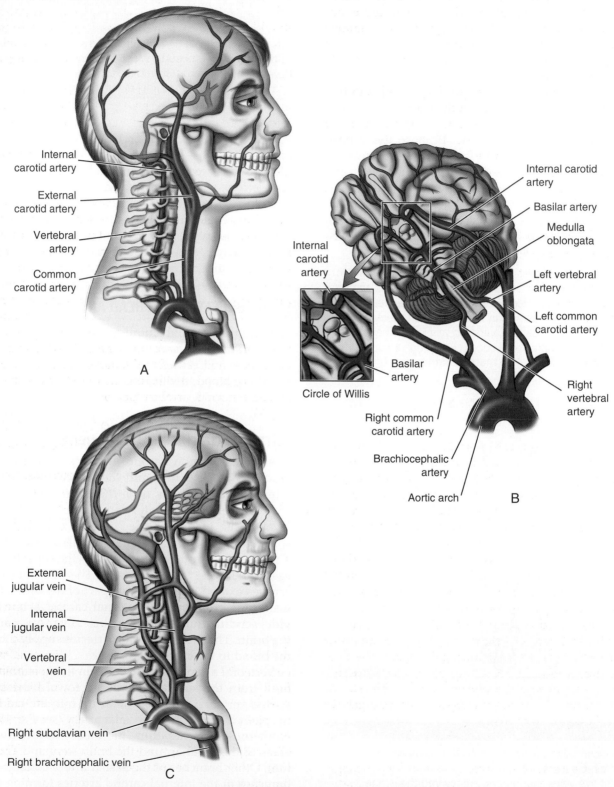

FIG. 18.7 Blood supply to the head and the brain. (A) The head is supplied by the common carotid and the vertebral arteries. (B) The circle of Willis. (C) Venous drainage of the brain and head.

Most of the blood supply to the brain runs through the internal carotid arteries. What about knotted or clotted carotids? If the carotid arteries become blocked, the brain receives insufficient blood because the vertebral arteries cannot make up for the deficit. This deficit results in impaired brain function, most often observed as a cognitive (thinking) impairment and dizziness.

VENOUS DRAINAGE OF THE HEAD AND BRAIN

The external and internal jugular veins are the two major veins that drain blood from the head and neck (see Fig. 18.7C). The external jugular veins are more superficial and drain blood from the posterior head and neck region. They empty into the subclavian veins. The internal jugular veins drain the anterior head, face, and neck. The deep internal jugular veins drain most of the blood from the venous sinuses of the brain. The internal jugular veins on each side of the neck join with the subclavian veins to form the brachiocephalic veins (then to the SVC).

Re-Think

1. Explain the formation of the circle of Willis by the carotid and vertebral arteries.
2. What is the clinical consequence of a blocked carotid artery?
3. What is the role of the jugular veins?

BLOOD SUPPLY TO THE LIVER AND THE HEPATIC PORTAL CIRCULATION

The purpose of the hepatic portal circulation is to carry blood rich in digestive end products from the organs of digestion to the liver. Because it plays such a critical role in metabolism, the liver needs easy access to the digestive end products. As the blood flows through the liver, many of the nutrients are extracted from the blood and modified in some way. For example, the liver prevents nitrogen from entering the general circulation as ammonia. Instead, the nitrogen is excreted by the liver into the blood in the form of urea. Urea is less toxic than ammonia and is easily eliminated by the kidneys. In addition to its handling of nitrogen, the liver also has immediate access to the large amounts of glucose that is absorbed during digestion. The liver stores the excess glucose as glycogen; when needed, the liver can release the glucose into the blood. For many reasons it is crucial that blood from the digestive organs first goes to the liver!

HEPATIC BLOOD VESSELS

The blood vessels of the liver have a unique arrangement. Three groups of blood vessels are associated with hepatic circulation: the portal vein, the hepatic veins, and the hepatic artery.

The portal vein is a large vein that carries blood from the organs of digestion to the liver (Fig. 18.8). It is formed by the union of two large veins: the superior mesenteric vein and the splenic vein. The superior mesenteric vein receives blood from the small intestine (where most digestion and absorption occur) and the first part of the large intestine. The splenic vein receives blood from the stomach, spleen, and pancreas. In addition, the splenic vein receives blood from the inferior mesenteric vein, which drains the distal part of the large intestine. This unique venous arrangement is called the **hepatic portal system**.

In addition to the portal vein, the liver has two other blood vessels: the hepatic artery and the hepatic veins. The hepatic artery is a branch of the celiac trunk (Fig. 18.5), a large artery that branches off the abdominal aorta. The hepatic artery carries oxygen-rich blood to the liver. The hepatic veins drain blood from the liver and deliver it to the inferior vena cava.

Note that both the hepatic artery and portal vein carry blood toward the liver. The hepatic artery carries oxygen-rich blood, and the portal vein carries blood rich in the products of digestion to the liver but poor in oxygen content. Once in the liver, blood from the hepatic artery and portal vein perfuses the capillaries called *hepatic sinusoids*. The sinusoids have large pores that permit the mixing of arterial and venous blood, and facilitate the delivery of digestive end-products to the liver cells. The sinusoids are also lined with phagocytic cells called *Kupffer cells*; these cells remove bacteria from portal blood before the blood leaves the liver and enters the general circulation.

Re-Think

1. List the blood vessels through which blood is delivered to the liver.
2. Identify the blood vessels that carry blood away from the liver and deliver it to the inferior vena cava.
3. What is the role of the hepatic sinusoids?
4. What is the purpose of the hepatic portal system?

FETAL CIRCULATION

Look at your "belly button," or umbilicus. At one time, you had a long umbilical cord, a lifeline that attached you to a structure called the *placenta* embedded in the wall of your mother's uterus. Why was this attachment necessary? As a fetus, you were submerged in amniotic fluid and were unable to eat, breathe, and eliminate as you do now. All your nutrients and oxygen had to be supplied by your mother. Your mother also absorbed much of the waste produced by your tiny body and eliminated it through her excretory organs. The exchange of your nutrients, gases, and waste occurred at the placenta.

Because of these special needs, the fetal heart and **fetal circulation** have several modifications that make them different from "life on the outside" (Fig. 18.9). The following modifications are described and summarized in Table 18.2 on p. 355:

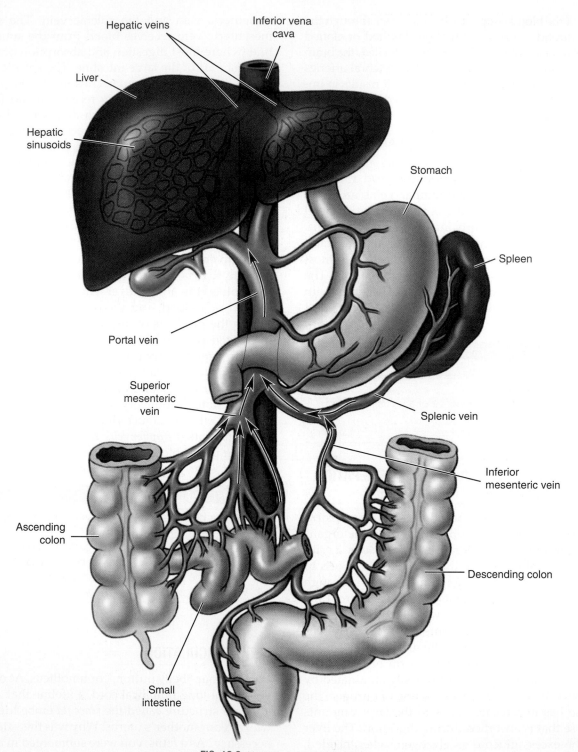

FIG. 18.8 **Hepatic portal circulation.**

- Umbilical blood vessels. The umbilical cord contains three blood vessels: one large umbilical vein and two smaller umbilical arteries. The **umbilical vein** carries blood rich in oxygen and nutrients from the placenta, embedded in the mother's uterine wall, to the fetus. The two **umbilical arteries** carry carbon dioxide and other waste from the fetus to the placenta. Note: In the fetal circulation, the umbilical vein carries oxygen-rich blood, whereas it is the umbilical arteries that carry oxygen-poor blood.

- **Ductus venosus**. Blood flows through the umbilical vein from the placenta into the fetus. Within the body of the fetus, the umbilical vein branches. Some blood flows through one branch to the fetal liver. Most of the blood, however, bypasses the liver and flows through the ductus venosus into the IVC. After birth, the ductus venosus closes and serves no further purpose.

Because the deflated fetal lungs are not used for gas exchange, they have no need for blood to be pumped

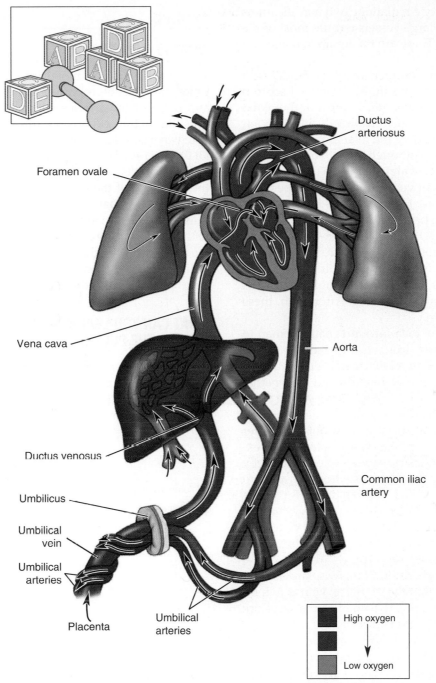

FIG. 18.9 Fetal circulation. Locate the ductus arteriosus, foramen ovale, and ductus venosus.

Table **18.2**	Special Features in the Fetal Circulation	
STRUCTURE	**LOCATION**	**FUNCTION**
Umbilical arteries (two)	Umbilical cord	Transport unoxygenated blood from fetus to the placenta
Umbilical vein (one)	Umbilical cord	Transports oxygenated blood from the placenta to the fetus
Ductus venosus	Between the umbilical vein and inferior vena cava	Carries blood from the umbilical vein to the inferior vena cava; allows some of the blood to bypass the liver
Foramen ovale	Septum between the right and left atria	Allows blood to flow directly from the right atrium into the left atrium to bypass the pulmonary circulation Permanent closure in about 1 year
Ductus arteriosus	Between the pulmonary artery and aorta	Allows blood in the pulmonary artery to flow directly into the descending aorta to bypass the pulmonary circulation Permanent closure in 2–3 months

through the pulmonary circulation. Two modifications in the fetal heart and large vessels reroute most of the blood past the lungs. These are the foramen ovale and the ductus arteriosus:

- **Foramen ovale**. The foramen ovale (foh-RAY-men oh-VAL-ee) is an opening in the interatrial septum of the heart. This opening allows most of the blood to flow from the right atrium directly into the left atrium thereby bypassing the fetal lungs
- **Ductus arteriosus**. Although most blood flows through the foramen ovale into the left atrium, some blood enters the right ventricle and is pumped into the pulmonary trunk. How does this blood bypass the lungs? The fetal heart has a short tube called the *ductus arteriosus* (DUK-tus ar-teer-ee-OH-sus) that connects the pulmonary trunk with the descending aorta. Blood pumped into the pulmonary trunk bypasses the lungs by flowing through the ductus arteriosus directly into the aorta. After birth, these fetal structures close.

Why is it not a good idea for a pregnant woman to take aspirin or a similar drug, such as indomethacin? Naturally secreted prostaglandins help keep the ductus arteriosus open. Drugs such as aspirin and indomethacin block prostaglandin synthesis, thereby causing a premature closure of the ductus arteriosus. Not good!

Occasionally, the fetal structures do not close after birth and appear as congenital heart defects. For example, the ductus arteriosus may fail to close, thereby allowing blood to shunt continuously from the aorta to the pulmonary trunk. This congenital defect is called a *patent ductus arteriosus* (PDA).

See Fig. 18.9 for color-coding of the fetal veins and arteries. Blood vessels carrying oxygenated blood are in red; these are usually the arteries. Vessels carrying unoxygenated blood are in blue; these are usually veins. Note, however, that the umbilical vein is red, indicating oxygenated blood. The umbilical arteries are blue, indicating unoxygenated blood.

Note the color of the upper portion of the vena cava. The adult venae cavae are colored blue because they contain unoxygenated blood. The fetal venae cavae, however, are violet, indicating that the blood is a mixture of unoxygenated blood (coming from the metabolizing fetal tissue) and oxygenated blood (coming from the umbilical vein). Note also the color of the blood in the fetal aorta; it is not the bright red that is characteristic of the adult aorta. The adult aorta carries only oxygenated blood, but the fetal aorta has a mixture of oxygenated and unoxygenated blood.

> **? Re-Think**
> 1. List three structural modifications of the fetal circulation.
> 2. Describe how the foramen ovale and ductus arteriosus allow the blood to bypass the fetal lungs.
> 3. To what maternal structure do the umbilical blood vessels attach?

PULSE

WHAT IS A PULSE?

The ventricles pump blood into the arteries about 72 times/min. The blood causes an alternating expansion and recoil of the arteries with each beat of the heart. This alternating expansion and recoil creates a pressure wave (similar to vibration), which travels through all the arteries. This wave is called the **pulse**.

Because it is caused by the rhythmic contraction of the ventricles of the heart, the pulse is often described as a "heartbeat that can be felt at the wrist." Although a pulse can be felt in any artery lying close to the surface of the body, the site most often used to feel the pulse is the radial artery in the wrist area. Determine your own radial pulse and then try feeling a pulse at any of the nine "pulse points" identified in Fig. 18.10.

WHAT CAN YOU LEARN ABOUT A PATIENT BY FEELING THE PULSE?

By feeling a person's pulse, you can determine the heart rate. A normal heart rate is about 72 beats/min. You can also determine if the heart is beating regularly (rhythmically) or irregularly.

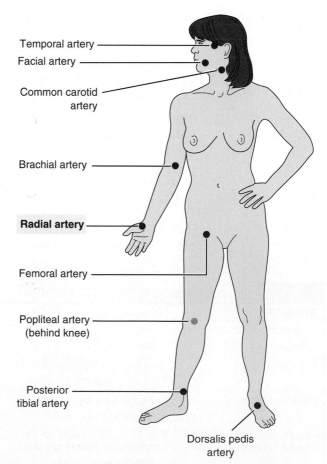

Temporal artery
Facial artery
Common carotid artery
Brachial artery
Radial artery
Femoral artery
Popliteal artery (behind knee)
Posterior tibial artery
Dorsalis pedis artery

FIG. 18.10 Pulse points. Radial pulse is most commonly used site.

You can also assess the pulse for its strength. Does the pulse feel strong or weak? At times, the heart contracts so weakly that the heartbeat cannot be felt over the radial artery; this happens in a person who has lost a lot of blood and is in shock. His pulse may be described as being "rapid and thready." A pulse may also be described as "full or bounding," as happens in a person with excess blood volume. It is also possible that you may not be able to detect a pulse in a particular artery. The pulse may be absent if the artery is blocked or occluded. For example, if a person has poor arterial circulation to the feet, as occurs with many diabetic persons, the dorsalis pedis pulse may be undetectable. Lastly, you may also be asked to assess for a pulse deficit. A pulse deficit is a difference between the heart rate as determined by auscultation at the apex of the heart and the heart rate as determined by palpation of the radial artery. In certain clinical conditions, such as atrial fibrillation, the heart beats, but it does so ineffectively. Consequently, the vibration set up in the arterial wall is too weak to be felt at the wrist (radial pulse). The underlying cause of a pulse deficit is easily detected with an electrocardiogram (ECG). Thus, a correct assessment of the pulse can provide much useful information about the patient's condition.

◎ Sum It Up!

There are three special circulations: circulation to the head and brain, the hepatic portal circulation, and the fetal circulation. The brain receives oxygen-rich blood from the circle of Willis, formed by branches of the internal carotid and the vertebral arteries. The purpose of the hepatic portal circulation is to deliver blood rich in digestive end products to the liver for metabolic processing. The portal vein is formed by the merger of the splenic and superior mesenteric veins, both of which receive blood from the organs of digestion. The fetal circulation has three modifications that allow the fetus to "live under water": the ductus venosus, foramen ovale, and ductus arteriosus. The fetus "breathes, feeds, and eliminates" at the placenta. The pulse is described as a "heartbeat that can be felt at the wrist." Numerous pulse points can be used to assess the pulse.

Note: The As You Age box and the Medical Terminology and Disorders table appear in Chapter 19.

Get Ready for Exams!

Summary Outline

The circulatory system is a series of blood vessels that begin and end in the heart. The circulatory system delivers blood to all the body's cells and then returns the blood to the heart.

I. **Circles, Circuits, and Circulations**
   A. The heart and blood vessels form a circle or circuit.
   B. There are two circulations: pulmonic and systemic.

II. **Blood Vessels**
   A. Naming the blood vessels
      1. Arteries carry blood away from the heart; the smallest arteries are the arterioles.
      2. Capillaries connect arteries and veins; a capillary is close to every cell in the body.
      3. Veins carry blood back to the heart; small veins are called *venules.*
   B. Layers of blood vessels
      1. The tunica intima is the smooth, innermost layer.
      2. The tunica media is the middle layer, which contains elastic tissue and smooth muscle.
      3. The tunica adventitia is the outermost layer of connective tissue.
   C. Blood vessels: what they do
      1. Arteries conduct blood from the heart to the organs and are called *conductance vessels.*
      2. The arterioles constrict and dilate, thereby determining resistance to the flow of blood. The arterioles are called *resistance vessels.*
      3. Capillaries are concerned with the exchange of water and dissolved substances between the blood and tissue fluid. Capillaries are called *exchange vessels.*
      4. Veins and venules return blood to the heart from the body. The veins also store blood and are therefore called *capacitance vessels.* Unlike arteries and capillaries, veins contain valves.

III. **Major Arteries of the Systemic Circulation**
   A. The major arteries include the aorta and the arteries arising directly and indirectly from the aorta.
   B. The aorta arises from the left ventricle.
   C. See Fig. 18.5 for the names and locations of the major arteries.

IV. **Major Veins of the Systemic Circulation**
   A. The major veins include the venae cavae and the veins that directly and indirectly empty into the superior and inferior venae cavae.
   B. The venae cavae carry blood to the right atrium.
   C. See Fig. 18.6 for the names and locations of the major veins.

V. **Special Circulations**
   A. The head and brain are supplied by two sets of arteries: the common carotid arteries and the vertebral arteries. The internal carotid arteries and the vertebral arteries form the circle of Willis. Blood from the head and brain drains into the jugular veins.
   B. The blood supply of the liver is composed of the portal vein, hepatic artery, and hepatic veins. The hepatic artery brings oxygen-rich blood to the liver. The portal vein carries blood from the organs of digestion to the liver. Blood flow through the portal vein to the liver is called the hepatic portal system. The hepatic veins carry blood from the liver to the inferior vena cava.

C. The fetal circulation has several unique features. The fetus uses the placenta as sites of nourishment and gas exchange (O_2 and CO_2). The umbilical blood vessels carry blood between the placenta and the fetus. Three special structures (modifications) are the ductus venosus, foramen ovale, and ductus arteriosus.

VI. The Pulse
A. The pulse is caused by the alternating expansion and recoil of the artery creating a pressure wave that can be palpated.
B. The pulse is often described as a "heartbeat that can be felt at the wrist."
C. Fig. 18.10 identifies the major pulse points.

Review Your Knowledge

Matching: Blood Vessels: Structure and Function
Directions: Match the following words with their descriptions. Some words may be used more than once.

a. large arteries
b. arterioles
c. capillaries
d. veins

1. __C__ Exchange vessels
2. __b__ Resistance vessels
3. __C__ Composed of a single layer of epithelium sitting on a basement membrane
4. __C__ The most numerous of the blood vessels
5. __d__ Capacitance vessels
6. __d__ Blood pressure is lowest in these blood vessels.
7. __d__ Generally colored blue and contain valves
8. __a__ These are the strongest of the blood vessels.
9. __a__ Blood pressure is highest in these blood vessels.
10. __C__ Connect the arteries and veins

Matching: Names of Blood Vessels
Directions: Match the following words with their descriptions below. Some words may be used more than once.

a. aorta
b. inferior vena cava
c. carotids
d. circle of Willis
e. portal vein
f. hepatic artery
g. jugular
h. brachial
i. renal artery
j. median cubital vein
k. saphenous
l. radial artery
m. coronaries

1. __F__ Carries oxygen-rich blood to the liver
2. __l__ Carries oxygen-rich blood to the kidneys
3. __e__ Carries blood that is rich in digestive end products to the liver
4. __a__ Classified as ascending, arch, and descending
5. __e__ The superior mesenteric and splenic veins merge to form this vein.
6. __a__ Classified as thoracic and abdominal
7. __J__ Vein in the arm that is used to "draw" a sample of blood
8. __g__ Main vein that drains the brain

9. ___ Arterial blood supply at the base of the brain
10. ___ Arteries that ascend along the anterolateral neck to the brain
11. ___ Longest superficial vein in the thigh and leg
12. ___ The common iliac veins drain into this blood vessel.
13. ___ Blood pressure is usually taken over this artery.
14. ___ This artery is usually used in "taking a pulse."
15. ___ These arteries supply the myocardium.

Matching: Fetal Circulation
Directions: Match the following words with their descriptions.

a. umbilical arteries
b. umbilical vein
c. ductus arteriosus
d. ductus venosus
e. foramen ovale

1. __a__ Carry blood from the fetus to the placenta
2. __e__ Opening that connects the right and left atria in the fetal circulation
3. __c__ Structure that connects the pulmonary trunk and the aorta in the fetal circulation
4. __d__ Structure that partially bypasses the fetal liver
5. __b__ Carries oxygen-rich blood from the placenta to the fetus

Multiple Choice
1. Which of the following is true about the capillaries?
   a. They are called the *resistance vessels.*
   b. Capillary membranes have multiple layers of smooth muscle.
   c. Capillary membranes are thin and contain numerous pores, thereby facilitating transport.
   d. Capillaries receive blood from the veins and venules.

2. The common carotid
   a. supplies oxygenated blood to the brain.
   b. is the main vein that drains the brain.
   c. is part of the hepatic portal system.
   d. ascends along the posterolateral neck to the brain to form the basilar artery.

3. The purpose of the hepatic portal system is to
   a. provide the fetus with oxygenated blood.
   b. deliver blood that is rich in digestive end products to the liver.
   c. drain unoxygenated blood from the brain.
   d. deliver oxygenated blood to the liver.

4. Which statement is true about the fetal circulation?
   a. The umbilical arteries deliver oxygenated blood to the fetus from the placenta.
   b. The umbilical vein delivers oxygenated blood to the fetus from the placenta.
   c. The ductus venosus forms an opening between the right and left fetal atria.
   d. The ductus arteriosus bypasses the fetal liver.

5. Which of the following is descriptive of the aorta?
   a. It is the largest and strongest of the arteries.
   b. It carries unoxygenated blood and is therefore color-coded blue.
   c. It is lined with large valves, ensuring a one-way flow of blood.
   d. Blood pressure in the aorta is lower than blood pressure in the veins.

6. The portal vein, hepatic veins, and celiac trunk are most associated with the
   a. kidneys.
   b. brain.
   c. diaphragm.
   d. liver.

7. The superior mesenteric vein and the splenic vein
   a. drain directly into the superior vena cava.
   b. form the circle of Willis.
   c. merge to form the portal vein.
   d. carry venous blood from the liver to the inferior vena cava.

8. Which of the following is true of the common iliac arteries, renal arteries, and celiac trunk?
   a. They are branches of the descending aorta.
   b. They are branches of the abdominal aorta.
   c. They carry oxygenated blood.
   d. All of the above are true.

9. The median cubital vein, brachial vein, and radial vein
   a. carry oxygenated blood.
   b. are color-coded red because they carry unoxygenated blood.
   c. are located in the upper extremities.
   d. deliver blood to the hepatic portal system.

10. Both the brachiocephalic artery and the left common carotid artery
    a. arise from the arch of the aorta.
    b. arise from the abdominal aorta.
    c. deliver unoxygenated blood into the superior vena cava.
    d. receive unoxygenated blood from the jugulars.

11. The femoral, popliteal, anterior tibial, and dorsalis pedis arteries
    a. deliver oxygenated blood to the aorta.
    b. deliver oxygenated blood to the lower extremities.
    c. receive oxygenated blood from the inferior vena cava.
    d. are part of the hepatic portal system.

12. Which of the following correctly maps blood flow?
    a. Ascending aorta→ thoracic aorta → the coronary arteries
    b. Splenic vein → the hepatic vein → the portal vein
    c. Descending aorta → the common iliac arteries → the great saphenous → the dorsalis pedis
    d. Subclavian vein → the brachiocephalic vein → the superior vena cava → the right atrium

13. The coronary arteries
    a. arise from the pulmonary artery.
    b. arise from the ascending aorta.
    c. receive blood from the venae cavae.
    d. deliver blood to the circle of Willis.

14. Which of the following blood vessels runs parallel to the femoral artery?
    a. Anterior tibial artery
    b. Popliteal artery
    c. Femoral vein
    d. Common iliac artery

15. A drop of blood flows from the superior mesenteric vein to the right atrium. Through which blood vessel must it flow on this path?
    a. Great saphenous vein
    b. Dorsalis pedis artery
    c. Portal vein
    d. Jugular vein

16. Which of the following is true?
    a. Blood flows from the superior vena cava to the right jugular.
    b. Blood flows from the inferior vena cava to the right renal vein.
    c. Blood flows from the abdominal aorta to the common iliac arteries.
    d. Blood flows from the hepatic veins to the portal vein.

17. Blood flows from the
    a. vertebral arteries to the basilar artery.
    b. circle of Willis to the internal common carotid arteries.
    c. abdominal aorta to the aortic arch.
    d. brachiocephalic artery to the left common carotid artery.

18. Blood flows from the
    a. right jugular to the right subclavian vein.
    b. inferior vena cava to the common iliac veins.
    c. subclavian veins to the jugulars.
    d. axillary arteries to the subclavian arteries.

19. Which of the following blood vessels contains valves?
    a. Aorta
    b. Circle of Willis
    c. Femoral vein
    d. Renal artery

20. The mixing of blood from the hepatic artery and the portal vein occurs within which porous structure?
    a. Hepatic bile ducts
    b. Celiac trunk
    c. Hepatic sinusoids
    d. Kupffer cells

Go Figure

1. Which of the following is correct according to Fig. 18.1?
   a. Blood is pumped by the heart along this route: → arteries → veins → capillaries → back to the right side of the heart.
   b. The capillaries are closer to the individual cells than is the aorta.
   c. Veins deliver blood to the left heart.
   d. The venae cavae deliver blood to the capillaries.

2. Which of the following is correct according to Fig. 18.2 and Table 18.1?
   a. The venae cavae are larger and structurally stronger than the aorta.
   b. The aorta is ideally structured for the diffusion of nutrients and oxygen into the interstitium.
   c. The color-coding of the capillaries is indicative of the amount of oxygen in the blood.
   d. The tunica intima, media, and adventitia are descriptive of capillary structure.

3. Which of the following is correct according to Fig. 18.3?
   a. Exercise causes the valves in the deep veins of the leg to close.
   b. Exercise causes blood to stagnate in the deep veins of the leg.
   c. Contraction of the muscles in the leg externally compresses the deep veins and enhances blood flow toward the heart.
   d. Blood returns to the heart because the valves in the deep veins pump blood out of the legs.

4. Which of the following is correct according to Figs. 18.4 and 18.5?
   a. The ascending aorta gives rise to the common iliac arteries.
   b. Both common carotid arteries arise directly from the arch of the aorta.
   c. The abdominal aorta is part of the descending aorta.
   d. The thoracic aorta gives rise to the renal arteries.

5. Which of the following is correct according to Fig. 18.5?
   a. The descending aorta bifurcates into the common iliac arteries.
   b. The right and left common carotid arteries emerge from the aortic arch.
   c. The celiac trunk emerges from the thoracic aorta.
   d. The subclavian arteries are extensions of the common carotid arteries.

6. Which of the following is correct according to Fig. 18.6?
   a. The femoral and the great saphenous veins deliver blood to the anterior and posterior tibial veins.
   b. The subclavian veins deliver blood to the jugular veins.
   c. The blue color-coding indicates that these veins are carrying unoxygenated blood.
   d. All of the above are true.

7. Which of the following is correct according to Fig. 18.7?
   a. The jugulars are part of the circle of Willis.
   b. The vertebral arteries carry blood to the facial structures.
   c. The internal carotid arteries and vertebral arteries deliver oxygenated blood to the circle of Willis.
   d. All blood delivered to the circle of Willis comes from the internal carotid arteries.

8. Which of the following is correct according to Fig. 18.8?
   a. The portal vein bypasses the liver and drains directly into the inferior vena cava.
   b. The superior mesenteric vein and splenic vein merge to form the portal vein.
   c. The hepatic vein delivers blood to the portal vein.
   d. The portal vein delivers blood to the organs of digestion.

9. Which of the following is correct according to Fig. 18.9?
   a. The ductus venosus is the hole in the fetal interatrial septum.
   b. The umbilical vein carries oxygenated blood from the placenta to the fetus.
   c. The foramen ovale is the fetal structure that connects the pulmonary artery with the aorta.
   d. The fetal heart has the same color-coding as the adult heart.

10. Which of the following is correct according to Fig. 18.10?
    a. A pulse can be palpated over most arteries and veins.
    b. The most accurate pulse is determined at the wrist (radial artery).
    c. The dorsalis pedis pulse is determined at the inguinal region.
    d. The radial artery is most often used to assess the pulse.

Functions of the Blood Vessels

Objectives

1. List the five functions of the blood vessels.
2. Discuss blood pressure, including the following:
   - Define *blood pressure, systolic pressure, diastolic pressure, and pulse pressure*.
   - Explain the variance of blood pressure in different blood vessels.
   - Describe the factors that determine blood pressure.
   - Explain the mechanisms involved in regulation of blood pressure, including the baroreceptor reflex.
3. Explain how blood vessels act as exchange vessels, including the following:
   - Describe the factors that determine capillary exchange.
   - Describe the mechanisms of edema formation.
4. Explain how the blood vessels respond to changing body needs.
5. Describe the role of the blood vessels in the regulation of body temperature.

Key Terms

baroreceptor reflex (p. 365)
blood pressure (p. 361)
capillary exchange (p. 367)
diastolic pressure (p. 361)
hypertension (p. 362)

hypotension (p. 362)
ischemia (p. 361)
oncotic pressure (p. 368)
pulse pressure (p. 361)
systemic vascular resistance (p. 362)

systolic pressure (p. 361)
vasoconstriction (p. 364)
vasodilation (p. 364)
vasopressor (p. 367)

As mentioned earlier in this text, it took seemingly forever for the ancients to "connect" the heart and the peripheral blood vessels. After that connection was made, scientists realized that blood was pumped out of the left heart, circulated around the body, and returned to the right side of the heart. However, we still had no real understanding of the functions (physiology) of the peripheral blood vessels.

Today, we know that the blood vessels do more than allow blood to run around in circles. The blood vessels perform five important functions:
1. Act as a delivery system
2. Regulate blood pressure
3. Engage in the exchange of nutrients and waste between the capillaries and cells
4. Redistribute blood in response to changing body needs
5. Help regulate body temperature

BLOOD VESSELS DELIVER

The primary purpose of the cardiovascular system is to deliver blood that is rich in oxygen, hormones, nutrients, and water to the cells; the blood also collects cellular waste and delivers it to organs of excretion, such as the kidneys. The delivery of oxygen is especially critical. All cells need oxygen; without oxygen, they die. Impaired blood flow and oxygen deprivation is called **ischemia**; the consequences of ischemia are tissue damage, pain, and gangrene.

BLOOD VESSELS REGULATE BLOOD PRESSURE

Blood pressure is the force that blood exerts against the walls of the blood vessels. Why do you need a blood pressure? Blood pressure is needed to push blood through the blood vessels to an organ. No blood pressure means no organ perfusion! The **systolic pressure** is the highest pressure recorded during systole (myocardial contraction). The **diastolic pressure** is the lowest pressure recorded during diastole (myocardial relaxation).

You just had a physical exam. The physician nodded approvingly that your blood pressure is 116/72 mm Hg. Although you are thrilled to be normotensive, what does it all mean? First, your blood pressure is normal; that is, you are normotensive. Second, your systolic pressure is 116 mm Hg (the top number), and your diastolic pressure is 72 mm Hg (bottom number). Your **pulse pressure** is the difference between the systolic and the diastolic pressures (44 mm Hg, or 116 minus 72).

Do You Know...
About the MABP?

A blood pressure is expressed as 120/80 mm Hg. What is the mean arterial blood pressure (MABP)? MABP is calculated as follows:

MABP = 2/3 diastolic pressure + 1/3 systolic pressure

or

MABP = diastolic pressure + 1/3 pulse pressure

For a blood pressure of 120/80 mm Hg, the MABP is 94 mm Hg. Why is the MABP important? It is important because the organs are perfused by or "feel" the MABP. Note that the MABP expresses more of the diastolic pressure than the systolic pressure. The dominance of the MABP by the diastolic pressure is the basis for the clinical concern for the diastolic reading.

BLOOD PRESSURE: NORMAL AND ABNORMAL

Blood pressure readings vary according to age, gender, and size (and don't discount your emotional state). For example, the normal blood pressure of a 2-year-old child is 95/65 mm Hg. The normal blood pressure for an adult is defined as a systolic pressure of less than 120 mm Hg and a diastolic pressure of less than 80 mm Hg. For many years, a blood pressure of 120/80 mm Hg was considered normal for an adult; today, it is classified as prehypertensive. The maintenance of normal blood pressure is extremely important. If blood pressure becomes too low (**hypotension**), blood flow to vital organs decreases, and the person is said to be in shock. Without immediate treatment, the person may die. If the blood pressure becomes elevated (**hypertension**), the blood vessels may burst, or rupture. A ruptured blood vessel in the brain, for example, is a major cause of stroke, resulting in loss of speech, paralysis, and possible death. Hypertension also puts added strain on the heart, damages the blood vessels in the kidneys, and damages the retina, causing loss of vision. You will spend much time "taking" blood pressures (Fig. 19.1) and will be expected to interpret abnormal readings.

Do You Know...
About "White Coat Hypertension"?

Often a patient's blood pressure elevates in response to a health care worker (wearing a white coat) recording his or her blood pressure—hence the term *white coat hypertension*. In fact, the person's blood pressure should be recorded a second or third time after he or she has relaxed. Emotions matter! Diagnosis and treatment are never based on a single blood pressure recording. There are other considerations in recording blood pressure, including proper cuff size and the patient's position (sitting with feet on the floor). The person should not be talking. One study has indicated that over 90% of blood pressure recordings in a single clinic violate proper procedure.

Re-Think

1. Define *systolic pressure*. Define *diastolic pressure*.
2. Your patient's blood pressure is 145/88 mm Hg. To what do the top and bottom numbers refer? Calculate his pulse pressure.
3. Your patient's initial blood pressure was 145/88 mm Hg. After 10 minutes, his blood pressure had declined to 122/76 mm Hg. What is a likely explanation for this spontaneous decline in blood pressure?

BLOOD PRESSURE IN DIFFERENT BLOOD VESSELS

Blood pressures vary from one type of blood vessel to the next (Fig. 19.2). Note that the blood pressure is highest in the aorta because it is closest to the left ventricle; the left ventricle pumps blood with great force. The blood pressure gradually declines as the blood flows from the large arteries into the arterioles, into the capillaries, into the venules and, finally, into the veins. This difference in pressure causes blood to flow from the arterial side of the circulation to the venous side. Note that a blood pressure of 116/72 mm Hg is normal only for large blood vessels. Capillary pressure is generally much lower. Pressure within the large veins is around 0 mm Hg.

Repeat! Blood flows from the arterial to the venous side of the circulation primarily because of the pressure difference between the two.

Sum It Up!

The blood vessels deliver blood to every organ in the body. The driving force for the movement of blood through the blood vessels is the blood pressure. Blood pressure is highest in the large arteries and lowest in the veins, accounting for the flow of blood from arteries to veins. A typical normal blood pressure in an adult is 116/72 mm Hg. The upper number (116) is the systolic pressure, which is the highest pressure recorded during systole. The lower number is the diastolic pressure, which is the lowest number recorded during diastole.

WHAT DETERMINES BLOOD PRESSURE?

Blood pressure is determined by the heart (cardiac output) and the blood vessels (**systemic vascular resistance**).

Blood pressure = Cardiac output × Systemic vascular resistance

HEART AND BLOOD PRESSURE

How does myocardial function affect blood pressure? You probably have watched enough television to know that when the heart stops beating, the blood pressure drops to 0 mm Hg and the person dies, indicating an

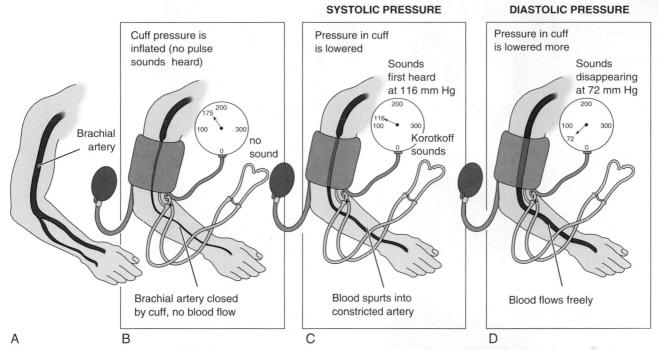

SYSTOLIC PRESSURE

DIASTOLIC PRESSURE

Cuff pressure is inflated (no pulse sounds heard)

Pressure in cuff is lowered

Pressure in cuff is lowered more

Brachial artery

Sounds first heard at 116 mm Hg

Sounds disappearing at 72 mm Hg

no sound

Korotkoff sounds

Brachial artery closed by cuff, no blood flow

Blood spurts into constricted artery

Blood flows freely

A   B   C   D

FIG. 19.1 Taking a blood pressure. The measurement of blood pressure requires a sphygmomanometer and a stethoscope. Follow the panels for an explanation of the systolic (116 mm Hg) and diastolic (72 mm Hg) pressures. **(A)** Identify the location of the brachial artery. **(B)** Inflate the cuff, thereby squeezing the upper arm. At this point, the cuff pressure has become greater than the blood pressure in the brachial artery. The cuff pressure collapses the brachial artery, thereby stopping the flow of blood. No sound can be heard through the stethoscope. **(C)** As you slowly lower the pressure in the cuff , the artery opens slightly, and blood spurts through the blood vessel in response to the pressure in the brachial artery. You can hear the spurting effect of the blood as soft tapping sounds (called *Korotkoff sounds*). The number on the sphygmomanometer that corresponds to the tapping sounds is recorded as the systolic blood pressure (116 mm Hg). With further reduction in cuff pressure, the brachial artery opens wider and allows blood flow through the artery to increase. **(D)** As cuff pressure declines even further, the brachial artery opens completely, and normal blood flow through the artery resumes. At this point, the sounds heard through the stethoscope disappear or sound muffled. The pressure at which the sounds disappear is read as the diastolic blood pressure (72 mm Hg).

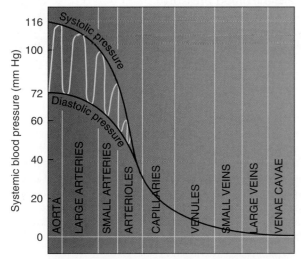

FIG. 19.2 Blood pressure in the different blood vessels.

obvious relationship between cardiac function and blood pressure.

What is the heart component of blood pressure? It is the cardiac output. Recall from Chapter 17 that cardiac output is determined by heart rate (HR) and stroke volume (SV). The stronger the force of contraction, the greater the SV, the greater the cardiac output, and the higher the blood pressure. The faster the heart rate, the greater the cardiac output, and the higher the blood pressure. Conversely, a decline in HR and/or SV decreases cardiac output and blood pressure.

BLOOD VESSELS AND BLOOD PRESSURE

How do the peripheral blood vessels affect blood pressure? A garden hose illustrates the blood vessels' effect on blood pressure. In Fig. 19.3A, the hose is hooked up to a faucet. When the faucet is turned on, water flows through the hose and falls to the ground in big droplets. In Fig. 19.3B, a nozzle has been attached to the end of the hose, thereby narrowing the end of the hose. The nozzle has increased the resistance to the flow of water. Because of the resistance of the nozzle, water does not fall out of the hose in big droplets, as in Fig. 19.3A; instead, water squirts out of the end of the hose. Notice how much further the squirted water travels. What is the reason for this difference? If you were to measure the pressures at point X, you would record a higher pressure in the hose with the nozzle on it. The nozzle increases resistance to

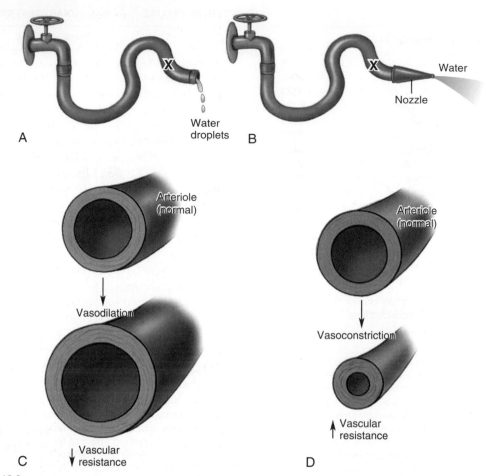

FIG. 19.3 Effect of resistance on pressure. (A) Low resistance and low pressure. (B) High resistance and high pressure. (C) Vasodilation, low resistance, and low pressure. (D) Vasoconstriction, high resistance, and high pressure.

the flow of water and causes the pressure behind the nozzle to increase. The increased pressure in the nozzled hose simply pushes the water further.

How does the example of the hose apply to blood pressure? The large blood vessels are similar to the hose. The smaller vessels, especially the arterioles, act as nozzles. Because the arterioles are composed largely of smooth muscle, the contraction and relaxation of the muscle allow the arterioles to change their diameter and therefore their resistance to blood flow. *Systemic vascular resistance* (SVR) is the clinical term that refers to the resistance offered by all the peripheral blood vessels; it is the same as *total peripheral resistance* (TPR).

Arteriolar smooth muscle determines resistance. **Vasodilation** occurs when arteriolar smooth muscle relaxes and increases the diameter of the blood vessels. The process is comparable to removing the nozzle from the end of the hose (see Fig. 19.3C). Vasodilation decreases resistance in the blood vessels and decreases blood pressure. When the smooth muscle contracts, the diameter of the arteriole becomes smaller. This process is known as **vasoconstriction** and is comparable to adding a nozzle to the hose (see Fig. 19.3D). Vasoconstriction increases SVR and raises blood pressure.

Thus, the arterioles' ability to dilate and constrict helps determine blood pressure.

Do You Know...

About Obesity and the Miles and Miles of New Blood Vessels?

Blood pressure is determined by cardiac output and systemic vascular resistance (SVR). SVR is usually determined by changes in the diameter of the arterioles. Other resistance terms such as *blood vessel length* and *blood viscosity* are normally ignored. However, the accumulation of excess fat tissue not only adds pounds; it also contributes miles of additional new blood vessels, making blood vessel length a significant contributor to SVR. Fat tissue also secretes hormones that narrow or constrict blood vessels. Excess fat therefore elevates SVR, making the person hypertensive. What to do to lower that blood pressure? Lose weight!

Re-Think

1. What are the two determinants of blood pressure?
2. Explain why a significant loss of blood or severe dehydration causes hypotension.
3. Why would excessive peripheral vasodilation cause dizziness and possibly syncope (fainting)?

Do You Know...

About Venodilation and This "Fainting" Balloon?

If a patient takes a drug that causes venodilation, the following events occur: blood "pools" in the veins; less blood returns to the heart (decreased venous return); myocardial contraction decreases (Starling effect); cardiac output decreases; and blood pressure decreases (hypotension). If the patient attempts to change position quickly, as in rising from a supine (lying down) to a standing position, insufficient blood is pumped to the brain, causing dizziness, fainting, and falling. This series of events is called *postural hypotension*, because it usually occurs when the patient assumes an upright posture. The water-filled balloon illustrates venodilation and pooling when the position of the balloon changes from a lying (horizontal) to standing (vertical) position. Lesson? Advise your patients to get up slowly from lying to sitting to upright. Other common causes of postural hypotension are blood volume depletion (dehydration), an aging cardiovascular system, and autonomic dysfunction. Elderly persons are especially prone to postural hypotension.

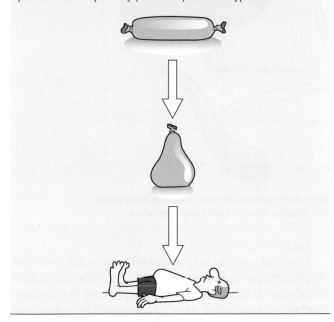

HOW BLOOD PRESSURE STAYS WITHIN NORMAL LIMITS

Under normal conditions, blood pressure remains relatively constant, at slightly less than 120/80 mm Hg. Regulation of blood pressure involves rapidly acting and slowly acting mechanisms.

RAPIDLY ACTING MECHANISMS

The most important of the rapidly acting mechanisms is a nervous reflex mechanism called the **baroreceptor reflex**. This reflex consists of the following structures: receptors, sensory nerves, medulla oblongata, and motor nerves. (Follow the arrows in Fig. 19.4 as you read about the components of the baroreceptor reflex.)
- *Receptors.* The special receptors, called *baroreceptors* (bar-oh-ree-SEP-tors), or pressure receptors, are located in the walls of the aortic arch and carotid

sinus. The baroreceptors sense sudden changes in blood pressure.
- *Sensory nerves.* Once the baroreceptors have been activated, the sensory information travels along the nerves to the brain. The nerves that carry the sensory information are cranial nerves (CNs) IX (glossopharyngeal) and X (vagus).
- *Medulla oblongata.* The medulla oblongata of the brain stem interprets sensory information coming from the baroreceptors. The medulla oblongata then decides what to do. If the blood pressure is low, the medulla oblongata tells the heart and blood vessels to increase blood pressure. If the medulla oblongata receives information that the blood pressure is high, it tells the heart and blood vessels to decrease blood pressure.
- *Motor nerves.* Once the medulla oblongata has identified adjustments needed to restore blood pressure to normal, the motor nerves carry information to the heart and blood vessels. The motor nerves involved are the nerves of the autonomic nervous system (sympathetic and parasympathetic nervous systems).

What happens if a person's blood pressure suddenly declines, as in hemorrhage? The decline in blood pressure is sensed by the baroreceptors and the information carried by sensory nerves (CNs IX and X) to the medulla oblongata. The motor response? Activation of the sympathetic nervous system. Stimulation of the sympathetic nerves causes the sinoatrial (SA) node to fire more quickly, thereby increasing heart rate. Sympathetic firing also causes the ventricular myocardium to contract more forcefully, increasing SV. Both of these responses increase cardiac output and blood pressure. Firing of the sympathetic nerves also causes vasoconstriction of the arterioles, thereby increasing SVR and blood pressure. In fact, many of the signs of shock are due to the firing of the sympathetic nerves as it tries to restore blood pressure.

The same series of events occurs in a person who suddenly experiences a sudden, drug-induced (e.g., nitroglycerin) decline in blood pressure. Activation of the baroreceptors causes an increase in HR, or reflex tachycardia. The tachycardia can overburden a damaged heart, causing angina (chest pain) and additional myocardial damage. The effect of drugs on baroreceptor responses is huge!

What happens if a person's blood pressure suddenly increases? The baroreceptor reflex is activated resulting in the stimulation of parasympathetic discharge. Parasympathetic (vagal) stimulation decreases HR and therefore decreases cardiac output and blood pressure. Blood pressure also decreases because the blood vessels dilate, thereby decreasing resistance. If the blood vessels do not contain parasympathetic nerves, why do they dilate? The vasodilation is not caused by parasympathetic activity; it occurs because the sympathetic nerves become less active when the parasympathetic nerves fire.

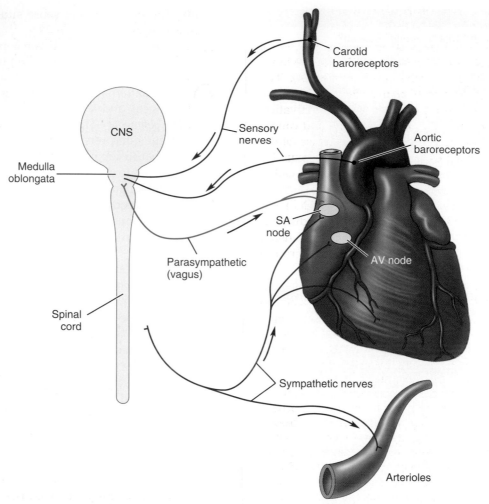

FIG. 19.4 Baroreceptor reflex. Locate the baroreceptors, afferent arm (sensory nerves), medulla oblongata, motor arm (sympathetic and parasympathetic nerves), and the effector organs (heart and arterioles)

Carotid sinus syncope also illustrates the baroreceptor response to a sudden increase in blood pressure. A tight collar exerts pressure over a hypersensitive carotid sinus, activating the baroreceptors. The medulla oblongata falsely interprets the blood pressure information as an elevation in blood pressure. Information sent from the brain to the heart and blood vessels lowers the blood pressure, so much so that the person faints (syncope). This response is called *carotid sinus syncope*. Other stimuli for carotid sinus syncope include shaving over the neck region, showering with strong spurts of water, and the use of shoulder strap seat belts.

Re-Think

1. What is the signal that initiates the baroreceptor reflex?
2. What is the afferent or sensory arm of the baroreceptor reflex?
3. What is the efferent or motor arm of the baroreceptor reflex?
4. What is the baroreceptor response to excess vasodilation, as often occurs in the pharmacological treatment of hypertension?

A second rapidly acting mechanism is the secretion of epinephrine and norepinephrine from the medulla of the adrenal gland. These hormones prolong the effects of the baroreceptor reflex; they increase cardiac output and cause vasoconstriction, thus increasing blood pressure.

Do You Know...

About Val Salva's Most Embarrassing Medical Moment?

Val was constipated! Sounds like an insignificant problem, but in a person with a history of coronary artery disease (CAD), constipation can prove fatal. While "straining at stools," Val suffered a near-fatal heart attack. Straining at stools initiates the Valsalva maneuver, which occurs when a person tries to force an exhalation with the mouth and nose closed (as in having a bowel movement). The forced exhalation increases pressure in the chest, which in turn increases blood pressure. The sudden increase in blood pressure activates the baroreceptor reflex, causing a sudden burst of parasympathetic activity that not only slows the heart rate but triggers a fatal dysrhythmia, leading to cardiac arrest. Unfortunately, it is a rather common occurrence that someone with a history of CAD has a heart attack while on the "porcelain throne." How embarrassing—and to think it might have been prevented by a stool softener or laxative.

SLOWER-ACTING MECHANISMS AND LONG-TERM REGULATION OF BLOOD PRESSURE

Several hormonal mechanisms act slowly to control blood pressure and are more concerned with the long-term regulation of blood pressure (Chapter 24). The most important of the slowly acting mechanisms is the renin–angiotensin–aldosterone mechanism. Activation of this mechanism increases blood volume and causes vasoconstriction. Both of these effects increase blood pressure. Other hormones that affect blood pressure include antidiuretic hormone (ADH). ADH is also called *vasopressin* because it exerts a **vasopressor** effect (increases blood pressure). Atrial natriuretic peptide (ANP) and brain natriuretic peptide (BNP), secreted by the distended walls of the heart, lower blood pressure by causing vasodilation and by decreasing blood volume through the renal (kidney) secretion of sodium and water.

◎ Sum It Up!

Blood pressure is defined as the force that blood exerts against the walls of the blood vessels. Blood pressure is determined by the activity of the heart (cardiac output) and blood vessels, especially the arterioles (systemic vascular resistance). Remember: blood pressure = cardiac output × systemic vascular resistance. Several mechanisms regulate blood pressure. The most important rapidly acting mechanism is the baroreceptor reflex; a sudden decline in blood pressure triggers a sympathetic discharge, whereas a sudden increase in blood pressure triggers parasympathetic or vagal discharge. The secretion of epinephrine and norepinephrine contributes to and prolongs the rapid-response system. Long-term mechanisms are hormonal and include the renin–angiotensin–aldosterone system, antidiuretic hormone (ADH), and the natriuretic peptides.

BLOOD VESSELS ACT AS EXCHANGE VESSELS

In **capillary exchange**, the capillaries engage in the exchange of nutrients and waste between the blood and cells. Accordingly, the capillaries are called *exchange vessels*. The capillaries are the most numerous of the blood vessels. If all the capillaries in the body were lined up end to end, they would encircle the earth 2.5 times.

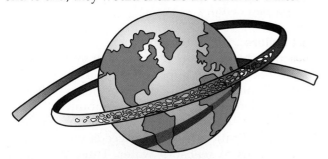

WHAT IS AN EXCHANGE VESSEL?

An exchange vessel exchanges or swaps substances, much like a waiter (Fig. 19.5A). For example, a waiter

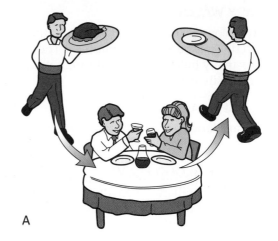

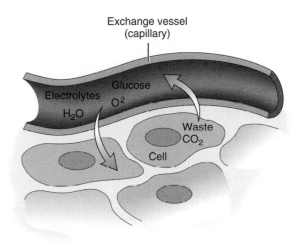

FIG. 19.5 Capillary exchange: deliveries and pickup. (A) Waiters delivering food and picking up empty trays. (B) Capillary exchange; delivering oxygen, nutrients, and water and picking up waste (CO_2) and excess water.

delivers food to hungry guests. After some time has passed, the waiter picks up the waste—the empty trays, dirty dishes, and leftover food. Note the exchange part: food is dropped off, and waste is picked up.

The capillaries work like the waiter (see Fig. 19.5B). As blood flows through the capillaries, substances move out of the capillary into the surrounding tissue spaces (interstitium). These substances include oxygen, water, electrolytes, and various nutrients such as glucose; they are the substances that the cell needs to live, work, and grow.

Oxygen and nutrients are taken up and used by the cells. As the cells carry on their work, they produce waste material such as carbon dioxide. The cellular waste diffuses out of the cell, into the interstitium, and then into the blood within the capillary. The blood carries the waste away from the capillary to the organs of excretion, such as the kidneys and the lungs.

WHY CAPILLARIES ARE GOOD EXCHANGE VESSELS

Three characteristics make the capillaries good exchange vessels: thin capillary walls, large numbers of capillaries, and slow blood flow through the capillaries.

THIN CAPILLARY WALLS

The capillary wall consists of a single layer of epithelium that sits on a delicate basement membrane. The epithelial layer has many holes, or pores, through which water and solute easily move.

MILLIONS OF CAPILLARIES

The millions of capillaries provide a huge surface area for exchange.

SLOW VELOCITY OF BLOOD FLOW

The large numbers of capillaries also affect the rate of blood flow. The greater the number of capillaries, the slower the flow of blood through the capillaries. The slow blood flow allows more time for exchange.

CAPILLARY FORCES: EXCHANGE

How do the water, nutrients and waste "know" where to go? There are forces that move water, nutrients, and waste in and out of the capillaries. These forces are diffusion and a filtration-osmosis balancing act.

EXCHANGE INVOLVING DIFFUSION

Diffusion is the primary process causing substances to move across the capillary wall. Diffusion means that a substance moves downhill from an area of high concentration to an area of low concentration. For example, the concentration of oxygen is higher in the capillary than in the tissue fluid. Thus, oxygen diffuses from the capillary into the interstitium and then into the cell. On the other hand, carbon dioxide concentration is higher in the interstitium than in the capillaries. Thus, carbon dioxide diffuses from the interstitium into the capillary.

EXCHANGE INVOLVING FILTRATION-OSMOSIS

A second process of exchange involves filtration-osmosis and is particularly important for water exchange. Filtration is illustrated in the syringe in Fig. 19.6A (upper). A syringe is loaded with water. When the plunger is pushed, the pressure within the barrel of the syringe increases and water is forced out of the syringe through the needle. What would happen if you were to punch holes in the side of the syringe and push on the plunger, as in Fig. 19.6A (lower)? Not only would water flow through the needle end, but it would also squirt out of the side of the syringe in response to the pressure.

The plunger and syringe are similar to the heart and capillaries (see Fig. 19.6B). The heart, like the plunger, creates a pressure that accomplishes two things. First, blood is pushed forward from the arterial end of the capillary to the venous end of the capillary. Second, because of the pores in the capillary wall, water and the smaller substances (electrolytes, glucose) squirt into the interstitium. Plasma proteins, such as albumin, are too large to fit through the capillary pores and therefore remain in the capillaries.

The pushing of the water and dissolved substances through the pores is filtration. Note that the cause of filtration is blood pressure. Note also the direction of filtration. In response to the pressure in the capillary, water and the dissolved substances are pushed out of the capillary into the interstitium.

What happens to all the substances pushed into the interstitium? The nutrients are used by the cells. What about the water that was filtered? The water is reabsorbed at the venous end of the capillary. The force that is responsible for the reabsorption of water is the oncotic pressure. The **oncotic pressure** is the plasma osmotic pressure that is due to the plasma proteins. Fig. 19.6C shows that the inward-pulling oncotic pressure in the capillary is higher than the outward-pushing filtration pressure The capillary oncotic pressure is higher because of the plasma proteins trapped within the capillaries. The high oncotic pressure causes the water to diffuse from the interstitium into the capillary.

A word about the lymphatic vessels described in Chapter 20. About 85% of the water that is filtered out of the arterial end of the capillary into the interstitium is reabsorbed at the venous end of the capillary. The remaining 15% is reabsorbed by the lymphatic vessels and returned to the general circulation. In the absence or occlusion of lymphatic vessels, the water remains in the interstitium, causing edema.

What is the balancing act? The exact amount of water filtered at the arterial end of the capillary is reabsorbed at the venous end of the capillary. The balancing act is important. If the amount of water filtered out of the capillary exceeds the amount reabsorbed from the interstitium , fluid collects in the interstitium. Excess fluid collection in the interstitium is called *edema*. Or, if more water is reabsorbed from the tissue space than was filtered, the tissue space becomes depleted, and the patient appears dehydrated. Fluid imbalances occur in many clinical conditions.

MECHANISMS OF EDEMA FORMATION

The forces that determine the movement of water across the capillary walls are disrupted in many clinical conditions. Some of the more common conditions are described here.

Heart Failure

A patient in heart failure retains water and develops excess blood volume (hypervolemia). The expanded blood volume, in turn, increases capillary filtration pressure, thereby increasing the amount of water filtered out of the capillaries into the interstitium. The excess filtration of water exceeds the ability of the capillaries to reabsorb water. Thus, the excess water remains in the interstitium, causing edema. Excess filtration of water into the lungs is called *pulmonary edema* and results in impaired oxygenation.

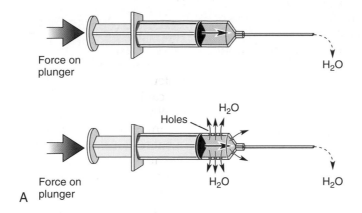

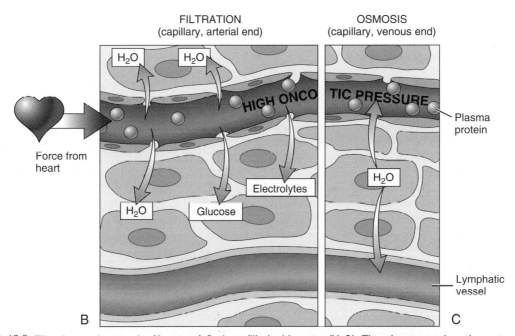

FIG. 19.6 Filtration and osmosis. **(A, upper)** Syringe filled with water (H_2O). The plunger pushes the water out of the syringe at the needle tip. **(A, lower)** Syringe, with holes in the barrel and filled with water. The plunger pushes the water out of the syringe at the needle tip; the plunger also pushes water through the holes in the syringe. **(B)** Capillary with many small pores and filled with blood. The heart pushes blood forward toward the venous end of the capillary; the heart also pushes water and dissolved substances out of the capillary through the pores into the interstitium. **(C)** Movement of water back into the capillary because of the oncotic pressure in the capillary. The oncotic pressure is due to the plasma proteins (albumin). Capillary reabsorption is aided by the lymphatic vessels.

Excess fluid accumulation in the feet is called *pedal edema*.

Severe Burn

A patient is admitted to the emergency room with severe burns on the lower extremities. In response to the thermal injury, the capillary pores dilate, thereby allowing the escape of excess water and plasma proteins into the interstitium. The "leaked" protein causes edema for two reasons. First, the reduction in plasma protein decreases oncotic pressure within the capillary; this, in turn, decreases the pulling-in pressure and decreases the reabsorption of water. Second, the leaked protein "holds" the water in the interstitium thereby slowing its reabsorption from the interstitium.

Kidney Disease

A child is diagnosed with a kidney disease called *nephrotic syndrome*. The child's mother first noticed edema around his eyes (periorbital edema) and difficulty in fastening the waist of his pants. Nephrotic syndrome is characterized by the excretion of large amounts of the plasma protein, albumin, in the urine (albuminuria); this results in low plasma levels of albumin (hypoalbuminemia). The edema of nephrotic syndrome is caused in part by the hypoalbuminemia, resulting in a decreased plasma oncotic pressure.

Blocked Lymphatic Drainage

A woman goes to a clinic complaining of a grossly swollen leg and is eventually diagnosed with a large tumor in her lower pelvis. The tumor has compressed the lymphatic vessels, thereby impairing the drainage of lymph; impaired lymph drainage causes the accumulation of fluid in the interstitium (edema).

Your understanding of capillary forces enables you to understand the mechanisms of edema formation.

 Re-Think

1. Why are capillaries good exchange vessels?
2. Why is water filtered at the arterial end of the capillary? Why is water reabsorbed at the venous end of the capillary?
3. Explain the capillary forces that enable the body to "borrow" water from the interstitium in a dehydrated person.

Sum It Up!

The capillaries are well suited for exchange because of three characteristics: thin capillary wall, large surface area of capillaries, and slow velocity of capillary blood flow. Most solute exchanges by simple diffusion. Water and dissolved solute exchange using the filtration–osmosis pressures (filtration at the arterial end and osmosis at the venous end of the capillary). Edema formation is due to an imbalance of the filtration-osmosis transport mechanisms at the capillary level.

BLOOD VESSELS DISTRIBUTE BLOOD

Blood vessels are also "in charge" of distributing blood according to changing body needs. As Fig. 19.7 shows, blood flow to a particular area of the body can change. For example, in the resting state, the skeletal muscle receives 20% of the total blood flow, and the kidney and abdomen receive 19% and 24%, respectively. Note what happens during strenuous exercise. Blood flow is redirected; the percentage of blood flow pumped to skeletal muscle greatly increases (to 71% of total flow). Why? Exercising muscle needs more oxygen and nutrients. In addition, the increased blood flow carries heat and waste products away from the exercising muscles. At the same time, the percentage of blood that flows through the kidney and abdomen decreases (3.5% of total flow). In other words, the blood is directed to sites where it is most needed, such as the skeletal muscle. Note also that the blood flow to the skin increases from 9% to 11% of total flow. The increased blood flow to the skin helps lose the excess heat, thereby helping regulate body temperature.

BLOOD VESSELS REGULATE BODY TEMPERATURE

The regulation of body temperature is described in Chapter 7. In essence, the blood vessels help dissipate (get rid of) or conserve heat. For example, with exercise and temperature elevation, the blood vessels dilate, thereby allowing more blood to flow to the skin. This activity transfers heat from the deeper tissues to the surface of the body. The heat radiates from the flushed skin, thereby lowering body temperature. Conversely, heat is conserved when the blood vessels of the skin constrict, diverting the warm blood from surface blood vessels into deeper parts of the body.

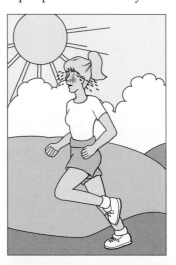

Sum It Up!

The circulatory system does more than run around in circles. It acts as a delivery system, regulates blood pressure, engages in the exchange of nutrients and waste, redistributes blood in response to changing body needs, and helps in the regulation of body temperature.

 As You Age

1. The circulatory system is one of the body systems most affected by age. The walls of the arteries thicken and become less elastic and stiffer. Two major consequences occur: blood flow to vital organs (e.g., the brain) decreases, and blood pressure increases, thereby increasing the work of the heart.
2. Changes occur in both the walls and the valves of the veins. As a result, older persons are more prone to the development of varicose veins.
3. The inner surface of the blood vessels becomes roughened because of age-related changes in the vessel wall and the development of fatty plaques. As a result, older persons are more prone to thrombus formation.
4. The baroreceptors become less sensitive. Cardiovascular adjustments to changes in position are slowed, and the person may become dizzy and tend to fall.
5. The permeability of the capillary membrane increases with age, thereby increasing edema formation in older persons.

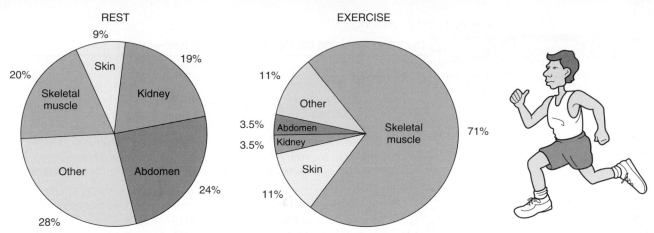

FIG. 19.7 Distribution of blood flow at rest and during exercise.

🔲 Medical Terminology and Disorders — Disorders Involving the Peripheral Vasculature

MEDICAL TERM	WORD PARTS	WORD PART MEANING OR DERIVATION	DESCRIPTION
Words			
angioplasty	angi/o-	vessel	An **angioplasty** is *the surgical repair of a blood vessel, either by the insertion of a balloon-tipped catheter or reconstruction of the vessel*. The widened blood vessel improves blood flow; angioplastic procedures most commonly involve the coronary arteries in an attempt to improve blood flow to the myocardium.
	-plasty	surgical repair of or reconstruction	
intravenous	intra-	within	Refers to *the space within a vein*. Access is achieved by a venipuncture, or the insertion of a needle into a vein. Fluids and drugs are often administered intravenously.
	-ven/o-	vein	
	-ous	pertaining to	
phlebotomy	phleb/o-	vein	A **phlebotomy** is *the entrance into a vein for the purpose of obtaining blood for analysis or treatment.*
	-otomy	incision into	
vascular	vascul/o-	vessel	A term that *refers to blood vessels,* as in vascular disease or vascular resistance.
	-ar	pertaining to	
Disorders			
aneurysm		From a Greek word meaning "dilation" or "wide"	An **aneurysm** is *an abnormal bulging or ballooning of the walls of blood vessels, especially the arteries.* Aneurysms have two shapes: fusiform and saccular. The **fusiform aneurysm** is a weakness along an extended section of the aorta and involves the entire circumference of the aorta. A **saccular aneurysm** is a small bulge or sac on one side of the aorta. There are three types of aneurysms based on location: aortic, cerebral (or berry), or peripheral aneurysm. The **aortic aneurysms** are classified as thoracic and abdominal. **Cerebral (or berry) aneurysms** occur in an artery of the brain and are often berry sized. **Peripheral aneurysms** are those that occur in arteries other than the aorta and brain. An aortic aneurysm can also occur with dissection **(dissecting aneurysm),** in which a small tear in the aortic wall allows the blood to flow through the layers, thereby extending the tear and occluding blood vessels supplying other organs.
angioma	angi/o-	blood vessel	An **angioma** is *a benign tumor composed of blood vessels or lymph vessels that usually appears at the surface of the skin.* There are many types of angiomas: a **hemangioma,** such as a **port-wine stain,** is a proliferation of endothelial cells lining a blood vessel. The angioma often looks like a stain created by spilled red wine.
	-oma	tumor	
claudication		From a Latin word, *claudicare,* meaning "limping"	**Claudication** is *a condition that usually occurs in the legs.* **Vascular claudication** refers to discomfort caused by poor circulation to the extremities and is common in persons with diabetes. **Spinal or neurogenic claudication** is due to nerve root compression (e.g., herniated disk, bone spurs, scar tissue) or stenosis of the spinal canal. Claudication usually presents as pain, discomfort, or tiredness in calf muscles while walking; it is often described in terms of city blocks. A "one-block claudication" refers to the onset of claudication when the person experiences discomfort after walking one city block. There is also two-block or three-block claudication. Claudication may occur intermittently with exercise or occur at rest. **Rest claudication** is usually indicative of more serious underlying pathology.

Continued

MEDICAL TERM	WORD PARTS	WORD PART MEANING OR DERIVATION	DESCRIPTION
hypertension	hyper-	excessive	*High blood pressure* (**hypertension**) is defined as a blood pressure >140/90 mm Hg. Hypertension can cause blood vessels to rupture with catastrophic results, such as a hemorrhage into brain tissue. Chronic hypertension increases the workload of the heart, gradually causing the heart to enlarge (ventricular hypertrophy) and fail. Hypertension also causes damage to other organs such as the kidneys, eyes, and brain.
	-tension	From a Latin word, *tendere,* meaning "to stretch"	
hypotension	hypo-	below	*Low blood pressure* (**hypotension**) is a blood pressure <90/60 mm Hg. Hypotension reduces blood flow to vital organs. Very low blood flow to the brain causes a loss of consciousness (syncope). Low blood flow to the heart may cause ischemic chest pain and necrosis (myocardial infarction).
	-tension	From a Latin word, *tendere,* meaning "to stretch"	
ischemia	isch/o-	blockage	**Ischemia** means *insufficient blood supply to a tissue or an organ.* The ischemic tissue is deprived of oxygen and nutrients. Examples include myocardial ischemia and an ischemic gut.
	-emia	blood condition	
peripheral arterial disease			**Peripheral arterial disease (PAD)** involves *an atherosclerotic narrowing and deterioration of the arteries of the neck, abdomen, and periphery.* The most significant risk factors are hypertension, elevated cholesterol, diabetes mellitus, and, chiefly, cigarette smoking. Although any artery can be affected, PAD most often involves the coronary, carotid, distal abdominal aorta, iliac, and femoral arteries.
Raynaud's phenomenon		Named for French physician Dr. Maurice Raynaud (1834–1881)	**Raynaud's phenomenon** is *an episodic vasospasm (involuntary contraction of the blood vessels), most often of the cutaneous blood vessels of the fingers and toes (also ears and nose).* Vasospastic episodes cause the digits to change color: pallor (white) to cyanosis (bluish-purple) to rubor (red). Poor perfusion to the digits causes pain and tissue changes and damage, including gangrene.
shock			**Shock** is a general term used to characterize *a hypoperfusion of tissues and impairment of cellular metabolism. Shock is caused by low blood flow or maldistribution of blood flow.* Low blood flow is caused by poor cardiac function **(cardiogenic shock)** or low blood volume **(hypovolemic shock).** Hypovolemia is a consequence of hemorrhage, pooling of blood, and systemic vasodilation. Maldistribution of blood flow is caused by **neurogenic shock** (spinal cord injury), **septic shock** (infection), and **anaphylactic shock** (severe allergic response).
thrombophlebitis	thromb/o-	From the Greek word *thrombos,* meaning "clot or curdled milk"	**Thrombophlebitis** is *the most common disorder of the veins; it is the formation of a thrombus (blood clot) in association with inflammation of the vein.* Classifications include **superficial thrombophlebitis** and the more clinically significant **deep vein thrombosis (DVT).** DVT is characterized by **Virchow's triad:** venous stasis, damage of the venous endothelium, and hypercoagulability. The thrombus most often forms in the deep veins of the legs; a piece of the thrombus may break off, becoming an embolus that lodges in the pulmonary circulation **(pulmonary embolus). Phlebothrombosis** refers to the development of a thrombus in the veins without the associated inflammation. It is usually caused by sluggish circulation in the legs, caused by prolonged bed rest, long car trips, or extended air travel.
	-phleb/o-	vein	
	-itis	inflammation	
varices		From a Latin word meaning "raised area," a reference to the bulging area of the legs associated with varicose veins	**Varices** are *abnormally dilated and lengthened arteries, veins, or lymph nodes.* In the lower extremities, varices are known as **varicose veins.** These are large, tortuous veins; they are of cosmetic concern and cause discomfort and a feeling of heaviness while standing. Other veins throughout the body can be affected. In the digestive system, esophageal varices develop in the lower esophagus in response to elevated portal pressure caused by cirrhosis of the liver. The concern is that the varices will rupture and bleed. In the rectal area, varices are called *hemorrhoids.* **Hemorrhoids** may be external or internal. **External hemorrhoids** are often painful, are accompanied by irritation and itching, and are prone to thrombosis. **Internal hemorrhoids** are generally not painful but may bleed when irritated. A scrotal varicosity is called a **varicocele. Telangiectasia** is an enlargement of superficial cutaneous blood vessels that are most visible on the face and thighs.

Get Ready for Exams!

Summary Outline

The blood vessels perform five main functions.

I. Functions as a Delivery System
  A. The blood vessels deliver oxygen, nutrients, and hormones to the cells.
  B. The blood vessels pick up waste from the cells and deliver it to the organs of excretion.

II. Regulates Blood Pressure
  A. The blood vessels maintain a blood pressure to ensure an adequate flow of blood to the body.
  B. The normal blood pressure is slightly less than 120/80 mm Hg; 116/72 mm Hg is a normal blood pressure—116 is the systolic reading, and 72 is the diastolic reading.
  C. Blood pressure varies throughout the circulatory system; it is highest in the aorta and lowest in the venae cavae. This pressure difference is responsible for the flow of blood from the aorta to the venae cavae and right heart.
  D. Blood pressure is determined by the action of the heart and blood vessels. The heart affects blood pressure by increasing or decreasing cardiac output. The blood vessels affect blood pressure by constricting or dilating the arterioles (systemic vascular resistance).
  E. Blood pressure is regulated acutely by the baroreceptor reflex. A sudden decline in blood pressure causes the sympathetic nerves to fire. A sudden increase in blood pressure causes the parasympathetic (vagus) nerves to fire. The participation of the adrenal medullary hormones (epinephrine and norepinephrine) accompany and amplify the effects of sympathetic activity.
  F. Other hormonal mechanisms can correct blood pressure more slowly. The most important is the renin–angiotensin–aldosterone system.

III. Acts as Exchange Vessels
  A. The capillaries are the site of exchange of nutrients and waste between the blood and tissue fluid.
  B. Factors that make the capillaries ideal exchange vessels are the thin capillary walls with many pores, millions of capillaries, and a slow rate of blood flow through the capillaries.
  C. Most exchange occurs by diffusion.
  D. Water and dissolved substances exchange by filtration–osmosis. The capillary pressure pushes (filtration) water out of the capillary at its arterial end. Water and dissolved waste move from the tissue fluid into the capillaries in response to plasma oncotic pressure. Lymphatic vessels assist with reabsorption.

IV. Distributes Blood According to Need
  A. Fig. 19.7 compares the distribution of blood during rest and exercise.
  B. Note the change in skeletal muscle blood flow during rest (20%) and exercise (71%).

V. Regulates Body Temperature
  A. Vasodilation of the blood vessels of the skin encourages heat loss.
  B. Vasoconstriction of the blood vessels of the skin decreases heat loss.

Review Your Knowledge

Matching: Blood Pressure Terms
Directions: Match the following words with their descriptions. Some of the words may be used more than once.

a. systolic pressure
b. diastolic pressure
c. pulse pressure
d. mean arterial blood pressure (MABP)
e. reflex tachycardia
f. Korotkoff sounds
g. brachial artery
h. baroreceptors

1. ___d___ ⅔ diastolic pressure + ⅓ systolic pressure
2. ___f___ Silent...tap...tap...tap...tap...muffle
3. ___a___ Pressure reading that reflects myocardial contraction
4. ___h___ Cells in the carotid sinus and aortic arch that detect changes in blood pressure
5. ___g___ Usual site of blood pressure recording
6. ___a___ The top number of a blood pressure recording
7. ___b___ The bottom number of a blood pressure recording
8. ___c___ The difference between the systolic and diastolic pressures
9. ___b___ Pressure reading that reflects myocardial relaxation
10. ___e___ A cardiac consequence of a sudden drop in blood pressure

Matching: Blood Pressure Readings
Directions: Match the following blood pressure readings with their descriptions.

a. 116/72 mm Hg
b. 70/40 mm Hg
c. 220/120 mm Hg

1. ___a___ Normal blood pressure recorded in the aorta
2. ___a___ Normal blood pressure recorded in the brachial artery
3. ___b___ A "shocky" blood pressure
4. ___c___ A hypertensive blood pressure
5. ___b___ A hypotensive blood pressure
6. ___a___ Normotensive reading
7. ___b___ A postoperative blood pressure that may require a vasopressor drug
8. ___c___ A blood pressure that requires immediate treatment with an antihypertensive drug
9. ___a___ Has a pulse pressure of 44
10. ___b___ Blood pressure that is most likely to cause a reflex tachycardia

Matching: Changes in Blood Pressure

Directions: Indicate if each of the following (a) increases blood pressure or (b) decreases blood pressure.

1. _a_ Sympathetic nerve stimulation
2. _b_ Vagal discharge
3. _a_ Effects of a vasopressor agent
4. _a_ Effects of epinephrine and angiotensin II
5. _a_ Increased systemic vascular resistance (SVR)
6. _b_ Decreased cardiac output
7. _a_ Arteriolar constriction
8. _b_ Administration of an alpha$_1$-adrenergic blocker
9. _a_ IV infusion of Levophed (norepinephrine)
10. _a_ Administration of a beta$_1$-adrenergic agonist

Multiple Choice

1. Which of the following is true of a blood pressure reading of 116/72 mm Hg for a 20-year-old adult female?
   a. It is a hypertensive reading.
   b. The 116 mm Hg is the diastolic pressure.
   c. The 72 mm Hg is the systolic pressure.
   d. The pulse pressure is 44 mm Hg.
2. The ability of the arterioles to contract and relax allows them to
   a. regulate heart rate.
   b. prevent the backflow of venous blood.
   c. function as resistance vessels.
   d. function as exchange vessels.
3. Which of the following is a consequence of sympathetic nerve stimulation?
   a. Decreased cardiac output
   b. Peripheral vasodilation
   c. Elevation of blood pressure
   d. Decreased systemic vascular resistance
4. A sudden decrease in blood pressure is most likely to cause
   a. edema.
   b. reflex tachycardia.
   c. increase in the synthesis of albumin.
   d. arteriolar dilation.
5. Which of the following is true of an increase in systemic vascular resistance?
   a. Increases blood pressure
   b. Is caused by vagal discharge
   c. Is caused by peripheral vasodilation
   d. Is due to the relaxation of the aorta
6. In which blood vessel is blood pressure highest?
   a. Superior vena cava
   b. Aorta
   c. Renal artery
   d. Jugular vein
7. In which of the following vessels is blood flow slowest?
   a. Aorta
   b. Arterioles
   c. Capillaries
   d. Veins
8. Which of the following is most apt to lower plasma oncotic pressure?
   a. Dehydration and decreased intravascular volume
   b. Hypoalbuminemia
   c. Hypertension
   d. Blood transfusion

9. Which of the following is responsible for the plasma oncotic pressure?
   a. Plasma sodium concentration
   b. RBCs
   c. Plasma proteins such as albumin
   d. Urea
10. Which of the following is most apt to cause edema?
    a. Decreased filtration pressure as in dehydration
    b. Increased plasma oncotic pressure
    c. Accumulation of albumin in the interstitium (tissue space)
    d. Hypotension
11. Which of the following occurs in the dehydrated state?
    a. The capillary oncotic pressure decreases, and fluid accumulates in the tissue spaces.
    b. Tissue fluid is absorbed into the capillaries.
    c. The capillary filtration rate increases, thereby increasing lymph formation.
    d. Plasma protein is filtered into the tissue spaces, thereby causing edema.
12. Which of the following is true of the baroreceptor reflex?
    a. Baroreceptors are located in the SA and AV nodes of the heart.
    b. Sensory information from the baroreceptors is carried to the CNS by sympathetic and parasympathetic nerves.
    c. Motor information elicited by the baroreceptor reflex is carried by autonomic nerves from the CNS to the heart and blood vessels.
    d. Motor information elicited by the baroreceptor reflex is carried by sympathetic nerves from the CNS to the baroreceptors in the aortic arch and carotid sinus.
13. Baroreceptors are located within the
    a. SA and AV nodes.
    b. medulla oblongata.
    c. venae cavae and arterioles.
    d. aortic arch and carotid sinus.
14. Which of the following is most apt to induce postural hypotension?
    a. Anxiety
    b. sudden change of position (from lying supine to standing)
    c. Ingestion of a fatty meal
    d. Forced exhalation with nose and mouth closed
15. Which of the following is most apt to elicit the Valsalva maneuver?
    a. Anxiety
    b. Sudden change of position (from lying supine to standing)
    c. Walking
    d. Straining at stool

Go Figure...

1. According to Fig. 19.1B, neither the systolic pressure nor diastolic pressure can be heard because
   a. the cuff has not been inflated sufficiently.
   b. the brachial artery is compressed, thereby blocking any flow of blood.
   c. the stethoscope is in the wrong place; it should be proximal to the cuff.
   d. Korotkoff sounds can only be heard when the cuff is inflated to more than 200 mm Hg.

2. Which of the following is correct according to Fig. 19.2?
   a. The pressure within the capillaries is less than the pressure within the venae cavae.
   b. The pulse pressure within the capillaries is equal to the pulse pressure within the large arteries.
   c. Arteriolar pressure is greater than venous pressure.
   d. Pressure is lowest in the arterioles.

3. Which of the following is correct according to Fig. 19.3?
   a. Resistance is greater in panel A than in panel B.
   b. The radius of the arterioles in panels C and D determines the resistance to flow (of blood).
   c. Vasoconstriction decreases the resistance to flow.
   d. Vasodilation increases the resistance to flow.

4. Which of the following is correct according to Fig. 19.4?
   a. The baroreceptors are located in the SA and AV nodes.
   b. Sensory neurons of cranial nerves IX and X carry pressure information from the SA and AV nodes to the aortic arch and the carotid sinus.
   c. Motor information regarding the adjustment of blood pressure is transmitted to the heart and blood vessels by autonomic nerves.
   d. Motor information regarding the adjustment of blood pressure is transmitted to the carotid sinus and the aortic arch by sympathetic nerves.

5. Which of the following is correct according to Fig. 19.6?
   a. In panel B, water is oncotically reabsorbed into the capillary.
   b. In panel B, the plasma proteins (albumin) are filtered into the interstitium.
   c. In panel C, water is oncotically reabsorbed from the interstitium into the capillary.
   d. Oncotic pressure is primarily caused by the plasma electrolytes and glucose.

6. Which of the following is correct according to Fig. 19.6?
   a. Albumin is filtered at the arterial end of the capillary.
   b. Water is reabsorbed by both the venous end of the capillary and the lymphatic vessels.
   c. The capillary membrane is impermeable to water, electrolytes, and plasma protein.
   d. The lymphatic vessel is impermeable to albumin, electrolytes, and water.

7. According to Fig. 19.7, in response to exercise, blood is diverted
   a. to skeletal muscles.
   b. to the skin.
   c. away from the kidneys.
   d. All of the above

Lymphatic System

Objectives

1. List three functions of the lymphatic system.
2. Describe the composition and flow of lymph.
3. List the lymphatic organs and lymphatic nodules

4. Describe the lymph nodes, and state the location of the cervical nodes, axillary nodes, and inguinal nodes.

Key Terms

appendix (p. 381)
lymph (p. 376)
lymph nodes (p. 378)
lymphatic ducts (p. 377)
lymphatic nodules (p. 381)

lymphatic vessels (p. 376)
MALT (mucosal-associated lymphatic tissue) (p. 381)
Peyer's patches (p. 381)
right lymphatic duct (p. 377)

spleen (p. 379)
thoracic duct (p. 377)
thymosins (p. 379)
thymus gland (p. 379)
tonsils (p. 381)

The woman in Fig. 20.1 has a condition called *elephantiasis*. The name is an obvious reference to the size and shape of her leg. Elephantiasis is caused by the invasion and blockage of the lymphatic vessels by small worms called *filariae*. The amount of swelling illustrates the importance of the lymphatic system, which drains fluid from our tissue spaces.

The lymphatic system contains lymph, lymphatic vessels, and lymphatic tissues and organs, which are widely scattered throughout the body. The three main functions of the lymphatic system are as follows:

• The lymphatic vessels absorb fluid from the tissue spaces and return it to the blood.

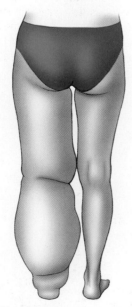

FIG. 20.1 Elephantiasis, a form of lymphedema.

• Specialized lymphatic vessels play an important role in the intestinal absorption of fats and fat-soluble vitamins (further explained in Chapter 23).
• Lymphatic tissue helps the body defend itself against disease.

LYMPH AND LYMPHATIC CIRCULATION

LYMPH: WHAT IT IS, WHERE IT COMES FROM

Lymph (limf) is a clear pale yellow fluid that resembles plasma. Lymph is composed primarily of water, electrolytes, waste from metabolizing cells, and some protein that leaks out of the capillaries into the tissue space.

Where does lymph come from? Water and dissolved substances are continuously filtered out of the blood capillaries into the interstitium to form tissue fluid. Approximately 85% of this tissue fluid moves back into the blood capillaries and is carried away as part of the venous blood. What about the 15% of the tissue fluid that is not reabsorbed into the blood capillaries? This remaining fluid (about 3 L/day) is drained by the lymphatic capillaries that surround the blood capillaries (Fig. 20.2). The tissue fluid entering the lymphatic vessels is called *lymph*.

LYMPHATIC VESSELS

The **lymphatic vessels** include lymphatic capillaries and several larger lymphatic vessels. Like the blood vessels, the lymphatic vessels form an extensive network. The distribution of lymphatic vessels is similar to the distribution of veins. With the exception of

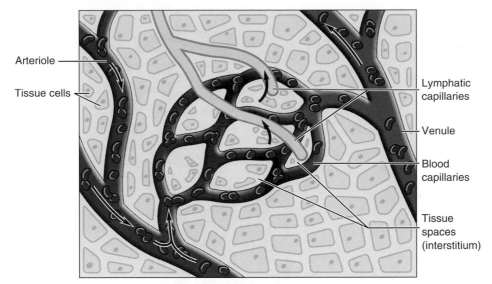

FIG. 20.2 Lymphatic capillaries and blood capillaries.

the central nervous system (CNS), every organ in the body has a rich supply of lymphatic vessels. These pick up tissue fluid and transport it toward the heart. Fig. 20.3 shows the relationship between the circulatory system and the lymphatic system. Note especially the close relationship of the lymphatic vessels with the veins.

The walls of the lymphatic capillaries are made up of a single layer of epithelium and have large pores. This large-pore structure allows the lymphatic capillaries to drain tissue fluid and proteins, thereby forming lymph. Lymph flows from the lymphatic capillaries toward the heart through a series of larger and larger lymphatic vessels until it reaches the two largest **lymphatic ducts**.

For example, lymph from the right arm and right side of the head and thorax drains into the right lymphatic duct. Lymph from the rest of the body drains into the thoracic duct (Fig. 20.4). Both ducts empty the lymph into the subclavian veins. The **right lymphatic duct** drains lymph into the right subclavian vein; the **thoracic duct** drains lymph into the left subclavian vein. The circulation of lymph is summarized in Fig. 20.5. Lymph comes from the blood and returns to the blood.

WHAT CAUSES LYMPH TO MOVE?

Whereas blood moves because it is pumped by the heart, lymph depends on other means for movement. Lymph moves in response to the following:

- *The "milking" action of the skeletal muscles.* As the skeletal muscles contract, they squeeze the surrounding lymphatic vessels, thereby pushing lymph toward the heart.
- *The movement of the chest during respiration.* Contraction and relaxation of the chest muscles cause changes in the pressure within the thoracic cavity. The changes in intrathoracic pressure increase the flow of lymph toward the subclavian veins.

Do You Know...

Why the Axillary Lymph Nodes Are Removed During a Mastectomy (Surgical Breast Removal)?

Many cancers metastasize, or spread, by way of the lymphatic vessels. Cancer of the breast commonly metastasizes to the axillary lymph nodes. In an attempt to rid the body of all cancer cells, the surgeon removes the breast and associated axillary lymph nodes. The lymph nodes are then biopsied; further treatment often depends on how many of the lymph nodes are positive (i.e., are cancerous, or malignant). Removal of the axillary lymph nodes frequently impairs lymphatic drainage. Consequently, the woman may develop edema of the affected arm and shoulder. Because the edema develops in response to impaired drainage of lymph, it is called *lymphedema*.

A new technique is the sentinel node biopsy. The procedure was developed to determine if a cancer has spread without doing the traditional and extensive lymph node dissection. It is based on the following observation. Lymphatic vessels of the breast usually drain to one lymph node first and then to the others in the axillary region. The lymph node that receives the initial drainage is called the *sentinel lymph node* and is identified by the injection of dye. If the sentinel node biopsy is negative, it is assumed that the cancer has not spread to the axillary lymph nodes.

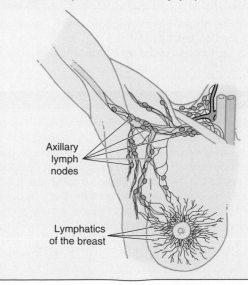

Axillary lymph nodes

Lymphatics of the breast

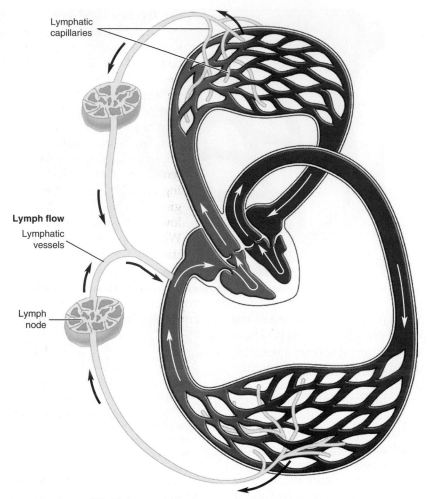

Lymphatic capillaries

Lymph flow

Lymphatic vessels

Lymph node

FIG. 20.3 **Lymphatic vessels accompany the veins.**

- *The rhythmic contraction of the smooth muscle in the lymphatic vessels.* The alternating contraction and relaxation of the smooth muscle cause lymph to flow.
- *The presence of valves.* Like the veins, the lymphatic vessels contain valves. Valves prevent any backflow of lymph; if lymph moves at all, it must move toward the heart.

? Re-Think

1. Why are the lymphatic vessels aligned with the venous side of the circulation?
2. What is the function of the right lymphatic and thoracic ducts?

◎ Sum It Up!

Lymphatic vessels accompany venous blood vessels throughout the body. They drain fluid and protein from tissue spaces; the lymph drains into the main lymphatic ducts (right lymphatic duct and thoracic duct). The main lymphatic ducts drain into the general circulation through the subclavian veins. Lymph is not pumped by the heart; it moves in response to skeletal and smooth muscle activity and the movement of the chest during respiration.

LYMPHATIC TISSUE

Lymphatic tissue includes lymphatic organs and lymphatic nodules; the lymphatic organs are encapsulated masses of lymphatic tissue while the lymphatic nodules are partially or non-encapsulated. It is called *lymphatic tissue* because it contains lymphocytes and related cells. In general, lymphatic tissue helps defend the body against disease; it filters particles such as pathogens and cancer cells from the lymph, tissue fluid, and blood and supports the immune activities of the lymphocytes.

LYMPHATIC ORGANS

The lymphatic organs are the lymph nodes, thymus gland, and spleen (Fig. 20.6).

LYMPH NODES

Lymph nodes are small pea-shaped patches of lymphatic tissue strategically located to filter the lymph as it flows through the lymphatic vessels. Lymph nodes

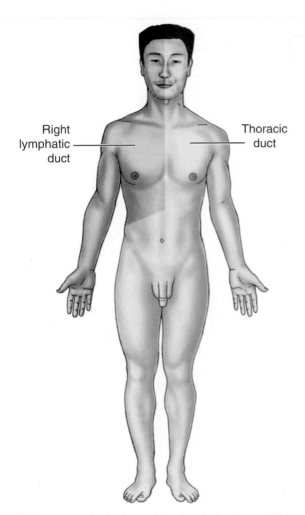

FIG. 20.4 Main lymphatic ducts: right lymphatic duct and thoracic duct.

Flow of Lymph

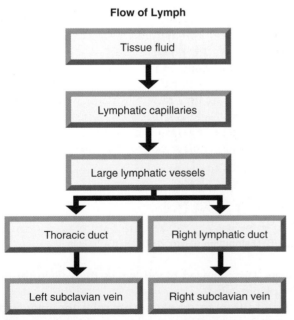

FIG. 20.5 Flow of lymph from the lymphatic capillaries to the subclavian veins.

tend to appear in clusters (see Fig. 20.6B). Three of the larger clusters include the following:

- Cervical lymph nodes drain and cleanse lymph coming from the head and neck areas. Enlarged, tender cervical lymph nodes often accompany upper respiratory infections.
- Axillary lymph nodes are located in the axillary area, or armpit. These nodes drain and cleanse lymph coming from the upper extremities, shoulders, and breast area. Cancer cells that leave the breast are often found in the axillary lymph nodes.
- Inguinal lymph nodes are located in the groin region. These nodes drain and cleanse lymph from the lower extremities and external genitalia.

What does a lymph node look like? A lymph node contains several compartments, called *lymph nodules,* that are separated by lymph sinuses (Fig. 20.7). The lymph nodules are masses of lymphocytes and macrophages. These cells are defensive cells and are concerned with immunity and phagocytosis; they protect the body against disease. The lymph nodules are separated by lymph sinuses; these are lymph-filled spaces. Afferent lymphatic vessels carry lymph into the node for cleansing. The lymph leaves the node through the efferent lymphatic vessels as it continues its journey through the lymphatic vessels toward the heart.

THYMUS GLAND

The **thymus gland** is located in the mediastinum of the thoracic cavity (see Fig. 20.6A). The thymus gland is relatively large in infancy and early childhood and shrinks after puberty. With advancing age, thymus tissue is gradually replaced with adipose and connective tissue, but the thymus still retains an age-related role in immune function. The thymus gland is the home of many lymphocytes; many are inactive, whereas others mature into T lymphocytes, which leave the thymus and travel throughout the body, engaging in immune activity. The thymus gland also secretes hormones called *thymosins.* **Thymosins** promote the proliferation and maturation of special lymphocytes (T cells) in lymphatic tissue throughout the body (see Chapter 21).

SPLEEN

The **spleen** is the largest lymphatic organ in the body. It is located in the left upper quadrant of the abdominal cavity, just beneath the diaphragm, and is normally protected by the lower rib cage (Fig. 20.8). Although the spleen is much larger, it resembles a lymph node.

The spleen filters blood rather than lymph. The spleen is composed of two types of tissue: white pulp and red pulp. The white pulp is lymphatic tissue consisting primarily of lymphocytes surrounding arteries. The red pulp contains venous sinuses filled with blood

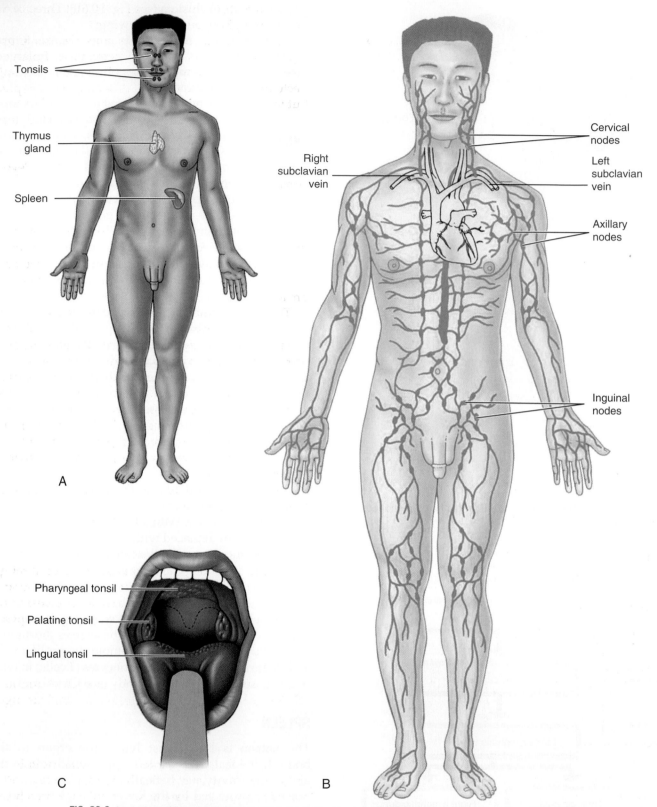

FIG. 20.6 Location of lymphatic tissue. (A) Lymphatic organs. (B) Distribution of lymph nodes. (C) Tonsils.

and disease-preventing cells such as lymphocytes and macrophages. Blood enters the spleen through the splenic artery. The blood is cleansed as it slowly flows through the spleen. Microorganisms trapped by the spleen are destroyed by the leukocytes in the

spleen. The cleansed blood leaves the spleen through the splenic vein.

In addition to its cleansing role, the spleen has other functions. The spleen stores blood, especially platelets. (As much as 30% of the platelets are

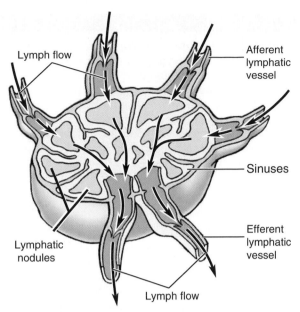

FIG. 20.7 **Cross-section of a lymph node.**

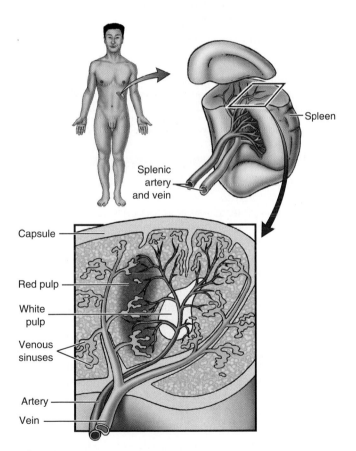

FIG. 20.8 **Spleen: lymphatic nodules and sinuses; white pulp and red pulp.**

stored in the spleen.) The spleen also destroys and phagocytoses old, worn-out red blood cells (RBCs). Therefore, the spleen is called the "graveyard" of the RBCs. Finally, the spleen plays a role in fetal erythropoiesis. After birth, the spleen stops producing RBCs but continues its lifelong production of lymphocytes.

Because of its location, the spleen is commonly injured. Because it is difficult to repair and prone to bleed, the spleen may be removed surgically. The splenectomized patient can live quite well without a spleen but may be more prone to infection.

LYMPHATIC NODULES

Lymphatic nodules include the tonsils, MALT, Peyer's patches, and the appendix.

TONSILS

Tonsils are partially encapsulated lymph nodes in the throat area (see Fig. 20.6A and C). They filter tissue fluid contaminated by pathogens that enter the body through the nose and mouth. The names of the tonsils are as follows:

- The palatine tonsils (there are two) are small masses of lymphoid tissue located at the opening of the oral cavity into the pharynx. A tonsillectomy is most often performed on this particular set of tonsils.
- The pharyngeal tonsil is also called the *adenoid* and is located near the opening of the nasal cavity in the upper pharynx. The adenoid atrophies during adolescence. Enlargement of the adenoid may interfere with breathing and may require surgical removal, a procedure known as *adenoidectomy.*
- The lingual tonsils (there are two) are located at the back of the tongue.

MALT

MALT refers to **mucosal-associated lymphatic tissue**; it is lymphatic tissue that is diffusely scattered throughout the body in its mucous membranes. It is found in the organs of the respiratory, digestive, urinary, and reproductive tracts—all organ systems that are open to the external environment.

PEYER'S PATCHES

Peyer's patches refer to lymphatic nodules found in the lower part of the small intestine (part of the digestive tract).

APPENDIX

The **appendix** is an outpouching located within the large intestine that contains lymphatic nodules. Both lymphatic structures are busily involved with a heavy load of microorganisms.

 Re-Think

1. What is the primary function of lymphatic tissue?
2. List three lymphatic organs.
3. List three functions of the spleen.
4. Why are the tonsils referred to as lymphatic nodules?

Sum It Up!

Lymphatic tissue includes lymphatic organs and lymphatic nodules. Lymphatic tissue contains lymphocytes and related cells and plays an important role in immune function and the prevention of disease. The lymphatic organs are the lymph nodes, thymus gland, and spleen. The lymphatic nodules include the tonsils (palatine, pharyngeal, and lingual), MALT (mucosal-associated lymphatic tissue), Peyer's patches, and appendix.

 As You Age

1. Lymphatic tissue reaches its peak development at puberty and then progressively shrinks with age.
2. After puberty, the thymus gland involutes, or shrivels up, and is replaced by adipose and connective tissue. The gland, however, retains a reduced ability to function in immune activity. This process involves a decrease in the amount of thymosins produced. Because of these changes, the defense mechanisms of the body diminish with age.

Medical Terminology and Disorders | Disorders of the Lymphatic System

MEDICAL TERM	WORD PARTS	WORD PART MEANING OR DERIVATION	DESCRIPTION
Words			
hypersplenism	hyper-	excessive	**Hypersplenism** is *a disorder in which an overactive spleen prematurely destroys red blood cells, white blood cells, and platelets, thereby causing anemia, leukopenia, and thrombocytopenia.*
	-splen/o-	spleen	
	-ism	condition of	
lingual	lingul/o-	tongue	The **lingual** tonsils are located on the posterior tongue.
	-al	pertaining to	
splenomegaly	splen/o-	spleen	**Splenomegaly** is *an enlarged spleen; it usually accompanies hypersplenism and the excessive destruction of blood cells.*
	-megaly	enlargement	
tonsillectomy	tonsil/o-	tonsil	A **tonsillectomy** is *the removal of the tonsils,* usually the palatine tonsils.
	-ectomy	removal of	
Disorders			
lymphadenopathy	lymph/o-	lymph	Means *disease of the lymph nodes,* but is used synonymously with "swollen or enlarged lymph nodes." Lymph nodes swell in response to a number of conditions, both localized and systemic (infectious mononucleosis), autoimmune diseases and malignancies. Rarely is the distinction made between lymphadenopathy and **lymphadenitis,** *an inflammation of the lymph nodes.*
	-aden/o-	gland	
	-pathy	disease	
lymphedema	lymph/o-	lymph	Also called **lymphatic obstruction**; it is *a condition in which there is localized tissue swelling caused by damaged lymphatic vessels and poor drainage of tissue fluid.* The most common cause of lymphedema in the United States is related to the treatment of cancer: lymph node dissection, cancer surgery, and radiation therapy. In tropical regions of the world a common cause of severe lymphedema is filariasis, a parasitic infection.
	-edema	From a Greek word meaning a "swelling tumor"	
lymphoma	lymph/o-	lymph	*A solid malignant tumor of lymphoid cells, specifically the lymphocytes.* Abnormal lymphocytes collect and grow in lymph nodes or in lymphatic organs/nodules such as the spleen and tonsils, forming tumors that eventually metastasize throughout the body. There are two main categories of lymphomas: Hodgkin lymphoma (HL) and non-Hodgkin lymphoma (NHL).
	-oma	tumor	

Get Ready for Exams!

Summary Outline

The main functions of the lymphatic system are defense of the body against infection, return of fluid from the tissue spaces to the blood, and absorption of fat and fat-soluble vitamins from the digestive tract.

I. The Lymphatic System
   A. Lymph
     1. Lymph is a clear fluid containing water, electrolytes, waste, and some protein.
     2. Water and electrolytes are filtered from the plasma into the tissue spaces. Tissue fluid leaves the interstitium by way of the lymphatic vessels; in the lymphatic vessels, the fluid is known as *lymph.*
   B. Lymphatic vessels
     1. Lymphatic vessels are similar to the blood capillaries and the veins. The large holes in the lymphatic capillaries absorb fluid and protein from the tissue spaces.
     2. Lymph is carried by lymphatic capillaries to larger lymphatic vessels and finally to the right lymphatic duct and thoracic duct; both ducts drain into the subclavian veins.
   C. Movement of lymph
     1. Lymph is not pumped by the heart like blood.
     2. Lymph moves in response to skeletal muscle contraction (through milking action), chest movement, and contraction of smooth muscle in the lymphatic vessels. Valves in the lymphatic vessels ensure a one-way flow of lymph.

II. Lymphatic Organs
   A. Lymph nodes
     1. The major clusters of lymph nodes are the cervical, axillary, and inguinal nodes.
     2. Lymph nodes help protect the body against infection.
   B. Thymus gland
     1. The thymus gland produces and helps differentiate T lymphocytes.
     2. The thymus gland secretes thymosins.
   C. Spleen
     1. It functions as a large lymph node.
     2. It has a store of WBCs that phagocytose microorganisms and participate in the immune process.
     3. It stores blood and removes worn-out red blood cells and platelets.
     4. It engages in fetal erythropoiesis.

III. Lymphatic nodules
   A. Tonsils
     1. Filter tissue fluid that is contaminated by pathogens that enter via the nose and mouth
     2. Include the palatine, lingual, and pharyngeal tonsils
   B. MALT (mucosal-associated lymphatic tissue): diffusely distributed throughout the mucous membranes of the body
   C. Peyer's patches: lymphatic nodules that are located in the mucous membrane of the small intestine
   D. Appendix: a small outpouching of the large intestine that contains lymphatic nodules

Review Your Knowledge

Matching: Lymph Terms
Directions: Match the following words with their descriptions.

a. lymph nodes
b. subclavian veins
c. thoracic duct
d. spleen
e. tonsils

1. __e__ Pharyngeal, lingual, palatine
2. __c__ Most of the lymph drains into this large duct
3. __b__ The large lymphatic ducts empty lymph into these blood vessels
4. __d__ Contains red pulp and white pulp; it is the largest lymphatic organ in the body
5. __a__ Small, pea-shaped lymphatic structures that filter lymph as it flows through the lymphatic vessels

Multiple Choice

1. With which of the following are lymph nodes populated?
   a. Granulocytes and Kupffer cells
   b. Lymphocytes and macrophages
   c. Reticulocytes and eosinophils
   d. Only granulocytes

2. The spleen
   a. is located in the right upper quadrant.
   b. receives lymph from the thoracic duct.
   c. engages in phagocytosis and removes worn-out RBCs and platelets from the circulation.
   d. pumps lymph throughout the body, much like the heart pumps blood.

3. An overly active spleen may prematurely remove platelets from the circulation, thereby
   a. making the person hypertensive.
   b. predisposing the person to infection.
   c. predisposing the person to bleeding.
   d. causing hyperbilirubinemia and jaundice.

4. Which complication is most apt to develop in the patient who has had a breast removed (mastectomy) and lymph node dissection?
   a. Lymphoma
   b. Bleeding
   c. Lymphedema
   d. Jaundice

5. Which of the following statements is true about the palatine, pharyngeal, and lingual lymphatic nodules?
   a. They are composed of red pulp and white pulp.
   b. They are called tonsils.
   c. They receive lymph from the thoracic duct.
   d. They drain lymph from all cervical and axillary lymph nodes.

6. The right lymphatic duct and the thoracic duct deliver
   a. blood to the lymphatic organs.
   b. venous blood to the right heart.
   c. lymph to the subclavian veins.
   d. lymph to the axillary lymph nodes.

7. The term MALT
   a. refers to lymphatic tissue in the mucosal membranes of many organs.
   b. is the medical term for lymph.
   c. refers to pools of lymph stored within the spleen.
   d. is lymphatic tissue that is restricted to the thoracic cavity.

8. Which of the following is *not* true of lymph?
   a. It is formed from tissue or interstitial fluid.
   b. It is pumped into the main lymphatic ducts by the heart.
   c. It drains from the right lymphatic and thoracic ducts into the subclavian veins.
   d. It is cleansed by phagocytes as it flows through lymphatic organs.

9. The lymphatic circulation
   a. is most closely associated with the venous side of the circulation.
   b. accompanies the aorta and its branches.
   c. is concerned primarily with the transport of oxygen.
   d. plays a vital role in hemostasis.

10. Which lymphatic structure is composed of red pulp and white pulp and is called the "graveyard" of the red blood cells?
    a. Thymus gland
    b. Peyer's patches
    c. Spleen
    d. Appendix

Go Figure

1. Which of the following is correct according to Fig. 20.2?
   a. Lymph is filtered from the lymphatic vessels into the interstitium.
   b. Oxygenated blood is pumped from the interstitium into the lymphatic vessels.
   c. Lymphatic vessels drain fluid and proteins from the interstitium.
   d. Fluid is filtered by veins into the interstitium.

2. Which of the following is correct according to Fig. 20.3?
   a. The lymphatic vessels accompany the distribution of the veins.
   b. Lymph nodes act as pumps to move the lymph from node to node.
   c. Lymph is emptied into the large arteries to circulate as blood.
   d. Lymph is formed within the lymph nodes and filtered into the interstitium.

3. Which of the following is correct according to Fig. 20.4?
   a. Most lymph drains into the right lymphatic duct.
   b. Most lymph drains into the thoracic duct.
   c. The right lymphatic duct pumps lymph into the arteries that supply the upper right thorax and head.
   d. The thoracic duct pumps lymph into the arteries that supply most of the body, with the exception of the upper right thorax and head.

4. Which of the following is correct according to Fig. 20.6?
   a. The cervical, axillary, and inguinal lymph nodes receive lymph from the upper torso.
   b. The thoracic and right lymphatic ducts empty lymph into the subclavian veins.
   c. The left subclavian vein pumps lymph into the thoracic duct.
   d. Lymphatic tissue is found only in lymph nodes.

5. According to Fig. 20.6, which of the following is true of the tonsils?
   a. Classified as pharyngeal, palatine, and lingual
   b. Masses of lymphatic tissue
   c. Concerned with fighting pathogens that enter through the nose and mouth
   d. All of the above

6. Which of the following is correct according to Figs. 20.7 and 20.8?
   a. Each lymph node is composed of red and white pulp.
   b. The spleen is located within the mediastinum of the thoracic cavity.
   c. All lymph nodes receive oxygenated blood from the splenic artery.
   d. The spleen is composed of red and white pulp.

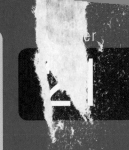

Immune System

Objectives

1. Discuss nonspecific immunity, including the following:
   - Describe the process of phagocytosis.
   - Explain the causes of the signs of inflammation.
   - Explain the role of fever in fighting infection.
   - Explain the role of interferons, complement proteins, and natural killer cells in the defense of the body.
2. Discuss specific immunity, including the following:
   - Differentiate between specific and nonspecific immunity.
   - Explain the role of T cells in cell-mediated immunity.
   - Explain the role of B cells in antibody-mediated immunity.
3. Differentiate between genetic immunity and acquired immunity.
4. Describe naturally and artificially acquired active and passive immunity.
5. Describe other immune responses, including the following:
   - Identify the steps in the development of anaphylaxis.
   - Define *autoimmunity*.

Key Terms

active immunity (p. 395)
adaptive immunity (p. 389)
allergen (p. 396)
antibodies (p. 392)
antibody-mediated immunity (AMI) (p. 391)
antigen presentation (p. 392)
antigens (p. 390)
artificially acquired immunity (p. 395)
autoimmunity (p. 390)
B lymphocytes (B cells) (p. 390)

cell-mediated immunity (CMI) (p. 391)
clone (p. 392)
complement proteins (p. 389)
fever (p. 388)
immunity (p. 385)
immunization (p. 395)
immunoglobulins (p. 392)
immunotolerance (p. 390)
inflammation (p. 388)
innate immunity (p. 385)
interferons (p. 389)

macrophages (p. 392)
natural killer (NK) cells (p. 386)
naturally acquired immunity (p. 395)
nonspecific immunity (p. 385)
passive immunity (p. 395)
phagocytosis (p. 387)
pyrogen (p. 388)
specific immunity (p. 385)
T lymphocytes (T cells) (p. 390)
vaccine (p. 395)
vaccination (p. 395)

If there is one system that has achieved immense clinical significance today it is the immune system. Recent developments have ended the need for the lifetime isolation of a child with a primary immunodeficiency disorder. Today we are more apt to encounter persons who are immunosuppressed because of human immunodeficiency (HIV) infection or treatment for cancer in the form of chemotherapy or radiation. This is a new day of bone marrow transplants, vaccinations, immunotherapies, and recognition of the scope of autoimmune diseases. The term *immune system* refers to the defensive mechanisms that protect us from pathogens, foreign substances such as pollens, and cancer cells. The immunity provided by this system is not restricted to a single organ or tissue; rather, it is diffusely scattered throughout the body. There is a multitude of moving parts that work together to provide such protection. The study of the immune system is called *immunology*.

CLASSIFICATION OF THE IMMUNE SYSTEM

The defense mechanisms of the immune system are classified as nonspecific and specific immunity. **Nonspecific immunity** protects the body against many different types of foreign agents. With nonspecific immunity, the body need not recognize the specific foreign agent.

Specific immunity, on the other hand, hones in on a specific substance.

NONSPECIFIC IMMUNITY

Nonspecific immunity is also called **innate immunity** because we are born with certain defensive mechanisms that do not require prior exposure to the pathogen or foreign agent. A number of defense mechanisms are included in the category of nonspecific immunity

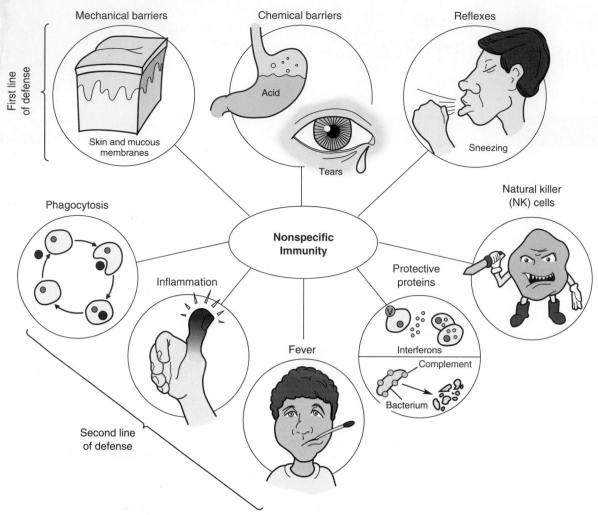

FIG. 21.1 Nonspecific immunity. First line of defense: mechanical barriers, chemical barriers, and reflexes. Second line of defense: phagocytosis, inflammation, fever, protective proteins, and natural killer (NK) cells.

(Fig. 21.1). Nonspecific immunity can be divided into two lines of defense. The first line of defense includes mechanical barriers, chemical barriers, and reflexes. The second line of defense includes phagocytosis, inflammation, fever, protective proteins (interferons and complement proteins), and **natural killer (NK) cells.** Remember that the nonspecific defense mechanisms work against all foreign agents or type of injury; no recognition of a specific agent or injury is necessary. Table 21.1 lists the many types of cells involved in the immune response.

FIRST LINE OF DEFENSE

The first line of defense includes mechanical barriers, chemical barriers, and reflexes. Intact skin and mucous membranes serve as mechanical barriers; pathogens cannot cross these structures and enter the body. Destruction of mechanical barriers is an invitation to microbial invasion and subsequent infection (see Fig. 21.1). Assisting the skin and mucous membranes with their mechanical defensive functions are their chemical secretions. For example, the secretions of the sebaceous and sweat glands of the skin form an acid coating that

inhibits bacterial growth while the external layer of the skin continuously sloughs off, thereby shedding microorganisms from the skin surface. Other chemical barriers include stomach secretions, saliva, sweat, and enzymes such as lysozyme. The acid and digestive enzymes secreted by the cells of the stomach kill most of the microorganisms that are swallowed. Perspiration, tears, and saliva contain *lysozyme,* an enzyme that discourages the growth of pathogens.

Other secretions make the environment sticky and so provide another type of barrier. The mucus secreted by the mucous membranes of the respiratory tract traps inhaled foreign material. Then the cilia, which line most of the respiratory structures, sweep the entrapped material toward the throat so that the material can eventually be coughed up or swallowed. In addition to the mechanical and chemical barriers, reflexes assist in the removal of pathogens. Sneezing and coughing help remove pathogens from the respiratory tract, whereas vomiting and diarrhea help remove pathogens from the digestive tract.

Mechanical barriers, chemical barriers, and reflexes are not an adequate defense against all pathogens,

Table 21.1	Cells Involved in Immunity	
CELL TYPE	**PRODUCTION SITE**	**FUNCTION**
Granular Leukocytes		
Neutrophils	Bone marrow	Phagocytosis
Basophils	Bone marrow	Secrete histamine, leukotrienes, and heparin
Eosinophils	Bone marrow	Destroy parasites
Nongranular Leukocytes		
Monocytes	Bone marrow	Phagocytosis; they enter tissues and are transformed into macrophages
Lymphocytes		
• B cells	Bone marrow	Antibody-mediated immunity; accounts for 20% to 30% of blood lymphocytes
Plasma cells		Secrete antibodies
Memory B cells		Remember the antigens
• T cells	Bone marrow and lymphoid tissue	Cell-mediated immunity; accounts for 70% to 80% of blood lymphocytes
Cytotoxic T cells		Kill cells in cell-to-cell combat
Helper T cells		Secrete cytokines, which activate T and B and other cells
Suppressor T cells		Inhibit B- and T-cell activity (help control immune response)
Memory T cells		Remember the antigens and respond quickly to a second encounter
• Natural killer (NK) cells	Lymphoid tissue	Kill cells
Other Cells		
Macrophages	Almost all organs and tissues	Phagocytosis; present antigens to lymphocytes
Mast cells	Almost all organs and tissues, especially liver and lungs	Release histamine and other chemicals involved in inflammation

however. If a pathogen penetrates this first line of defense, it encounters processes that make up the second line of defense.

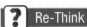 Re-Think

1. List the three mechanisms that make up the first line of defense.
2. Describe three ways that the skin acts as a barrier to the entrance of pathogens.
3. How does mucus assist the respiratory system in avoiding the inhalation of pathogens and other particulate matter?
4. Why do health care workers wear gloves while handling the body secretions of patients?

SECOND LINE OF DEFENSE

The second line of defense includes phagocytosis, inflammation, fever, protective proteins, and NK cells.

Phagocytosis

The leukocytes ingest and digest pathogens and other foreign substances by **phagocytosis**. Two important phagocytes are the neutrophils and monocytes. The neutrophils are small and motile, and they travel to the site of infection quickly. There they engage the pathogen aggressively, and most die in battle, becoming part of the cellular debris and pus. The neutrophils are also active in the absence of infection; they constantly wander throughout the connective tissue, killing bacteria before they have a chance to grow and multiply. Adding to its phagocytic bag of tricks, the neutrophil, when prompted to phagocytose, secretes and surrounds itself in a cloud of bactericidal chemicals. The neutrophil thus feasts away in a phagocytic-friendly chemical killing zone.

The second group of phagocytes consists of the agranulocytic monocytes. Some monocytes circulate within the blood; they are described as free and motile. Other monocytes leave the blood, develop into macrophages, and become fixed in lymphatic tissue throughout the body. Macrophages that become fixed in specific organs are stationary or nonmotile. They can, however, divide and produce new macrophages in their fixed sites. The macrophages that become fixed in a particular organ often take on a variety of names. For instance, the Kupffer cells in the liver are fixed to the walls of the large capillaries called *sinusoids*. As blood flows through the sinusoids, pathogens and other foreign substances are removed from the blood and phagocytosed. The liver, spleen, lungs, and lymph nodes have a particularly rich supply of phagocytes. Some fixed macrophages in the lungs are called "dust cells" because they phagocytose inhaled solid particles in the air…better known as *dust*. Thus, the macrophages function as phagocytes—"big eaters," as their name implies. The macrophages play another important defensive role. They assist the lymphocytes as antigen-presenting cells in mounting an immune response (described later in the chapter).

Asking Directions: How Phagocytes "Find" the Site of Infection. As they travel through the blood to the site of infection, the neutrophils and monocytes can squeeze through the tiny gaps between the endothelial cells of the capillary walls and enter the tissue spaces at the site of infection. The process of squeezing through the tiny gaps is called *diapedesis* (dye-ah-peh-DEE-sis). How do the neutrophils and monocytes know where to go? Chemicals released by injured cells attract them to the injured site. The signaling is called *chemotaxis* (kee-moh-TAK-sis). This process is similar to a bloodhound tracking a scent; the hound picks up the signal (odor), which identifies its source.

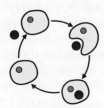

What Does a Phagocyte Do? What exactly does the phagocyte do? A phagocyte engulfs, or eats, particles or pathogens, much like an ameba does. The phagocyte's plasma membrane sends out pseudopods ("false feet") that surround the pathogen. The surfaces of the pseudopods then fuse, thereby enclosing the pathogen within the phagocyte. The trapped pathogen encounters a lysosome; the lysosomal membrane fuses with the pathogen, releasing potent enzymes that destroy the pathogen. The process of phagocytosis can be summarized as "ingested (eaten) and digested."

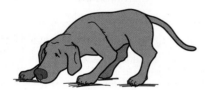

? Re-Think

1. List two important phagocytes.
2. Describe how phagocytosis occurs.
3. What point is the bloodhound making about white blood cells?
4. Define *diapedesis* and *chemotaxis*.

Inflammation

Inflammation refers to the responses the body makes when confronted by an irritant. The irritant can be almost anything; common irritants include pathogens, friction, excessive heat or cold, radiation, injuries, and chemicals. If the irritant is caused by a pathogen, the inflammation is called an *infection*.

Inflammation is characterized by redness, heat, swelling, and pain (see Fig. 21.1). What are the causes of these symptoms? When the tissues are injured or irritated, injured cells release histamine and other chemicals. These chemicals cause the blood vessels in the injured tissue to dilate. The dilated blood vessels bring more blood to the area; the increased blood flow causes redness and heat. The histamine causes the blood vessel walls to leak fluid and dissolved substances into the tissue spaces, causing swelling. Fluid and irritating chemicals accumulating at the injured site also stimulate pain receptors; therefore, the person experiences pain. Redness, heat, swelling, and pain are the classic signs of inflammation.

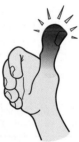

🦉 Do You Know…

How and Why the Body "Walls Off the Pus"?

When an area becomes infected, the cells involved in the inflammatory response do two things. First, they kill the pathogens. As the war continues, dead cells (including phagocytes, injured cells, and pathogens) and secretions accumulate in the area as pus. Second, the cells build a wall of tissue around the infected debris. This walled-off area is an abscess. An abscess performs a beneficial role in that it restricts the spread of the infection throughout the body. A large abscess may require a surgical procedure in which the abscess is lanced and drained.

? Re-Think

1. Differentiate between infection and inflammation.
2. List the four signs of inflammation, and explain the physiological basis of each.
3. What makes up pus?
4. What is the purpose of abscess formation?

Fever

Fever, also known as *pyrexia* (pye-REK-see-ah), is an abnormal elevation in body temperature. As phagocytes perform their duty, they release fever-producing substances called **pyrogens** (from the Latin word for "fire"). The pyrogens stimulate the hypothalamus in the brain to reset the body's temperature, producing a fever. The elevation in temperature is thought to be beneficial in two ways: a fever stimulates phagocytosis and decreases the ability of certain pathogens to multiply.

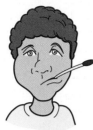

What happens physiologically when the hypothalamus resets the body temperature? First, the person shivers in an attempt to generate heat; the heat is conserved as the blood vessels of the skin constrict. The person may have chills and feel cold and clammy, even though the body temperature is rising. The elevated temperature hovers around the new set point while the pathogen is active, but when the infection is contained and the secretion of pyrogens diminishes, the hypothalamus resets its thermostat back to normal. Heat-losing mechanisms are activated; the blood vessels of the skin dilate, and the person sweats.

Evidence suggests that the reduction of fever prolongs an infection. Note, however, that a very high fever must be reduced because high body temperature may cause severe and irreversible brain damage. High fever, especially in children, is frequently accompanied by seizures. Seizures resulting from an elevated body temperature are called *febrile (fever) seizures*.

Protective Proteins

Two groups of protective proteins, the interferons and complement proteins, act nonspecifically to protect the body (see Fig. 21.1). **Interferons** (in-ter-FEER-ons) are a group of proteins secreted by cells infected by a virus. The interferons diffuse to surrounding cells where they prevent viral replication, thereby protecting neighboring cells. Researchers first found interferons in cells infected by the influenza virus and named them accordingly because they interfered with viral replication. Interferons also activate NK cells and macrophages, thus boosting the immune system.

A second group of proteins that protect the body is the complement proteins. **Complement proteins** circulate in the blood in their inactive form. When the complement proteins are activated against a bacterium, they swarm over it. The complement attaches to the bacterium's outer membrane and punches holes in it. The holes in the membrane allow fluid and electrolytes to flow into the bacterium, causing it to burst and die. The activated complement proteins perform other functions that enhance phagocytosis and the inflammatory response.

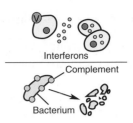

Interferons

Complement

Bacterium

Natural Killer Cells

NK cells are a small population of a special type of lymphocyte that acts nonspecifically to kill a variety of cells. NK cells are effective against many microbes and certain cancer cells. NK cells cooperate with the specific defense mechanisms to mount the most effective defense possible.

 Re-Think

1. Explain how a pathogen causes a fever.
2. Explain why pyrexia, but not hyperthermia, is considered the second line of defense. (Refer back to Chapter 7, if needed.)
3. What is a febrile seizure?
4. Explain how the interferons and complement proteins participate in the destruction of pathogens and fight infection.

 Sum It Up!

Fig. 21.2 summarizes the functions of the nonspecific defense mechanisms in defense against pathogens, pollens, and cancer. The wall of the fortress is the first line of defense; it includes mechanical barriers, chemical barriers, and reflexes. Behind the wall of the fortress is the second line of defense: phagocytosis, inflammation, fever, protective proteins, and NK cells. The third line of defense includes lymphocytes that are concerned with specific immunity, the topic of the next section.

SPECIFIC IMMUNITY: THIRD LINE OF DEFENSE

Specific immunity is also called **adaptive immunity** because the immune cells are able to respond or adapt to newly encountered pathogens or foreign agents. There are two characteristics that distinguish specific immunity from nonspecific immunity: specificity and memory.

- *Specificity.* As stated earlier, with nonspecific immunity, the body need not recognize the specific foreign agent. Specific immunity homes in on a foreign substance, such as the measles virus or ragweed pollen, and provides protection against one specific substance but not others.
- *Memory.* Memory refers to the ability to respond faster and more robustly to re-exposure to the same pathogen or foreign agent.

The cells that play key roles in specific immunity are the lymphocytes (B lymphocytes and T lymphocytes) and the macrophages. Understanding the

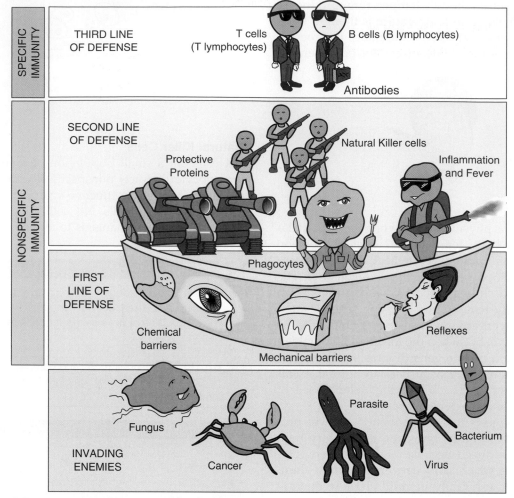

FIG. 21.2 The immune system wages its battle with three lines of defense. (Read from bottom to top.)

function of lymphocytes requires an understanding of antigens.

ANTIGENS

An **antigen** is a substance that stimulates the formation of antibodies. In fact, the word *antigen* is made up of words that refer to *anti*body *gen*erating. Antigens are generally large molecules; most are proteins, but a few are polysaccharides and lipids. Antigens are found on the surface of many substances, such as pathogens, red blood cells, pollens, foods, toxins, and cancer cells. Foreign substances that display antigens are described as antigenic. Antigenic substances are attacked by macrophages and lymphocytes.

SELF AND NONSELF: IS THAT ME?

Before birth, your lymphocytes somehow get to know who belongs and who does not. In effect, your lymphocytes learn to recognize "you" (self) and take steps to eliminate "not you" (nonself, or foreign agent). Your body perceives your own cells and secretions as non-antigenic and other cells as antigenic. The antigenic cells are subsequently eliminated. Recognition of self is called **immunotolerance**. Sometimes, a person's

immune system fails to identify self and mounts an immune attack against its own cells. This attack is the basis of **autoimmune** diseases, such as rheumatoid arthritis.

 Re-Think

1. Why is specific immunity referred to as adaptive immunity?
2. What is the origin of the word *antigen*?
3. Define *immunotolerance*.
4. What is a consequence of the failure of the immune system to "recognize self"?

LYMPHOCYTES

The two types of lymphocytes are **T lymphocytes (T cells)** and **B lymphocytes (B cells)**. Although both come from the stem cells in the bone marrow, they differ in their development and functions (Table 21.1).

Why the Names "T" and "B" Cells?

During fetal development, stem cells in bone marrow produce lymphocytes. The blood carries lymphocytes throughout the body. About half of the lymphocytes travel to the thymus gland, where they mature and

T Cell Activation

Step 1   Origin, maturation, seeding

Step 2   Antigen presentation

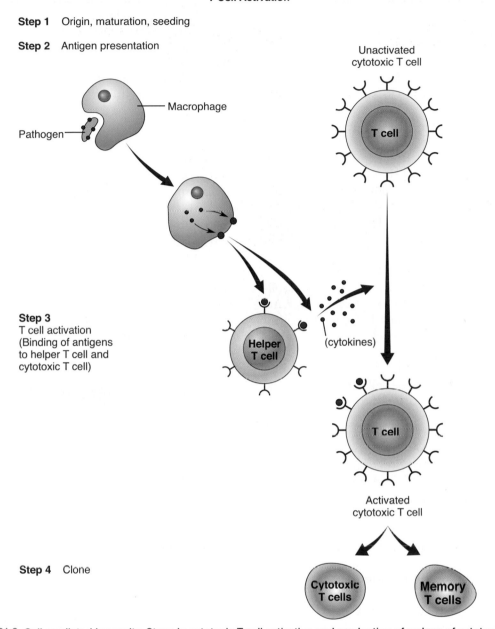

Step 3
T cell activation
(Binding of antigens
to helper T cell and
cytotoxic T cell)

Step 4   Clone

FIG. 21.3 Cell-mediated immunity. Steps in cytotoxic T-cell activation and production of a clone of cytotoxic T cells and memory T cells.

differentiate into T cells (the "T" is for *t*hymus-derived lymphocytes). Eventually, the blood carries T cells away from the thymus gland to various lymphatic tissues, particularly the lymph nodes, liver, and spleen. T cells live, work, and reproduce in the lymphatic tissue as well as circulate in the blood, making up 70% to 80% of the blood's lymphocytes.

What about the B lymphocytes? B cells differentiate in the fetal liver and bone marrow (the "B" is for *b*one. Like the T cells, the B cells take up residence in lymphatic tissue, chiefly the lymph nodes. B cells make up 20% to 30% of the circulating lymphocytes.

Both T cells and B cells attack antigens, but they do so in different ways. T cells attack antigens directly, through cell-to-cell contact. This immune response is called **cell-mediated immunity (CMI)**. B cells, on the other hand, interact with the antigen indirectly, through the secretion of antibodies. This response is called **antibody-mediated immunity (AMI)**. Because the antibodies are carried by the blood and other tissue fluid (the body "humors"), this type of immunity is also called *humoral immunity*.

T-Cell Activation and Cell-Mediated Immunity

T cells are effective against many pathogens, tumor cells, and foreign tissue such as organ transplants. Refer to Fig. 21.3 as you read about the following steps in CMI:

- Step 1. T cells originate in the red bone marrow and migrate to the thymus gland, where they mature;

they then seed other lymphatic tissue, where they eventually encounter an antigen.

- Step 2—antigen presentation. The antigen, on the surface of the pathogen, is phagocytosed by a **macrophage**. The macrophage digests the pathogen and pushes the antigen to its surface. The macrophage's ability to push the antigen to its surface is called **antigen presentation**.
- Step 3—T- cell activation. The antigen binds to the receptor sites on both the helper T cells and the inactivated cytotoxic T cell. The helper T cell then secretes cytokines, chemicals that activate cytotoxic T cells. Activated cytotoxic T cells bind to pathogens and destroy them.
- Step 4—production of a clone. The activated T cells divide repeatedly, creating clones of cytotoxic T cells and memory T cells. (A **clone** is a group of identical cells formed from the same parent cell.)

The cytotoxic T cells are killer cells, engaging in cell-to-cell combat. They destroy the pathogen through the use of two mechanisms, punching holes in the pathogen's cell membrane and secreting substances called *cytokines,* which enhance phagocytic activity. The memory T cells do not participate in the destruction of the pathogen (antigen). These cells "remember" the initial encounter with the antigen. If the antigen is presented at some future time, the memory cells quickly reproduce and thus allow a faster immune response to occur.

We have described the function of three T cells (cytotoxic T cells, helper T cells, and memory T cells). A fourth T cell, called a *suppressor T cell,* inhibits or dampens the immune response when the antigen has been destroyed. (The origin and development of the helper T cell and suppressor T cell are not shown in Fig. 21.3.)

B-Cell Activation and Antibody-Mediated Immunity

B cells engage in AMI. Activated B cells produce antibody-secreting plasma cells. The antibodies are carried by the blood and body fluids to the antigen-bearing pathogens (antigens) that usually reside in the plasma or other extracellular fluid. B cells can produce over 10 million different antibodies; each B cell interacts with a specific antigen and produces its own antibody. The large numbers of antibodies allow the body to develop immunity against many different diseases. Follow Fig. 21.4 as you read about the following steps in AMI:

- Step 1. The B cell originates and matures in the red bone marrow; it then seeds other lymphatic tissue where it eventually encounters an antigen.
- Step 2—antigen presentation. A macrophage engulfs and processes an antigen. The antigen is pushed to the surface of the macrophage.
- Step 3—B-cell and helper T-cell activation. The presented antigens bind to the B cell and helper T cell. Cytokines from the activated helper T cells participate in B-cell activation.

- Step 4—production of a clone. The B cells reproduce, creating clones of plasma cells and memory B cells. Plasma cells secrete large quantities of antibodies that travel through the blood to the foreign antigens (pathogens). The memory B cells do not participate in the attack; they remember the specific antigen during future encounters and allow a quicker response to the invading pathogen (antigen).

Note that B- and T-cell activation depends on helper T-cell activity. HIV attacks the helper T cells, thereby producing severe impairment of both B- and T-cell function. HIV infection may progress to a syndrome called *acquired immunodeficiency syndrome* (AIDS). Because of the widespread impairment of their immune system, persons with HIV infection and AIDS experience numerous and serious bouts of infection.

Another name for the helper T cell. The helper T cell is also called the *CD4$^+$ T cell* (because of a surface protein called CD4). The CD4$^+$ T cell is a marker for immune function, and the progression of HIV infection is monitored by the CD4$^+$ T-cell count. The CD4$^+$ T cell count decreases as the infection progresses.

 Re-Think

1. List two lymphocytes that engage in specific immunity.
2. Describe the activation of the cytotoxic T cell.
3. Describe the activation of the B cell.
4. Explain why helper T cells are crucial for both T-cell and B-cell function.

ANTIBODIES

What Antibodies Are

The **antibodies** secreted by the B cells are proteins called **immunoglobulins** and constitute the gamma globulin fraction of plasma proteins. There are five major types of immunoglobulins:

- Immunoglobulin G (IgG) is an antibody found in plasma and tissue fluids. It is particularly effective against certain bacteria, viruses, and toxins.
- Immunoglobulin A (IgA) is an antibody found primarily in the secretions of exocrine glands. IgA in milk, tears, and gastric juice helps protect against infection. Breast milk contains IgA antibodies and helps the infant ward off infection.
- Immunoglobulin M (IgM) is an antibody found in blood plasma. The anti-A and anti-B antibodies associated with red blood cells are a type of IgM antibody.
- Immunoglobulin D (IgD) is an antibody found on the surface of B cells and participates in the activation of B cells.
- Immunoglobulin E (IgE) is an antibody that appears in the exocrine secretions such as breast milk, tears, gastrointestinal secretions, and urine. The IgE antibody participates in allergic reactions and is described further later in the chapter.

B-Cell Activation

Step 1   Origin, maturation, seeding

Step 2   Antigen presentation

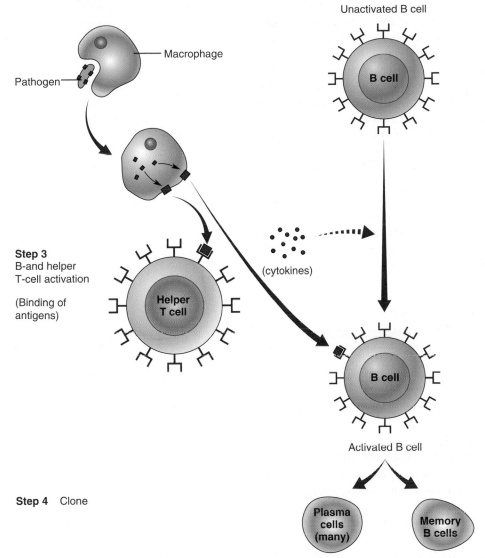

Step 3
B-and helper
T-cell activation

(Binding of
antigens)

Step 4   Clone

FIG. 21.4 **Antibody-mediated immunity. Steps in B-cell activation and production of a clone of antibody-secreting plasma cells and memory B cells.**

What Antibodies Do

Antibodies destroy antigens. They accomplish this task directly by attacking the antigen and indirectly by activating complement proteins that in turn facilitate the attack on the antigens.

When antibodies react with antigens directly, the antibodies bind to antigens in a process called an *antigen–antibody reaction*. By engaging in an antigen–antibody reaction, the antigen–antibody components clump together, or agglutinate (ah-GLOO-tin-ate). Agglutination makes it easier for the phagocytic cells to destroy the antigen. Under normal conditions, direct attack by the antibodies is not very helpful in protecting the body against invasion by pathogens.

A more effective way for antibodies to attack an antigen is through activation of the complement proteins.

These activated complement proteins cause a variety of effects: they stimulate chemotaxis (attract more phagocytes), promote agglutination, make pathogens more susceptible to phagocytosis, and encourage lysis, or rupture of the pathogen's cell membrane. Direct and indirect attacks by antibodies provide an effective defense against foreign agents.

Remember Me? Primary and Secondary Responses

When exposed to an antigen, B cells are activated and produce many antibody-secreting plasma cells and memory cells. Note the primary and secondary responses in Fig. 21.5. The primary response is due to the initial exposure to the antigen; it develops slowly and produces a small number of antibodies. Note what happens to antibody production with a second exposure to the antigen. The immune system responds quickly and produces a large number of antibodies. This second challenge is called the *secondary response.*

Why is the secondary response so much greater? The initial exposure to the antigen has stimulated the formation of antibody-secreting plasma cells and memory cells. The memory cells, which live for a long time in the plasma, are activated very quickly on the second exposure. The activated memory cells, in turn, induce the formation of many antibody-secreting plasma cells.

What does the secondary response mean for you? It means that you won't get the disease a second time; you are immune to that disease. For example, if you had measles as a child, you developed measles antibodies and many memory cells. If you are then exposed to the measles virus later in life, the memory cells "remember" the first exposure and produce antibody-secreting plasma cells very quickly. The measles antibodies, in turn, attack the measles virus and prevent you from becoming ill.

The level of antibodies in your blood is called an *antibody titer.* If you have had measles, for example, your measles antibody titer is higher than the titer of someone who has never had measles.

 Re-Think

1. List the five immunoglobulins.
2. Define *agglutination*, and explain how it facilitates phagocytosis and cell death.
3. List two differences between the primary and secondary responses.

◎ Sum It Up!

Specific immunity or adaptive immunity forms the third line of defense of the immune response. It allows the immune system to recognize and destroy specific substances called *antigens.* The B and T lymphocytes and the macrophages are the most important cells associated with specific immunity. T cells engage in cell-to-cell combat (CMI—cell-mediated immunity), whereas B cells fight indirectly through the mediation of antibodies (AMI—antibody-mediated immunity). Macrophages engage in both phagocytosis and antigen presentation, a process necessary for B and T cell activation. Antibodies are called *immunoglobulins* (IgG, IgA, IgM, IgD, and IgE); they engage antigens causing agglutination. Agglutination, in turn, facilitates phagocytosis and results in the death of the pathogen. The primary and secondary responses refer to the secretion of antibodies by plasma cells and memory cells in response to antigen stimulation.

TYPES OF IMMUNITY

The two main categories of immunity are genetic immunity and acquired immunity (Fig. 21.6).

GENETIC IMMUNITY

Do you ever wonder why you have never gotten heartworms from your dog or why your dog did not pick

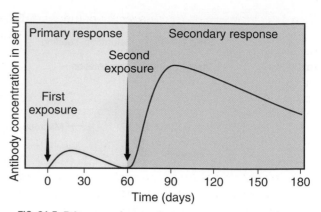

FIG. 21.5 Primary and secondary responses to an antigen.

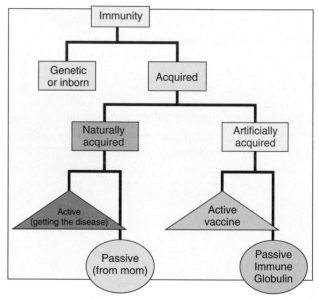

FIG. 21.6 Types of immunity.

up chickenpox from you? As a human, you have inherited immunity to certain diseases such as canine heartworm; you are immunologically protected from your pet. Similarly, your dog will never contract chickenpox; Rover is immunologically protected from you. Another comforting thought is that neither you nor your dog is in danger of contracting Dutch elm disease from your tree. Each of you was born with genetic information that provides immunity to certain diseases. Genetic immunity is also called *inborn, innate,* or *species immunity.* As you can see, your species protects you from many diseases that afflict other species.

ACQUIRED IMMUNITY

Unlike genetic immunity, acquired immunity is received during a person's lifetime. Acquired immunity comes either naturally or artificially.

NATURALLY ACQUIRED IMMUNITY

You can acquire immunity naturally in two ways. The first is by getting the disease. As a child, you probably had one of the childhood diseases such as chickenpox.

Your body responded to the specific pathogen by developing antibodies. After that first exposure, you never became ill with chickenpox again because your immune system had a ready supply of antibodies and memory cells with which to respond quickly to the second invasion of the chickenpox virus. Because your own body produced the antibodies, this type of **naturally acquired immunity** is called **active immunity**. Active immunity is generally long-lasting.

The second way to acquire immunity naturally is by receiving antibodies from your mother. Some antibodies (IgG) crossed the placenta from your mother into you as a fetus. Your mother developed these antibodies in response to the pathogens that she encountered throughout her lifetime. Because your immune system did not produce these antibodies (you received them as a gift from your mother), this type of immunity is called **passive immunity**. Antibodies can also be transferred passively from mother to infant through breast milk. Breast milk contains IgA antibodies.

Unlike active immunity, which often lasts a lifetime, passive immunity is short-lived. The antibodies that are acquired passively are broken down and eliminated from the baby's body. The mother's antibodies afford protection to the infant for about the first 6 months after birth. Breast-feeding may extend the length of immunoprotection.

ARTIFICIALLY ACQUIRED IMMUNITY

You can also acquire immunity artificially in two ways. The first is by a vaccine; the second is by injection of immune globulin. Both provide **artificially acquired immunity**.

A **vaccine** is an antigen-bearing substance, such as a pathogen, injected into a person in an attempt to stimulate antibody production. For example, the measles virus is first killed or weakened or attenuated (ay-TEN-yoo-ayt-ed). The attenuated virus cannot cause the disease (measles) when injected into the person, but it can still act as an antigen and stimulate the person's immune system to produce antibodies. The use of a dead or attenuated pathogen to stimulate antibody production is called **vaccination**, or **immunization**. The solution of dead or attenuated pathogens is the vaccine. Because the use of a vaccine stimulates the body to produce its own antibodies, vaccines induce active immunity.

A vaccine can also be made from the toxin secreted by the pathogen. The toxin is altered to reduce its harmfulness, but it can still act as an antigen to induce immunity. The altered toxin is called a *toxoid*. Because a toxoid stimulates the production of antibodies, it causes active immunity.

The purpose of vaccination is to provide an initial exposure and stimulate the formation of memory cells (the primary response). The purpose of a booster shot is to stimulate the secondary response by administering another dose of the vaccine (antigen).

Vaccines have almost eradicated certain diseases. For example, infants routinely receive a series of DTP injections. DTP injections stimulate active immunity for *d*iphtheria (diphtheria toxoid), *t*etanus (tetanus toxoid), and *p*ertussis, or whooping cough (pertussis vaccine). The MMR vaccine (*m*easles-rubeola, *m*umps, and *r*ubella) is also used preventively during early childhood.

Immune globulin differs from a vaccine. Immune globulin is obtained from a donor (human or animal) and contains antibodies (immune globulins). The antibodies are formed in the donor in response to a specific antigen. These preformed antibodies are taken from the donor and injected into a recipient, thereby conveying passive immunity.

 Do You Know...

Why Joey Is Mooing?

Here's the story. Vaccination against smallpox was originally accomplished by injecting the cowpox virus, a cousin to the smallpox virus. Although Edward Jenner (circa 1850) had demonstrated some success with vaccination, many doctors opposed the procedure. His fellow doctors therefore spread a nasty rumor designed to scare the peasant population. The rumor claimed that the injection of the cowpox virus makes the child take on the characteristics of a cow…Mooooo! Pictures were widely distributed of Joey mooing, swatting flies with his tail, and clanging a cowbell hung around his neck.

Fortunately, the peasants weren't duped because they knew that milkmaids rarely came down with smallpox. Most attributed the immunity of the milkmaids to the cowpox lesions that developed when the milkmaid milked the cows infected with the cowpox virus. (Holy cow—this sounds like bull!) Just remember, the Latin word for *cow* is *vacca*, the root word for *vaccination*.

Why might you receive an injection of immune globulin? Assume for the moment that you are not immune to hepatitis B and so do not have antibodies against the hepatitis B virus. You are then exposed to the virus. Because you have no immunity to the virus, you may receive immune globulin (antibodies) in an attempt to provide immediate protection against the virus. Because this is a form of passive immunity, the immunity is short-lived. Immune globulins are available for rubella (German measles), hepatitis A and B, rabies, and tetanus. A comparison of the different types of acquired immunity appears in Table 21.2.

Other forms of passive immunity are commonly used to prevent the disease or the development of severe symptoms of the disease. Antitoxins contain antibodies that neutralize the toxins secreted by the pathogens but have no effect on the pathogens themselves. Examples of antitoxins include tetanus antitoxin (TAT) and the antitoxins for diphtheria and botulism. Antivenoms contain antibodies that combat the effects of the poisonous venom of snakes.

Table 21.2   Types of Acquired Immunity

TYPE	STIMULUS	RESULT
Naturally Acquired		
Active immunity	Exposed to live pathogens (e.g., get the disease)	Long-term immunity; makes antibodies
Passive immunity	Antibodies are passed from mother to infant (across placenta and/or by breast-feeding)	Short-term immunity (lasts approximately for the first 6 months and for duration of breast-feeding); does not stimulate the production of antibodies
Artificially Acquired		
Active immunity	Vaccination	Long-term immunity; makes antibodies
Passive immunity	Injection with gamma globulin (antibodies)	Short-term immunity; does not stimulate the production of antibodies

Do You Know...

Why the Ancient "Charmers" Ate Snake Venom?

Long ago, Indian snake charmers squeezed the venom from their cobras and drank it. Why? They realized that by eating the venom, they developed resistance to the bite of the family pet. This practice was observed by a number of physicians, and the concept eventually evolved into our modern-day immunology.

Re-Think

1. Differentiate between active and passive immunity. Give an example of each.
2. Differentiate between naturally and artificially acquired immunity. Give an example of each.
3. What is a vaccine? Why is it necessary to attenuate the pathogen used in a vaccine?

OTHER IMMUNE RESPONSES

Normally the immune system protects the body from nonself; foreign agents are recognized and eliminated. Sometimes, however, the immune system goes awry: it attacks the self, causing autoimmune disease, or it overreacts, causing allergies.

ALLERGIC REACTIONS

The immune system sometimes forms antibodies to substances not usually recognized as foreign. This response forms the basis of allergic reactions. The two common allergic reactions are the delayed-reaction allergy and the immediate-reaction allergy.

The *delayed-reaction allergy* is so named because it usually takes about 48 hours to occur; its onset is delayed. This type of allergic response can occur in anyone. It usually results from the repeated exposure of the skin to chemicals such as household detergents. Repeated exposure to the chemical activates T cells, which eventually accumulate in the skin. Local tissue response to T-cell activity causes skin eruptions and other signs of inflammation. This skin response is called *contact dermatitis*. Other forms of contact dermatitis are associated with poison ivy, poison oak, certain cosmetics, and soaps.

The *immediate-reaction allergy*, as its name implies, occurs rapidly in response to its stimulus. It is more commonly called *immediate hypersensitivity reaction* and involves immunoglobulin E, the IgE antibodies. **Allergens** are antigens capable of inducing allergy. Allergens that are apt to be involved in this acute type of allergic response include insect venom, drugs such as penicillin, and foods such as peanuts. The following steps are involved in the development of an immediate hypersensitivity reaction (Fig. 21.7):

- Step 1. An allergen (red dot) activates a B cell.
- Step 2. The activated B cell forms a clone of antibody-secreting plasma cells and memory B cells.
- Step 3. The plasma cells secrete large amounts of IgE antibodies against the specific allergen.
- Step 4. The IgE antibodies bind to the mast cells in body tissues.
- Step 5. More of the allergen invades the body. The allergen binds with the IgE antibodies on the mast cells. The mast cells release large amounts of histamine, leukotrienes, and other chemicals that cause systemic effects, especially issues regarding blood pressure and impaired breathing.

The systemic effects can be severe; they include a massive vasodilation, which causes a sharp drop in blood pressure and severe constriction of the respiratory passages (bronchoconstriction), making breathing extremely difficult and, in some cases, impossible. This severe form of the immediate hypersensitivity reaction is called *anaphylaxis* or *anaphylactic shock*. Persons allergic to penicillin are at particular risk for anaphylaxis. As a result, always ask a person about allergies to medications before administering any type of drug, particularly antibiotics. (Some persons are even allergic to aspirin.) The immediate administration of a drug such as epinephrine (adrenalin) is particularly effective because it "opens up" breathing passages and elevates blood pressure. Most persons who are prone to anaphylactic responses carry a source of injectable epinephrine.

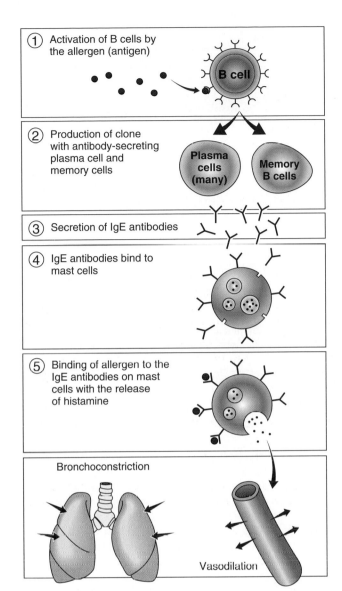

1. Activation of B cells by the allergen (antigen)

B cell

2. Production of clone with antibody-secreting plasma cell and memory cells

Plasma cells (many) Memory B cells

3. Secretion of IgE antibodies

4. IgE antibodies bind to mast cells

5. Binding of allergen to the IgE antibodies on mast cells with the release of histamine

Bronchoconstriction

Vasodilation

FIG. 21.7 Immediate hypersensitivity reaction.

Re-Think

1. What is the stimulus for the secretion of IgE antibodies?
2. What is the stimulus for the release of histamine and leukotrienes?
3. What are the effects of histamine on blood pressure and breathing?
4. Explain how epinephrine relieves anaphylaxis.

Do You Know...
About Rejection? It Can Go Either Way!

When dealing with transplant patients, we watch closely for signs of organ rejection by the host (recipient). The recipient's immune system recognizes the donated organ such as a kidney as foreign and mounts an immune attack against it. When the immune attack is successful, the organ is destroyed and is said to be rejected. Following organ transplant, the recipient usually receives drugs that suppress the immune system thereby preserving the donated organ. However, some patients experience the opposite effect—the transplanted organ (or blood) rejects the host. This response is called *graft-versus-host disease* (GVHD); GVHD usually occurs in immunodeficient patients and is caused in part by transplanted T cells. The target organs for rejection are the skin, digestive tract, and liver. The biggest clinical problem is a variety of infections that gradually overwhelm the granulocytopenic patient. So the transplant recipient faces two huge clinical challenges: his body can reject the donated organ, or the donated organ can reject the recipient.

Sum It Up!

Immunity is classified as genetic or acquired. Immunity may be acquired naturally or artificially. Immunity is also classified as active or passive. If a person makes antibodies in his or her own body, the immunity is active. If the person merely receives antibodies that were made by another person or animal, the immunity is passive. Active immunity is generally long-lasting, whereas passive immunity is short-lasting. Although the immune system normally works to protect the body, it can go awry, causing allergic reactions and autoimmune disease. Anaphylaxis is a serious IgE hypersensitivity reaction that is life threatening.

As You Age

1. T cell and B cell function are somewhat deficient in older adults. Depressed lymphocyte function is accompanied by a decrease in macrophage activity. Consequently, older adults are more prone to develop infections, and they recover more slowly. Depressed lymphocyte function might also explain the higher incidence of cancer in older adults.
2. Older adults often have a reduced fever response to infection and may therefore have difficulty in combating infection.
3. Older adults have increased levels of circulating autoantibodies (antibodies directed against self). This increase explains, in part, why they are more prone to the development of autoimmune disease.
4. Older adults often take drugs or undergo treatment that depresses the immune system. For example, the use of steroids in the treatment of arthritis and the use of drugs and radiation in the treatment of cancer all cause immunosuppression.

Medical Terminology and Disorders   Disorders of the Immune System

MEDICAL TERM	WORD PARTS	WORD PART MEANING OR DERIVATION	DESCRIPTION
Words			
anaphylaxis	ana-	up	**Anaphylaxis** is *a life-threatening hypersensitivity reaction mediated by IgE antibodies.*
	-phylaxis	From a Greek word meaning "watching or guarding"	
immune	immune/o-	From a Latin word meaning "exempt from"	To be **immune** is *to be exempt or protected from a particular disease.*
lymphocyte	lymph/o-	lymph	A **lymphocyte** is *a nongranular white blood cell.* There are T lymphocytes (T cells) and B lymphocytes (B cells).
	-cyte	cell	
macrophage	macro-	large	A **macrophage** (fixed or wandering) is *a type of white blood cell that digests foreign materials, including pathogens.*
	-phage	eat	
wheal and flare reaction			A **wheal and flare reaction** is *a skin reaction to an allergen or antigen.* The response is a circular (wheal) blanched area surrounded by an area of redness.
Disorders			
hypersensitivity reactions			A **hypersensitivity reaction** is *the immune system response to a foreign substance, or what is perceived as "foreign" in the case of autoimmune disease. Hypersensitivity reactions include allergies and autoimmune diseases.*
allergies			An **allergy** occurs when the immune system reacts to a foreign substance. Allergies are described in many ways: atopic, bacterial, contact, cold, drug, immediate, delayed, etc. The symptoms vary in intensity from mild to life threatening. An **atopic allergy** is genetic and refers to the development of a hypersensitivity reaction to an environmental allergen (e.g., pollen, bee venom, dander, food, environmental chemicals). Atopic reactions generally include eczema (atopic dermatitis), allergic rhinitis (hay fever), allergic conjunctivitis, or allergic asthma. A **latex allergy** is an allergic reaction to proteins found in natural rubber latex. Latex is found in many articles, such as shoes, balloons, condoms, medical equipment, drugs, paints, and adhesives, and for some is considered a major occupational hazard. About 50% of persons with latex allergy have allergic reactions to certain foods: avocado, banana, plum, strawberry, and tomato. **Anaphylaxis** is a severe and life-threatening hypersensitivity reaction, mediated by IgE antibodies.
autoimmune diseases	auto-	self	**Autoimmune system disorders** occur when a person's immune system produces antibodies against its own cells; the immune system no longer recognizes self from nonself. There are many **autoimmune diseases,** including rheumatoid arthritis, Hashimoto thyroiditis, diabetes mellitus (type 1), and rheumatic fever. **Rheumatic fever** is an immune disorder in which the antibodies produced in response to a streptococcal infection attack the heart muscle and its valves. Many of the autoimmune diseases are described in other chapters.
	-immun/o-	immunity	

Medical Terminology and Disorders   Disorders of the Immune System—cont'd

MEDICAL TERM	WORD PARTS	WORD PART MEANING OR DERIVATION	DESCRIPTION
Disorders			
immunodeficiency disorders	immun/o- -deficiency		*Disorders caused by an impaired immune response.* Immunodeficiency disorders are classified as primary or secondary. **Primary immunodeficiency disorders** are rare, an example being **severe combined immunodeficiency disease (SCID). Secondary immunodeficiency disorders** are common, the most common cause being a drug-induced immune deficiency such as the granulocytopenia resulting from cancer chemotherapy. Other causes include radiation therapy, steroid therapy, stress, malignancies, aging, and many diseases, especially infection with the human immunodeficiency virus (HIV). **HIV infection** is usually transmitted sexually. Because it is also transmitted through accidental or intended sharing of injection equipment, HIV is a serious threat to hospital workers and others who routinely handle blood or blood-related products or equipment. Initial infection with HIV causes **viremia** (virus in the blood), which persists for many years and which targets the immune system, particularly the CD4+ T cells (helper T cells). The late and severe manifestation of HIV infection is called **acquired immunodeficiency syndrome (AIDS).** At this stage all organ systems are adversely affected, and death is most often caused by infection.
scleroderma	scler/o- -derm/o	hard skin	*A chronic autoimmune disease characterized by a hardening of the skin or other organs.* The systemic form of the disease may be fatal because of heart, kidney, lung, and intestinal involvement. The limited form of the disease is called **CREST,** an acronym for the five main signs: *c*alcinosis, *R*aynaud's syndrome, *es*ophageal dysfunction, *s*clerodactyly (hardness of fingers or toes), *t*elangiectasia. CREST usually spares the lungs and kidneys.
systemic lupus erythematosus (SLE)		From the Latin word meaning "wolf" (lupus)	**SLE** is a chronic autoimmune disorder. Symptoms are due to inflammation and are highly variable, but all persons experience joint pain (especially fingers, hands, wrist, and knees). A "butterfly" rash over the bridge of the nose and patchy skin color are characteristic of SLE. Persons who experience only the skin symptoms have **discoid erythematosus.** A **drug-induced lupus erythematosus (DIL)** can develop in response to certain medications; symptoms gradually disappear when the medication is stopped.

Get Ready for Exams!

Summary Outline

The immune system is a defense system that protects the body from foreign agents such as pathogens, pollens, toxins, and cancer cells.

I. Nonspecific Immunity
A. Nonspecific immune mechanisms (innate immunity) protect the body against many different types of foreign agents and do not require recognition of the specific agent.
B. Lines of defense
   1. The first line of defense includes mechanical barriers, chemical barriers, and reflexes.
   2. The second line of defense includes phagocytosis, inflammation, fever, protective proteins, and natural killer (NK) cells.

II. Immunity
A. Specific immunity (adaptive) protects the body against specific foreign agents and requires recognition of the specific agent involved.
B. T cells, or T lymphocytes
   1. The T cells make up 70% to 80% of the blood's lymphocytes.
   2. T cells engage in cell-mediated immunity (CMI).
   3. Activated cytotoxic T cells produce a clone (cytotoxic T cells and memory T cells).
   4. Helper T cells secrete cytokines and are necessary for activation of the cytotoxic T cells.
C. B cells, or B lymphocytes
   1. B cells make up 20% to 30% of the blood's lymphocytes.
   2. B cells engage in antibody-mediated immunity (AMI).

3. Activated B cells produce a clone of (memory cells and plasma cells). The plasma cells secrete antibodies that travel through the blood to the antigens located primarily in extracellular fluids.
4. The antibodies are called immunoglobulins (IgG, IgA, IgM, IgD, and IgE).
5. Immunoglobulin E (IgE) presents a serious problem with regard to an acute allergic response.

III. Types of Immunity
A. Genetic or acquired immunity
1. With genetic immunity, a person is genetically immune to an antigen.
2. A person can acquire immunity naturally or artificially.
3. A person can acquire immunity naturally in two ways: by getting the disease or by receiving antibodies from the mother across the placenta and/or through breast milk.
4. Immunity can be acquired artificially in two ways: by the use of a vaccine or by injection of immune globulin made by another person or animal.
B. Active or passive immunity
1. Active immunity means that a person's body makes the antibodies (usually long-lasting).
2. Passive immunity means that the antibodies are made by another animal and then injected into a patient's body (usually short-lasting).

IV. Other Immune Responses
A. Allergic reactions
1. Allergic reactions are caused by the formation of antibodies to substances usually not recognized as foreign.
2. There are two types of allergic reactions: delayed-onset allergy and immediate-reaction allergy.
3. A delayed-onset allergy takes about 48 hours to develop. Contact dermatitis to a household chemical is a common example.
4. An immediate-reaction allergy (also called an immediate hypersensitivity reaction) is often caused by exposure to pollens and drugs such as penicillin. The most severe form is anaphylaxis.

Review Your Knowledge

Matching: Nonspecific Immunity
Directions: Match the following words with their descriptions. Some words may be used more than once.
a. protective proteins
b. phagocytosis
c. inflammation
d. fever
1. ___ Caused by pyrogens
2. ___ Eats debris and pathogens
3. ___ Redness, heat, swelling, and pain
4. ___ Neutrophils and monocytes
5. ___ Complement and interferons

Matching: Specific Immunity
Directions: Match the following words with their descriptions.
a. immunotolerance
b. cell-mediated immunity
c. antibody-mediated immunity
d. macrophage
e. plasma cells
1. ___ Subgroup of the B cell clone that secretes antibodies
2. ___ Recognition of self
3. ___ The cell responsible for antigen presentation
4. ___ Also called humoral immunity
5. ___ T cell immunity

Matching: Active and Passive Immunity
Directions: Indicate whether each of the following conveys active immunity (a) or passive immunity (b).
1. ___ Vaccine
2. ___ Antivenom
3. ___ Antitoxin
4. ___ Toxoid
5. ___ Gamma globulin
6. ___ Getting the disease

Multiple Choice
1. Complement and interferons are
   a. considered to be specific or adaptive immunity.
   b. protective proteins engaged in nonspecific immunity.
   c. secreted by B cells and T cells.
   d. vaccines, conveying active immunity.
2. T and B cells
   a. engage in nonspecific or innate immunity.
   b. are granulocytic neutrophils.
   c. both secrete immunoglobulins.
   d. are lymphocytes that are responsible for specific or adaptive immunity.
3. Which of the following is *not* related to cell-mediated immunity?
   a. Cell-to-cell combat
   b. Cytotoxic T cells
   c. Immunoglobulins
   d. Antigen presentation by a macrophage
4. Pyrexia, pyrogens, and febrile seizures are most related to which nonspecific form of immunity?
   a. Inflammation
   b. Fever
   c. Anaphylaxis
   d. Diapedesis, chemotaxis, and phagocytosis
5. Plasma cells
   a. are activated T cells.
   b. are the same as NK cells.
   c. secrete antibodies.
   d. secrete interferons and complement proteins.

6. With which of the following is anaphylaxis most associated?
   a. Interferons
   b. Phagocytosis
   c. IgE antibodies
   d. Contact dermatitis

7. What is the primary concern regarding the care of a person experiencing an anaphylactic reaction?
   a. Inability to breathe and hypotension
   b. Development of hives (urticaria) and intense itching (pruritus)
   c. Development of a high fever and febrile seizures
   d. Development of jaundice and itching

8. Which of the following is most characteristic of a vaccine?
   a. Artificially acquired active immunity
   b. Passive immunity and short-lived immunity
   c. Innate nonspecific immunity
   d. Administration of antibodies formed by another person or animal

9. Inflammation is
   a. a form of specific or adaptive immunity.
   b. characterized by redness, heat, swelling, and pain.
   c. known as cell-mediated immunity.
   d. synonymous with *infection.*

10. Specificity and memory are characteristic of
    a. interferons and complement proteins.
    b. B and T lymphocytes.
    c. innate or nonspecific immunity.
    d. myelocytic phagocytes.

11. Which words most accurately describe phagocytosis?
    a. Chemotaxis and diapedesis
    b. B cell and T cell activation
    c. Antigen presentation and agglutination
    d. Ingestion and digestion

12. Which of the following is true of the person who develops measles?
    a. She should receive the measles vaccine immediately.
    b. She should be started on a 7-day course of a broad-spectrum antibiotic.
    c. She will develop a naturally acquired active immunity.
    d. She will require a weekly a dose of gamma globulin to maintain her measles antibody titer.

13. Which of the following is characterized by redness, heat, swelling, and pain?
    a. Anaphylaxis
    b. Pyrexia
    c. Phagocytosis
    d. Inflammation

14. A deficiency of helper T cells
    a. causes anaphylaxis.
    b. affects B cell and T cell function.
    c. affects only cell-mediated immunity; antibody-mediated immunity is unaffected.
    d. affects only T cell activation.

15. Which of the following is descriptive of the protection offered by an intact skin and mucous membranes?
    a. Mechanical barriers
    b. Specific or adaptive immunity
    c. B cell and T cell activation
    d. Diapedesis and chemotaxis

Go Figure

1. Which of the following is correct according to Fig. 21.1?
   a. The second line of defense mechanisms is only activated in response to viral pathogens.
   b. The skin and mucous membrane are described as the second line of defense because they house interferons and complement proteins.
   c. Interferons and complement proteins are considered chemical barriers.
   d. Nonspecific immunity includes mechanical barriers, the inflammatory response, fever, and phagocytosis.

2. Which of the following is correct according to Fig. 21.2?
   a. The natural killer cell is a lymphocyte and is therefore considered a type of specific immunity.
   b. Phagocytosis, inflammation, and fever occur only in response to invasion by a pathogen.
   c. Interferons are lymphocytes.
   d. T and B cells are lymphocytes and are considered a form of specific immunity.

3. According to Fig. 21.3, the cytotoxic T cell is
   a. also called a plasma cell.
   b. engaged in dampening the immune response.
   c. the killer T cell that engages in cell-to-cell combat.
   d. antigen-presenting.

4. Which of the following is correct according to Fig. 21.3?
   a. Macrophages engage in antigen presentation.
   b. Cytotoxic T cell activation requires cytokines secreted by helper T cells.
   c. Activated cytotoxic T cells produce clones, including cytotoxic T cells and memory T cells.
   d. All of the above are true.

5. According to Fig. 21.4, the antibody-secreting cell is the
   a. antigen-secreting macrophage.
   b. plasma cell.
   c. helper T cell.
   d. cytotoxic T lymphocyte.

6. Which of the following is correct according to Fig. 21.4?
   a. Only T cells have memory cells in their clones.
   b. A deficiency of helper T cells, as in HIV infection, depresses B-cell activity.
   c. Activated B cells engage in cell-to-cell combat.
   d. Helper T cells secrete cytokines, which in turn suppress B cell activity.

7. According to Fig. 21.5, the surge in antibody production on the second exposure is primarily due to
   a. the killer activity of the cytotoxic T cells.
   b. phagocytosis.
   c. the rapid response of memory cells to the antigen.
   d. the activity of suppressor T cells.

8. Which of the following is correct according to Fig. 21.6?
   a. Active immunity can be acquired only through vaccination.
   b. "Getting the disease" is a form of artificially acquired active immunity.
   c. Naturally acquired passive immunity describes the immunity of a breast-fed infant.
   d. A vaccine conveys long-lasting passive immunity.

9. Which of the following is correct according to Fig. 21.7?
   a. The allergen (antigen) is phagocytized by the plasma cell.
   b. The antibodies activate the B lymphocyte.
   c. The plasma cell merges with the mast cell, thereby releasing histamine.
   d. Antigens bind to antibodies on the mast cells, thereby releasing histamine.

Respiratory System

Objectives

1. Describe the structure and functions of the organs of the respiratory system, and trace the movement of air from the nostrils to the alveoli.
2. Describe why lungs collapse or expand and the role of pulmonary surfactants.
3. Discuss the three steps in respiration, including the following:
   - Describe the relationship of Boyle's law to ventilation.
   - Explain how respiratory muscles affect thoracic volume.

- List three conditions that make the alveoli well suited for the exchange of oxygen and carbon dioxide.
4. List lung volumes and capacities.
5. Discuss the voluntary and involuntary control of breathing, including the following:
   - Explain the neural and chemical control of breathing.
   - Describe common variations and abnormalities of breathing.

Key Terms

alveolus (p. 410)
Boyle's law (p. 415)
bronchial tree (p. 408)
bronchioles (p. 410)
bronchus (p. 408)
compliance (p. 414)
diaphragm (p. 416)
epiglottis (p. 407)
exhalation (p. 415)
glottis (p. 407)

inhalation (p. 415)
intercostal muscles (p. 416)
intrapleural pressure (p. 412)
larynx (p. 405)
lower respiratory tract (p. 403)
partial pressure (p. 419)
pharynx (p. 405)
phrenic nerve (p. 417)
pleurae (p. 411)
pleural cavity (p. 410)

surface tension (p. 411)
surfactants (p. 412)
tidal volume (p. 421)
trachea (p. 408)
upper respiratory tract (p. 403)
ventilation (p. 415)
vital capacity (p. 422)
vocal cords (p. 407)

Is he breathing? This is the first question asked about a person who has been seriously injured. The question indicates the importance of each breath. To breathe is to live; not to breathe is to die. Each breath is a breath of life.

Because of its close connection with life, ancient peoples attributed the act of breathing to the divine. Even the phases of breathing are called *inspiration* and *expiration,* references to a divine spirit moving into and out of our lungs. The creation story in Genesis, in which God breathes life into the little clay figure of Adam, vividly expresses an image of divine breath. Poetry also describes breathing as the life force. For example, the great Persian poet Sa'di echoed the sacredness of breath in a prayer: "Each respiration holds two blessings. Life is inhaled, and stale, foul air is exhaled. Therefore, thank God twice every breath you take."

In a more physiologic tone the respiratory system performs the following functions:
- Delivery of oxygen-rich air into the body and excretion of carbon dioxide–rich air out of the body

- Filtration and humidification of inhaled air
- **Regulation of acid-base balance**
- Production and modulation of various sounds, including the voice
- Olfaction…the nasal home of the olfactory chemoreceptors

STRUCTURE: ORGANS OF THE RESPIRATORY SYSTEM

UPPER AND LOWER RESPIRATORY TRACTS

The respiratory system contains the upper and lower respiratory tracts (Fig. 22.1). The **upper respiratory tract** contains the respiratory organs located outside the chest cavity: the nose and nasal cavities, pharynx, larynx, and upper trachea. The **lower respiratory tract** consists of organs located in the chest cavity: the lower trachea, bronchi, bronchioles, and alveoli. The lower parts of the bronchi, bronchioles, and alveoli are located in the lungs. The pleural membranes and the

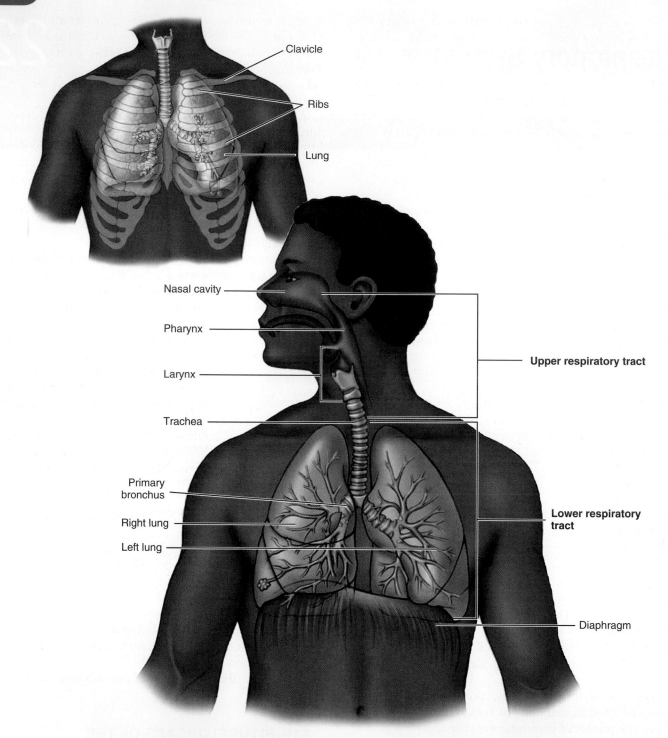

FIG. 22.1 Organs of the respiratory system: upper respiratory tract and lower respiratory tract.

muscles that form the chest cavity are also part of the lower respiratory tract.

Most of the respiratory organs are concerned with conduction, or movement, of air through the respiratory passages. The alveoli are the tiny air sacs located at the distal end of the respiratory passages. They are concerned with the exchange of oxygen and carbon dioxide, the respiratory gases, between the air and the blood across the walls of the pulmonary capillaries.

It is critical that the airway remains open; airway obstruction is life-threatening!

NOSE AND NASAL CAVITIES

The nose includes an external portion that forms part of the face and an internal portion called the *nasal cavities*. The nasal cavities are separated into right and left halves by a partition called the *nasal septum*, which is made of bone and cartilage. Air enters the nasal cavities through two openings called the *nostrils*, or *nares*. Nasal hairs in the nostrils filter large particles of dust that might otherwise be inhaled. In addition to its respiratory function, the nasal cavity contains the receptor cells for the sense of smell. The olfactory receptors cover the mucous membrane of the upper parts of the nasal cavity and a part of the nasal septum.

Three bony projections called *nasal conchae* (KONCH-ay) appear on the lateral walls of the nasal cavities. The conchae increase the surface area of the nasal cavities and support the ciliated mucous membranes, which line the nasal cavities. Mucous membranes contain many blood vessels and mucus-secreting cells. The rich supply of blood warms and moistens the air, and the sticky mucus traps dust, pollen, and other small particles, thereby cleansing the air as it is inhaled. Because the nose helps warm, moisten, and cleanse the air, breathing through the nose is better than mouth breathing.

 Do You Know...

That Your Nose Is More Than Just a Smeller?

The nose does a few things really well; as you know, the nose knows smells. It also "nose" how to clean and humidify air. Equally important, the nose plays a big cosmetic role: it makes us look good, and if it doesn't, we simply rearrange it surgically until it is fashioned into a great-looking nose. Nose-related medical conditions or procedures are named after the rhino, who sports the mother of all noses. For instance, a *rhinoplasty* (RYE-no-PLASS-tee) refers to the surgical reshaping, resizing, or realigning of the nose. *Rhinorrhea* refers to a runny nose, as in the common cold or the discharge of cerebrospinal fluid from the nose. *Rhinokyphosis* (RYF-no-ky-FOH-sis) is a humpback nose, and, of course, you can have a pain in the nose—*rhinodynia* (RYF-no-DIN-ee-uh). It is interesting that the rhino has captured the nose words because the rhino's nose is merely hardened hair; it doesn't sniff or drip, and it certainly doesn't check itself in for a nose job.

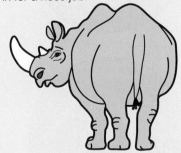

The nasal cavities contain several drainage openings. Mucus from the paranasal sinuses (see Fig. 8.8) drains into the nasal cavities. The paranasal sinuses include the maxillary, frontal, ethmoidal, and sphenoidal sinuses. Tears from the nasolacrimal ducts also drain into the nasal cavities. (Cry and your nose runs.)

In some persons, the nasal septum may bend toward one side or the other, thereby obstructing the flow of air and making breathing difficult. This abnormal positioning of the septum is called a *deviated septum*. Surgical repair of the deviated septum (septoplasty) corrects the problem.

And for the nose that snorts cocaine? Chronic exposure to the drug causes intense vasoconstriction of the blood vessels that supply the septum. The septal cartilage dies, thereby creating a hole in the septum and giving the nose a collapsed or "caved-in" appearance. Not a good look!

PHARYNX

The **pharynx** (FAIR-inks), or throat, is located behind the oral cavity and between the nasal cavities and the larynx (Fig. 22.2). The pharynx includes three parts: the nasopharynx (upper section), the oropharynx (middle section), and the laryngopharynx (lower section). The oropharynx and the laryngopharynx are part of both the digestive and respiratory systems and function as a passageway for both food and air. The pharynx conducts food toward the esophagus (tube for food to enter the stomach). The pharynx also conducts air to the larynx as it moves toward the lungs.

The pharynx contains two other structures: the openings from the eustachian tubes (auditory tubes) and the tonsils. The eustachian tube connects the nasopharynx with the middle ear.

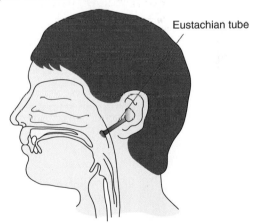

Eustachian tube

LARYNX

WHERE AND WHAT IS YOUR VOICEBOX?

The **larynx** (LAIR-inks), also called the *voicebox*, is located between the pharynx and trachea (see Fig. 22.2A). The larynx has three functions: it acts as a passageway for air during breathing, it produces sound (your voice), and it prevents food and other foreign objects from entering the distal respiratory structures. The larynx is a triangular structure made primarily of cartilage, muscles, and ligaments (see Fig. 22.2C and D).

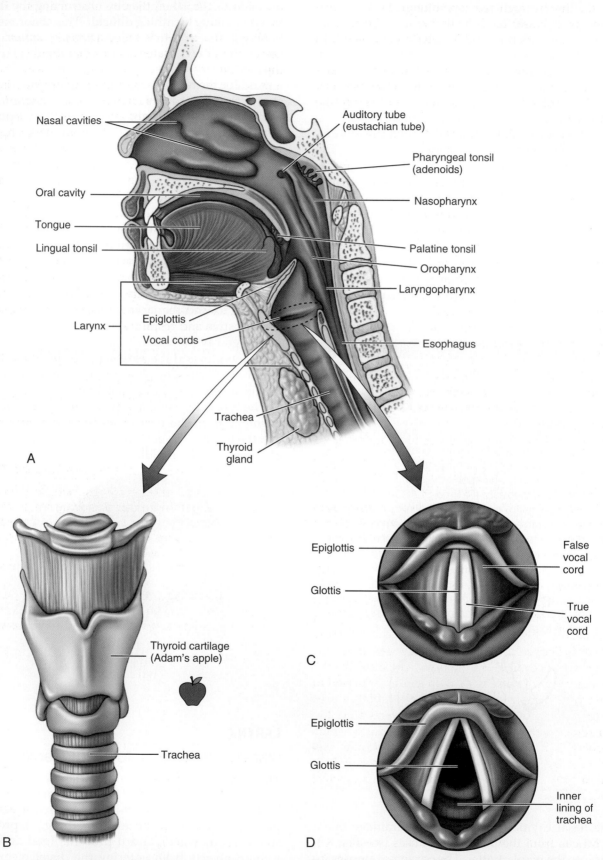

FIG. 22.2 (A) Organs of the upper respiratory tract. (B) Larynx, showing the thyroid cartilage (Adam's apple). (C) Vocal cords and glottis (closed). (D) Vocal cords and glottis (open).

The largest of the cartilaginous structures in the larynx is the thyroid cartilage. It is a tough hyaline cartilage and protrudes in the front of the neck. The thyroid cartilage is larger in men and is called the *Adam's apple* (see Fig. 22.2B).

The **epiglottis** (ep-i-GLOT-iss) is another cartilaginous structure, located at the top of the larynx (see Fig. 22.2A). The epiglottis acts as a flap, a very important flap. It covers the opening of the trachea during swallowing so that food does not enter the lungs.

VOCAL CORDS

The larynx is called the *voicebox* because it contains the vocal cords (see Fig. 22.2A and C). The **vocal cords** are folds of tissue composed of muscle and elastic ligaments and covered by mucous membrane. The cords stretch across the upper part of the larynx. The **glottis** is the space between the vocal cords.

TRUE OR FALSE

The two types of vocal cords are the false and true vocal cords. The false vocal cords are called "false" because they do not produce sounds. Instead, the muscles in this structure help to close the airway during swallowing. The true vocal cords produce sound. Air flowing from the lungs through the glottis during exhalation causes the true vocal cords to vibrate, thereby producing sound.

The loudness of your voice depends on the force with which the air moves past the true vocal cords. The pitch of your voice depends on the tension exerted on the muscles of the true vocal cords. You form sound into words with your pharynx, oral cavity, tongue, and lip movement. The nasal cavities, sinuses, and pharynx act as resonating chambers, thereby altering the quality of your voice. Listen to the different voices of your friends. One voice may sound high and squeaky, whereas another may sound low and booming.

From boy to young man. At puberty, under the influence of testosterone, the male larynx enlarges, and the vocal cords become longer and thicker. The larger vocal cords deepen the male voice. Changes in the larynx and vocal cords cause the boy's voice to "break" as he matures into a young man. In an earlier period in history, young choir boys with beautiful, high voices were castrated. Castration, the surgical excision of the testes, removes the source of testosterone and prevents thickening of the vocal cords. These unfortunate castrated boys continued to sing beautifully as members of the castrati choir. For obvious reasons, this practice eventually disappeared.

DOWN THE WRONG WAY

As shown in Fig. 22.2A, the pharynx acts as a passageway for food, water, and air. Food and water in the pharynx, however, should not enter the larynx. How are food and water normally kept out of the larynx?

When you breathe in air, the glottis opens, and air moves through the glottis into tubes that carry it to the lungs.

When you swallow food, however, the epiglottis covers the glottis, thereby preventing food from entering the lower respiratory passages. Instead, the food enters the esophagus, the tube that empties into the stomach. How does this happen? During swallowing, the larynx moves upward and forward while the epiglottis moves downward. If you place your fingers on your larynx as you swallow, you can feel the larynx move upward and forward. In addition to the movement of the epiglottis, the glottis closes. Compare the size of the glottis in Fig. 22.2C and D.

Note that swallowing plays a key role in preventing the entrance of food or water into the respiratory tubes. Some patients develop difficulty in swallowing, particularly those who have suffered neurological damage such as cerebral palsy or a stroke. Any patient who experiences difficulty in swallowing is at risk for aspiration (entrance of food or water into the lungs). Aspiration is a large clinical problem.

Re-Think

1. Trace the flow of air from the nose to the trachea.
2. Explain why food and water do not enter the respiratory structures during swallowing.

Do You Know...
Why You Should Know How to Perform the Abdominal Thrust?

The abdominal thrust is a simple life-saving technique that was designed to dislodge an obstructing object from the throat of a choking person. The "bear hug" procedure is demonstrated on an adult in the accompanying illustration. Here are the steps for the adult:

1. Stand behind the choking person and wrap your arms around the person's waist.
2. Position your hands (fist position) between the person's navel and the bottom of the rib cage.
3. Press your fist into the abdomen with a quick upward movement.
4. Repeat several times as necessary.

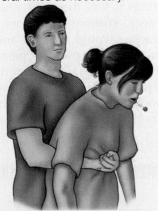
Abdominal thrust (adult)

Do You Know...

How "Dumb Plant" Was Used to Control Gossip (Without, of Course, Killing the Gossiper)?

A tea made from dieffenbachia ("dumb plant") was given to Roman slaves before they were sent to the market to shop. The tea caused the slave's tongue and mouth to swell and paralyzed the throat. The slave was therefore unable to speak and gossip about household affairs. It is still used by some African tribes as a punishment for gossip. An overdose of the poison causes excessive swelling, obstruction of the respiratory passageways, and death by suffocation. On an updated note, acute respiratory obstruction can be induced when a patient is given a drug or food to which she is allergic. "Dumb plant ingestion" may be dead, but the anaphylactic response (respiratory obstruction) is very much alive and well.

TRACHEA

WHERE IT SITS AND WHERE IT SPLITS

The **trachea** (TRAY-kee-ah), or windpipe, is a tube 4 to 5 inches (10 to 12.5 cm) long and 1 inch (2.5 cm) in diameter (Fig. 22.3). The trachea extends from the larynx downward into the thoracic cavity, where it splits into the right and left bronchi (sing., **bronchus**). The trachea splits, or bifurcates, at a point called the *carina* (kah-RYE-nah) at the manubriosternal junction (where the manubrium of the sternum meets the sternal body). Why is the carina so important clinically? The carina is very sensitive; touching it during suctioning causes vigorous coughing. The purpose of the trachea? It conducts air to and from the lungs.

KEEPING IT OPEN

The trachea lies in front of the esophagus, the food tube. C-shaped rings of cartilage partially surround the trachea for its entire length and serve to keep it open. The rings are open on the back side of the trachea so that the esophagus can bulge forward as food moves along the esophagus to the stomach. You can feel the cartilaginous rings if you run your fingers along the front of your neck. Without this strong cartilaginous support, the trachea would collapse and shut off the flow of air through the respiratory passages. Because of the cartilaginous rings, a tight collar or necktie does not collapse the trachea. A severe blow to the anterior neck, however, can crush the trachea and cause an acute respiratory obstruction. The trachea must be kept open.

BRONCHIAL TREE: BRONCHI, BRONCHIOLES, AND ALVEOLI

The **bronchial tree** consists of the bronchi, the bronchioles, and the alveoli. It is called a *tree* because the

 Do You Know...

What a Tracheostomy Is?

Sometimes a part of the upper respiratory tract becomes blocked, thereby obstructing the flow of air into the lungs. To restore airflow, an emergency tracheostomy may be performed. This procedure is the insertion of a tube through a surgical incision into the trachea below the level of the obstruction. The tracheostomy bypasses the obstruction and allows air to flow through the tube into the lungs.

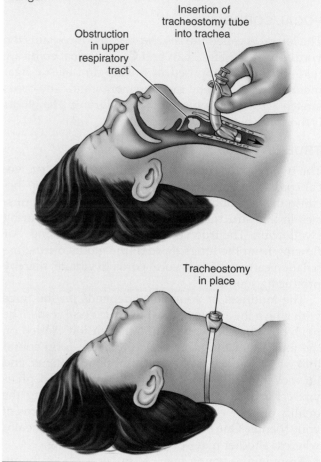

bronchi and their many branches resemble an upside-down tree. Most of the bronchial tree is in the lungs.

BRONCHI

The right and left primary bronchi are formed as the lower part of the trachea divides into two tubes. The primary bronchi enter the lungs at a region called the *hilus*. The primary bronchi branch into secondary bronchi, which branch into smaller tertiary bronchi. Because the heart lies toward the left side of the chest, the left bronchus is narrower and positioned more horizontally than the right bronchus. The right bronchus is shorter and wider than the left bronchus and extends downward in a more vertical direction. Because of the differences in the size and positioning of the bronchi, food particles and small objects

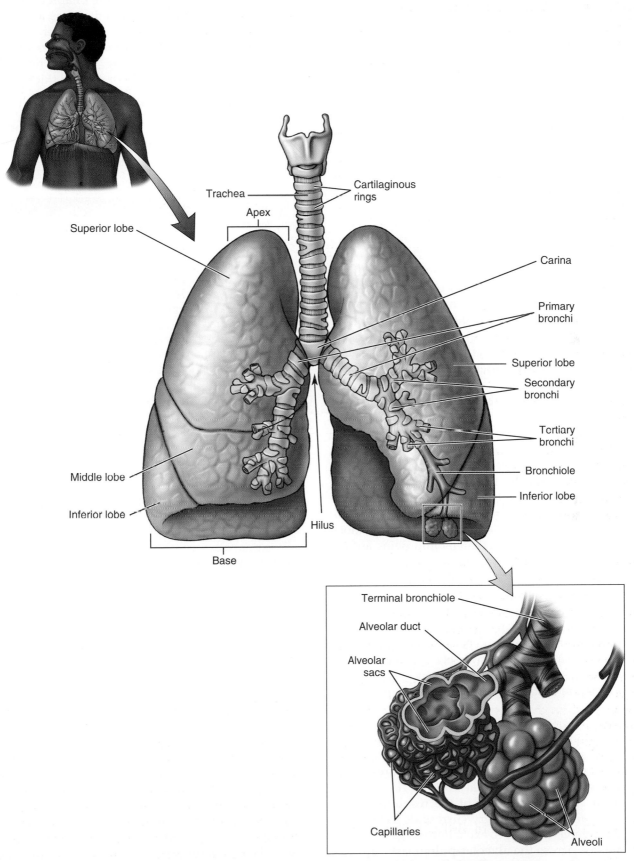

FIG. 22.3 Trachea and bronchial tree (bronchi, bronchioles, and alveoli).

are more easily inhaled, or aspirated, into the right bronchus.

Why are tiny toys not good for tiny tots? Young children generally put toys in their mouths. The tiny toy may become lodged in the larynx or bronchus, causing an acute respiratory obstruction. Unless relieved immediately, the obstruction can be fatal. Tiny toys are responsible for many toy recalls.

The upper segments of the bronchi have C-shaped cartilaginous rings, which help keep the bronchi open. As the bronchi extend into the lungs, however, the amount of cartilage decreases and finally disappears. The finer and more distal branches of the bronchi contain no cartilage.

BRONCHIOLES

The bronchi divide repeatedly into smaller tubes called **bronchioles** (BRON-kee-ohls). The walls of the bronchioles contain smooth muscle and no cartilage. The bronchioles regulate the flow of air to the alveoli. Contraction of the bronchiolar smooth muscle causes the bronchioles to constrict, thereby decreasing the bronchiolar lumen (opening) and thus decreasing the flow of air. Relaxation of the bronchioles causes the lumen to increase, thereby increasing the flow of air.

An asthma attack illustrates the effect of bronchiolar smooth muscle constriction. In a person with asthma, the bronchioles hyperrespond to a particular stimulus. The bronchiolar smooth muscle then constricts, decreasing the flow of air into the lungs. The person complains of a tight chest and expends much energy trying to force air through the constricted bronchioles into the lungs. Forced air causes a wheezing sound. Bronchiolar smooth muscle relaxants are medications that cause bronchodilation, thereby improving airflow and relieving the wheezing.

Let's translate this into autonomic pharmacology. The bronchioles contain beta$_2$-adrenergic receptors. Stimulation of these receptors causes relaxation of the bronchiolar smooth muscle, thus inducing bronchodilation and improved airflow. Albuterol, a beta$_2$-adrenergic agonist, is a bronchodilator drug. Conversely, a beta-adrenergic blocker, such as propranolol, causes bronchoconstriction and is therefore contraindicated in asthmatic patients.

ALVEOLI

The bronchioles continue to divide and give rise to many tubes called *alveolar ducts* (see Fig. 22.3). These ducts end in very small, grapelike structures called *alveoli* (sing., **alveolus**). The alveoli are tiny air sacs that form at the distal ends of the respiratory passages. A pulmonary capillary surrounds each alveolus. The alveoli function to exchange oxygen and carbon dioxide across the alveolar-pulmonary capillary membrane. Oxygen diffuses from the alveoli into the blood; carbon dioxide diffuses from the blood into

the alveoli. Alveolar characteristics that favor gas exchange are described later in the chapter. The term *atelectasis* refers to collapsed and airless alveoli. Atelectasis occurs commonly as a postoperative complication and as a result of conditions such as pneumonia and cancer of the lung. Certain respiratory diseases may destroy alveoli or cause a thickening of the alveolar wall. As a result, the exchange of gases is slowed. Oxygenation of the blood may decrease, causing hypoxemia and cyanosis, and the blood may retain carbon dioxide, causing a disturbance in acid–base balance (acidosis).

 Do You Know...

Why You May Diagnose Cystic Fibrosis by Kissing Your Baby's Face?

Cystic fibrosis (CF) is a hereditary disease that is characterized by thickened secretions of most exocrine glands. Consequently, CF affects many organs, including the liver, pancreas, and especially the lungs. The production of thick bronchial secretions is of particular concern because the secretions block narrow breathing passages, causing atelectasis and pulmonary infections. Eventually, lung tissue is destroyed; for this reason, the clinical picture of CF is dominated by pulmonary dysfunction. In addition, sweat glands and salivary glands produce a very salty secretion because of a hereditary defect of the cellular chloride pumps. Mothers often notice the salty taste of their infants upon kissing them; this observation is often the stimulus for the visit to the pediatrician.

 Do You Know...

How You Spot "Clubbed" Fingers?

Patients who experience chronic hypoxemia, such as those with impaired lung and heart function, often develop clubbing of the fingers and toes. Clubbing is characterized by enlarged fingertips and toes and changes in the thickness and shape of the nails. The enlargement is due to the formation of additional capillaries and tissue hypertrophy in an attempt to deliver additional oxygen to the oxygen-deprived cells.

LUNGS

RIGHT AND LEFT

The two lungs, located in the **pleural cavities**, extend from an area just above the clavicles to the diaphragm. The lungs are soft cone-shaped organs so large that they occupy most of the space in the thoracic cavity (see Fig. 22.3). The lungs are subdivided into lobes. The right lung has three lobes: the superior, middle, and inferior lobes. Because of the location of the heart in the left side of the chest, the left lung has only two lobes: the superior lobe and the inferior lobe.

The upper rounded part of the lung is called the *apex*, and the lower portion is called the *base*. The base of the lung rests on the diaphragm. The amount of air the lungs can hold varies with a person's body build, age, and physical conditioning. For instance, a tall person has larger lungs than a short person. A swimmer generally has larger lungs than a "couch potato," and the trained singer has larger lungs than the typical "shower singer."

Re-Think

1. Explain why the trachea remains open.
2. What structures make up the bronchial tree?
3. What is the "problem" caused by bronchoconstriction?
4. What is the primary function of the alveoli?

PLEURAL MEMBRANES

PLEURA

The outside of each lung and the inner chest wall are lined with a continuous serous membrane called the **pleurae** (Fig. 22.4). The pleurae are named according to their location. The membrane on the outer surface of each lung is called the *visceral pleura;* the membrane lining the chest wall is called the *parietal pleura*. The visceral pleura and the parietal pleura are attracted to each other like two flat plates of glass whose surfaces are wet. The plates of glass can slide past one another but offer some resistance when you try to pull them apart.

PLEURAL CAVITY: A POTENTIAL SPACE

Between the visceral pleura and the parietal pleura is a space called the *intrapleural space*. The pleural membranes secrete a small amount of serous fluid (approximately 25 mL). The fluid lubricates the pleural membranes and allows them to slide past one another with little friction or discomfort. Under abnormal conditions, the intrapleural space has the potential to accumulate excess fluid, blood, and air. An excess secretion of pleural fluid is called *pleural effusion*. Purulent (pus) pleural effusion is called *empyema*.

Sum It Up!

Air moves through the following structures—from the nasal cavities, to the pharynx, to the larynx, to the trachea, to the bronchi, to the bronchioles, and finally to the alveoli. When the air reaches the alveoli (the tiny air sacs at the end of the bronchial tree), the respiratory gases oxygen and carbon dioxide diffuse across the alveolar–pulmonary capillary membrane. Most of the respiratory structures conduct air to and from the alveoli in the lungs. Only the alveoli function in the exchange of the respiratory gases between the outside air and the blood. The lungs contain the structures of the lower respiratory tract. Pleural membranes surround the lungs and line the thoracic cavity, creating the intrapleural space or pleural cavity.

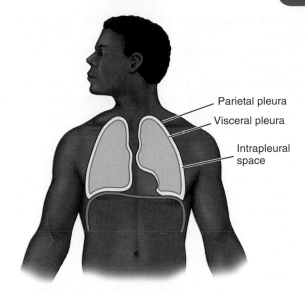

FIG. 22.4 Lungs, pleural membranes, and the intrapleural space.

COLLAPSED AND EXPANDED LUNGS

Fig. 22.1 shows that the lungs occupy most of the thoracic cage, but this statement must be qualified: the *expanded* lungs occupy most of the thoracic cage. Under normal conditions, the lungs expand like inflated balloons. Under abnormal conditions, however, a lung may collapse. What determines whether or not the lungs collapse or expand?

WHY LUNGS COLLAPSE

If the pleural cavity is entered surgically or in response to a penetrating chest injury, the lungs collapse. There are two reasons why the lungs collapse: elastic recoil and surface tension.

ELASTIC RECOIL

Consider a balloon and a lung (Fig. 22.5A). If you blow up a balloon but fail to tie off the open end, the air rushes out, and the balloon collapses. It collapses because of the arrangement of its elastic fibers. When these fibers stretch, they remain stretched only when tension is applied (the air blown into the balloon stretches the balloon). If the end of the balloon is not tied off, the elastic fibers recoil, forcing air out and collapsing the balloon. The same can be said of the lung. The arrangement of the lung's elastic tissue is similar to the arrangement of the elastic fibers in the balloon. The elastic tissue of the lung can stretch, but it recoils and returns to its unstretched position if tension is released (see Fig. 22.5B). This is called *elastic recoil*.

SURFACE TENSION

The lung also collapses for a second reason, a force called **surface tension**. The single alveolus in Fig. 22.5C illustrates surface tension. A thin layer of water lines

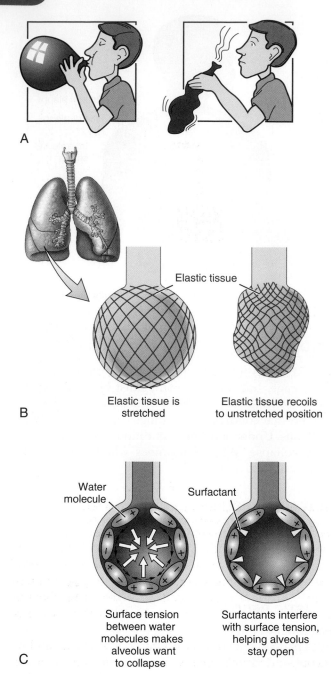

A

Elastic tissue

Elastic tissue is stretched | Elastic tissue recoils to unstretched position

B

Water molecule | Surfactant

Surface tension between water molecules makes alveolus want to collapse | Surfactants interfere with surface tension, helping alveolus stay open

C

FIG. 22.5 (A and B) Elastic recoil. (C) Surface tension: water and the effect of surfactants.

the inside of the alveolus. Water is a polar molecule; one end of the water molecule has a positive (+) charge, whereas the other end of the molecule has a negative (−) charge. Note how the water molecules line up. The positive (+) end of one water molecule is attracted to the negative (−) charge on the second water molecule. Each water molecule pulls on the other and on the water molecules beneath them. The electrical attraction of the water molecules is the surface tension. As the water molecules pull on one another, they tend to make the alveolus smaller; in other words, they tend to collapse the alveoli.

NOTE: The surface tension of pure water is normally very high. In the mature normal lung, special alveolar cells secrete pulmonary surfactants. **Surfactants** (sur-FAK-tants) are detergent-like lipoproteins that decrease surface tension by interfering with the electrical attraction between the water molecules on the inner surface of the alveolus (see Fig. 22.5C). The secretion of surfactant is stimulated by a sigh. After every five or six breaths, a person takes a larger-than-normal breath (a sigh); the sigh stretches the alveoli, promoting the secretion of surfactant. Surfactants lower surface tension but do not eliminate it. Surface tension remains a force that acts to collapse the alveoli.

Do You Know...

Why a Premature Infant Is More Apt Than a Full-Term Infant to Develop Respiratory Distress Syndrome?

Surfactant-secreting cells appear only during the later stages of fetal development. An infant born 2 to 3 months prematurely generally has insufficient surfactant-secreting cells. As a result, surface tension within the alveoli is excessively high, the alveoli collapse, and the infant experiences respiratory distress. The infant may die in respiratory failure or heart failure. The heart literally fails because it is "worked to death" providing the energy necessary for ventilation. This condition is commonly called *respiratory distress syndrome*. Before delivery, the mother may be given steroids to hasten the development of surfactant-secreting cells. In addition, a premature infant is given surfactants through inhalation in an attempt to prevent this life-threatening condition.

Re-Think

1. List two reasons that the lungs want to collapse.
2. Why does water have a high surface tension?
3. Why does a deficiency of surfactants increase the "work" of breathing?

WHY LUNGS EXPAND

If elastic recoil and surface tension collapse the lungs, why do they remain expanded in the normal closed thorax? Lung expansion depends on pressure within the intrapleural space. A series of diagrams in Fig. 22.6 illustrates this point. In Fig. 22.6A, the three pressures are labeled P1, P2, and P3. P1 is the pressure outside the chest (the pressure in the room), also called the *atmospheric pressure*. P2 is the pressure in the lung, also called the *intrapulmonic pressure*. P3 is the pressure in the intrapleural space, also called the **intrapleural pressure**. Note in Fig. 22.6A that the lungs are normally expanded.

Fig. 22.6B and C show why the lungs expand. To illustrate this point, a hole is created in the right chest wall so that the right lung collapses. Note the pressures. Because of the hole in the chest wall, all the pressures are equal. In other words, P1 = P2 = P3. In

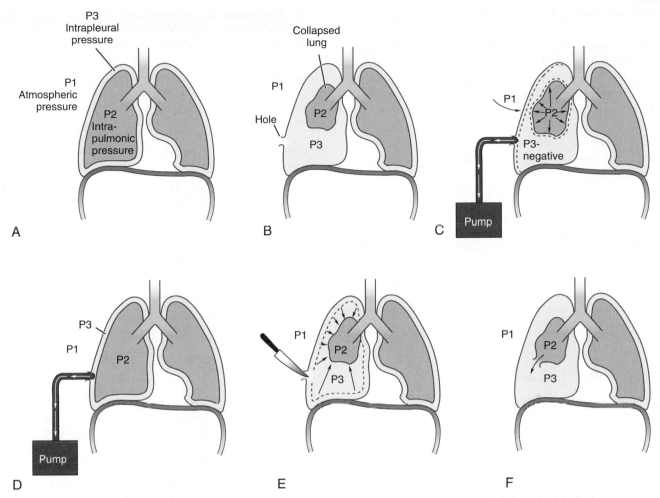

FIG. 22.6 Lung expansion and collapse. (A) The lungs expand. (B) The right lung collapses because of the hole in the chest wall. (C) Air is pumped out of the intrapleural space, creating a negative intrapleural pressure. (D) The lung expands because of the negative intrapleural pressure. (E) The lung collapses because of the hole (knife wound) in the chest wall. (F) The lung collapses because of a hole in the lung.

Fig. 22.6C, a tube is inserted through the hole of the right chest wall into the intrapleural space. The tube is attached to a pump, which removes air from the intrapleural space. As air moves from the intrapleural space, the intrapleural pressure (P3) decreases and becomes negative. This negative intrapleural pressure (P3) merely means that it is lower than the atmospheric pressure (P1) or the intrapulmonic pressure (P2).

What is the effect of a negative intrapleural pressure? Because P2 (intrapulmonic pressure) is greater than P3 (intrapleural pressure), the lung is pushed toward the chest wall, causing the lung to expand. Also, because P1 (atmospheric pressure) is higher than P3, the chest wall is pushed inward toward the lung. When the chest wall and the lungs meet, the lung is expanded (see Fig. 22.6C and D). The important point is that the lung expands and remains expanded because the intrapleural pressure is negative.

What happens if the pump is removed, thereby recreating the hole in the chest wall? Because P1 is higher than P3, air rushes into the intrapleural space through

the hole and eliminates the negative intrapleural pressure. As a result, the lung collapses. Remember that the lung expands only when the intrapleural pressure is negative.

Fig. 22.6E, illustrates the effects of a stab wound to the chest. The hole created by the knife allows the air to rush into the intrapleural space and eliminate the negative intrapleural pressure. The introduction of air into the intrapleural space and subsequent collapse of the lung is called a *pneumothorax* (*pneumo-* means "air"; *thorax* means "chest"). Air in the intrapleural space is also why the lungs collapse when a surgical incision is made through the chest wall into the pleural cavity.

Fig. 22.6F shows the effect of a hole in the lung. Because the intrapulmonic pressure (P2) is higher than the intrapleural pressure (P3), air rushes into the intrapleural space through the hole in the lung, thereby eliminating the negative intrapleural pressure and collapsing the lung. Sometimes, people with emphysema develop blebs, or blisters, on the outer surface of their lungs. The blebs rupture and create a hole between the intrapulmonic and intrapleural spaces, causing air to rush into the intrapleural space and collapsing the lung.

What can be done for a collapsed lung? The physician inserts a tube through the chest wall into the intrapleural space and pulls air out of the intrapleural space. As the air leaves the intrapleural space, negative pressure is reestablished, and the lung expands. Sometimes, the physician inserts a large needle into the intrapleural space to aspirate, or withdraw, air, blood, and pus in a procedure called a *thoracentesis*. It facilitates lung expansion.

NOTE: The intrapleural pressure remains negative only when no hole exists in the chest wall or the lungs.

? Re-Think

1. Explain why the lungs remain expanded. Use the terms *atmospheric pressure, intrapleural pressure,* and *intrapulmonic* pressure in your explanation.
2. Explain why a hole in the chest wall causes the lung to collapse.

SAYING IT ANOTHER WAY: COMPLIANCE

Compliance is the measure of elastic recoil and can be illustrated by two balloons. One balloon has never been inflated and is stiff. A second balloon has been inflated many times and has lost some of its elasticity (elastic recoil); it appears baggy. Which balloon is easier to inflate? The baggy balloon is easier to inflate because it has lost some of its elasticity and is less stiff. Translation: The baggy balloon is more compliant (stretchy). The new balloon is less compliant (stiff) and is therefore more difficult to inflate.

The same is true for the lungs. When lung compliance decreases (stiff lungs), the lungs are more difficult to inflate. Some conditions associated with decreased lung compliance are pulmonary edema, respiratory distress syndrome (deficiency of surfactants), and pulmonary fibrosis. Decreased lung compliance is not good!

What about increased lung compliance? Lungs that are too stretchy also cause problems. For example, the patient with emphysema has damaged lung structure and reduced elastic recoil. Lung compliance has increased too much; there is not enough elastic recoil to completely expel air on exhalation. The increased compliance also contributes to the formation of the barrel chest appearance that characterizes a person with chronic lung disease.

? Re-Think

1. Explain compliance using the example of two springs: a heavy-duty spring used on garage doors and the tiny springs found in ballpoint pens.
2. Explain why an increase in lung compliance causes barrel-chestedness.

 Do You Know...

Why This Person's Chest Looks Like a Barrel?

This person has emphysema, a condition characterized by damaged tissue in the lower respiratory structures and overinflated alveoli. As a result, the lungs cannot exhale the proper amount of air, and the air remains trapped in the alveoli. (*Emphysema* means "puffed up" alveoli.) Consequently, the alveoli and lungs become overinflated and cause the chest to be shaped like a barrel, so a person with severe emphysema is described as barrel-chested.

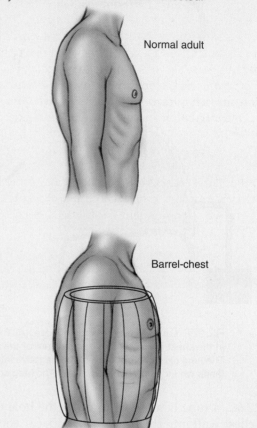

Normal adult

Barrel-chest

◎ Sum It Up!

The expanded lungs normally fill the thoracic cavity. Unless pressure conditions in the pleural cavity are correct, the lungs collapse. The tendency of the lungs to collapse is due to the result of two factors: elastic recoil and alveolar surface tension. The expansion of the lungs is caused by a negative intrapleural pressure within the intrapleural space. If the negative intrapleural pressure is eliminated, the lungs collapse.

RESPIRATORY FUNCTION

THREE STEPS IN RESPIRATION

Most of us equate breathing with respiration. Respiration includes breathing, but it is more than breathing; it involves the entire process of gas exchange between the atmosphere and the body's cells. Respiration includes the following three steps:

- Ventilation, or breathing
- Exchange of oxygen and carbon dioxide
- Transport of oxygen and carbon dioxide by the blood

STEP 1: VENTILATION OR BREATHING

What It Is

Movement of air into and out of the lungs is called **ventilation**; it is more commonly called *breathing*. The two phases of ventilation are inhalation and exhalation. **Inhalation**, also called *inspiration,* is the breathing-in phase. During inhalation, oxygen-rich air moves into tiny air sacs (alveoli) in the lungs. **Exhalation**, also called *expiration,* is the breathing-out phase. During exhalation, air rich in carbon dioxide is moved out of the lungs. One inhalation and one exhalation make up one respiratory cycle.

Boyle's Law: Pressure and Volume

To understand ventilation, you need some background information. You need to know the relationship between pressure and volume, a relationship called **Boyle's law**. Note the two tubes in Fig. 22.7. Tube A is a small tube that fits into a bicycle tire. When filled, the tube can hold 1 liter (L) of air. Tube B is larger and fits into a truck tire. When filled, it can hold 10 L of air. Thus, the volume of the truck tube (B) is 10 times greater than the volume of the bicycle tube.

In the upper panel of Fig. 22.7, both tubes are empty. Let's add 1 L of air to each tube and measure the pressure in each tube. By touching the surfaces of the tubes, you can get a rough estimate of the pressures. Tube A feels firm, whereas tube B feels soft. In other words, the pressure in tube A is higher than the pressure in tube B. Both tubes received the same amount of air, so why are the pressures different? The different volumes of the tubes cause the different pressures. The pressure is higher in tube A because the volume of tube A is small; 1 L of air completely fills the tube. The pressure in tube B is lower because its volume is large (10 L). One liter of air only partially fills the truck tube. The smaller the volume, the higher the pressure; the greater the volume, the lower the pressure. If volume changes, the pressure changes. This is Boyle's law, the principle on which ventilation is based.

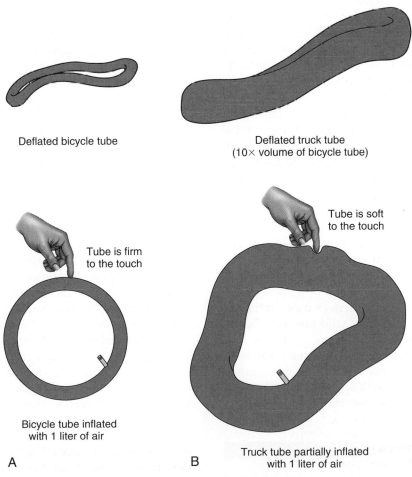

Deflated bicycle tube

Deflated truck tube
(10× volume of bicycle tube)

Tube is firm
to the touch

Tube is soft
to the touch

Bicycle tube inflated
with 1 liter of air

Truck tube partially inflated
with 1 liter of air

A   B

FIG. 22.7 Boyle's law: relationship between pressure and volume.

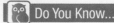

Do You Know...

About the Pink Puffers and Blue Bloaters?

Both Pink Puffers and Blue Bloaters suffer from breathing difficulties, such as asthma, emphysema, or chronic obstructive pulmonary disease (COPD). Pink Puffers gasp for breath and, in doing so, turn red in the face. Blue Bloaters, having suffered from poor pulmonary function for a longer time, are accustomed to struggling for air and so don't gasp and struggle like the Pink Puffers. The Blue Bloaters, with weakened respiratory muscles, don't have the energy to puff away and turn red; rather, they tend to inhale a large volume of air, hold it, and become bloated. This type of respiratory activity causes their oxygen levels to decline, thereby causing hypoxemia and cyanosis. Complicating the hypoxemia is an accumulation of carbon dioxide in the blood, which in turn causes respiratory acidosis. Of the two, Blue Bloaters are generally the most seriously ill and in need of treatment. Furthermore, their already depleted oxygen levels decline quickly if they develop an acute complication such as pneumonia.

Boyle's Law and Breathing

What does Boyle's law have to do with ventilation? On inhalation (breathing in), air flows into the lungs. What is the force that causes the air to flow in? Place your hands on your rib cage. Inhale. Notice that the thoracic cage moves up and out on inhalation (Fig. 22.8A and C). This movement increases the volume of the thoracic cavity and lungs. As the volume in the lung increases, the pressure in the lung (P2) decreases (satisfying Boyle's law). As a result, P2 becomes less than P1 (atmospheric pressure, the air you breathe). Air flows from higher pressure to lower pressure, through the nose into the lungs.

What happens on exhalation? Another change in lung volume. Place your hands on your rib cage and exhale. The thoracic and lung volumes decrease as the rib cage returns to its resting position (see Fig. 22.8B and D). The decreased lung volume causes the pressure within the lungs (P2) to increase. Now P2 is higher than P1, and air flows out of the lungs through the nose. Let us clarify the relationship between Boyle's law and ventilation:

- Air flows in response to changes in pressure. As the lung volume increases on inhalation, the intrapulmonic pressure (P2) decreases, and air flows into the lungs.
- On exhalation, lung volume decreases, intrapulmonic pressure (P2) increases, and air flows out of the lungs.
- Air flows in response to pressure changes. Pressure changes occur in response to changes in volume. Inhalation is associated with an increase in thoracic volume; exhalation is associated with a decrease in thoracic volume.

Re-Think

1. List the two phases of ventilation.
2. Explain ventilation in terms of Boyle's law.

The Muscles of Respiration

What causes the thoracic volume to change? The change in thoracic volume is caused by the contraction and relaxation of the respiratory muscles. On inhalation, the respiratory muscles, diaphragm, and intercostal muscles contract (see Fig. 22.8A and C). The **diaphragm** is a dome-shaped muscle that forms the floor of the thoracic cavity and separates the thoracic cavity from the abdominal cavity. The diaphragm is the chief muscle of inhalation. Contraction of the diaphragm flattens the muscle and pulls it downward, toward the abdomen. This movement increases the length of the thoracic cavity. During quiet breathing, the diaphragm accounts for most of the increase in the thoracic volume.

The two **intercostal muscles**, the external and internal intercostals, are located between the ribs. When the external intercostal muscles contract, the rib cage moves up and out, thereby increasing the width of the thoracic cavity. Note that the size of the thoracic cavity increases in three directions: from front to back, from side to side, and lengthwise. Why is this increase in thoracic volume so important? As the thoracic volume increases, so does the volume of the lungs. According to Boyle's law, the increase in volume decreases the pressure in the lungs and, as a result, air flows into the lungs. Some of the accessory muscles of respiration, located in the neck and chest, can move the rib cage even farther during exertion.

On exhalation, the muscles of respiration relax and allow the ribs and diaphragm to return to their original positions (see Fig. 22.8B and D). This movement decreases thoracic and lung volume and increases pressure in the lungs. Consequently, air flows out of the lungs. Elastic recoil of lung tissue and surface tension within the alveoli aid with exhalation. Forced exhalation uses the accessory muscles of respiration. These include the muscles of the abdominal wall and the internal intercostal muscles. Contraction of the accessory muscles of respiration pulls the bottom of the rib cage down and in, and it forces the abdominal viscera upward toward the relaxed diaphragm. These actions force additional air out of the lungs.

How much energy does it take to breathe? Inhalation is a result of the contraction of the respiratory muscles, so it is an active process. The muscles use up energy (ATP) as they contract. Exhalation associated with normal quiet breathing is passive. Exhalation is caused by muscle relaxation; no energy is required for muscle relaxation. Thus, in normal, quiet breathing, we use up energy during half of the respiratory cycle (inhalation). We rest on exhalation. During forced exhalation (as in exercise), however, the accessory muscles of respiration must contract, and exhalation becomes energy using, or active.

With certain lung diseases such as emphysema, exhalation can be achieved only when the accessory muscles of respiration are used. The patient with emphysema therefore uses energy during both inhalation and exhalation. This process is physically exhausting, and these patients usually complain of being very tired.

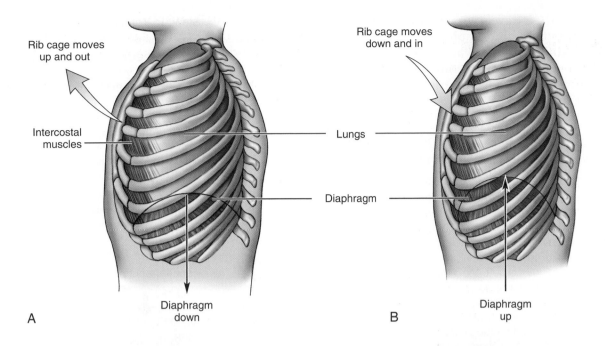

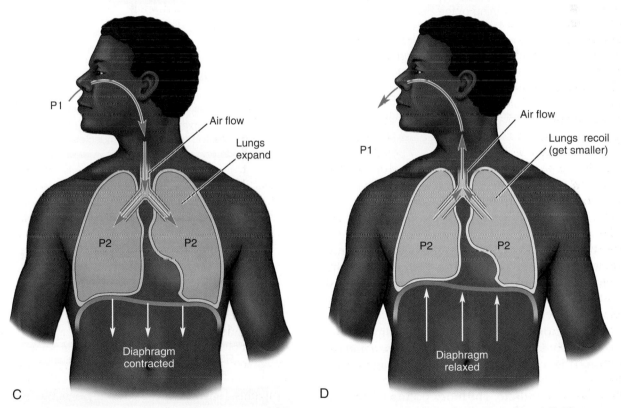

FIG. 22.8 Inhalation and exhalation. The thoracic volume increases, and air rushes into the lungs (A and C). The thoracic volume decreases, and air rushes out of the lungs (B and D).

? Re-Think

1. What muscles are used for inhalation?
2. Using the term *Boyle's law*, explain how contraction of the respiratory muscles causes air to move into the lungs.
3. Using the term *Boyle's law*, explain how relaxation of the respiratory muscles causes air to move out of the lungs.
4. What is meant by *forced exhalation*? How do the abdominal muscles assist with forced exhalation?

Nerves That Supply the Respiratory Muscles

Ventilation occurs in response to changes in the thoracic volume, and the changes in thoracic volume are caused by muscle contraction and relaxation. The respiratory muscles, being skeletal muscles, must be stimulated by motor nerves to contract. The motor nerves supplying the respiratory muscles are the **phrenic nerve** and intercostal nerves. The phrenic nerve exits from the spinal cord at the level of C4, travels within the cervical plexus, and is distributed to the diaphragm. Firing of the phrenic nerve stimulates the diaphragm to contract. The intercostal nerves supply the intercostal muscles. Thus, inhalation is initiated by the firing of the phrenic and intercostal nerves.

Do You Know...

That a Boa Constrictor Knows More About Boyle's Law Than the Early Corset Makers?

The boa fully appreciates Boyle's law! It knows that by wrapping itself around an animal's chest, it can suffocate the victim by preventing chest expansion and inhalation. Early corset makers, however, ignored this basic information. Corsets were designed to constrict the waist—the tighter the corset, the smaller the waist. A successfully corseted young lady might boast of a 12-inch–diameter waist! Problem was, the upper part of the corset included the lower part of the rib cage. What was the result of this constant binding? The corset prevented adequate ventilation and caused a permanent deformity of the rib cage, to say nothing of the displaced abdominal organs. The corseted young lovely couldn't breathe and often fainted. Herein lies the physiological basis of the "swoon" and delicate weakness that characterized wealthy young women. They were not weak because of their female X chromosomes; they were merely hypoxemic—no oxygen going to the brain. Fortunately, only the wealthiest could make a fashion statement by fainting.

You will be caring for patients whose nerve and muscle function are impaired. For example, if the spinal cord is severed above C4, the phrenic nerve cannot fire. As a result, the skeletal muscles (diaphragm and intercostals) cannot contract. The person not only is a quadriplegic, but also can breathe only with the assistance of a ventilator. Other patients experience difficulty in breathing because of the effects of certain drugs. (Review the N_M receptors at the neuromuscular junction, p. 149.) Curare, for example, is a drug commonly used during surgery to cause muscle relaxation. It is a neuromuscular blocking agent that interferes with the transmission of the electrical signal from nerve to muscle. The block occurs within the neuromuscular junction, including the neuromuscular junction of the phrenic nerve and diaphragm. The patient is not only unable to move the body voluntarily but also is unable to breathe.

Re-Think

1. What is the respiratory consequence of an injured or severed phrenic nerve?
2. Explain how blockade at the neuromuscular junction (phrenic nerve/diaphragm) impairs ventilation.

Steps in Ventilation

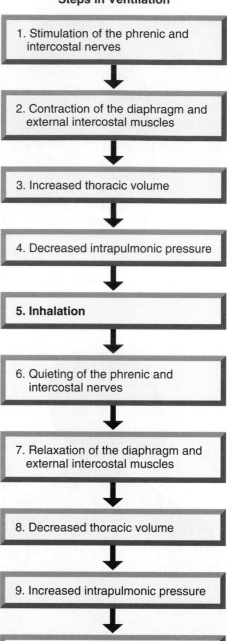

1. Stimulation of the phrenic and intercostal nerves
2. Contraction of the diaphragm and external intercostal muscles
3. Increased thoracic volume
4. Decreased intrapulmonic pressure
5. **Inhalation**
6. Quieting of the phrenic and intercostal nerves
7. Relaxation of the diaphragm and external intercostal muscles
8. Decreased thoracic volume
9. Increased intrapulmonic pressure
10. **Exhalation**

FIG. 22.9 Flowchart: Steps in ventilation.

Sum It Up!

The three steps in respiration are ventilation, exchange of oxygen and carbon dioxide in the lungs and cells, and transport of oxygen and carbon dioxide by the blood. Ventilation occurs in response to changes in thoracic volumes, which in turn cause changes in intrapulmonic pressures (Boyle's law). Inhalation occurs when the respiratory muscles, primarily the diaphragm) contract and enlarge the thoracic cage. Exhalation occurs when the respiratory muscles relax, allowing the thorax to return to its smaller, resting thoracic volume. The muscles of respiration are skeletal muscles and contract in response to stimulation of the phrenic and intercostal nerves. The steps involved in ventilation are summarized in Fig. 22.9.

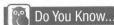

Do You Know...

That Charles Dickens "Nailed It" in His Novel *The Pickwick Papers*?

Yup, the creator of our beloved Tiny Tim in *A Christmas Carol* was the first to accurately describe (but not name) the syndrome of obesity-associated alveolar hypoventilation, or Pickwickian syndrome. In Dickens's description in *Pickwick Papers*, he refers to "a fat boy and red-faced boy in a state of somnolency" (extreme sleepiness). He subsequently addresses the boy as "Young Dropsy" (a reference to his obesity), Young Opium-eater (a reference to his somnolency), and Young Boa Constrictor (a reference to his excessive appetite). Physiologically, this is what Dickens meant to say: The boy's immense abdominal girth causes ventilatory insufficiency (periodic respirations and hypoventilation) and hypoxemia, explaining his extreme sleepiness (somnolence). The hypoxemia also stimulates RBC production and polycythemia (through erythropoietin) in an attempt to increase oxygen in the blood; this accounts for the boy's red appearance. Had Dickens known a little pathophysiology, he would have thrown into the mix a probable hematocrit of 65, expanded blood volume, hypercapnia with mild respiratory acidosis, alveolar hypoventilation, and an enlarged right heart. He would have explained that right heart failure, in turn, causes distention of the neck veins (JVD), hepatomegaly, and pedal edema.

Although Dickens didn't throw around much medical terminology, Young Dropsy's appearance described the syndrome quite accurately. So why is Pickwickian syndrome of such concern today? Because of the prevalence of obesity in our society and the wide varieties of obesity-related health conditions! Our increasing girth continues to "expand" upward. The short-term solution may be to increase the size of clothes, chairs, and caskets, but the real solution is to waste the waist. The good news? Weight loss appears to reverse the signs and symptoms of Pickwickian syndrome, including the "obesity heart disease."

STEP 2: EXCHANGE OF OXYGEN AND CARBON DIOXIDE

Inhalation delivers fresh oxygen-rich air to the alveoli and exhalation removes carbon dioxide–laden air from the alveoli. The second step of respiration is the exchange of the respiratory gases. Exchange occurs at two sites: in the lungs and at the cells (Fig. 22.10).

Why the Lungs Are Good Gas Exchangers

Gas exchange occurs in the lungs, specifically across the membranes of the alveoli and pulmonary capillaries. Three conditions make the alveoli well suited for the exchange of oxygen and carbon dioxide: a large surface area, thin alveolar and pulmonary capillary walls, and a short distance between the alveoli and pulmonary capillaries.

- *Large surface area.* Millions of alveoli, approximately 350 million per lung, create a total surface area about half the size of a tennis court. The large surface increases the amount of oxygen and carbon dioxide exchanged across the alveolar membranes.

- *Thin alveolar and pulmonary capillary walls.* The thin walls favor diffusion because they do not offer much resistance to the movement of oxygen and carbon dioxide across the membranes.

- *Closeness of the alveoli to the pulmonary capillaries.* Each alveolus is very close to a pulmonary capillary. For diffusion, closeness ensures a high rate of diffusion.

Partial Pressures and the Diffusion of Gases
What Causes the Respiratory Gases to Diffuse?

Chapter 3 describes how molecules diffuse from an area of higher concentration to an area of lower concentration. For gases such as oxygen and carbon dioxide, however, concentration is related to pressure. When the molecules of a gas are highly concentrated, the gas creates a high pressure. Consequently, we can talk about diffusion from areas of higher pressure to areas of lower pressure.

Ordinary room air is a gas composed of 78% nitrogen, 21% oxygen, and 0.04% carbon dioxide. Each part of the gas contributes to the total pressure. The amount of pressure each gas contributes is called the **partial pressure**. The symbol for the partial pressure of oxygen is PO_2; the symbol for the partial pressure of carbon dioxide is PCO_2. (Because the body does not use nitrogen gas, we can ignore it.)

Partial Pressures Within the Lungs. Fig. 22.10 illustrates the diffusion of the respiratory gases at two sites: the lungs and the tissues. Let us analyze the partial pressures of the respiratory gases in the alveoli and pulmonary capillaries. The PO_2 of air in the alveoli is 104 mm Hg, whereas the PO_2 of venous blood (the blue end of the pulmonary capillary) is 40 mm Hg. Oxygen diffuses from the area of higher pressure (the alveolus) to the area of lower pressure (the pulmonary capillary). Note that the PO_2 in the blood increases from 40 mm Hg (blue) to 95 mm Hg (red). The partial pressure of oxygen increases because the blood has been oxygenated.

As for the waste, the carbon dioxide, the PCO_2 in the blood (blue capillary) is 45 mm Hg, whereas the PCO_2 in the alveolus is only 40 mm Hg. Carbon dioxide diffuses from the capillary, the area of higher pressure, to the alveolus, the area of lower pressure. Because of the diffusion of carbon dioxide out of the blood, the PCO_2 of the blood decreases from 45 mm Hg at the blue end of the capillary to 40 mm Hg at the red end of the capillary. What has been accomplished? The blood coming from the right side of the heart (blue) has been oxygenated, and the oxygenated blood (red) eventually returns to the left side of the heart so that it can be pumped throughout the body. As oxygenation occurs, carbon dioxide has been removed; it leaves the lungs during exhalation.

Partial Pressure at the Cells. What happens to the gases at the tissues, or body cells? Two events occur.

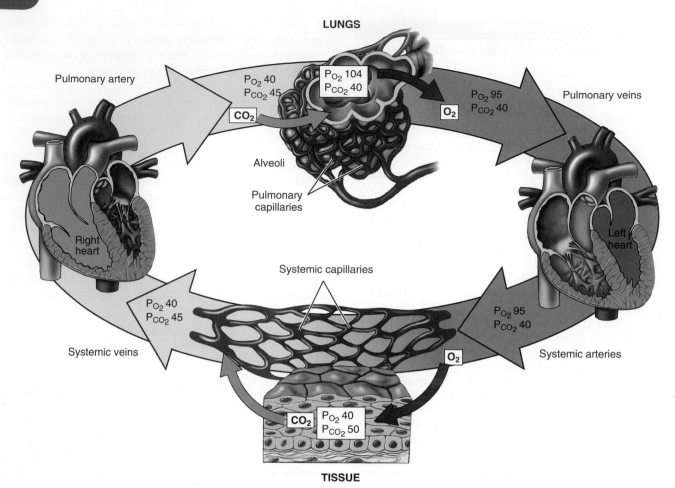

FIG. 22.10 Partial pressures of oxygen (PO_2) and carbon dioxide (PCO_2) within the lungs and at the cellular level (in mm Hg).

First, oxygen leaves the blood and diffuses into the cells, where it can be used during cell metabolism. Second, carbon dioxide, a consequence of cell metabolism, diffuses into the blood.

What partial pressures cause these events to happen? The PO_2 of the arterial blood is 95 mm Hg, whereas the cellular PO_2 is only 40 mm Hg. During gas exchange, oxygen diffuses from the blood into the space surrounding the cells. The PCO_2 of the cells is 50 mm Hg, and the arterial PCO_2 is only 40 mm Hg. Carbon dioxide therefore diffuses from the cells into the blood. The blood then carries the carbon dioxide to the lungs for excretion. Thus, oxygenated blood from the lungs carries the oxygen to the cells; the oxygen then diffuses from the blood into the cells. The carbon dioxide, or the waste produced by the metabolizing cells, diffuses into the blood, which carries it to the lungs for excretion. Note the venous blood leaving the cells. The PO_2 is 40 mm Hg because the oxygen has been used up by the cells. The PCO_2 is 45 mm Hg because the waste was removed from the cells.

STEP 3: TRANSPORT OF OXYGEN AND CARBON DIOXIDE

The third step in respiration is the blood's mechanism for transporting oxygen and carbon dioxide between the lungs and body cells. Although the blood transports both oxygen and carbon dioxide, the way in which blood transports each gas differs.

Oxygen Transport

Almost all the oxygen (98%) is transported by the hemoglobin in the red blood cells. The remaining 2% of the oxygen is dissolved in the plasma. As soon as oxygen enters the blood in the pulmonary capillaries, it immediately forms a loose bond with the iron portion of the hemoglobin molecule. This new molecule is oxyhemoglobin. As the oxygenated blood travels to the cells throughout the body, the oxygen unloads from the hemoglobin molecule and diffuses across the capillary walls to the cells. The oxygen is eventually used up by the metabolizing cells.

Carbon Dioxide Transport

Blood carries carbon dioxide from the metabolizing cells to the lungs, where it is exhaled. Blood carries carbon dioxide in the following three forms:

- Ten percent of the carbon dioxide is dissolved in plasma.
- Twenty percent of the carbon dioxide combines with hemoglobin to form carbaminohemoglobin. Note that the hemoglobin carries both oxygen and

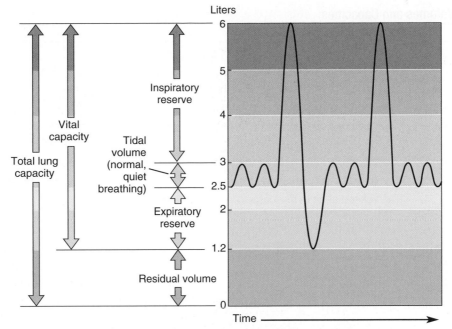

FIG. 22.11 Pulmonary volumes and capacities.

carbon dioxide but at different sites on the hemoglobin molecule. The oxygen forms a loose bond with the iron portion of the hemoglobin, whereas the carbon dioxide bonds with the globin, or protein (amino acids) portion, of the hemoglobin.

- Seventy percent of the carbon dioxide is converted to the bicarbonate ion (HCO_3^-). Note that the blood carries most of the carbon dioxide in the form of bicarbonate.

? Re-Think

1. What is the PO_2 in the alveoli, pulmonary veins, tissue, and vena cava?
2. What is the driving force for oxygen to move from the alveoli into the blood? From the blood into the tissues?
3. What is the primary way that blood transports oxygen? Carbon dioxide?

◎ Sum It Up!

The exchange of the respiratory gases occurs at two sites: the lungs and the cells. Oxygen diffuses from the alveoli into the pulmonary capillaries. Carbon dioxide diffuses from the pulmonary capillaries into the alveoli. At the cellular sites, oxygen diffuses from the capillaries into the cells; carbon dioxide diffuses from the cells into the capillaries. Blood transports oxygen and carbon dioxide. Hemoglobin carries most of the oxygen as oxyhemoglobin. The blood carries most of the carbon dioxide in the form of a bicarbonate ion (HCO_3^-).

AMOUNTS OF AIR

LUNG VOLUMES

Think about all the ways that you can vary the amount of air you breathe. For example, you can inhale a small amount of air, or you can take a deep breath. How are you breathing now? Probably slowly and effortlessly. With strenuous exercise, you breathe more rapidly and deeply. If you become anxious, your breathing pattern becomes more rapid and shallow. With certain diseases, your respirations might increase or decrease. In other words, the amount, or volume, of air you breathe can vary significantly.

The different volumes of air you breathe have names. The four pulmonary volumes are *tidal volume, inspiratory reserve volume, expiratory reserve volume,* and *residual volume.* A spirometer (spih-ROM-eh-ter) is a device that measures pulmonary volumes. The patient blows into the spirometer, which measures the amount of air and prints the results on graph paper. A recording of the volumes appears in Fig. 22.11 and is summarized in Table 22.1:

- Tidal volume. Breathe in and out. The amount of air moved into or out of the lungs with each breath is called the **tidal volume**. The average tidal volume during normal quiet breathing is about 500 mL. Tidal volume increases with exercise.
- Inspiratory reserve volume. Inhale a normal volume of air. Now, in addition to this normal amount of air, inhale as much as you possibly can. The additional volume of air is called the inspiratory reserve volume. This extra volume is approximately 3000 mL.
- Expiratory reserve volume. Exhale a normal amount of air. Now, in addition to this normal amount of air, exhale as much as you possibly can. The extra volume of exhaled air is called the expiratory reserve volume. It is about 1100 mL.
- Residual volume. Even after a forced exhalation, about 1200 mL of air remains in the lungs. This remaining air is the residual volume. Residual air

Table 22.1 Lung Volumes and Capacities

NAME	DESCRIPTION	AMOUNT (mL)
Volumes		
Tidal volume	The volume of air moved into or out of the lungs during one respiratory cycle	500
Residual volume	The volume of air that remains in the lungs after a forceful exhalation	1200
Inspiratory reserve volume	The volume of air that can be forcefully inhaled after normal inhalation	3000
Expiratory reserve volume	The volume of air that can be forcefully exhaled after normal exhalation	1100
Capacities		
Vital capacity	The maximum volume of air that can be exhaled following maximal inhalation	4600
Functional residual capacity	The volume of air remaining in the lungs following exhalation during quiet breathing	2300
Total lung capacity	The volume of air in the lungs following a maximal inhalation	5800

remains in the lungs at all times, even between breaths. Note in Fig. 22.11 that the four pulmonary volumes add up to the total lung capacity.

LUNG CAPACITIES

In addition to four pulmonary volumes, there are three pulmonary capacities (one described here). A pulmonary capacity is a combination of pulmonary volumes. For example, **vital capacity** (4600 mL) refers to the combination of tidal volume (500 mL), inspiratory reserve volume (3000 mL), and expiratory reserve volume (1100 mL). The measurement of vital capacity is a commonly used pulmonary function test.

You can measure vital capacity as follows. Take the deepest breath possible. Exhale all the air you possibly can into a spirometer. The spirometer measures the amount of air you forcibly exhale. The amount exhaled should be approximately 4600 mL. In other words, vital capacity is the maximal amount of air exhaled after a maximal inhalation. Vital capacity measures pulmonary function in patients with lung diseases such as emphysema and asthma. A more commonly used clinical term for forced vital capacity is the *forced expiratory volume* (FEV). The FEV is the fraction of the forced vital capacity exhaled in a specific number of seconds. The subscript in FEV_1 indicates the number of seconds that the measurement lasted. The term *peak expiratory flow rate* (PEFR) is another clinically useful respiratory measurement. It is defined as the maximal rate of airflow during expiration. PEFR is measured by a handheld flow meter. Asthmatic patients are taught to measure FEV_1 and/or PEFR in an attempt to manage their asthma. (Other pulmonary capacities are listed in Table 22.1.)

DEAD SPACE

Some of the air you inhale never reaches the alveoli. It stays in the conducting passageways of the trachea, bronchi, and bronchioles. Because this air does not reach the alveoli, it is not available for gas exchange and is said to occupy anatomical dead space. The dead space holds about 150 mL of air. Breathing slowly and deeply increases the amount of well-oxygenated air that reaches the alveoli. Conversely, rapid panting delivers a poorer quality of air to the alveoli because a greater percentage of the inhaled volume of air remains in the anatomical dead space. Therefore, when you encourage your patients to take deep breaths, you are also helping supply the alveoli with well-oxygenated air.

 Re-Think

1. Differentiate between tidal volume and vital capacity.
2. Explain to your postoperative patient why deep breathing is beneficial.
3. Explain to your patient in two to three sentences what to do in order to measure vital capacity.

CONTROL OF BREATHING

Normal breathing is rhythmic and involuntary. For example, as you read, you are breathing effortlessly, about 16 times/min. (The normal respiratory rate ranges from 12 to 20 breaths/min in an adult and from 20 to 40 breaths/min in a child, depending on the age and size of the child.) You do not have to remember to breathe in and out, nor do you have to calculate how deeply to breathe. Fortunately, breathing occurs automatically.

You can voluntarily control breathing up to a point. Hold your breath for 5 seconds. Now try to hold your breath for 3 minutes. You can't do it; you must breathe. The need to breathe means that Sammy should not hold you hostage with his temper tantrums. No matter how good his performance and how long he holds his breath, he will eventually take a really deep breath and live.

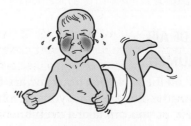

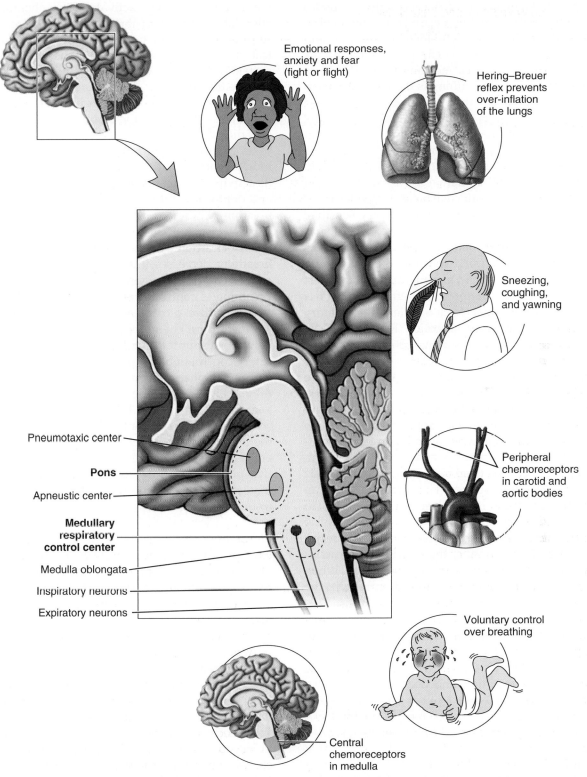

Emotional responses, anxiety and fear (fight or flight)

Hering–Breuer reflex prevents over-inflation of the lungs

Sneezing, coughing, and yawning

Pneumotaxic center

Pons

Apneustic center

Medullary respiratory control center

Medulla oblongata

Inspiratory neurons

Expiratory neurons

Peripheral chemoreceptors in carotid and aortic bodies

Voluntary control over breathing

Central chemoreceptors in medulla

FIG. 22.12 Neural and chemical factors that influence breathing.

NEURAL CONTROL OF BREATHING

How does the body control breathing? The two means of controlling breathing are nervous and chemical mechanisms. The nervous mechanism involves several areas of the brain, the most important being the brain stem. Special groups of neurons are widely scattered throughout the brain stem, particularly in the medulla oblongata and

the pons (Fig. 22.12). The main control center for breathing, in the medulla oblongata, is called the *medullary respiratory control center*. It sets the basic breathing rhythm.

Inhalation occurs when the inspiratory neurons in the medulla oblongata fire, giving rise to nerve impulses. The nerve impulses travel from the medulla oblongata along the phrenic and intercostal nerves to the muscles of respiration. Contraction of the respiratory muscles causes inhalation. Exhalation occurs when the expiratory neurons in the medulla oblongata fire and shut down the inspiratory neurons. This process inhibits the formation of nerve impulses and causes the respiratory muscles to relax. Thus, breathing is the result of the alternate firing of the inspiratory and expiratory neurons.

Although the medulla oblongata is the main control center for breathing, the pons also plays an important role. The pons contains the pneumotaxic center and the apneustic center. These areas in the pons modify and help control breathing patterns. Damage to these areas, as in stroke, produces some distinctive breathing patterns.

The medullary respiratory center is very sensitive to the effects of opioids (narcotics). Narcotics, such as morphine, depress the medulla oblongata and slow respirations. If the narcotic overdose is large enough, respirations may even cease, causing respiratory arrest and death. Because of the profound effect of narcotics on respirations, you must check a patient's respiratory rate before administering narcotics. Respiratory depression is always an issue with narcotic use.

Although the brain stem normally determines the basic rate and depth of breathing, other areas of the brain, including the hypothalamus and cerebral cortex, can also affect breathing patterns. For example, the hypothalamus processes our emotional responses, such as anxiety and fear. The hypothalamus, in turn, stimulates the brain stem and changes the breathing pattern. Rapid breathing, a response to anxiety or fear, is part of the fight-or-flight response. The cerebral cortex can also affect respiration; cortical activity allows us to control the depth and rate of breathing voluntarily.

Several other nervous pathways affect the respiratory system. For example, the vagus nerve carries nerve impulses from the lungs to the brain stem. When the lungs become inflated, nerve impulses travel to the brain stem, inhibiting the inspiratory neurons. This response is called the *Hering-Breuer reflex*. It prevents overinflation of the lungs. The nervous structures not only control breathing patterns but also affect several reflexes associated with the respiratory system. These include coughing, sneezing, and yawning.

> **? Re-Think**
>
> 1. What part of the brain stem exerts the greatest control of respiration?
> 2. What are inspiratory and expiratory neurons?
> 3. Explain how you would add information about inspiratory and expiratory neurons to Fig. 22.9 (flowchart).
> 4. Why will a downward herniation of the brain stem through the foramen magnum cause respiratory arrest?

CHEMICAL CONTROL OF BREATHING

Chemicals dissolved in the blood also affect breathing (see Fig. 22.12), including carbon dioxide, hydrogen ion (which determines the pH), and oxygen. These chemicals are detected by chemosensitive cells called *chemoreceptors*. When activated, the chemoreceptors stimulate the areas of the brain stem concerned with respiration. The two types of chemoreceptors are central chemoreceptors, located in the central nervous system (CNS), and peripheral chemoreceptors, located outside the CNS.

The central chemoreceptors in the medulla oblongata detect changes in the blood concentrations of carbon dioxide and hydrogen ions. If carbon dioxide or hydrogen ion concentration increases, the central chemoreceptors signal the respiratory center to increase its activity. This response causes an increase in the rate and depth of breathing. As a result of the increase in breathing, carbon dioxide is exhaled and the blood levels of carbon dioxide decrease. Conversely, if the blood levels of carbon dioxide and hydrogen ions decrease, breathing decreases, thereby allowing concentrations of both carbon dioxide and hydrogen ions to increase. Breathing is controlled primarily by blood concentrations of carbon dioxide and hydrogen ions, which trigger the central chemoreceptors. (Note the relationship between respiratory activity and blood pH; the respiratory control of blood pH is described in Chapter 25.)

The peripheral chemoreceptors are in the walls of the carotid arteries and the walls of the aorta in the neck and chest region. They are called the *carotid* and *aortic bodies*. (Do not confuse the chemoreceptors with the baroreceptors, which are located in the same general area.) The peripheral chemoreceptors are sensitive primarily to low concentrations of oxygen and increased hydrogen ion concentration. Blood concentrations of oxygen, however, must be very low to trigger the peripheral chemoreceptors. Thus, oxygen plays only a minor role in the regulation of breathing. *Remember: PCO_2 is the major regulator of respirations.*

There are two clinical concerns regarding PCO_2 as the major regulator of respiratory activity:

- The patient with obstructive lung disease who has a chronic elevation of PCO_2
- The dangerous practice of hyperventilation and free diving

As stated previously, PCO_2 is normally the major regulator of respiratory activity. In a patient with a chronic elevation in PCO_2, as in obstructive lung disease, the major regulator of respiratory activity shifts from PCO_2 to PO_2. This patient now breathes in response to declining levels of PO_2. This shift is of clinical concern for the following reason. If the COPD patient's PO_2 declines too acutely, he may require the administration of supplemental O_2 to correct the life-threatening hypoxemia. The critical point: The amount of O_2 must be sufficient to address the hypoxemia but not enough to "knock out" the new respiratory regulator (the low PO_2). If too much O_2 is administered, the PO_2 increases, and the patient's color improves. Unfortunately, he loses his stimulus to breathe and becomes apneic. The apnea causes a drastic increase in PCO_2, which in turn causes CNS depression and

Table 22.2 Common Respiratory Terms

TERM	DESCRIPTION
Apnea	Temporary cessation of breathing
Cheyne-Stokes respirations	An irregular breathing pattern characterized by a series of shallow breaths that gradually increase in depth and rate; the series of increased respirations is followed by breaths that gradually decrease in depth and rate. A period of apnea lasting 10 to 60 seconds follows; the cycle then repeats.
Cyanosis	A bluish color of the skin or mucous membrane caused by a low concentration of oxygen in the blood
Dyspnea	Difficult or labored breathing
Eupnea	Normal, quiet breathing
Hypercapnia	An abnormally high concentration of carbon dioxide in the blood
Hyperventilation	An increase in the rate and depth of respiration. Hyperventilation causes an excess exhalation of carbon dioxide and alkalosis.
Hypocapnia	An abnormally low concentration of carbon dioxide in the blood
Hypoventilation	A decrease in the rate and depth of respiration. Hypoventilation causes a retention of carbon dioxide and acidosis.
Hypoxemia	An abnormally low concentration of oxygen in the blood
Hypoxia	An abnormally low concentration of oxygen in the tissues
Kussmaul breathing	An increase in rate and depth of respiration stimulated by metabolic acidosis
Orthopnea	Difficulty in breathing that is relieved by a sitting-up position
Rales	Crackles (as in snap, crackle, and pop) are small clicking sounds in the lungs that resemble rubbing hair together next to the ear. They are typically inspiratory and are believed to occur when air opens closed air spaces. Rales or crackles can be further described as moist, dry, fine, and coarse.
Rhonchi	Snoring-like sounds that generally occur with obstruction of air in the large airways (trachea and bronchi)
Stridor	High-pitched, wheezelike sound that can be heard on both inhalation and/or exhalation. It is caused by an obstruction of airflow in the upper airway, such as the trachea, or in the back of the throat.
Tachypnea	Rapid breathing
Wheezes	High-pitched sounds typically on exhalation. Wheezing and other abnormal sounds can sometimes be heard without a stethoscope. Wheezing occurs when air is forced through narrow airways. Although commonly associated with asthma, wheezing may also be caused by other obstructing conditions (e.g., tumors, swelling, foreign bodies).

induces a stuporous state progressing to unconsciousness. This latter sequence of events is called "CO_2 narcosis." In response to supplemental O_2 the patient with obstructive lung disease literally "pinks up and dies."

The second point addresses a dangerous practice that is used by free divers to prolong time underwater. Like anyone else, the diver breathes normally in response to increasing PCO_2; as PCO_2 increases, he inhales. Here is the dangerous practice: The diver hyperventilates before the dive in an attempt to lower his PCO_2. The lower the PCO_2, the longer it takes for the PCO_2 to increase to the level that forces him to inhale. He thus prolongs the time he can remain submerged. With excessive hyperventilation, the PCO_2 declines. However, as the diver swims about underwater, he consumes O_2, and his PO_2 declines. The decline in PO_2 may be sufficient to cause hypoxemia and loss of consciousness. The unconscious diver resumes breathing underwater and drowns.

Respiratory patterns change, most often in response to changing body needs and sometimes in response to underlying pathology. Table 22.2 includes respiratory terms commonly used to describe altered respiratory activity.

 Re-Think

1. What is the major chemical regulator of breathing?
2. List and locate the chemoreceptors involved in the chemical regulation of breathing.
3. What stimulates the chemoreceptors?
4. The patient with obstructive lung disease has a chronically elevated PCO_2. Explain why the administration of oxygen can cause him to "pink up and die."

 Sum It Up!

Normal breathing is rhythmic and involuntary. Nervous and chemical mechanisms control breathing. The nervous mechanism involves several areas of the brain, the most important of which is the brain stem. The inspiratory and expiratory neurons in the medulla oblongata determine the basic breathing pattern, which can be modified by the apneustic center and pneumotaxic center in the pons. Chemicals in the blood help control respirations. The central chemoreceptors in the brain are sensitive to carbon dioxide and hydrogen ions, and the peripheral chemoreceptors are sensitive to low blood levels of oxygen and an increase in the hydrogen ion concentration. PCO_2 is the major regulator of respirations. The patient with obstructive lung disease has a chronically elevated PCO_2 and may shift his respiratory drive from PCO_2 to PO_2.

As You Age

1. As a person ages, lung capacity decreases. The decrease in lung capacity is caused by the loss of elasticity of the lung tissue and diminished efficiency of the respiratory muscles. By the age of 70 years, vital capacity has decreased 33%.

2. With aging, many of the protective mechanisms of the respiratory system decline. The ciliary activity of the mucosa decreases, for example, and the phagocytes in the lungs become less effective. As a result, older adults are at greater risk for respiratory infections, especially pneumonia and bronchitis.

3. With age-related structural changes, the number of alveoli diminishes. The resulting decrease in oxygenation ultimately diminishes the capacity for physical activity.

4. Respiratory control is altered; consequently, the PO_2 drops to a lower level, whereas the PCO_2 increases to a higher level.

5. Having breathed a lifetime's worth of various harmful substances (e.g., cigarette smoke, pollutants, pollens, pathogens), the lungs of an older person often show evidence of wear and tear, leading to emphysema and other respiratory disorders.

Medical Terminology and Disorders   Disorders of the Respiratory System

MEDICAL TERM	WORD PARTS	WORD PART MEANING OR DERIVATION	DESCRIPTION
Words			
epistaxis		From a Greek word meaning "to drip"	**Epistaxis** is *a nosebleed.*
eupnea (and other "-pnea" words)	eu-	normal	**Eupnea** means *normal breathing.* To contrast, **bradypnea** (brady- = slow) is slow breathing, whereas **tachypnea** (tachy- = rapid) means rapid breathing. **Apnea** (a- = without) refers to the temporary cessation of breathing, **dyspnea** (dys- = difficult) is difficulty in breathing, and **orthopnea** (ortho- = straight) is the inability to breathe unless in an upright position.
	-pnea	breathing	
inspiration	in-	in	**Inspiration** refers to *breathing in or inhalation;* **expiration** (ex- = out) refers to *breathing out or exhalation.*
	-spir/o	breathing	
oximeter	-ox/i-	oxygen	A pulse **oximeter** is *a mechanical device used to measure oxygen levels in the blood.*
	-meter	measure	
thoracentesis	thorac/o-	chest	A **thoracentesis** is *the incision through the chest wall in order to aspirate fluid or air for therapeutic or diagnostic purposes.*
	-centesis	surgical puncture	
Disorders			
influenza		From an Italian word meaning "influence of the cold"	*A respiratory infection (also known as* **the flu***) that can be caused by several influenza viruses.*
pharyngitis	pharyng/o-	pharynx or throat	*Also called a sore throat; refers to an inflammation of the pharynx or throat.* Approximately 70% of the cases are virally induced. Infection by beta-hemolytic streptococcus is called *strep throat.*
	-itis	inflammation of	
rhinitis	rhin/o-	nose	Refers to the inflammation of the nasal mucosa. **Allergic rhinitis** refers to the response of the nasal mucosa to an allergen. **Seasonal allergic rhinitis** is triggered by high pollen counts. **Perennial allergic rhinitis** is present constantly throughout the year and is triggered by pet dander, cockroaches, and dust mites. **Acute viral rhinitis** is the **common cold** or **acute coryza.**
	-itis	inflammation of	
sinusitis (acute)	sinus/o-	sinus	*Refers to inflammation of the sinuses and is most often due to a swelling and narrowing of passages that drain the sinuses.*
	-itis	inflammation of	
Lower Respiratory Disorders			
asthma		From a Greek word meaning "to breathe hard" or "to pant"	A chronic immune-mediated airway inflammation, characterized by breathlessness, tightness of the chest, dyspnea, wheezing, and coughing. The inflammatory process produces **bronchial hyper-reactivity,** so that milder stimuli, such as exercise, act as triggers.
bronchiectasis	bronch/o-	bronchus	*Refers to the permanent and abnormal dilation of the bronchi.* The characteristic sign of bronchiectasis is a persistent or recurrent cough and the production of purulent sputum.
	-ectasis	stretching or dilation	

Medical Terminology and Disorders   Disorders of the Respiratory System—cont'd

MEDICAL TERM	WORD PARTS	WORD PART MEANING OR DERIVATION	DESCRIPTION
bronchocarcinoma	bronch/o-	bronchus	A common cause of cancer-related deaths in the United States. It is especially common in persons >50 years with a long history of cigarette smoking. More than 90% of lung cancers are bronchogenic and arise from the bronchial epithelium.
	-carcin/o-	cancer	
	-oma	tumor	
tuberculosis	tubercul/o-	tubercle	Commonly called TB. It is known historically as "consumption" and was responsible for the "white plague." Globally TB is responsible for more deaths than any other infectious disease. TB is caused by *Mycobacterium tuberculosis,* or the "acid-fast" bacillus, and is generally spread by droplet infection through inhalation of the pathogen. It usually affects the upper lobes of the lungs, but can infect many other organs and spread or seed throughout the body (miliary TB). Following inhalation, the mycobacteria continue to multiply without any resistance from the host. In about 10 to 20 days a cellular immune response limits the growth and spread of the infection by the formation of a granuloma. The inner core of the granuloma is called the *Ghon tubercle;* it undergoes caseous necrosis, thereby forming a cheesy mass of dead cells and debris. The lesion may also liquefy and drain into surrounding bronchi, causing cavitation. The primary lesion often becomes fibrotic and calcifies. The infection enters a latent period during which mycobacteria become dormant. The activation of the dormant mycobacteria can occur at any time, particularly in an immunosuppressed person and in patients taking steroids.
	-osis	condition of	

Restrictive Lung Disorders

Disorders characterized by decreased "stretchiness" of the lungs and/or chest wall. They are classified as extrapulmonary and intrapulmonary disorders. Extrapulmonary causes of restrictive disorders include disorders of the CNS, the neuromuscular junction, and the chest wall. The intrapulmonary disorders are described as follows.

MEDICAL TERM	WORD PARTS	WORD PART MEANING OR DERIVATION	DESCRIPTION
pleuritis	pleur/o-	pleura	*Also called **pleurisy** and refers to an inflammation of the pleura.* Pleurisy is classified as **dry pleurisy** (fibrinous) and **wet pleurisy** (serofibrinous, with an increased secretion of pleural fluid).
	-itis	inflammation	
pleural effusion	pleur/o-	pleura	*Refers to the accumulation of excess fluid between the two pleural membranes.* (An effusion is an escape of a fluid into a body cavity.) The two types of pleural effusion are the transudative and the exudative.
	-al	pertaining to	
	effusion	From a Latin word meaning "to pour out"	
pneumothorax	pneum/o-	air or lung	*Refers to the accumulation of air within the pleural space, causing the lung to collapse.* A pneumothorax can be opened or closed. An open pneumothorax occurs when the chest wall is penetrated, as in stabbing or gunshot wounds. A **closed pneumothorax** is not caused by an external wound; its cause originates within, as in a ruptured bleb (air bubble or blister) in a person with emphysema, ventilator-induced lung injury, and lung injury from broken ribs. A **tension pneumothorax** is due to a rapid accumulation of air in the pleural space. In addition to air, the lung may also collapse in response to the accumulation of blood in the pleural space (**hemothorax;** hem/o- = blood) or lymph (**chylothorax;** chyl/o- = lymph).
	-thorac/o-	chest	
interstitial lung diseases (ILDs)			*A general term that includes many disorders characterized by inflammation and fibrosis.* The largest group of disorders appears in occupations and environments where there is significant inhalation of dust, gas, or fumes. ILDs also occur in response to infections and as a result of connective tissue disorders such as rheumatoid arthritis and scleroderma. **Sarcoidosis** and **idiopathic pulmonary fibrosis** are the two most common ILDs with an unknown etiology.

Continued

Medical Terminology and Disorders — Disorders of the Respiratory System—cont'd

MEDICAL TERM	WORD PARTS	WORD PART MEANING OR DERIVATION	DESCRIPTION
pneumonia	pneum/o-	air or lung	*Refers to an inflammation of lung tissue.* Pneumonia is the leading cause of death by infectious disease in the United States and has the highest mortality rate of all nosocomial (hospital-acquired) infections. There are many types of pneumonia. Pneumonia may be classified according to its cause: bacterium, virus, fungus, *Mycoplasma,* parasite, and chemical. Pneumonia is also classified according to whether it is community-acquired pneumonia or hospital-acquired pneumonia. **Community-acquired pneumonia (CAP)** is most commonly caused by *Streptococcus pneumoniae* and has its onset in the community or during the first 48 hours of hospitalization. **Hospital-acquired pneumonia (HAP)** occurs after 48 hours of admission to a hospital. The causative organisms of HAP are primarily bacterial, and differ from those involved with CAP. **Aspiration pneumonia** refers to the response of lung tissue to the entry of a foreign substance from the mouth or stomach. It usually occurs in persons with a diminished gag or cough reflex as occurs with loss of consciousness. **Opportunistic pneumonia** refers to pneumonia that develops in immunosuppressed persons. Immunosuppression is common in persons receiving cancer chemotherapy and radiation therapy.
	-ia	condition of	
acute respiratory distress syndrome (ARDS)			**Adult respiratory distress syndrome,** or ARDS, is *a syndrome that leads to multiple organ failure and death.* **Infant respiratory distress syndrome (IRDS)** occurs in the premature infant and is due to the lack of pulmonary surfactants. (IRDS was formerly called **hyaline membrane disease.**)

Chronic Obstructive Pulmonary Diseases

Called COPD and includes diseases (chronic bronchitis and emphysema) characterized by increased airflow obstruction. The major risk factor is cigarette smoking.

MEDICAL TERM	WORD PARTS	WORD PART MEANING OR DERIVATION	DESCRIPTION
emphysema		From a Greek word meaning "puffed up or bloated"	*Characterized by hyperinflation and destruction of the alveoli, obstruction of the small airways, and loss of elasticity of the lung tissue.*
chronic bronchitis	bronch/o-	bronchus	*The excessive production of mucus in the bronchi and the development of a recurrent and productive cough.* Chronic bronchitis is characterized by hyperplasia of the mucus-secreting cells in the trachea and bronchi; this causes narrowing of the airways and alters the functioning of the macrophages.
	-itis	inflammation of	

Vascular Lung Disorders

MEDICAL TERM	WORD PARTS	WORD PART MEANING OR DERIVATION	DESCRIPTION
pulmonary edema			*A collection of fluid within the alveolar and interstitial spaces of the lungs.* The presence of fluid impairs the diffusion of respiratory gases causing dyspnea, hypoxemia, CO_2 retention, and respiratory acidosis.
pulmonary embolism			*The lodging of an embolus or emboli in the pulmonary arterial circulation.* The affected part of the lung is therefore ventilated, but not perfused (with blood). The most common causes of pulmonary embolus are a blood clot arising from a thrombus in the deep veins of the legs or a clot originating in the right side of the heart in a person with atrial fibrillation.
pulmonary artery hypertension			*An elevation in pulmonary artery pressure.* Pulmonary hypertension increases the workload of the right ventricle, causing ventricular hypertrophy and cor pulmonale.

Get Ready for Exams!

Summary Outline

The respiratory system is primarily concerned with the delivery of oxygen to every cell in the body and the elimination of carbon dioxide.

I. **Structures: Organs of the Respiratory System**
   A. Consists of the upper and lower respiratory tracts
   B. Nose and nasal cavities
   1. The nose and nasal cavities warm and humidify inhaled air.
   2. Olfactory receptors are located in the nose.
   3. The nasal cavities receive drainage from the paranasal sinuses and tear ducts.
   C. Pharynx (throat)
   1. The nasopharynx forms a passage for air only.
   2. The oropharynx and laryngopharynx form passageways for both air and food.
   D. Larynx (voicebox)
   1. The larynx is a passage for air.
   2. The epiglottis is the uppermost cartilage and covers the larynx during swallowing.
   E. Trachea (windpipe)
   1. It bifurcates into the right and left bronchi and carries air to and from the lower respiratory structures.
   2. C-shaped rings of cartilage keep the trachea open.
   F. Bronchial tree
   1. The bronchial tree contains the bronchi, bronchioles, and alveoli.
   2. The bronchioles determine the radius of the respiratory air passages and therefore affect the amount of air that can enter the alveoli.
   3. The alveoli are tiny grapelike air sacs surrounded by pulmonary capillaries.
   4. Gas exchange occurs across the thin walls of the alveoli.
   G. Lungs
   1. The right lung has three lobes, and the left lung has only two lobes.
   2. The lungs contain the structures of the lower respiratory tract.
   H. Pleural membranes
   1. The serous membranes in the chest cavity are the parietal pleura and the visceral pleura.
   2. Serous fluid between the pleural membranes prevents friction.
   3. The intrapleural space is located between the visceral and parietal pleurae
   4. For the lungs to remain expanded, the pressure in the intrapleural space must be negative.

II. **Respiratory Function**
   A. Respiration includes three steps: ventilation, exchange of respiratory gases, and transport of respiratory gases in the blood.
   1. Ventilation (breathing)
      a. The two phases of ventilation are inhalation and exhalation.
      b. Ventilation occurs in response to changes in the thoracic volume (Boyle's law).
      c. Thoracic volume changes because of the contraction and relaxation of the respiratory muscles.
      d. The phrenic and intercostal nerves are motor nerves that supply the diaphragm and the intercostal muscles.
      e. Inhalation is an active process (ATP is used during muscle contraction). Unforced exhalation is passive (no ATP used).
   2. Exchange of gases
      a. Exchange of respiratory gases occurs by diffusion across the alveoli and pulmonary capillaries.
      b. Oxygen diffuses from the air in the alveoli into the blood while carbon dioxide diffuses from the blood into the alveoli.
      c. At the cellular layer, oxygen diffuses from the capillaries to the cells. Carbon dioxide diffuses from the cells into the capillaries, where it is transported to the lungs for excretion.
   3. Transport of gases in the blood
      a. Most of the oxygen is transported by the red blood cell (oxyhemoglobin).
      b. The blood transports most carbon dioxide in the form of bicarbonate ion (HCO_3^-).
   B. Amounts of air
   1. Pulmonary volumes
      a. Refers to the amounts of air moved into and out of the lungs
      b. Pulmonary volumes are illustrated in Fig. 22.11 and summarized in Table 22.1.
   2. Vital capacity and anatomical dead space
      a. Lung capacities are combinations of pulmonary volumes.
      b. Vital capacity is the amount of air that can be exhaled after a maximal inhalation.
      c. Anatomical dead space refers to air remaining in the large conducting passageways that is unavailable for gas exchange, approximately 150 mL of air.
   C. Control of breathing
   1. Neural control of breathing
      a. The respiratory center is located in the brain stem.
      b. The medullary respiratory center contains inspiratory and expiratory neurons. Nerve impulses travel along the phrenic and intercostal nerves to the muscles of respiration.
      c. The pneumotaxic center and apneustic center are in the pons. These centers help control the medullary respiratory center to produce a normal breathing pattern.
      d. Two other areas of the brain can affect respirations: the hypothalamus and cerebral cortex.
   2. Chemical control of breathing
      a. Central chemoreceptors are stimulated by carbon dioxide (PCO_2) and [H+].
      b. Peripheral chemoreceptors are sensitive to low concentrations of oxygen and increased hydrogen ion concentration in the blood.

Review Your Knowledge

Matching: Structures of the Respiratory Tract

Directions: Match the following words with their descriptions. Some words may be used more than once.

a. pharynx

b. trachea

c. larynx

d. bronchus

e. paranasal sinuses

f. bronchioles

g. carina

h. alveoli

1. __d__ The trachea branches into a right and left _____

2. __c__ Called the voicebox because it contains the vocal cords

3. __e__ Mucus drains from these mucous membrane-lined structures into the nasal passages.

4. __a__ The respiratory structure connected to the middle ear by the eustachian tube

5. __b__ Large tube supported by rings of cartilage; called the windpipe

6. __h__ The respiratory structure(s) concerned with the exchange of the respiratory gases

7. __h__ Structure closest to the pulmonary capillaries

8. __f__ Tiny respiratory passages that deliver air to the alveoli

9. __d__ Respiratory passage that delivers air to the bronchioles

10. __g__ The point at which the trachea splits; causes intense coughing when stimulated by a suction catheter

Matching: Thoracic Cavity and Ventilation

Directions: Match the following words with their descriptions. Some words may be used more than once.

a. parietal pleura

b. thoracic cavity

c. intrapleural space

d. visceral pleura

e. phrenic

f. diaphragm

1. __d__ Membrane on the outer surface of each lung

2. __b__ Contains the pleural cavity, pericardial cavity, and mediastinum

3. __c__ The lung collapses when air or fluid collects in this space

4. __e__ The motor neuron that innervates the diaphragm

5. __f__ Dome-shaped muscle that is the chief muscle of inhalation

6. __a__ Membrane that lines the walls of the pleural cavity

7. __c__ Must have a negative pressure here

Multiple Choice

1. Ventilation
   a. refers to transport of the respiratory gases by hemoglobin.
   b. is caused by the movement of expired air through the glottis.
   c. consists of inhalation and exhalation.
   d. consists of inhalation and inspiration.

2. The bronchi, bronchioles, and alveoli are
   a. the sites of the exchange of respiratory gases.
   b. upper respiratory structures.
   c. collectively referred to as the bronchial tree.
   d. surrounded by rings of cartilage.

3. The diameter of the bronchioles determines the
   a. amount of mucus secreted by the respiratory membranes.
   b. rate of surfactant secretion.
   c. airflow to the alveoli.
   d. ventilatory rate.

4. Firing of the phrenic nerve
   a. is responsible for exhalation.
   b. causes the diaphragm to contract.
   c. is responsible for the pumping of O_2 from the alveoli into the pulmonary capillaries.
   d. decreases thoracic volume.

5. Which of the following best describes the visceral and parietal pleura?
   a. They line the inner wall of the trachea, bronchi, and bronchioles.
   b. They line the mediastinum.
   c. They are serous membranes.
   d. They are surfactant-secreting membranes.

6. If intrapleural pressure equals or exceeds intrapulmonic pressure,
   a. surfactant secretion ceases.
   b. the lung collapses.
   c. the larynx can no longer generate sound.
   d. air is inhaled.

7. Which of the following does *not* occur on inhalation?
   a. Air moves into the lungs.
   b. Thoracic volume increases.
   c. The diaphragm contracts.
   d. Pressure within the intrapleural space becomes positive.

8. Which of the following is the normal drive for ventilation?
   a. Surfactants
   b. Bicarbonate
   c. Increasing PCO_2
   d. Increasing PO_2

9. A deficiency of surfactants in the neonate
   a. makes it difficult to expand the lungs.
   b. decreases alveolar surface tension.
   c. causes epiglottal swelling and laryngospasm.
   d. makes the central chemoreceptors unresponsive to increasing PCO_2.

10. When the muscles of ventilation relax, which of the following takes place?
    a. Thoracic volume increases, and air moves out of the lungs.
    b. Air is inhaled.
    c. Thoracic volume decreases, and air moves out of the lungs.
    d. Thoracic volume decreases, thereby decreasing intrapulmonic pressure.

11. A person exhales maximally after a maximal inhalation. The amount of air forcibly exhaled is called the
    a. total lung volume.
    b. tidal volume.
    c. residual volume.
    d. vital capacity.

12. The epiglottis
    a. prevents entrance of food and water into the respiratory passages.
    b. is a tube that connects the pharynx and the middle ear.
    c. is located within the pleural cavities.
    d. is innervated by the phrenic nerve.

13. The phrenic nerve
    a. exits the spinal cord at the level of C4 and travels within the cervical plexus.
    b. innervates the epiglottis.
    c. innervates the intercostal muscles.
    d. innervates the accessory muscles of exhalation.

14. Identify the names of the following: voicebox, throat, and windpipe.
    a. Larynx, vocal cords, and trachea
    b. Larynx, epiglottis, and eustachian tube
    c. Larynx, pharynx, trachea
    d. Bronchial tree, carina, and apex

15. Which of the following describes Boyle's law?
    a. An increase in thoracic volume causes an increase in intrapleural pressure.
    b. There is no relationship between intrapulmonic pressure and thoracic volume.
    c. An increase in thoracic volume decreases intrapulmonic pressure.
    d. A decrease in thoracic volume decreases intrapulmonic pressure.

Go Figure

1. Which of the following is correct according to Fig. 22.1?
   a. All respiratory structures distal to the larynx are located within the lung.
   b. The alveoli are the most distal of all bronchial tree structures.
   c. The distal bronchioles have cartilaginous rings similar to the trachea.
   d. Gas exchange occurs across all respiratory structures located in the lung.

2. Which of the following is correct according to Fig. 22.2?
   a. The glottis is also called the true vocal cords.
   b. The epiglottis prevents the entrance of food and water into the respiratory structures.
   c. The esophagus is "covered" by the epiglottis during swallowing.
   d. The larynx is part of both the respiratory system and the digestive system.

3. Which of the following is correct according to Fig. 22.3?
   a. Cartilaginous rings are primarily found in the lower bronchioles and alveoli.
   b. The carina is located at the bifurcation of the bronchus into **the bronchioles.**
   c. The alveoli are the sites of exchange for the respiratory gases.
   d. The trachea and bronchi are wrapped together by the pleural membranes.

4. Which of the following is correct according to Fig. 22.3?
   a. The carina is located within the larynx.
   b. Alveoli are composed of a single layer of cells held open by cartilaginous rings.
   c. The alveoli are proximal to the bronchioles.
   d. The left lung has two lobes, whereas the right lung has three lobes.

5. Which of the following is correct according to Fig. 22.4?
   a. The intrapleural space is formed by the visceral and parietal pleurae.
   b. The pleural membranes surround the **heart.**
   c. The heart and great vessels are located within the pleural cavities.
   d. All thoracic organs are located within the **pleural** cavity.

6. Which of the following is correct according to Fig. 22.5?
   a. Elastic recoil and surface tension want to collapse the lungs.
   b. Surfactants increase surface tension.
   c. Surfactants "work" within the intrapleural space.
   d. The effect of elastic recoil is to keep the alveoli open.

7. Which of the following is correct according to Fig. 22.6?
   a. The lung collapses when the intrapulmonic pressure exceeds intrapleural pressure.
   b. The lung collapses when intrapulmonic pressure exceeds atmospheric pressure.
   c. The lung collapses when intrapleural pressure is lower than intrapulmonic pressure.
   d. Pressure is normally negative in the space between the visceral and parietal pleurae.

8. Which of the following is correct according to Fig. 22.7?
   a. When volume increases, pressure increases.
   b. When volume decreases, pressure decreases.
   c. There is no relationship between volume and pressure.
   d. When volume increases, pressure decreases.

9. Which of the following is correct according to Fig. 22.8?
   a. Air moves into the lungs when thoracic volume decreases.
   b. Air moves out of the lungs when thoracic volume increases.
   c. Air moves out of the lungs when the diaphragm and intercostal muscles contract.
   d. Intrapulmonic pressure decreases when the diaphragm contracts; air moves into the lungs.

10. Which of the following is correct according to Fig. 22.10?
    a. Tissue PO_2 is 95 mm Hg.
    b. Venous PO_2 is 95 mm Hg, whereas PCO_2 is 45 mm Hg.
    c. Aortic blood PO_2 and PCO_2 are both 95 mm Hg.
    d. Arterial PO_2 is higher than tissue PO_2.

11. Which of the following is correct according to Fig. 22.11?
    a. Tidal volume plus vital capacity equals the total lung capacity.
    b. Vital capacity is equal to the sum of the resting tidal volume and expiratory reserve volume.
    c. Vital capacity is equal to the tidal volume, inspiratory reserve volume, and expiratory reserve volume.
    d. Expiratory reserve volume is the same as residual volume.

12. Which of the following is correct according to Fig. 22.12?
    a. Inspiratory and expiratory neurons are located within the respiratory control center of the medulla oblongata.
    b. All respiratory control is located within the brain stem.
    c. All respiratory control is voluntary.
    d. The medulla oblongata is the only brain stem structure that affects respirations.

Digestive System

Objectives

1. Discuss the basic anatomy and physiology of the digestive system, including the following:
   - List four functions of the digestive system.
   - Explain the processes of digestion and absorption.
   - Describe the four layers, nerves, and membranes of the digestive tract.
2. Describe the structure and functions of the organs and accessory organs of the digestive tract.
3. Explain the physiology of digestion and absorption, including the following:
   - Describe the effects of amylases, proteases, and lipases.

- Describe the role of bile in the digestion of fats.
- Describe the effects of the hormones gastrin, cholecystokinin, and secretin.
4. Discuss nutrition concepts, including the following:
   - Describe five categories of nutrients.
   - Discuss the importance of a balanced diet.

Key Terms

absorption (p. 433)
alimentary canal (p. 433)
amylase (p. 449)
appendix (p. 442)
bile (p. 447)
biliary tree (p. 447)
cecum (p. 442)
cholecystokinin (p. 441)
chyle (p. 441)
chyme (p. 440)
colon (p. 442)
common bile duct (p. 447)
deglutition (p. 437)
digestion (p. 433)

digestive tract (p. 433)
disaccharides (p. 449)
duodenum (p. 441)
emulsification (p. 450)
enteric nervous system (p. 435)
esophagus (p. 438)
gallbladder (p. 448)
gastric juice (p. 438)
gastrin (p. 440)
gastrointestinal (GI) tract (p. 433)
glycemic index (p. 453)
ileum (p. 441)
jejunum (p. 441)
lipase (p. 450)

liver lobule (p. 447)
mastication (p. 435)
microbiota (p. 444)
minerals (p. 455)
pancreas (p. 448)
peristalsis (p. 434)
protease (p. 449)
salivary glands (p. 433)
secretin (p. 441)
segmentation (p. 434)
stomach (p. 438)
villus (p. 441)
vitamins (p. 454)

Most of us have no difficulty eating our way through the Thanksgiving holiday turkey dinner, although the hours after the feeding frenzy can be a digestive challenge. Our digestive systems work very efficiently to digest and absorb as much of the food as possible. Before the holiday is over, the turkey dinner will be a part of every cell in your body.

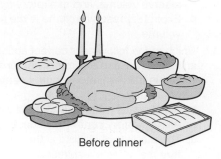

Before dinner

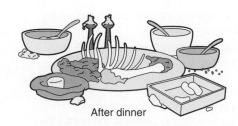

After dinner

Cells require a constant supply of nutrients and energy. Food is their source. The purpose of the digestive system is to break down or digest the food into particles that are small and simple enough to be absorbed. Thus, the digestive system ingests food, digests it, absorbs the end-products of digestion, and eliminates the waste. The study of the digestive tract is called *gastroenterology*.

OVERVIEW OF THE DIGESTIVE SYSTEM

The digestive tract and the accessory organs of digestion make up the digestive system. The **digestive tract**, also called the **alimentary canal** or the **gastrointestinal (GI) tract**, is a hollow tube extending from the mouth to the anus (Fig. 23.1). The structures of the digestive or GI tract include the mouth, pharynx, esophagus, stomach, small intestine, large intestine, rectum, and anus.

The accessory organs of digestion include the **salivary glands**, teeth, liver, gallbladder, and pancreas. The salivary glands empty their secretions into the mouth;

the liver, gallbladder, and pancreas empty their secretions into the small intestine.

DIGESTION AND ABSORPTION

Digestion is the process by which food is broken down into smaller particles suitable for absorption. Digestion takes place within the digestive tract. **Absorption** is the process whereby the end-products of digestion move across the walls of the digestive tract into the blood and lymph for distribution throughout the body.

The two forms of digestion are mechanical and chemical. Mechanical digestion is the breakdown of large food particles into smaller pieces by physical means. This process is usually achieved by chewing and by the mashing actions of the muscles in the digestive tract. Chemical digestion is the chemical alteration of food. For example, a protein is chemically digested into amino acids. Digestive enzymes, stomach acid, and bile accomplish chemical digestion.

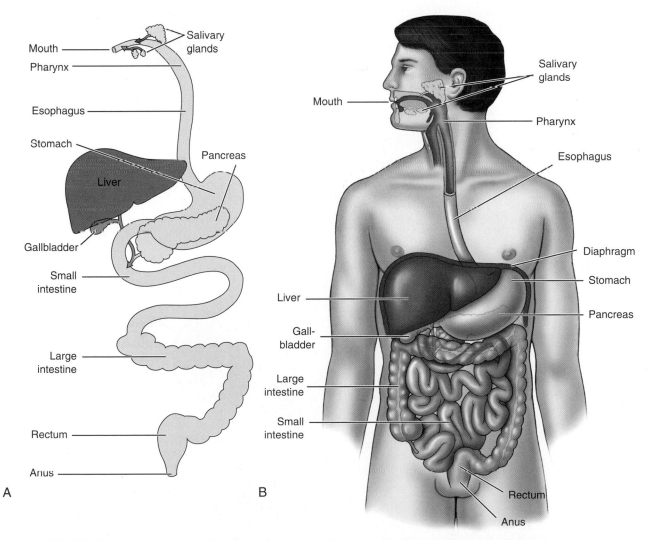

FIG. 23.1 The digestive system. (A) Hollow tube from mouth to anus. (B) Anatomical arrangement of organs of the digestive system.

The end-products of digestion are absorbed by moving across the lining of the digestive tract into the blood and lymph and eventually reach every cell in the body. The food that cannot be digested and absorbed is eliminated from the body as feces. Elimination of waste products is the last stage of the digestive process.

> ### ? Re-Think
> 1. Differentiate between digestion and absorption.
> 2. Differentiate between mechanical and chemical digestion.

LAYERS AND MEMBRANES OF THE DIGESTIVE TRACT

Although modified for specific functions in different organs, the wall of the digestive tract has a similar structure throughout its length (Fig. 23.2). The wall of the digestive tract has four layers: the mucosa, the submucosa, the muscle layer, and the serosa.

MUCOSA

The innermost layer of the digestive tract, the mucosa, consists of the mucous membrane, a small amount of connective tissue and smooth muscle. In parts of the digestive tract, especially the small intestine, the mucosa is folded so as to increase the surface area for absorption. Glands secrete mucus, digestive enzymes, and hormones. In general, the mucosa is concerned with digestion and absorption.

SUBMUCOSA

A thick layer of loose connective tissue, the submucosa, lies beneath the mucosa. The submucosa contains blood vessels, nerves, glands, and lymphatic vessels.

MUSCLE LAYER

The third layer of the digestive tract is the muscle layer. Two layers of smooth muscles are an inner circular layer and an outer longitudinal layer. The muscle layer is responsible for several types of movements in the digestive tract. Alternate contraction and relaxation of the stomach muscles digest the food mechanically and mix the particles with digestive juices. This type of muscle activity is called **segmentation**.

A second type of muscle movement is **peristalsis** (pair-i-STAL-sis), a rhythmic alternating contraction and relaxation of the muscles that pushes the food in a forward direction through the digestive tract. Peristalsis moves food in the same way that toothpaste squirts

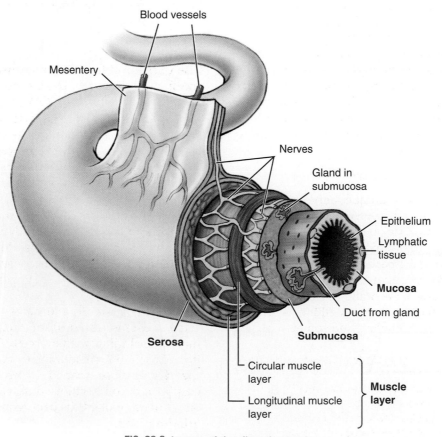

FIG. 23.2 **Layers of the digestive tract.**

from a tube, as illustrated here by G.I. Joe. The tooth-paste squirts in a forward direction because the bottom of the tube is squeezed. Peristaltic waves squeeze the food from behind and push it forward. Peristaltic waves are stimulated by the presence of food.

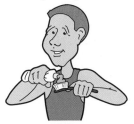

What happens if peristalsis stops? After surgery, intestinal peristalsis is often sluggish and may actually cease. This condition is called *paralytic ileus*. When this happens, food, gas, and liquid accumulate within the digestive tract, creating a life-threatening situation that demands immediate intervention.

Muscle activity is also responsible for other types of movement, such as swallowing and defecation (the elimination of waste from the digestive tract).

SEROSA

The outermost lining of the digestive tract is the serosa. The serosa extends as peritoneal membranes: the mesentery, mesocolon, and omentum. These form large, flat, folded structures that perform several important functions. They help anchor the digestive organs in place; carry blood vessels, lymph vessels, and nerves to the abdominal organs; and help restrict the spread of infection in the abdominal cavity.

The peritoneal membranes, located behind the digestive organs, are called the *mesentery* and *mesocolon*. When located in front of the organs, they are called the *greater* and *lesser omentum*. The greater omentum is a double layer of peritoneum that contains a considerable amount of fat and resembles an apron draped over the abdominal organs.

INNERVATION OF THE DIGESTIVE TRACT

The digestive tract has a unique nervous network called the **enteric nervous system** (ENS). The ENS regulates GI (gut) motility and secretion; its activity is modulated by autonomic nerves, especially the parasympathetic (vagal) fibers. Some refer to the gut as a second brain. Why? Because so many of the neurotransmitters that affect the brain also affect the gut. Ever have a "gut" feeling that something is wrong? Your "gut brain" might be telling you something!

? Re-Think

1. What are the four layers of the digestive tract?
2. What are the two types and functions of muscle movement achieved by gastrointestinal smooth muscle?
3. What is the role of the enteric nervous system?

 Sum It Up!

The digestive system is made up of a hollow tube (digestive tract alimentary canal, gastrointestinal tract) that extends from the mouth to the anus and the accessory organs of digestion. The digestive system has four functions: ingestion, digestion, absorption, and elimination. The wall of the digestive tract has four layers: mucosa, submucosa, muscle layer, and serosa. The muscle layer enables the digestive tract to mix, mash, and move food through the tract; the mixing and mashing are achieved by segmentation while the forward movement of food is caused by peristalsis. The enteric nervous system regulates gastrointestinal (gut) motility and secretion; its activity is modulated by autonomic nerves, especially the parasympathetic (vagal) fibers. Large, flat peritoneal membranes in the abdominal cavity help anchor the digestive organs in place.

STRUCTURES AND ORGANS

MOUTH

The digestive tract begins with the mouth, also known as the *oral cavity*. Food is ingested into the mouth where digestion begins immediately. The mouth is lined with mucous membrane and contains structures that assist in the digestive process. These include the teeth, tongue, salivary glands, and several other structures. The buccal cavity, as part of the oral cavity, refers to the area between the gums and the cheek or lips.

TEETH

The purpose of the teeth is to chew food and to begin mechanical digestion. During the process of chewing, or **mastication** (mass-ti-KAY-shun), the teeth break down large pieces of food into smaller pieces. Once moistened by the secretions in the mouth, the small pieces of food are easily swallowed.

During a lifetime, a person will have two sets of teeth: deciduous and permanent. The deciduous (deh-SID-yoo-us) teeth are also called *baby teeth* or *milk teeth*. There are 20 deciduous teeth. They begin to appear at the age of 6 months and are generally in place by the age of 2½ years. Between the ages of 6 and 12 years, these teeth are pushed out and replaced by the permanent teeth. There are 32 permanent teeth (Fig. 23.3A).

Note the positions and names of the teeth: the incisors, cuspids (canines), premolars (bicuspids), and molars, including wisdom teeth. The shape and location of each tooth determine its function. For example, the sharp, chisel-shaped incisors and cone-shaped cuspids are front teeth used to tear or grasp food. The larger flatter molars, the back teeth, are more suited for grinding food.

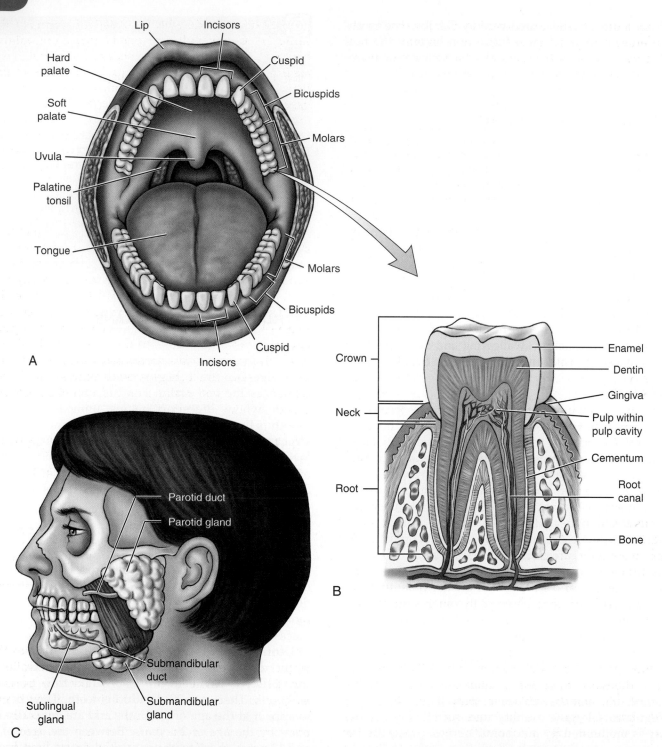

FIG. 23.3 Oral cavity. (A) Structures in the mouth. (B) Longitudinal view of a tooth. (C) Location of the salivary glands.

A tooth has three parts: the crown, the neck, and the root (see Fig. 23.3B). The crown of the tooth is above the level of the gum, or gingiva (JIN-ji-vah), and is covered with hard, brittle enamel. The neck connects the crown with the root of the tooth. The root is that part of the tooth embedded in the jawbone. The outer surface of the root is anchored to the periodontal membrane by cementum. The bulk of the tooth consists of a bonelike material called *dentin*. Nerves, blood vessels, and connective tissue, called *pulp,* penetrate the dentin through the pulp cavity and supply the tooth with sensation and nutrients. As the pulp cavity extends into the root, it is called the *root canal.* The *periodontium* is the name given to the tissues that surround the teeth and include the gums, soft tissue, and bone. Gingivitis and stomatitis are mouth conditions that are often drug induced. Both cause considerable discomfort and interfere with nutrition. Gingivitis is inflammation of the gums. Stomatitis refers to inflammation or ulcers of the oral mucosa of the mouth area.

Do You Know...

The Meaning of These Tooth Words?

Four back molars can appear later in life (at 17 to 25 years of age, when you have "become wiser") and are therefore called *wisdom teeth*. In many individuals, the wisdom teeth remain embedded in the jawbone and are said to be impacted. Because impacted teeth serve no function and are often a source of infection, they are frequently removed.

Lacking some naming creativity, the canine teeth are commonly called *eyeteeth* because they are positioned under the eyes. To be "long in the tooth" is a not-too-flattering reference to advanced age; the gums recede with aging, thereby exposing more of the tooth.

TONGUE

The tongue is a muscular organ that occupies the floor of the mouth and serves two major roles in the digestive process. First, it facilitates chewing and swallowing by continuously repositioning the food in the mouth. As swallowing begins, the tongue pushes the food, which it has molded into a ball-like mass called a *bolus* (BOH-luss), toward the pharynx. Second, the tongue contains the taste buds and allows us to taste food.

If you look under your tongue in the mirror, you will notice two structures. One is a small piece of mucous membrane called the *frenulum*, which anchors the tongue to the floor of the mouth. The second structure is an extensive capillary network that provides the sublingual (under the tongue) area with a rich supply of blood. Because the blood supply is so good, medications are absorbed rapidly when administered sublingually.

SALIVARY GLANDS

Three pairs of salivary glands secrete their contents into the mouth: the parotid glands, the submandibular glands, and the sublingual glands (see Fig. 23.3C). The parotid glands are the largest of the three glands and lie below and anterior to the ears. These are the glands infected by the mumps virus, which results in a chipmunk-like appearance. The submandibular glands are located on the floor of the mouth. The sublingual glands are located under the tongue and are the smallest of the salivary glands. The salivary glands are exocrine glands that secrete saliva (from a Greek word meaning "spittle"), a watery fluid that contains mucus and one digestive enzyme called *salivary amylase*, or *ptyalin*. Approximately 1 L of saliva is secreted each day. Saliva reaches the mouth by way of tiny ducts. The most important function of saliva is to soften and moisten food and thereby facilitate swallowing.

What does one do with 1 L of saliva? Normally, the saliva is swallowed. If someone is unable to swallow, however, the saliva must be suctioned so that it is not aspirated into the lungs. This problem occurs in patients who experience inflammation, tumors, or surgery of structures of the upper digestive tract.

Occasionally, one of the salivary ducts becomes obstructed by a stone. The condition is called *sialolithiasis* (si-ah-lo-li-THI-ah-sis) and is characterized by intense pain on eating when the salivary juices start to flow.

OTHER STRUCTURES WITHIN THE MOUTH

The hard and soft palates form the roof of the mouth (see Fig. 23.3A). The anterior hard palate separates the oral cavity from the nasal passages, and the posterior soft palate separates the oral cavity from the nasopharynx. The soft palate extends toward the back of the oral cavity as the uvula (YOO-vyoo-lah), the V-shaped piece of soft tissue that hangs down from the upper back region of the mouth. The uvula prevents food and water from entering the nasal passages during the act of swallowing. The palatine tonsils are masses of lymphatic tissue located along the sides of the posterior oral cavity (see Chapter 20).

Re-Think

1. Explain how the teeth, tongue, and salivary glands begin the process of digestion.
2. List the three salivary glands.
3. List the three parts of a tooth.
4. A patient is taking three medications: one by the oral route, the second by the buccal route, and the third to be administered sublingually. Explain the difference between the three routes of administration.

PHARYNX

The tongue pushes the food from the mouth into the pharynx (throat). The pharynx is involved in swallowing (**deglutition** [DEE-gloo-tih-shin]). The three parts of the pharynx are the nasopharynx, the oropharynx, and the laryngopharynx (Fig. 23.4). Only the oropharynx and laryngopharynx are part of the digestive tract.

The act of swallowing normally directs food from the pharynx (throat) into the esophagus, a long tube that empties into the stomach. Food does not normally enter the nasal or respiratory passages because swallowing temporarily closes off the openings to both. For example, during swallowing, the soft palate moves toward the opening to the nasopharynx. Similarly, the laryngeal opening is closed when the trachea moves upward and allows the epiglottis to cover the entrance to the respiratory passages. You can see this process as the up-and-down movement of the Adam's apple, part of the larynx or voicebox.

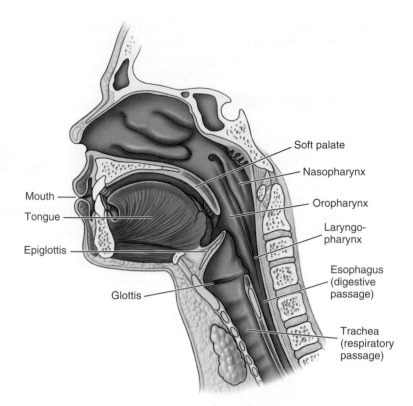

Mouth

Tongue

Epiglottis

Glottis

Soft palate

Nasopharynx

Oropharynx

Laryngo-
pharynx

Esophagus
(digestive
passage)

Trachea
(respiratory
passage)

FIG. 23.4 Eating and swallowing structures: from mouth to pharynx to esophagus.

ESOPHAGUS

The **esophagus** (eh-SOF-ah-gus) is the food tube that carries food from the pharynx to the stomach (see Fig. 23.1). The esophagus, which is approximately 10 inches (25 cm) in length, descends through the chest cavity and penetrates the diaphragm. The act of swallowing pushes the bolus of food into the esophagus. The presence of food in the esophagus stimulates peristaltic activity and causes the food to move through the esophagus into the stomach. Glands within the mucosa of the esophagus secrete mucus, which lubricates the bolus and facilitates its passage along the esophagus.

The two esophageal sphincters are the pharyngoesophageal sphincter located at the top of the esophagus, and the gastroesophageal, or lower esophageal sphincter (LES), located at the base of the esophagus (Fig. 23.5). Swallowing pushes food past the pharyngoesophageal sphincter into the esophagus. Relaxation of the LES keeps the base of the esophagus open, thereby allowing the passage of food into the stomach. When contracted, however, the LES closes the base of the esophagus, thereby preventing reflux, or regurgitation, of acidic stomach contents back into the esophagus.

In some persons, a poorly functioning LES allows for reflux of stomach contents into the esophagus. The condition is called *gastroesophageal reflux disease* (GERD) and is characterized by a burning sensation called *heartburn* or *pyrosis*. The burning sensation is a result of the high acidity of stomach contents.

 Re-Think

1. Explain how food and water are directed into the esophagus during the act of swallowing.
2. What structures are connected by the esophagus?
3. What is the location and purpose of the LES?

STOMACH

WHAT IT DOES

The **stomach** is a pouchlike organ that lies in the upper left part of the abdominal cavity under the diaphragm (see Fig. 23.1) and receives food from the esophagus. It performs five important digestive functions:

- Secretion of **gastric juice**, which includes digestive enzymes, hydrochloric acid (HCl), and intrinsic factor.
- Digestion of food. The stomach plays an important role in the mechanical digestion (mixing and mashing) of food. Chemical digestion is limited.
- Absorption of small quantities of water and dissolved substances. The stomach is not well suited for an absorptive role, so absorption is limited. It can, however, absorb alcohol efficiently. Therefore, the consumption of alcoholic beverages on an empty stomach can quickly increase blood levels of alcohol.
- Secretion of gastric hormones.
- Regulation of the rate at which the partially digested food is delivered to the small intestine. This is the most important function of the stomach.

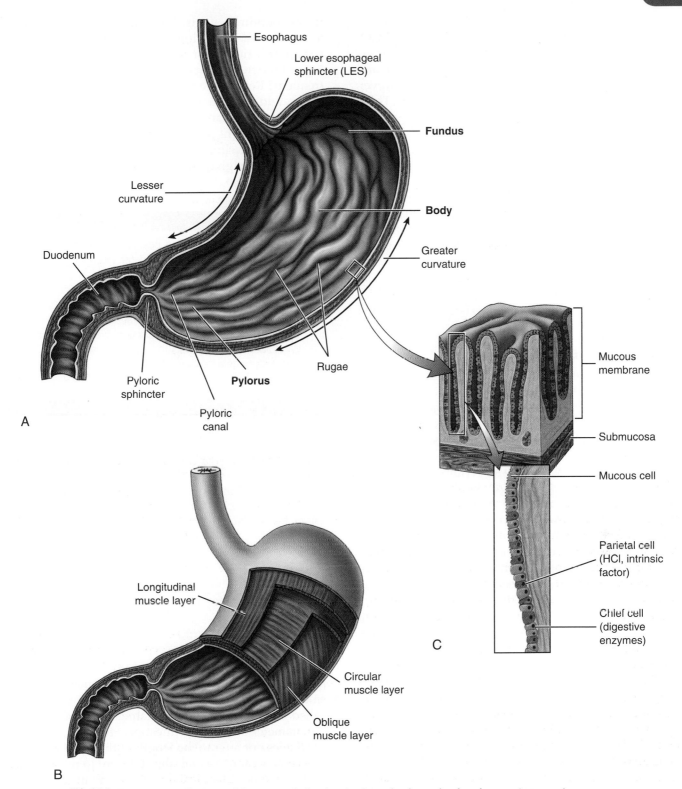

FIG. 23.5 Stomach. (A) Regions of the stomach: fundus, body, and pylorus; landmarks: greater curvature, lesser curvature. (B) Three muscle layers of the stomach. (C) Mucosa of the stomach, showing the mucus, parietal, and chief cells.

REGIONS OF THE STOMACH

The major regions of the stomach include the fundus, the body, and the pylorus (see Fig. 23.5A). The pylorus, which literally means "gatekeeper," continues as the pyloric canal. A pyloric sphincter is located at the end of the pyloric canal and performs two functions. First, the sphincter remains closed most of the time and therefore holds the food in the stomach long enough to allow the stomach to mix and mash its contents into a paste. Second. The pyloric sphincter helps regulate the rate at which gastric contents are delivered to the small intestine. Other landmarks of the stomach include the greater curvature and the lesser curvature.

How big can your stomach get? The empty stomach lies in thick accordion-like folds called *rugae* (ROO-gay). The rugae allow the stomach to expand. For example, when the stomach is empty, it is the size and shape of a sausage. Following a large meal, however, the stomach may expand to approximately 1 L. Think of your turkey dinner sitting in your very expanded stomach—it feels like you are going to pop! Sadly, the stomach can keep stretching in response to continued overeating.

MUSCLES OF THE STOMACH

The stomach has three layers of muscles that lie in three directions: longitudinal, oblique, and circular (see Fig. 23.5B). This arrangement allows the stomach to churn and mix the food with gastric juice to create a thick, pastelike mixture called **chyme** (kime). The stomach is your personal organ grinder. The muscles of the stomach also generate peristaltic waves that squeeze the food toward the pylorus.

GLANDS OF THE STOMACH

The mucous membranes of the stomach contain two types of glands: exocrine and neuroendocrine glands (see Fig. 23.5C). The exocrine glands contain three types of secretory cells: (1) the mucous cells, which secrete mucus; (2) the chief cells, which secrete digestive enzymes; and (3) the parietal cells, which secrete HCl and intrinsic factor. The secretions of the gastric glands are called *gastric juice*. An interesting note: the HCl in gastric juice is strong enough to eat the varnish off furniture. So why doesn't the acid eat a hole in your stomach? In addition to the gastric juice, other cells secrete thicker mucus and bicarbonate that adheres closely to the stomach lining. This secretion forms a protective coating for the stomach lining and prevents the acidic gastric juices from digesting the stomach itself. This also explains the burning sensation caused by the reflux of acidic chyme into the base of the esophagus. Unlike the stomach, the esophagus does not have this protective bicarbonate coating.

One of the neuroendocrine glands, the G cells, secretes **gastrin,** which is released in response to vagus nerve stimulation and the presence of amino acids and small peptides in the stomach. Gastrin stimulates secretion of the gastric glands.

VOMITING

Vomiting, or emesis, is and is not a stomach event. It is a stomach event in that the stomach is emptied on vomiting. However, vomiting is not a stomach event in terms of mechanism. Vomiting is part of the emetic reflex controlled by the medulla oblongata. In response to stimuli sent to the medullary vomiting center, the LES relaxes, and the diaphragm and abdominal muscles contract, thereby compressing the stomach and ejecting its contents. You should become a keen observer of vomited stomach contents and its surrounding events. For example, you will want to know if the vomiting was preceded by nausea or vertigo (dizziness), or related to food or drug intake. Record the frequency—is it an isolated event or more frequent? Record the amount and contents, including drugs, and note the color and any evidence of blood (blood that is changed because of the stomach acid can have a bright red or coffee grounds–like appearance). A lot of clinically valuable information can be obtained through your observations. Don't rush to flush!

Re-Think

1. Locate the following structures: LES, fundus of the stomach, pylorus, pyloric sphincter, and the greater and lesser curvatures of the stomach.
2. Describe the muscular layers and arrangement of the muscles of the stomach enabling it to generate chyme.
3. List four gastric glands and their secretions.
4. What is the most important function of the stomach?
5. What "burns" the base of the esophagus in patients with esophageal reflux (GERD)?

Sum It Up!

The mouth begins the process of mechanical and chemical digestion. The bolus of food is swallowed and moves from the mouth, through the pharynx and esophagus, and into the stomach. The stomach continues the digestive process by mixing the food with gastric juice and mashing it into a paste called chyme. Gastric juice contains the secretions from the gastric glands: mucus, pepsinogen (protease), HCl, intrinsic factor, and a hormone called gastrin. Digestion within the stomach is primarily mechanical; chemical digestion is minimal, as is absorption. An important function of the stomach is to deliver chyme to the duodenum (small intestine) at the proper rate.

SMALL INTESTINE

LOCATION AND PARTS

An acidic chyme is ejected by the stomach into the small intestine (see Fig. 23.1). The small intestine is called "small" because its diameter is smaller than the diameter of the large intestine. However, the word *small* does not refer to the length of the small intestine; it is considerably longer (about 20 feet [6 m]) than the large intestine (5 feet [1.5 m]). The small intestine is located in the central and lower abdominal cavity and is held in place by the mesentery. The small intestine performs three functions:

- It receives chyme from the stomach and digestive juices from the liver (bile) and pancreas (digestive enzymes); the process of digestion is completed within the small intestine
- It absorbs the end-products of digestion and key substances such as iron and vitamins.
- It moves the unabsorbed content into the large intestine.

The small intestine consists of three parts: the duodenum, the jejunum, and the ileum. Although the stock market can make your guts churn, it can also help you remember the parts of the small intestine:

Dow	Duodenum
Jones	Jejunum
Industrials	Ileum

SEGMENTS OF THE SMALL INTESTINE

The **duodenum** (doo-oh-DEE-num) is the first segment of the small intestine. The word *duodenum* literally means "twelve" (*duo* means "two"; *denum* means "ten"). In this case, the reference is to the width of 12 fingers. Thus, the length of the duodenum is 12 fingerbreadths or approximately 10 inches (25 cm).

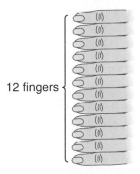

12 fingers

Why is the duodenum considered the meeting point for digestion? In addition to receiving chyme from the stomach, the duodenum also receives secretions from several accessory organs of digestion such as the liver, gallbladder, and pancreas (see Fig. 23.1). These secretions, in addition to those from the mouth, stomach, and duodenum, are responsible for the digestion of all food. Most digestion and absorption occur in the duodenum and the first third of the jejunum, the next segment. *To repeat: Most digestion and absorption occur in the duodenum and first third of the jejunum.*

The **jejunum** (jeh-JOO-num) is the second segment of the small intestine. It is approximately 8 feet (2.4 m) in length. Digestion and absorption of food occur in the first third of the jejunum.

 Do You Know...

What Borborygmus Is?

"Gurgle, gurgle," growls your guts. How embarrassing is this as you look around the room! This gurgling sound that eminently emanates from your intestines is caused by the rapid movement of gas and liquid through the intestines. The sounds are louder and more noticeable when you are hungry because you tend to salivate more and swallow more air. "Gurgle, gurgle" is called *borborygmus* (bor-bor-IG-mus) and comes from the Greek word meaning "to rumble." Despite this long and ugly name, borborygmus is embarrassing but normal.

The **ileum** (IL-ee-um) is the third segment of the small intestine and is approximately 12 feet (3.6 m) in length. It extends from the jejunum distally to the ileocecal sphincter. The ileocecal sphincter prevents the reflux of contents from the cecum (first part of the large intestine) back into the ileum. The function of the ileum is to complete the process of absorption of digestive end-products, vitamin B_{12}, and bile salts. The lining of the ileum contains numerous patches of lymphatic tissue called *Peyer's patches* that participate in the immune response to a heavy bacterial load. The ileum performs another important role as an "ileal brake." Through a reflex mechanism, the presence of fatty acids in the ileum slows gut motility. What you eat affects gut motility and secretions.

THE WALL OF THE SMALL INTESTINE AND ABSORPTION

What is so special about the wall of the small intestine? The wall of the small intestine forms circular folds with finger-like projections called *villi* (sing., **villus**) (Fig. 23.6). The epithelial cells of each villus form extensions called *microvilli*. The large number of villi and microvilli increases the amount of digested food and water that can be absorbed.

What is a villus? Each villus consists of a layer of epithelial tissue that surrounds a network of blood capillaries and a lymphatic capillary called a *lacteal* (see Fig. 23.6B). The villus absorbs the end-products of digestion from the small intestine into the blood capillaries or the lacteal. The capillary blood within the villus drains into the hepatic portal system and then into the liver. Thus, the end-products of carbohydrate and protein digestion first go to the liver for processing before being distributed throughout the body. The end-products of fat digestion enter the lacteal, forming a milky-white lymph called **chyle** (kile). The chyle empties directly into the lymphatic system and eventually into the general circulation. (Do not confuse the words *chyle* and *chyme*.)

In addition to forming a site for absorption, the cells of the intestinal wall also secrete several digestive enzymes and two important hormones: **secretin** and **cholecystokinin** (CCK). Table 23.1 lists the major intestinal enzymes and hormones.

Peristalsis and Absorption in the Small Intestine

Like other parts of the digestive tract, peristalsis moves its digestive contents through the small intestines. The peristalsis in the small intestine, however, is unique. Instead of merely pushing the digestive contents forward, the muscle activity also generates a swishing and swaying motion. This motion continually washes the nutrient-rich digestive contents across the villi, thereby increasing absorption. That which is not absorbed is moved forward by peristaltic waves toward the large intestine.

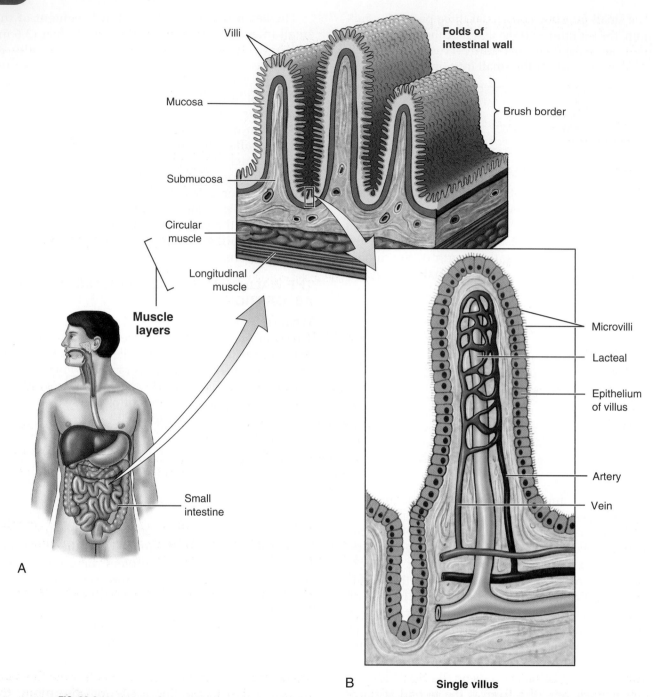

FIG. 23.6 Small intestine. (A) Folds of the intestinal wall. (B) Single villus showing the blood capillaries and the lacteal.

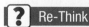 Re-Think

1. List the three segments of the small intestine.
2. Where does most digestion and absorption take place?
3. Describe the structure and function of the villus.
4. What is the role of the lacteal in absorption?

LARGE INTESTINE

The large intestine is approximately 5 feet (1.5 m) long and extends from the ileocecal sphincter to the anus (Fig. 23.7). The cecum, colon, rectum, and anal canal are parts of the large intestine.

SEGMENTS OF THE LARGE INTESTINE

The first part of the large intestine is the **cecum**. The cecum is located in the right lower quadrant (RLQ) and ascends on the right side as the ascending **colon**. Attached to the cecum is the **appendix,** a wormlike structure that contains lymphatic tissue and is a source of immune cells.

Occasionally, the appendix becomes inflamed, causing appendicitis, and must be surgically removed through an appendectomy. Failure to remove an inflamed appendix may cause it to rupture, discharging fecal material into the peritoneal cavity and causing a life-threatening infection called *peritonitis*. RLQ pain? Think appendicitis.

Table 23.1 Major Secretions of the Digestive System

NAME	SOURCE	DIGESTIVE FUNCTION
Enzymes		
Salivary Enzyme		
Amylase (ptyalin)	Salivary glands	Begins carbohydrate digestion to disaccharides
Gastric Enzyme		
Pepsin	Gastric glands	Begins digestion of protein
Pancreatic Enzymes		
Amylase	Pancreas	Digests polysaccharides to disaccharides
Lipase	Pancreas	Digests fats to fatty acids and glycerol
Proteases	Pancreas	Digests proteins to peptides and amino acids
Trypsin		
Chymotrypsin		
Carboxypeptidase		
Intestinal Enzymes		
Peptidases	Intestine	Digests peptides to amino acids
Disaccharidases	Intestine	Digests disaccharides to monosaccharides
Sucrase		
Lactase		
Maltase		
Lipase	Intestine	Digests fats to fatty acids and glycerol
Enterokinase	Intestine	Activates trypsinogen to trypsin
Digestive Aids		
Hydrochloric acid	Stomach	Helps unravel proteins; kills microorganisms that are ingested in food
Intrinsic factor	Stomach	Assists in the absorption of vitamin B_{12}
Bile	Liver	Emulsifies fats; aids in the absorption of fatty acids and the fat-soluble vitamins (A, D, E, K)
Mucus	Entire digestive tract	Softens food; lubricates food and eases its passage through the digestive tract. Forms a mucus barrier for protection against acid erosion
Hormones		
Gastrin	Stomach	Stimulates gastric glands to secrete gastric juice; increases gastric motility
Cholecystokinin	Duodenum	Stimulates the gallbladder to contract and release bile; stimulates release of pancreatic digestive enzymes; slows gastric emptying
Secretin	Duodenum	Stimulates the pancreas to secrete sodium bicarbonate; called "nature's own antacid"; makes chyme alkaline

The ascending colon ascends on the right side and curves acutely near the liver at the hepatic flexure. As it crosses the upper abdomen, it is known as the *transverse colon*. The colon then bends near the spleen at the splenic flexure to become the descending colon. The descending colon descends on the left side of the abdomen into an S-shaped segment called the *sigmoid colon*. Structures distal to the sigmoid colon include the rectum, anal canal, and anus. The anal canal ends at the anus, a structure composed primarily of two sphincter muscles (an involuntary internal sphincter and a voluntary external sphincter). The sphincters are closed except during the expulsion of the feces. Feces (FEE-seez) is waste composed primarily of nondigestible food residue, shed intestinal cells, and a host of microorganisms; it forms the stool, or bowel movement (BM). Expulsion of feces is called

defecation. In addition to the segments, note the band of connective tissue running lengthwise along the large intestine. It is called the *tenia coli*, and it causes the large intestine to pucker, thereby forming pouches called *haustra*.

FUNCTIONS OF THE LARGE INTESTINE

The four functions of the large intestine are as follows:
- Absorption of water and electrolytes
- Synthesis of certain vitamins by the intestinal bacteria (especially vitamin K and some B vitamins)
- Temporary storage site of waste (feces)
- Elimination of waste from the body (defecation)

Peristalsis and Absorption

Intermittent and well-spaced muscle movements slowly move the fecal material from the cecum

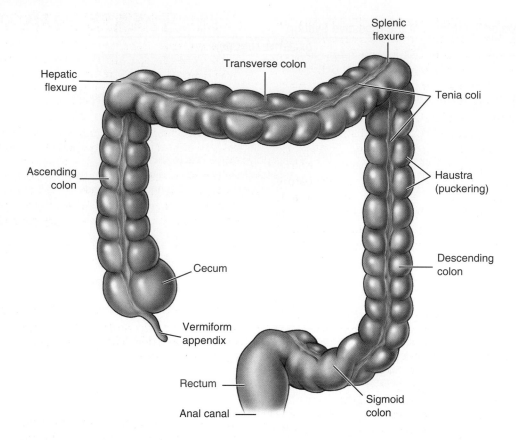

FIG. 23.7 **Large intestine: cecum with appendix; ascending colon, transverse colon, descending colon, and sigmoid colon; rectum and anal canal.**

through the colon. Forceful peristaltic waves occur only two to three times per day producing mass movements which finally move the feces into the rectum for expulsion. As the fecal material moves through the colon, water is continuously reabsorbed from the feces, across the intestinal wall, into the capillaries. Consequently, as the feces enter the rectum, it has changed from a watery consistency to a semisolid mass. Feces that remain in the large intestine for an extended period lose excess water, and the person experiences constipation. Rapid movement through the intestine allows insufficient time for water reabsorption, causing diarrhea.

Inside the Gut: Microbiota. Inside the gut and throughout the much-maligned waste there is a lot going on. Your gut **microbiota** (AKA...normal flora), mostly bacteria, viruses, and protozoa, are toiling away 24/7. There are 3 pounds' worth of mostly unidentified tiny critters. In fact, we have 10 times more microbes in our gut and on our skin than we have human cells. For this reason, some investigators actually refer to the microbiota as a functioning organ. For sure, we are a microbial lot!

The gut microbiota are doing all sorts of things for us, and no, it is not all nasty! The microbiota contribute to our physical and mental well-being. They synthesize vitamins, participate in our immune response,

modify hormonal activity, affect appetite, and assist with learning, memory, and mood... Yes, learning, memory, and mood! The medical literature is already exploding with regard to gut microbiota and conditions such as autism, multiple sclerosis, obesity, and depression. Although much is still unknown, we know for sure that the microbiota talk to the body and that the body is responsive.

 Do You Know...

About the Clinical Concern for *Clostridium Difficile*?

Clostridium difficile, a gram-positive bacillus, is a part of the intestinal microbiota or normal flora; it normally causes no problems. If the intestinal flora is disrupted, as may occur with antibiotic therapy, the number of *C. difficile* increases, causing a serious antibiotic-associated colitis. The combination of antibiotic therapy and severe diarrhea should send up a red flag: the possibility of superinfection with *C. difficile*. How did *C. difficile* get its name? From its uncooperative nature; it is difficult to grow in the lab.

Intestinal Gas

We have our own natural gas line! The average person expels about 500 mL of gas/day (always a crowd pleaser). The expelled gas is called *flatus* (FLAY-tus), and the process is called *flatulence* (FLATCH-yoo-lints). From a Ms. Manners perspective, most episodes of flatulence can be controlled, a much-appreciated act of kindness. Gas is normally produced from air that is swallowed and as a by-product of digestion, especially of gassy foods. Post-surgically, you will often hear surgeons ask patients if they have been "passing gas." A barely audible and embarrassed "yes" indicates that peristaltic activity, which often diminishes during surgery, has resumed. Passing gas after surgery is a good thing. Another interesting gas issue: The intestinal gases include methane and hydrogen gas, both of which are flammable. This is a concern in the operating room, where the use of electrical equipment (cautery) can cause the intestinal gas to explode.

 Do You Know....

That What's in Your Intestine May Be What's on Your Mind?

Gut microbes function as natural antidepressants. These microbes secrete the same neurotransmitters that are found in the brain...GABA, serotonin, dopamine, norepinephrine... and more. These neurotransmitters play a significant role in memory, mood, and learning. A new field called *psychobiotics* is studying the relationship of these mind-altering gut microbes to anxiety and depression. And why not? These microbes secrete neurotransmitters that resemble the effects of commonly prescribed psychiatric drugs, such as the benzodiazepines (e.g., Xanax) and the selective serotonin reuptake inhibitors (SSRIs), such as fluoxetine (Prozac). Take care of those intestinal critters. Feed them wisely... they don't like processed junk food. And stop killing them... they don't like chemical additives, antibiotics, and antibiotic-laced foods. The foods you choose may be the latest drug-free mental health breakthrough!

 Re Think

1. List the parts of the large intestine.
2. Why is the feces in the ascending colon more watery than the feces in the rectum?
3. Why is it important to assess your patient's bowel sounds postoperatively?
4. List three functions of the gut microbiota.

 Do You Know...

That the "Shepherd of the Anus" Was a High-Profile "Ca-rear"?

Ancient Egyptian medicine was divided into many specialties. Each area of the body had its own physician, or shepherd. The physician of the rectal area, comparable to today's proctologist, was called the "shepherd of the anus." Given the ancients' preoccupation with bowel irregularity and the popularity of emetics and purges, this shepherd was a very busy person—not too different from today if you note the staggering numbers of over-the-counter gastrointestinal drugs.

 Sum It Up!

Chyme is discharged from the stomach into the small intestine: duodenum, jejunum, and ileum. Most digestion and absorption occur in the duodenum and first third of the jejunum. The end-products of digestion and water are absorbed across the duodenal and jejunal walls into the villi of the small intestine. Glucose and amino acids are absorbed into the capillaries of the villi. The fats and fat-soluble vitamins are absorbed into the lacteals. Water and electrolytes are absorbed as the contents move through the small and large intestines (cecum, colon, and rectum). Digestive waste is eliminated as feces. The inside of the gut is alive and well with millions of microbes (microbiota) that are busily interacting in a largely beneficial way in our pursuit of health.

ACCESSORY DIGESTIVE ORGANS

Three important organs—the liver, the gallbladder, and the pancreas—empty their secretions into the duodenum (Fig. 23.8). These secretions are necessary for the digestion of food.

LIVER

The liver is a large reddish-brown organ located in the mid and right upper abdominal cavity (see Fig. 23.8A). It lies immediately below the diaphragm; much of the liver is tucked up under the right rib cage. The liver is the largest gland in the body, weighing about three pounds, and has two main lobes: a larger right lobe and a smaller left lobe separated by a ligament. This ligament secures the liver to surrounding structures. The liver is surrounded by a fibrous membrane called a *capsule*. The word *hepatic* refers to the liver.

WHAT THE LIVER DOES

The liver is essential for life and performs many vital functions:

- *Synthesis of bile salts and secretion of bile.* Bile salts play an important role in fat digestion and in the absorption of fat-soluble vitamins. Bile secretion is the main digestive function of the liver.
- *Synthesis of plasma proteins.* The plasma proteins play an important role in maintaining blood volume and controlling blood coagulation. With inadequate production of albumin, water cannot be retained within the blood vessels, and generalized edema develops. With inadequate production of blood coagulation factors, hemostasis is impaired, and the person is at risk for bleeding.
- *Storage.* The liver stores many substances: glucose in the form of glycogen, the fat-soluble vitamins (A, D, E, and K), and vitamin B_{12}.
- *Detoxification.* The liver plays an important role in the detoxification of drugs and other harmful substances. The liver changes these toxic substances

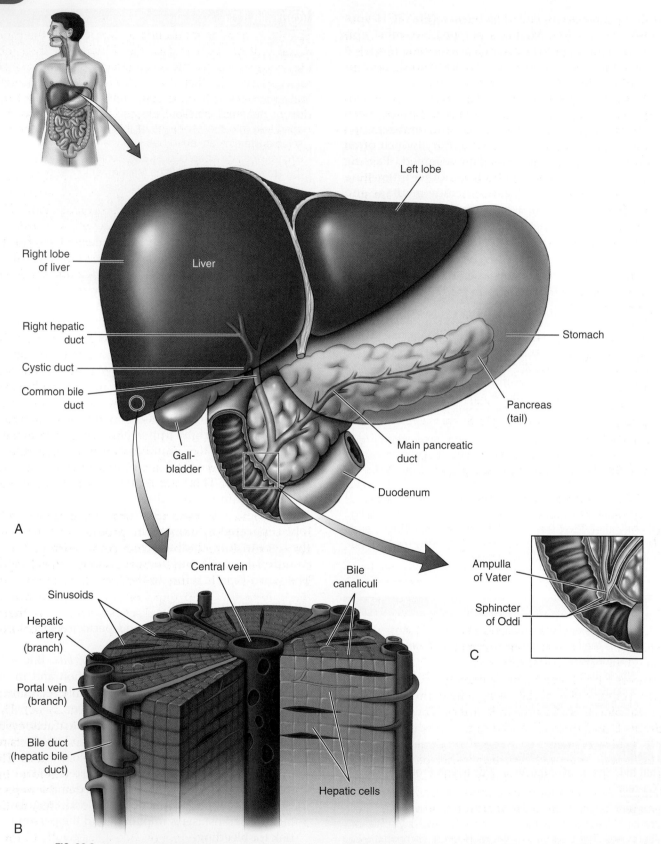

Left lobe

Right lobe
of liver

Liver

Right hepatic
duct

Cystic duct

Common bile
duct

Stomach

Pancreas
(tail)

Main pancreatic
duct

Gall-
bladder

Duodenum

A

Central vein

Bile
canaliculi

Sinusoids

Hepatic
artery
(branch)

Portal vein
(branch)

Bile duct
(hepatic bile
duct)

Hepatic cells

Ampulla
of Vater

Sphincter
of Oddi

C

B

FIG. 23.8 (A) Liver, gallbladder, bile ducts, and pancreas. (B) Liver lobule. (C) The entrance of the common bile
duct into the duodenum (ampulla of Vater and sphincter of Oddi).

into substances that can be more easily eliminated from the body by the kidneys. The liver is the most important organ in the biotransformation of drugs!

- *Excretion.* The liver excretes many substances, including bilirubin, cholesterol, and drugs.
- *Metabolism of carbohydrates.* The liver plays an important role in the regulation of blood glucose levels. If blood glucose levels rise above normal, the liver removes glucose from the blood, converts it to glycogen, and then stores it for future use. If the blood glucose levels decline below normal, the liver makes glucose from glycogen and nonglucose substances (gluconeogenesis) and releases it into the blood.
- *Metabolism of protein.* The liver can make a variety of different amino acids. Also, because only the liver contains the urea cycle enzymes, nitrogen (from ammonia) is converted to urea in the liver for eventual excretion by the kidneys. Free ammonia in the blood is toxic to humans.
- *Metabolism of fats.* The liver can break down fatty acids, synthesize cholesterol and phospholipids, and convert excess dietary protein and carbohydrates to fat.
- *Phagocytosis.* The Kupffer cells are hepatic macrophages and can phagocytose bacteria and other substances.

? Re-Think

1. What is the most important digestive function of the liver?
2. Explain how the liver helps regulate blood glucose.
3. Explain why a person with poor hepatic function requires a smaller dose of a drug.
4. Explain the role of Kupffer cells.

BLOOD SUPPLY TO THE LIVER

Blood Supply and the Hepatic Portal System

The liver has a unique arrangement of blood vessels called the *hepatic portal system* (see Fig. 18.8). The liver receives a lot of blood, approximately 1.5 L/min, from two sources: the portal vein, which provides most of the blood, and the hepatic artery. The portal vein drains blood from all of the organs of digestion and brings blood rich in digestive end-products to the liver. The hepatic artery delivers oxygen-rich blood from the aorta to the liver. Blood leaves the liver through the hepatic veins and empties into the inferior vena cava, where it is returned to the heart for recirculation.

? Re-Think

1. Why does the liver require a blood supply from both the hepatic artery and the portal vein?
2. What two large veins merge to form the portal vein?
3. Identify the blood vessels that carry the blood from the liver to the vena cava.

LIVER LOBULES

The liver contains thousands of **liver lobules**, the functional unit of the liver (see Fig. 23.8B). The liver lobules consist of a special arrangement of blood vessels and hepatic cells (hepatocytes). Note the central vein and the rows of hepatic cells that radiate away from the central vein. These cells are bathed by blood that enters the lobule from both the hepatic artery and the portal vein.

Blood from these two blood vessels mixes in the liver in spaces called *sinusoids* (SINE-u-soids), or large pore capillaries. The hepatic cells extract water and dissolved substances from the sinusoidal blood. Hepatic cells then secrete a greenish-yellow substance called *bile* into tiny canals called *canaliculi* (kan-ah-LIK-yoo-lye). These tiny bile canals merge with canals from other lobules to form larger hepatic bile ducts. Bile exits from the liver through two hepatic bile ducts.

BILE

Bile is a greenish-yellow secretion produced by the liver and stored in the gallbladder. Bile is composed primarily of water, electrolytes, cholesterol, bile pigments, and bile salts. The bile pigments bilirubin and biliverdin are formed from the hemoglobin of worn-out red blood cells. The bile salts are the most abundant constituents of the bile. Only the bile salts have a digestive function; they play an important role in fat digestion and in the absorption of fat-soluble vitamins. Between 800 and 1000 mL of bile is secreted per day.

Bile pigments, especially urobilinogen (yoo-roh-bil-IN-oh-jen) (a breakdown product of bilirubin), also give the stool a brownish color. With gallbladder disease, a gallstone sometimes becomes lodged in the common bile duct, blocks the flow of bile into the duodenum, and deprives the stools of brown pigments. Common bile duct obstruction is therefore characterized by colorless, gray, or clay-colored stools.

BILIARY TREE

The ducts that connect the liver, gallbladder, and duodenum are called the **biliary tree** (see Fig. 23.8A). This network of ducts includes the hepatic bile ducts, cystic duct, and common bile duct. The hepatic bile ducts receive bile from the canaliculi in the liver lobules. The hepatic ducts merge with the cystic duct to form the **common bile duct**, which carries bile from the hepatic ducts (liver) and the cystic duct (gallbladder) to the duodenum.

The base of the common bile duct swells to form the hepatopancreatic ampulla (ampulla of Vater; see Fig. 23.8C). The main pancreatic duct joins the common bile duct at this point. The hepatopancreatic sphincter (sphincter of Oddi) encircles the base of the ampulla, where it enters the duodenum. This sphincter helps regulate the delivery of bile to the duodenum and is sensitive to nervous, hormonal, and pharmacological control. (Do not confuse the ducts of the biliary tree with the hepatic blood vessels.)

GALLBLADDER

The **gallbladder** is a pear-shaped sac attached to the underside of the liver (see Fig. 23.8A). The cystic duct connects the gallbladder with the common bile duct. Bile, produced in the liver, flows through the hepatic ducts and into the cystic duct and gallbladder. The function of the gallbladder is to concentrate and store bile. The gallbladder concentrates about 1200 mL of bile/day.

The presence of dietary fat in the duodenum stimulates the release of a hormone, cholecystokinin (koh-lee-sis-toh-KYE-nin) (CCK). This hormone enters the bloodstream and circulates to the gallbladder, where it causes the smooth muscle of the gallbladder to contract. When the gallbladder contracts, the bile is ejected into the cystic duct and then into the common bile duct and duodenum.

For unknown reasons, bile components often form stones. The larger stones remain in the gallbladder. However, the smaller stones can be pushed out of the gallbladder when bile is ejected. The stones then lodge in the common bile duct. Bile that backs up behind the stones causes jaundice and impairs hepatic function. Also, the stagnant bile can also be forced into the main pancreatic duct, causing a life-threatening pancreatitis. The presence of stones in the gallbladder often causes an inflammation called *cholecystitis*. The presence of stones in the common bile duct is called *choledocholithiasis*. Both conditions may cause biliary colic, midepigastric pain that often radiates to the right subscapular area

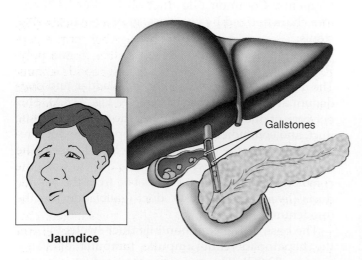

Jaundice

Gallstones

How can a fatty meal trigger biliary colic in a person with cholecystitis? When the fat enters the duodenum, it causes the release of CCK. The CCK travels via the blood to the gallbladder and stimulates the inflamed gallbladder to contract. Ouch!

 Re-Think

1. How does a liver lobule make bile?
2. What is the digestive role of bile?
3. Trace the flow of bile from its source to the gallbladder, and then to the duodenum.
4. Explain the difference in function between the hepatic portal system and the hepatobiliary system.

PANCREAS

The **pancreas** is an accessory organ of digestion located just below the stomach (see Fig. 23.8A). The head of the pancreas rests in the curve of the duodenum, and the tail lies near the spleen in the left upper quadrant of the abdominal cavity. The main pancreatic duct, which travels the length of the pancreas, joins with the common bile duct at the ampulla of Vater. The pancreatic duct carries digestive enzymes from the pancreas to the duodenum—the meeting point for digestion.

The pancreas secretes both endocrine and exocrine substances. The exocrine secretions include the digestive enzymes and an alkaline secretion. Acinar cells secrete the pancreatic enzymes in their inactive form. The enzymes travel through the main pancreatic duct to the duodenum and are activated in the duodenum. These secretions form the pancreatic juice; the pancreas secretes about 1400 mL/day. Premature activation of proteolytic enzymes within the pancreas causes autodigestion of the pancreas itself, a very painful and potentially lethal condition. *Note: The pancreatic enzymes are the most important of all the digestive enzymes.*

In addition to the digestive enzymes, the pancreas also secretes an alkaline juice rich in bicarbonate. The bicarbonate neutralizes the highly acidic chyme coming from the stomach into the duodenum. This neutralization is important because the digestive enzymes in the duodenum work best in an alkaline environment.

The secretion of the digestive enzymes and bicarbonate is under nervous (vagus) and hormonal control. The presence of food in the stomach and duodenum is the stimulus for the nervous and hormonal responses. For example, the presence of chyme in the duodenum stimulates the release of the hormone CCK from the duodenal walls. CCK travels by way of the blood to the pancreas, stimulating the release of pancreatic digestive enzymes. Note that CCK affects the gallbladder, pancreas, and stomach (see Table 23.1). It stimulates the gallbladder to contract and release bile, it stimulates the pancreas to secrete digestive enzymes, and it slows gastric emptying…activities that all encourage digestion and absorption. The acid chyme in the duodenum stimulates the release of a second hormone, secretin, from the duodenal walls. Secretin travels by way of the blood to the pancreas, stimulating release of the bicarbonate-rich juice. Bicarbonate neutralizes the gastric acid thereby creating an alkaline environment in which the digestive enzymes work best.

Re-Think

1. How does the pancreas get its digestive enzymes into the duodenum?
2. What are the stimuli for the release of CCK and secretin? List the ways in which CCK and secretin facilitate digestion.
3. From a dietary perspective, how does the gallbladder "know" when to release bile into the common bile duct?

Sum It Up!

The liver, gallbladder, and pancreas are accessory digestive organs. These organs secrete substances that enter the duodenum, the meeting place for digestion. The liver performs many functions. The liver's primary digestive role is the secretion of bile. Bile is concentrated and stored in the gallbladder; it is released into the bile ducts in response to cholecystokinin (CCK). The pancreatic acinar cells secrete the most potent digestive enzymes; pancreatic enzymes are secreted in response to CCK. The pancreatic enzymes enter the duodenum, where they mix with chyme from the stomach. CCK and secretion are two hormones that are secreted by the duodenal walls in response to the presence of acidic chyme in the duodenum. These hormones cause the release of bile, the secretion of pancreatic enzymes, the secretion of bicarbonate, and a decrease in gastric activity.

DIGESTION AND ABSORPTION

The primary purpose of the digestive system is to break down large pieces of food into small particles suitable for absorption. Food is digested mechanically and chemically. Mechanical digestion is the physical breakdown of food into small pieces. It is achieved by the chewing activity of the mouth and by the mixing and churning activities of the muscles of the digestive organs. Chemical digestion is the chemical change occurring primarily in response to the digestive enzymes and other digestive aids.

Food is made up of carbohydrates, proteins, and fats. Digestive enzymes and several digestive agents (mucus, HCl, and bile) play key roles in chemical digestion. Specific enzymes digest each type of food (see Table 23.1). (Review the structures of carbohydrates, protein, and fat in Chapter 4.)

CARBOHYDRATES AND CARBOHYDRATE-SPLITTING ENZYMES

Carbohydrates are classified according to size (see Fig. 4-2). Monosaccharides are single (*mono*) sugars (*saccharides*). The three monosaccharides are glucose, fructose, and galactose. Glucose is the most important of the three monosaccharides. **Disaccharides** are double (*di*) sugars. The three disaccharides are sucrose (table sugar), lactose, and maltose. Polysaccharides are many (*poly*) glucose molecules linked together. The shorter monosaccharides and disaccharides are called *sugars;* the longer-chain polysaccharides are *starches*.

A polysaccharide is digested in two stages: Fig. 23.9. First, enzymes called **amylases** (AM-eh-lays-ez) degrade the polysaccharide into disaccharides (sucrose, maltose, and lactose). The two amylases are salivary amylase (ptyalin [TIE-uh-lin]) and pancreatic amylase. Second, disaccharidases (sucrose, maltase, lactase) degrade disaccharides into monosaccharides. The three disaccharidases, located within the intestinal mucosal cells, are sucrase, lactase, and maltase. (The ending -*ase* indicates an enzyme.) Disaccharides therefore are split into monosaccharides in the duodenum and jejunum at the surface of the villi. The monosaccharides are immediately absorbed into the blood capillaries of the villus.

Certain carbohydrates, such as cellulose, cannot be digested and therefore remain in the lumen of the digestive system. Although providing no direct nourishment, dietary cellulose is beneficial in that it provides fiber and bulk to the stool.

Many persons suffer from a deficiency of the enzyme lactase. They are unable to digest the sugar found in milk (lactose) and are said to be lactose intolerant. This enzyme deficiency prevents lactose-intolerant people from digesting milk and many milk products. An interesting note: Most people worldwide are lactose intolerant!

PROTEINS AND PROTEIN-SPLITTING ENZYMES

The building blocks of proteins are amino acids (Fig. 4.5). Several amino acids linked together form a peptide. Many amino acids linked together form a polypeptide. Proteins are very long polypeptide chains; some proteins contain more than one polypeptide chain. To be absorbed across the wall of the digestive tract, these chains must be uncoiled and degraded into small peptides and amino acids.

Enzymes called **proteases**, or proteolytic enzymes, digest proteins (Fig. 23.10). Proteases are secreted by three organs: the stomach secretes pepsinogen, the intestinal cells secrete peptidase, and the pancreas secretes several proteases, including trypsinogen, chymotrypsinogen, and carboxypeptidase. The pancreatic proteases, once activated within the duodenum, are the most potent proteases. Proteins are broken down into small peptides and amino acids and are absorbed across the intestinal villi into the blood capillaries. (Interesting fact: Because it was thought to aid digestion, Pepsi was named after the enzyme pepsin.)

Carbohydrates: Digestion and Absorption

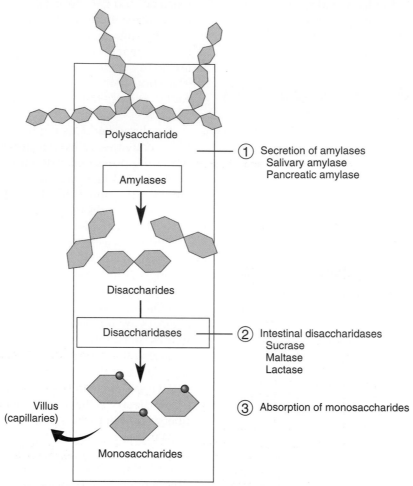

FIG. 23.9 **Carbohydrate digestion.**

Proteolytic activity is enhanced by both HCl and enterokinase. Although not an enzyme, HCl aids protein digestion. First, the HCl unravels the strands of protein, making the protein fragments more sensitive to the proteases. Second, the HCl activates a gastric proteolytic enzyme, pepsinogen, into pepsin. Pepsin then facilitates breaking protein into small peptides. Enterokinase, located within the intestinal mucosa, activates trypsinogen into trypsin, a powerful proteolytic enzyme.

FATS, BILE, AND FAT-SPLITTING ENZYMES

Fats are long-chain fatty acids attached to glycerol (Fig. 4.4). Enzymes called **lipases** (LYE-pays-ez) digest fats. The most important is pancreatic lipase (Fig. 23.11). The end-products of fat digestion are fatty acids and glycerol; fat is absorbed into the lacteals of the villi.

Why is bile necessary for fat digestion? Fats, unlike carbohydrates or proteins, are not soluble in water; they tend to clump together into large fat globules when added to water. If, for example, oil and water are placed in a test tube, the oil and water separate; the oil rises to the surface, and the water settles at the bottom. Oil and water simply do not mix. The same separation occurs in the digestive tract. Dietary fat tends to form large fat globules. The lipase cannot readily digest the fat; it can attack only the outside surface of the fat globule.

Bile solves the large fat globule problem. Bile can split the large fat globule into thousands of tiny fat globules. This process is **emulsification** (ee-MULL-seh-feh-KAY-shun). Because of emulsification, the lipases can work on the surfaces of all the tiny fat globules, thereby digesting more fat. Bile performs two other important roles. Bile salts prevent the fatty acids (end-products of fat digestion) from re-forming large fat globules in the intestine before they can be absorbed across the intestinal villi. Bile salts also help the absorption of the fat-soluble vitamins A, D, E, and K.

> **? Re-Think**
>
> 1. List the enzymes needed for carbohydrate, protein, and fat digestion.
> 2. Why does fat digestion require bile, whereas carbohydrate and protein digestion do not?
> 3. What gland secretes the most potent digestive enzymes?

Proteins: Digestion and Absorption

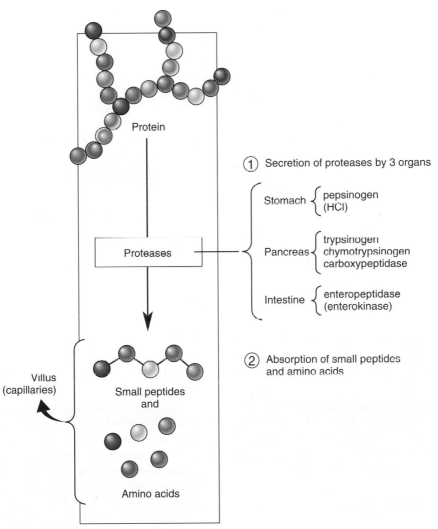

FIG. 23.10 **Protein digestion.**

Fat: Digestion and Absorption

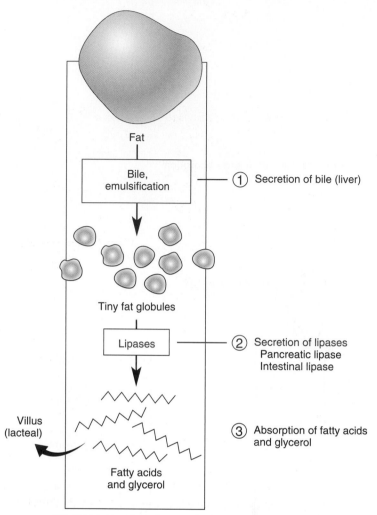

FIG. 23.11 **Fat digestion: emulsification and digestion.**

◎ Sum It Up!

How is a turkey dinner digested and absorbed (Fig. 23.12)?

1. In the mouth, food is chewed into tiny pieces and mixed with saliva (mechanical digestion). Minimal chemical carbohydrate digestion begins with salivary amylase (ptyalin).
2. The smaller pieces of food are swallowed and moved by peristalsis through the esophagus to the stomach; the pieces of food are mixed with gastric juice and churned into an acidic chyme. Pepsin begins the chemical digestion of protein.
3. The partially digested food (chyme) is ejected into the duodenum, where it mixes with bile and the pancreatic and intestinal digestive enzymes. Pancreatic amylase and the disaccharidases digest the polysaccharides to monosaccharides. The pancreatic proteases (trypsin and chymotrypsin) and the intestinal proteases digest the proteins to small peptides and amino acids. Bile emulsifies the fats, and the pancreatic and intestinal lipases digest them. The end-products of fat digestion

are fatty acids and glycerol. A pendulum-like peristaltic motion washes the digested food across each villus, thereby enhancing absorption.

4. The simple sugars and the amino acids are absorbed into the blood capillaries of the villi. These capillaries eventually empty into the portal vein for transport to the liver. The fat products are absorbed into the lacteals of the villi. Most of the digestion of food and the absorption of digestive end-products and water occurs in the duodenum and the proximal jejunum. A large amount of water is also absorbed into the blood capillaries from the intestines.
5. The unabsorbed food material, water, and some electrolytes continue along the jejunum and ileum and into the large intestine.
6. Water and certain electrolytes are absorbed along this route, and a semisolid stool is formed.
7. The presence of the fecal material in the rectum gives rise to an urge to defecate.

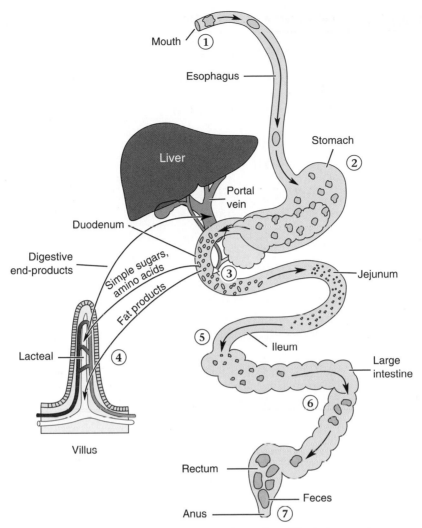

FIG. 23.12 **Summary: digestion and absorption of the turkey meal.**

NUTRITION: CONCEPTS TO KNOW

Nutrition is the science that studies the relationship of food to the functioning of the body. Food consists of nutrients, substances the body uses to promote normal growth, maintenance, and repair. The five categories of nutrients are carbohydrates, proteins, lipids, vitamins, and minerals.

CARBOHYDRATES

Dietary carbohydrates are classified as simple sugars and complex carbohydrates. A simple sugar is composed of monosaccharides and disaccharides. Glucose, the simplest carbohydrate, is the major fuel used to make ATP in most body cells. Most of the carbohydrates come from plants. The sugars are derived primarily from fruit, sugar cane, and milk.

The complex carbohydrates are larger sugar molecules (polysaccharides) and consist primarily of starch and fiber. Starch is found in cereal grains (wheat, oats, corn, barley), legumes (peas, beans), and root vegetables, such as potatoes. Fiber, or cellulose, is found primarily in vegetables.

Most dietary carbohydrate should be in the form of complex carbohydrates for two reasons. First, complex carbohydrates usually provide other nutrients, whereas simple sugars provide "empty calories" (nothing but calories). Second, complex carbohydrates are absorbed at a slower rate than sugars, thereby preventing a sudden spike in blood glucose. The spiking of blood glucose has been linked to an oversecretion of insulin, impaired cellular uptake of glucose, and hypertension. Our excessive intake of high fructose corn syrup is fattening us up and raising our blood pressures. Is it also creating a nation of diabetics?

The **glycemic index** is an excellent guide for the selection of dietary carbohydrate; it is a term that identifies the effects that foods exert on blood sugar. For example, rice and "peeps" are foods that have a high glycemic index, meaning that they are digested and absorbed rapidly, thereby spiking blood sugar. String beans have a low glycemic index; they are digested and absorbed more slowly and do not spike the blood

Table 23.2   **Selected Vitamins**

VITAMIN	FUNCTION	DEFICIENCY
Fat-Soluble Vitamins		
Vitamin A	Necessary for skin, mucous membranes, and night vision	Night blindness; dry, scaly skin; disorders of mucous membranes
Vitamin D (calciferol)	Necessary for the absorption of calcium and phosphorus	Rickets in children; osteomalacia in adults
Vitamin E	Necessary for health of cell membrane	None defined
Vitamin K	Needed for the synthesis of prothrombin and other clotting factors	Bleeding
Water-Soluble Vitamins		
Thiamine (vitamin B_1)	Helps release energy from carbohydrates and amino acids; needed for growth	Beriberi; alcohol-induced Wernicke's syndrome
Riboflavin (vitamin B_2)	Essential for growth	Skin and tongue disorders; dermatitis
Niacin (vitamin B_3)	Helps release energy from nutrients	Pellagra with dermatitis, diarrhea, mental disorders
Pyridoxine (vitamin B_6)	Participates in the metabolism of amino acids and proteins	Nervous system and skin disorders
Vitamin B_{12}	Helps form red blood cells and deoxyribonucleic acid (DNA)	Anemias, particularly pernicious anemia
Folic acid	Participates in the formation of hemoglobin and DNA	Anemia; neural tube defects in embryo
Ascorbic acid (vitamin C)	Necessary for synthesis of collagen; helps maintain capillaries; aids in the absorption of iron	Scurvy; poor bone and wound healing

sugar. The carbohydrates with a lower glycemic index are better dietary choices.

PROTEINS

Dietary proteins supply the body with amino acids. Because the body cannot store amino acids, a daily supply is necessary.

Proteins are classified as complete or incomplete. A complete protein contains all essential amino acids. Complete proteins are found in animal sources such as meat, eggs, and dairy products. Incomplete proteins do not contain all of the essential amino acids, and these proteins include vegetable proteins such as nuts, grains, and legumes. Vegetable proteins, if eaten in combinations, can supply a complete complement of amino acids. For example, a favorite Mexican dish containing rice and beans is complete in that it supplies all the essential amino acids, even though both the rice and the beans are incomplete proteins.

FATS (LIPIDS)

Most dietary lipids are triglycerides, or molecules that contain glycerol and fatty acids. Fatty acids are classified as saturated or unsaturated. A saturated fatty acid (e.g., butter, lard), which come primarily from animal sources, is solid at room temperature. Also included in this group are artificially hardened, or hydrogenated, fats such as vegetable shortening and margarine. An

unsaturated fat is liquid at room temperature and is called an *oil*.

The body can synthesize all fatty acids, with one exception: linoleic acid, an important component of cell membranes. Because the body cannot synthesize it, linoleic acid is an essential fatty acid and therefore must be included in the diet.

Foods high in fat come from both animal and plant sources. Animal sources, however, tend to contain more saturated fat. They include meat, eggs, butter, and whole-milk products such as cheese. Plant sources include coconut oil and palm oil. Hydrogenated vegetable oils in shortening and margarine are also high in saturated fat.

 Re-Think

1. How may the use of the glycemic index help avoid spikes in blood sugar?
2. What is the difference between a complete and incomplete protein?
3. Why is it important to ingest linoleic acid as a dietary fat?

VITAMINS

Vitamins are small organic molecules that help regulate cell metabolism (Table 23.2). Vitamins are parts of enzymes or other organic substances essential for normal cell function and are classified as fat soluble or water soluble. The fat-soluble vitamins include vitamins A,

Table 23.3	Selected Minerals	
MINERALS	**FUNCTION**	**DEFICIENCY**
Potassium (K)	Nerve and muscle activity	Nerve and muscle disorders
Sodium (Na)	Water balance; nerve impulse conduction	Weakness, cramps, diarrhea, dehydration, confusion
Calcium (Ca)	Component of bones and teeth, nerve conduction, muscle contraction, blood clotting	Rickets, tetany, bone softening
Phosphorus (P)	Component of bones and teeth; component of ATP, nucleic acids, and cell membranes	Bone demineralization
Iron (Fe)	Component of hemoglobin (red blood cells)	Anemia, dry skin
Iodine (I)	Necessary for synthesis of thyroid hormones	Hypothyroidism; iodine-deficient goiter
Magnesium (Mg)	Component of some enzymes; important in carbohydrate metabolism	Muscle spasm, dysrhythmias, vasodilation
Fluorine (F)	Component of bones and teeth	Dental caries
Trace minerals Zinc (Zn)	Small amounts required for certain specific functions Nerve and muscle activity	Nerve and muscle disorders Weakness, cramps, diarrhea, dehydration, confusion
Copper (Cu)	Activates many enzymes	Loss of structural support resulting from a deficiency of connective tissues in many organs and blood vessels
Manganese (Mn)	Component of bones and teeth; nerve conduction, muscle contraction, blood clotting	Bone demineralization
Selenium (Se)	Not determined, plays a significant role in many enzymes, thereby affecting metabolism	Cardiomyopathy; other conditions not yet identified

D, E, and K. Because the body stores fat-soluble vitamins, excess intake may result in symptoms of toxicity (hypervitaminosis).

The water-soluble vitamins include vitamins B and C. These vitamins, for the most part, are not stored by the body. Excess water-soluble vitamins are generally excreted in the urine. Excretion, however, does not rule out the possibility of toxicity in response to megadosing with water-soluble vitamins.

You can best appreciate the roles vitamins play by observing the effects of specific vitamin deficiencies. For example, vitamin A is necessary for healthy skin and night vision. Vitamin A deficiency is characterized by various skin lesions and by night blindness, or the inability to see in a darkened room. Vitamin D is necessary for the absorption of calcium and the development and formation of strong bones. Vitamin D deficiency causes rickets in children, a condition in which the bones are soft and often bow in response to weight-bearing. Because the skin can synthesize vitamin D in response to exposure to ultraviolet radiation, the incidence of rickets is higher in places with little sunlight. Vitamin D deficiency in adults results in a bone-softening condition called *osteomalacia*.

Vitamin K plays a crucial role in hemostasis. It is necessary for the synthesis of prothrombin and several other hepatic clotting factors. A deficiency of vitamin K causes hypoprothrombinemia and a tendency to bleed excessively.

Finally, vitamin C is necessary for the integrity of the skin and mucous membranes. A deficiency of vitamin C causes scurvy, a condition involving skin lesions and inability of the tissues to heal. Historically, scurvy was common on ships that were at sea for months at a time. Having determined that limes prevented scurvy, the British sailors traveled around the world sipping lime juice. In response to this habit, they were dubbed "limeys." Other vitamin deficiencies are included in Table 23.2.

MINERALS

Minerals are inorganic substances necessary for normal body function (Table 23.3). Minerals have numerous functions, ranging from regulation of plasma volume (sodium, chloride) to bone growth (calcium) to oxygen transport (iron) to the regulation of metabolic rate (iodine).

Mineral deficiencies can cause serious health problems. For example, because iodine is necessary for the synthesis of the thyroid hormone thyroxine, iodine deficiency can cause an enlarged thyroid gland (goiter) and hypothyroidism. Because iron is necessary for the synthesis of hemoglobin, iron deficiency can cause anemia. This anemic state is characterized by fatigue and, depending on its severity, a diminished ability to transport oxygen around the body.

Do You Know....

About Lead-Laced Painted Pottery Parts for Dinner?

Yummers! For unknown and puzzling reasons, some persons crave and compulsively eat nonfood substances. This condition is called *pica*, the Latin name for the magpie, a bird famous for its unusual and sometimes outrageous eating habits. Pica commonly involves the eating of cornstarch or laundry starch (amylophagia); earth, soil, or clay (geophagia); or ice (pagophagia). Pica or not, a significant number of women crave ice chips during pregnancy, a behavior usually attributed to iron deficiency (maybe, maybe not).

Although most instances of pica are harmless, the ingestion of some substances can be life-threatening. For instance, the ingestion of laundry starch during pregnancy can cause symptoms that mimic gestational diabetes, adversely affecting both mother and infant. Or, the ingestion of lead-painted pottery parts during pregnancy can induce a neurotoxic lead poisoning in the newborn. Overall, the causes and treatment for pica are unknown.

HEALTH AND A BALANCED DIET

A BALANCED DIET

A balanced diet contains all the essential nutrients and includes a variety of foods. The balanced diet has often been displayed in the form of food wheels or food pyramids. The latest design issued by the U.S. Department of Agriculture is MyPlate (MyPlate.gov) in which five food groups are organized so as to emphasize the relative proportions of each group.

POORLY BALANCED DIET AND DISEASE

Many health problems are thought to originate in poor dietary choices. Although overeating and obesity have been linked with health problems, a number of health problems are also related to a deficiency of certain foods. For example, a diet high in cholesterol or fat, or both, has been implicated in coronary artery disease, stroke, diabetes, and cancer. Our huge consumption of sugar is also a factor in obesity and high incidence of diabetes mellitus (and all its complications). Deficient diets are also problematic. For example, infants who are fed fat-poor diets (fat-free milk) may become deficient in fats essential for the development of nervous tissue resulting in nerve damage and developmental delay. In poverty-stricken areas of the world, protein deficiency diseases are common. Refer to Tables 23.2 and 23.3 for the consequences of vitamin and mineral deficiencies. Overnutrition and undernutrition are both forms of malnutrition.

 Do You Know...

That Kwashiorkor Refers to a "Displaced" Child?

Kwashiorkor is a condition of severe protein deficiency resulting in emaciation, edema formation, and ascites. The African word *kwashiorkor* (displaced or deposed) indicates the cause of the condition. A breast-fed infant is prematurely weaned from breast milk and placed on a protein-poor cereal diet. Why the premature weaning? To make room for baby brother. The 9-month-old infant is displaced or deposed by the newborn.

APPETITE CONTROL AND THE COUCH POTATO

Our couch potato would like to know: What makes us eat and stop eating? Don't know. We know that the hypothalamus plays an important role. There is an area of the lateral hypothalamus called the *feeding center*. When destroyed, it leads to anorexia and starvation. Another hypothalamic area is called the *satiety center*; damage to it causes overeating and morbid obesity. There are numerous theories about what satisfies (satiety [SAY-she-eh-tee]) and therefore suppresses appetite. The glucostat hypothesis states that the satiety center contains neurons called *glucostats* that absorb glucose and send inhibitory information to the feeding center. In response, appetite diminishes. The lipostat hypothesis states that adipocytes (fat cells) secrete an appetite-suppressing hormone called *leptin*. Alas! Couch Potato keeps eating, apparently ignoring the "stop eating" signals from his blitzed hypothalamus.

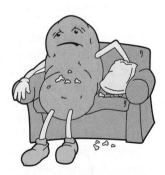

 Re-Think

1. What are the names of the deficiency states associated with iron, iodine, vitamin A, vitamin B_{12}, and vitamin D?
2. Explain two mechanisms whereby appetite is thought to be controlled.

 Sum It Up!

The body uses food for energy, repair, and maintenance. A balanced diet contains specific amounts and types of nutrients: carbohydrates, proteins, fats, vitamins, and minerals. Malnutrition includes overnutrition and undernutrition states; both are responsible for many diseases and disorders. Appetite control is not fully understood. The hypothalamus plays an important role containing a feeding center and a satiety center. Two theories include the glucostat theory and lipostat theory.

As You Age

1. The muscular wall of the digestive tract loses tone, causing constipation because of a slowing of peristalsis.
2. Secretion of saliva and digestive enzymes decreases, thereby decreasing digestion. The decrease in secretions also impairs the absorption of vitamins (vitamin B$_{12}$) and minerals (iron and calcium).
3. The sensations of taste and smell diminish with age. Consequently, food tastes different, and appetite may be affected.
4. The loss of teeth and an inability to chew food effectively makes eating difficult. The loss of teeth may also affect the choice of food, causing the older person to select a less nutritious diet, such as tea and toast.
5. Peristalsis in the esophagus is no longer triggered with each swallow, and the lower esophageal sphincter relaxes more slowly. These changes hamper swallowing and cause an early feeling of fullness.
6. A weakened gag reflex increases the risk of aspiration.
7. The liver shrinks and receives a smaller supply of blood. The rate of drug detoxification by the liver declines, thereby prolonging the effects of drugs and predisposing the person to a drug overdose. (Remember that the liver is the chief organ of drug inactivation or biotransformation.)

Medical Terminology and Disorders   Disorders of the Digestive System

MEDICAL TERM	WORD PARTS	WORD PART MEANING OR DERIVATION	DESCRIPTION
Words			
amylase	amyl/o-	starch	An **amylase** is *an enzyme that digests starch, a carbohydrate.* A **lipase** (lip/o- = fat) is *an enzyme that digests fat.* A **protease** is *an enzyme that digests protein.*
	-ase	enzyme	
buccal	bucc/o-	cheek	The **buccal** cavity is located between the teeth and cheeks.
	-al	pertaining to	
colonoscopy	colon/o-	colon, large intestine	A **colonoscopy** is *the visual examination of the colon using a scope.*
	-scopy	examination	
dyspepsia	dys-	difficult or faulty	**Dyspepsia** is *difficult or disturbed digestion.*
	-pepsia	digestion	
gastroenterology	gastr/o-	stomach	**Gastroenterology** is *the study of the digestive tract, made up largely of the stomach and intestines.*
	-enter/o-	intestines	
	-logy	study	
hematemesis	hemat/o-	blood	**Hematemesis** means *the vomiting of blood.*
	-emesis	vomiting	
melena	melan/o-	black	**Melena** *refers to dark-colored stools and is an indication of bleeding within the gastrointestinal tract.*
oral	or/o-	mouth	The **oral** cavity is the mouth. Many drugs are administered orally.
	-al	pertaining to	
postprandial	post-	after	**Postprandial** means *after a meal,* whereas **preprandial** means *before a meal.*
	-prand(ium)-	From a Latin word meaning "meal"	
	-al	pertaining to	
stomatitis	stomat/o-	mouth	**Stomatitis** means *inflammation of the oral mucosa (mouth).*
	-itis	inflammation	
sublingual	sub-	underneath	*Means underneath the tongue or hypoglossal.* Some drugs are administered **sublingually.**
	-lingul/o-	tongue	
Disorders			
diverticulitis	diverticul/o-	diverticulum	A **diverticulum** is *a sac formed by mucous membrane that herniates through a weakened muscular wall of the colon, especially the sigmoid colon.* **Diverticulitis** refers to *inflammation of the diverticula and surrounding tissue.* **Diverticulosis** refers to *the condition of having diverticula in the colon.*
	-itis	inflammation	
dysentery	dys-	difficult or abnormal	**Dysentery** is *a group of disorders characterized by inflammation of the intestines, especially the large intestine; it is characterized by cramping and the passage of bloody diarrhea.*
	-enter/o-	intestine	
	-ery	pertaining to	

Continued

Medical Terminology and Disorders   Disorders of the Digestive System—cont'd

MEDICAL TERM	WORD PARTS	WORD PART MEANING OR DERIVATION	DESCRIPTION
gastroenteritis	gastr/o-	stomach	*Inflammation of the stomach and the intestine.* It can be caused by a variety of pathogens, including viruses, bacteria, and parasites.
	-enter/o-	intestine	
	-itis	inflammation	
gastroparesis	gastr/o-	stomach	**Gastroparesis** is *paralysis of the stomach causing slow gastric emptying and esophageal reflux.*
	-paresis	paralysis	
gastroesophageal reflux disease (GERD)	gastr/o-	stomach	**GERD** *refers to the backflow (reflux) of stomach contents into the esophagus.* Relaxation of the lower esophageal sphincter (LES) commonly occurs with GERD and is thought to be the chief cause of reflux and heartburn, also known as **pyrosis** (pyr/o- = fire, burning).
	-esophagi/o-	esophagus	
gingivitis	gingiv/o-	gums	*Inflammation of the gums surrounding the teeth.* Gingivitis is a **periodontal disease.**
	-itis	inflammation	
hernia	hernia	Related to two Latin words meaning "rupture" and "intestine"	*A protrusion of an organ or part of an organ out of the cavity in which it is normally contained.* A hernia may be described as **incarcerated** *(the herniated intestine swells and becomes trapped),* **strangulated** *(the herniated intestine is trapped, swollen, and necrotic because its blood supply has been cut off),* **reducible** *(the herniated intestine can be pushed back into its proper cavity),* or **irreducible** *(the herniated intestine is not able to be pushed back into place).* Hernias develop in many different locations. An **inguinal hernia** refers to *the herniation of the intestine in the groin area.* A **femoral hernia** is *the herniation of intestine along a path used by the femoral artery as it leaves the abdomen and enters the thigh.* An **umbilical hernia** is *a herniation of intestine through the abdominal wall surrounding the umbilicus (belly button).* An **incisional hernia** is *the herniation of intestine through a surgically induced weakened abdominal wall.* Organs other than the intestine can herniate. A **hiatal hernia** refers to *the herniation of a part of the stomach into the thoracic cavity. Surgical repair of a hernia is called a* **herniorrhaphy.**
inflammatory bowel disease			Abbreviated as **IBD,** but also known as **ileitis** and **enteritis.** The two most common types of IBD are Crohn's disease and ulcerative colitis. **Crohn's disease** is *an inflammatory condition that can affect any part of the GI tract, most commonly the ileum.* **Ulcerative colitis** is *a chronic inflammatory condition that usually affects the inner lining of the colon and rectum.* **Irritable bowel syndrome (IBS)** *refers to periodic episodes of altered bowel function, diarrhea or constipation, and abdominal pain.*
intestinal obstruction			Also called a **bowel obstruction.** It is *a partial or complete blockage of the intestines that prevents the passage of food or fluid.* The obstruction may be mechanical, meaning that something is in the way. The obstruction may also be due to **paralytic ileus,** whereby *the intestinal or bowel muscles do not contract effectively to propel its contents forward.* There are many causes of intestinal obstruction: tumors, twisting, telescoping, hernias, and adhesions. Other conditions include **volvulus,** *a twisted intestine (like a twisted garden hose);* an **intussusception,** *a telescoped intestine;* **hernias,** *"trapped" intestines;* and **adhesions,** *bands of connective tissue that wrap around intestinal organs, such as the intestines, causing occlusion.*

Medical Terminology and Disorders   Disorders of the Digestive System—cont'd

MEDICAL TERM	WORD PARTS	WORD PART MEANING OR DERIVATION	DESCRIPTION
peptic ulcer disease (PUD)			**Peptic ulcer disease (PUD)** *refers to a mucosal erosion (ulcer) in an area of the gastrointestinal tract that has acidic contents.* Most often the cause of PUD is due to *Helicobacter pylori;* the ulcers develop within the duodenum (duodenal ulcer) and/or stomach (gastric ulcer).
Liver, Gallbladder, Pancreas			
cholecystitis	chol/e-	bile	*Inflammation of the gallbladder; characterized by nausea, vomiting, and severe RUQ pain that radiates to the right subscapular region.* The pain is called **biliary colic. Cholecystitis** is most often caused by gallstones in the gallbladder, a condition called **cholelithiasis** (chol/e- = bile; -lith/o- = stone). Sometimes the small gallstones escape from the gallbladder and become lodged in the common bile duct, called **choledocholithiasis** (chol/e- = bile; -doch/o- = duct; -lith/o- = stone), causing inflammation of the bile ducts, or **cholangitis** (chol/e- = bile; -angio- = vessel; -itis = inflammation), biliary obstruction, hyperbilirubinemia, and jaundice.
	-cyst/o-	bladder	
	-itis	inflammation	
cirrhosis of the liver	cirrh-	From the Greek word *kirrhos,* meaning "tawny"	*Scarring of the liver in response to repeated destruction and regeneration of the liver cells.* Despite hepatic regeneration, the architecture of the liver is altered so as to impair hepatic function and blood flow. Because of the obstruction of blood flow, blood bypasses the liver, eventually causing **hepatic encephalopathy.** Obstruction of blood flow also increases portal vein pressure, causing **portal vein hypertension,** which in turn causes ascites and esophageal varices.
	-osis	condition	
hepatitis	hepat/o-	liver	*An inflammation of the liver, usually caused by viral infection.* (There are nonviral causes of hepatitis.) There are five main types: A, B, C, D, and E. Hepatitis X is hepatitis caused by an unidentified virus. Hepatitis A and E are commonly transmitted by contaminated food or water. Hepatitis B and D are transmitted by contact with body fluids. Hepatitis C is transmitted by contact with contaminated blood and increases the patient's risk for cancer of the liver.
	-itis	inflammation	
pancreatitis	pancreat/o-	pancreas	**Pancreatitis** *is inflammation of the pancreas.* Approximately 70% of cases are caused by excess alcohol ingestion. **Acute pancreatitis** *is an emergency condition with severe abdominal pain as the most common symptom.* **Chronic pancreatitis** may persist for many years.
	-itis	inflammation	

Get Ready for Exams!

Summary Outline

I. Overview of the Digestive System
  A. Functions of the digestive system
   1. Ingestion (eating)
   2. Digestion
   3. Absorption
   4. Elimination
  B. The wall of the digestive tract and membranes
   1. Four layers: mucosa, submucosa, muscle, and serosa
   2. Peritoneal membranes: mesentery, mesocolon, and greater and lesser omentum

II. Structures and Organs of the Digestive System
  A. Mouth
   1. Teeth and tongue
   2. Salivary glands
     a. Parotid, submandibular, and sublingual glands
     b. Secretes saliva
  B. Pharynx (oropharynx and laryngopharynx)
  C. Esophagus
   1. The esophagus is a long tube that connects the pharynx to the stomach.
   2. There are two sphincters: pharyngoesophageal and LES.

D. Stomach
1. The three parts of the stomach are the fundus, body, and pylorus.
2. The stomach functions in digestion; its most important role is to regulate the rate at which chyme is delivered to the small intestine.
3. It secretes hormones, few digestive enzymes, HCl, and intrinsic factor.

E. Small intestine
1. The three segments of the small intestine are the duodenum, jejunum, and ileum.
2. Most of the digestion and absorption occurs within the duodenum and first third of the jejunum.
3. The end-products of digestion are absorbed into villi (capillaries and lacteal).
4. The common bile duct enters the small intestine at the duodenum.

F. Large intestine
1. The large intestine consists of the cecum, ascending colon, transverse colon, descending colon, sigmoid colon, rectum, and anus.
2. The large intestine functions in absorption of water and electrolytes.

III. Accessory Digestive Organs

A. Liver
1. The liver has many functions; its most important digestive function is the secretion of bile.
2. The liver receives most of its blood from the portal vein; portal blood is rich in digestive end-products.
3. The arterial blood is delivered by the hepatic artery (from the celiac trunk).

B. Biliary tree
1. The biliary tree is composed of the bile ducts that connect the liver, gallbladder, and duodenum.
2. The bile ducts are the hepatic ducts, cystic duct, and common bile duct.
3. The common bile duct empties into the duodenum.

C. Gallbladder
1. The gallbladder functions to store and concentrate bile.
2. The gallbladder contracts and releases bile into the bile ducts in response to the hormone cholecystokinin (CCK).

D. Pancreas
1. The pancreas secretes the most important digestive enzymes.
2. The pancreatic enzymes empty into the base of the common bile duct and then into the duodenum.
3. The pancreas is responsive to both cholecystokinin and secretin.

IV. Digestion and Absorption

A. Carbohydrate digestion
1. To be absorbed, carbohydrates must be broken down into monosaccharides, especially glucose.
2. Carbohydrates are digested by enzymes called amylases and disaccharidases.

B. Protein digestion
1. To be absorbed, proteins must be broken down into small peptides and amino acids.
2. Proteins are broken down by proteolytic enzymes or proteases.

C. Fat digestion
1. To be absorbed, fats must be broken down into fatty acids and glycerol.
2. Fats are emulsified by bile and then digested by enzymes called lipases.

V. Nutrition

A. Carbohydrates
1. Carbohydrates are simple or complex.
2. Glucose, the simplest carbohydrate, is the major fuel used by the body for energy.

B. Protein
1. The body needs essential amino acids, which it cannot synthesize; and nonessential amino acids, which it can synthesize.
2. Dietary proteins are complete or incomplete.

C. Fats (lipids)
1. Most dietary lipids are triglycerides.
2. Fats are saturated fats (like butter) or unsaturated fats (like oils).

D. Vitamins
1. Vitamins are small organic molecules that help regulate cell metabolism. Dietary vitamin deficiencies give rise to many diseases (see Table 23.2).
2. Vitamins are water soluble (vitamins B and C) or fat soluble (vitamins A, D, E, and K).

E. Minerals
1. Minerals are inorganic substances necessary for normal body function.
2. Mineral deficiencies can cause serious health problems (see Table 23.3).

Review Your Knowledge

Matching: Structures: Making the Connections
Directions: Match the following words with their descriptions.
a. ileum
b. sigmoid colon
c. jejunum
d. common bile duct
e. transverse colon
f. duodenum
g. esophagus
h. stomach

1. _c_ Connects the duodenum to the ileum
2. _d_ Connects the cystic and hepatic ducts to the duodenum
3. _b_ Connects the rectum to the descending colon
4. _e_ Connects the ascending colon to the descending colon
5. _h_ Connects the esophagus to the duodenum
6. _g_ Connects the pharynx to the stomach
7. _f_ Connects the stomach to the jejunum
8. _a_ Connects the jejunum to the cecum

Matching: Enzymes, Hormones, and Digestive Aids
Directions: Match the following words with their descriptions. Some words may be used more than once.
a. amylases
b. hydrochloric acid

c. disaccharidases

d. secretin

e. bile

f. proteases

g. cholecystokinin (CCK)

h. intrinsic factor

i. lipase

1. _f_ Classification of trypsin and chymotrypsin

2. _b_ Secreted by the parietal cells of the stomach; lowers gastric pH

3. _c_ Digests sucrose, maltose, and lactose

4. _e_ An emulsifying agent

5. _i_ Digest fats to fatty acids and glycerol

6. _g_ Hormone secreted by the duodenum in response to the presence of fat

7. _a_ Digest starch and polysaccharides to disaccharides

8. _d_ Hormone that stimulates the pancreas to secrete a bicarbonate-rich secretion

9. _g_ Hormone that stimulates the gallbladder to contract

10. _f_ Digest protein to small peptides and amino acids

11. _e_ Secreted by the liver and stored in the gallbladder

12. _h_ Necessary for the absorption of vitamin B_{12}

13. _c_ Classification of sucrase, maltase, and lactase

Multiple Choice

1. The esophagus
   a. secretes potent proteolytic enzymes.
   b. secretes intrinsic factor that is necessary for the absorption of vitamin B_{12}.
   c. is a tube that carries food from the pharynx to the stomach.
   d. is the primary site of digestion and absorption.

2. *Parotid, submandibular,* and *sublingual* are words that describe
   a. structures confined to the sphincters in the stomach.
   b. salivary glands.
   c. endocrine glands that regulate gastric motility.
   d. lipase-secreting exocrine glands.

3. Which of the autonomic nerves is the most important with regard to gastrointestinal secretion and motility?
   a. Olfactory
   b. Vagus
   c. Phrenic
   d. Hypoglossal

4. Which of the following is true regarding the stomach?
   a. Its most important function is the digestion of fat.
   b. It is lined with microvilli to maximize absorption.
   c. It is attached distally to the jejunum and proximally to the esophagus.
   d. The most important function is to deliver chyme to the duodenum at the proper rate.

5. Which of the following is *not* descriptive of bile?
   a. Aids in fat digestion
   b. Is an emulsifying agent
   c. Is classified as a lipase
   d. Is stored in the gallbladder

6. Lipases, proteases, and amylases are
   a. gastric hormones.
   b. synthesized by the liver and stored in the gallbladder.
   c. digestive enzymes.
   d. bile-dependent digestive enzymes.

7. Which of the following is *not* a function of the liver?
   a. Makes blood-clotting factors such as prothrombin
   b. Makes bile
   c. Secretes cholecystokinin and secretin
   d. Stores fat-soluble vitamins

8. Which of the following best describes emulsification?
   a. A fat is chemically digested to fatty acids and glycerol.
   b. The fatty acids are absorbed into the lacteal, becoming chyle.
   c. A large fat globule is mechanically broken into smaller fat globules.
   d. A large protein forms ammonia.

9. The pancreas
   a. secretes the most potent digestive enzymes.
   b. secretes CCK and secretin.
   c. is only important because of its endocrine (insulin) function.
   d. empties its digestive enzymes into the appendix.

10. The duodenum and proximal jejunum are most concerned with
    a. the secretion of intrinsic factor and the absorption of vitamin B_{12}.
    b. digestion and absorption.
    c. the synthesis of clotting factors and plasma proteins.
    d. the synthesis of bile and emulsification.

11. Which of the following is true of trypsinogen, chymotrypsinogen, and pepsinogen?
    a. They are secreted by the gastric lining.
    b. They are inactive proteases.
    c. They are pancreatic lipases.
    d. They are emulsifying agents.

12. Gastrin, cholecystokinin (CCK), and secretin are
    a. secretions of the salivary glands.
    b. digestive enzymes.
    c. emulsifying agents.
    d. gastrointestinal hormones.

13. Which of the following are found in gastric juice?
    a. Bile, trypsin, and secretin.
    b. HCl, pepsinogen, and intrinsic factor.
    c. HCl, CCK, bile, and ptyalin.
    d. Trypsin, enterokinase, and bile.

14. With which of the following are chyle and lacteal most associated?
    a. Appendix
    b. Gastric juice
    c. Villus
    d. Microbiota

15. This hormone is secreted by the walls of the duodenum; it slows gastric emptying, stimulates the secretion of pancreatic enzymes, and stimulates the release of bile by the gallbladder.
    a. Pepsinogen
    b. Trypsinogen
    c. Secretin
    d. Cholecystokinin

16. Which of the following is correct regarding the presence of dietary fat in the duodenum?
    a. Slows gastric motility
    b. Suppresses the secretion of CCK
    c. Increases peristalsis in both the stomach and duodenum
    d. All of the above

Go Figure

1. Which of the following is correct according to Fig. 23.1?
   a. All GI structures are located in the abdominopelvic cavity.
   b. The esophagus is located between the stomach and small intestine.
   c. The small intestine is distal to the large intestine.
   d. The liver and pancreas empty their digestive secretions into the upper part of the small intestine.

2. Which of the following is correct according to Fig. 23.2?
   a. The inner lining of the GI tract is composed of mesentery.
   b. GI smooth muscle is well innervated.
   c. The outermost serosal layer of the digestive tract is responsible for peristalsis.
   d. All smooth muscle fibers are oriented in a circular arrangement.

3. Which of the following is correct according to Fig. 23.3?
   a. The salivary glands are endocrine glands.
   b. The secretions of the parotid, submandibular, and sublingual glands are carried to the mouth by salivary ducts.
   c. The parotid duct delivers saliva to the parotid gland from the uvula.
   d. The uvula is a salivary gland.

4. Which of the following is correct according to Fig. 23.4?
   a. The epiglottis is a lid that prevents the entrance of food and water into the larynx and respiratory structures.
   b. The nasopharynx conducts air, water, and food.
   c. The epiglottis prevents the entrance of food and water into the esophagus during deglutition.
   d. The glottis is a large opening for the passage of food and water.

5. Which of the following is correct according to Fig. 23.5?
   a. The fundus, body, and pylorus are sphincters.
   b. The words *circular, longitudinal,* and *oblique* refer to gastric glands.
   c. Gastric contents can reflux from the stomach through the LES and into the base of the esophagus.
   d. The lesser and greater curvatures refer to stomach muscles.

6. Which of the following is correct according to Fig. 23.5?
   a. Parietal cells are located in the stomach lining.
   b. Chief cells secrete HCl and intrinsic factor.
   c. Rugae are found only within the pylorus.
   d. The greater curvature is a gastric structure, and the lesser curvature is a duodenal structure.

7. Which of the following is correct according to Fig. 23.6?
   a. Each villus contains capillaries that all empty into a lacteal.
   b. Villi are widely spread throughout the entire GI tract.
   c. Villi are found only in the stomach.
   d. Villi are found primarily in the small intestine, especially in the duodenum and proximal jejunum

8. Which of the following is correct according to Fig. 23.7?
   a. The hepatic and splenic flexures are parts of the cecum.
   b. The appendix is attached to the cecum in the RLQ.
   c. The sigmoid colon is located between the cecum and the ascending colon.
   d. Haustra are confined to the transverse colon.

9. Which of the following is correct according to Fig. 23.8?
   a. Both the common bile duct and the main pancreatic duct drain into the duodenum.
   b. The gallbladder ejects bile into the hepatic ducts, where it is pumped into the liver.
   c. The tail of the pancreas is closer to the ampulla of Vater than is the head of the pancreas.
   d. The green vessels in Fig. 23.8B carry blood from the portal vein to the hepatic veins.

10. Which of the following is correct according to Fig. 23.9?
    a. Amylases and lipases digest carbohydrates.
    b. Disaccharides are synthesized from amino acids.
    c. Monosaccharides, such as glucose, are the end-products of carbohydrate digestion.
    d. Sucrase, maltase, and lactase are disaccharides.

11. Which of the following is correct according to Fig. 23.12?
    a. The pancreas is located within the stomach.
    b. Most digestive end-products are absorbed across the wall of the small intestine into the villi.
    c. The common bile duct empties into the portal vein.
    d. Villi are found primarily in the large intestine.

12. Which of the following is correct according to Table 23.2?
    a. Thiamine, riboflavin, niacin, and pyridoxine are B vitamins.
    b. Vitamins A, D, E, and K are fat-soluble vitamins.
    c. Thiamine, riboflavin, niacin, and pyridoxine are water-soluble vitamins.
    d. All of the above are true.

13. Which of the following is correct according to Table 23.3?
    a. Iodine is necessary for the synthesis of T_3 and T_4.
    b. Iron, iodine, and calcium are trace minerals.
    c. A deficiency of iodine causes rickets.
    d. Rickets, osteomalacia, and goiters are calcium-deficient states.

Urinary System

Objectives

1. List four organs of excretion.
2. Describe the major organs of the urinary system.
3. Describe the location, structure, blood supply, nerve supply, and functions of the kidneys.
4. Explain the role of the nephron unit in the formation of urine.
5. Explain the three processes involved in the formation of urine: filtration, reabsorption, and secretion.
6. Describe the hormonal control of water and electrolytes by the kidneys.
7. List the normal constituents of urine.
8. Describe the structure and function of the ureters, urinary bladder, and urethra.

Key Terms

aldosterone (p. 468)
angiotensin II (p. 469)
antidiuretic hormone (ADH) (p. 470)
collecting duct (p. 466)
converting enzyme (p. 469)
creatinine (p. 468)
detrusor muscle (p. 473)
dialysis (p. 472)
diuresis (p. 468)
glomerulus (p. 466)

glomerular filtration rate (GFR) (p. 466)
juxtaglomerular apparatus (p. 469)
kidneys (p. 463)
loop of Henle (p. 466)
micturition (p. 475)
natriuresis (p. 470)
natriuretic peptides (p. 470)
nephron unit (p. 465)
peritubular capillaries (p. 466)

renal artery (p. 465)
renal tubules (p. 466)
renal vein (p. 465)
renin (p. 469)
specific gravity (p. 471)
ureter (p. 464)
urethra (p. 464)
urinary bladder (p. 464)
urinary specific gravity (p. 471)
urine (p. 463)

Sammy with his soggy diaper is a friendly reminder of our hardworking urinary system. Sammy may be a bundle of joy, but he is generally a wet bundle. What makes Sammy wet? Like a round-the-clock factory, Sammy eats, drinks, burns fuel, and produces waste products. To remain healthy, his kidneys must remove the waste and constantly adjust the amount of water and the concentration of electrolytes in his body. The kidneys work hard to do this; a wet Sammy is a healthy Sammy.

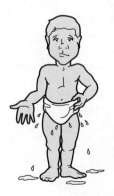

EXCRETION

ORGANS OF EXCRETION

The kidneys are the most important excretory organs. They eliminate nitrogenous waste, water, electrolytes, toxins, and drugs. Other organs perform excretory functions; the sweat glands secrete small amounts of nitrogen compounds, water, and electrolytes; the lungs eliminate carbon dioxide and water; and the intestines excrete digestive wastes, bile pigments, and other minerals (Table 24.1). Whereas the skin, lungs, and intestines eliminate waste, only the kidneys can fine-tune the excretion of water and electrolytes to maintain the normal volume and composition of body fluids.

URINARY SYSTEM ORGANS

The urinary system, shown in Fig. 24.1, makes urine, temporarily stores it, and finally eliminates it from the body. The major organs of the urinary system include the following:

- Two kidneys. The kidneys form urine from the blood.

Table 24.1	Organs of Excretion
ORGAN	**SUBSTANCES EXCRETED**
Kidneys	Water Electrolytes Nitrogenous waste
Skin (sweat glands)	Water Electrolytes Nitrogenous waste
Lungs	Carbon dioxide Water
Intestines	Digestive waste (feces) Bile pigments

- Two ureters. The **ureters** (YOOR-eh-ters) are tubes that conduct urine from the kidneys to the urinary bladder.
- One urinary bladder. The **urinary bladder** acts as a temporary reservoir; it receives urine from the ureters and stores the urine until it can be eliminated.
- One urethra. The **urethra** (yoo-REE-thrah) is a tube that conducts urine from the bladder to the outside for elimination. (Do not confuse the ureters with the urethra.)

URINARY SYSTEM TERMS

There are several words that refer to the urinary system and specifically to the kidneys. The word *renal* (REE-null) refers to the kidney. Thus, *renal physiology*

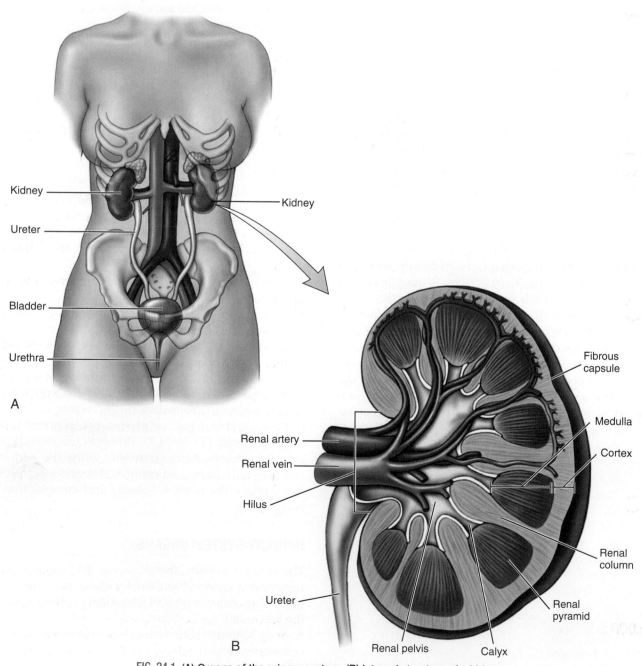

FIG. 24.1 **(A)** Organs of the urinary system. **(B)** Internal structure of a kidney.

refers to the study of kidney function. *Nephrology* (neh-FRALL-oh-jee) also refers to the study of kidney function. The term comes from the nephron unit—the unit in the kidney that makes urine. *Urology* (yur-ALL-oh-jee) is the study of the urinary system.

 Do You Know...

About Urine as a First-Aid Wash?

A scene from the old war stories journal! A soldier is seriously wounded in battle. He is propped up against a charred tree stump as the battle rages on. As his fellow soldiers pass by, they note a large gaping wound in his thigh. Each soldier stops and urinates on the wounded area. Seems rather hostile! However, urine is sterile and acidic. Given the unsanitary wartime conditions, the "cleansing" of the wounded area with urine helped prevent lethal wound infections. A urine wash—not recommended today, but it was better than nothing in the good ol' days.

KIDNEYS

LOCATION

The kidneys are located high on the posterior wall of the abdominal cavity, behind the parietal peritoneum (retroperitoneal; see Fig. 24.1A). The kidneys are cushioned and protected by the renal fascia, adipose tissue pads, and lower rib cage.

STRUCTURE

The kidney is a reddish-brown, beanlike structure enclosed in a tough fibrous capsule. Each kidney is about 4 inches (10 cm) long, 2 inches (5 cm) wide, and 1 inch (2.5 cm) thick. The indentation of the bean-shaped kidney is called the *hilus*. It is the point at which the blood vessels, ureter, and nerves enter and exit the kidney.

What do you see when you cut open a kidney? As shown in Fig. 24.1B, a kidney has three distinct regions: the renal cortex, the renal medulla, and the renal pelvis. The lighter, outer region is the renal cortex. The darker triangular structure, the renal medulla, is located deeper within the kidney. The renal medulla forms striped, cone-shaped regions called *renal pyramids*. Each pyramid is separated by a renal column, an extension of the outer renal cortex. The lower ends of the pyramids point toward the renal pelvis, a basin that collects the urine made by the kidney and helps form the upper end of the ureter. The cuplike edges of the renal pelvis, closest to the pyramids, are calyces. Calyces (KAY-liss-ees) (sing., calyx) collect the urine formed in the kidney.

BLOOD SUPPLY

Blood is brought to the kidney by the **renal artery**, which arises from the abdominal aorta (see Fig. 24.1B).

The renal arteries deliver a large amount of blood to the kidneys, averaging about 20% to 25% of the cardiac output. After entering the kidney, the renal artery branches into a series of smaller and smaller arteries, which deliver blood to the nephron units, the urine-making structures of the kidney. Blood leaves the kidney through a series of veins that finally merge to form the **renal vein**. The renal vein empties into the inferior vena cava.

NERVE SUPPLY

The renal nerves travel with the renal blood vessels to the kidney. The nerves are primarily sympathetic nerves that help control blood flow to the kidney and regulate the release of a blood pressure–regulating enzyme.

 Re-Think

1. List the major organs of the urinary system.
2. What is the name of the artery that supplies the kidney?
3. Explain why a physician may thump a patient in the upper left and right lumbar areas when assessing for evidence of a kidney infection.
4. Define: renal physiologist, nephrologist, and urologist.

FUNCTIONS OF THE KIDNEYS

In general, the kidneys cleanse the blood of waste products, help regulate the volume and composition of body fluids, and help regulate the pH of body fluids. Specifically, the kidneys perform the following tasks:

* Excrete nitrogenous waste such as urea, uric acid, ammonia, and creatinine
* Regulate blood volume by determining the amount of water excreted
* Help regulate the electrolyte content of the blood
* Play a major role in the regulation of acid–base balance (blood pH) by controlling the excretion of hydrogen ions (H^+). (See Chapter 25 for the renal regulation of acid–base balance.)
* Play a role in the long-term regulation of blood pressure
* Play a role in the regulation of red blood cell production through the secretion of erythropoietin

URINE MAKING: THE NEPHRON UNIT

STRUCTURES

The **nephron unit** is the functional unit, or urine-making unit, of the kidney. Each kidney contains about 1 million nephron units. The number of nephron units does not increase after birth, and they cannot be replaced if damaged. Each nephron unit has two parts: a tubular component (renal tubules) and a vascular component (blood vessels).

RENAL TUBULES

The **renal tubules** consist of a number of tubular structures. The glomerular capsule, called *Bowman's capsule,* is a C-shaped structure that partially surrounds a cluster of filtering capillaries called a **glomerulus** (gloh-MAIR-yoo-lus). Note that Fig. 24.2 shows two views of a nephron unit: an anatomical view (lower panel) and a schematic view (upper panel). You should become familiar with both.

Bowman's capsule extends from the glomerulus as a highly coiled tubule called the *proximal convoluted tubule.* The proximal convoluted tubule dips toward the renal pelvis to form a hairpin-shaped structure called the *loop of Henle.* The **loop of Henle** (HEN-lee) contains a descending and ascending limb. The ascending limb becomes the distal convoluted tubule. The distal convoluted tubules of several nephron units empty into a **collecting duct**. The collecting ducts run through the renal medulla to the calyx of the renal pelvis. Urine is formed and modified in these tubules.

RENAL BLOOD VESSELS (VASCULAR STRUCTURES)

The kidney receives blood from the renal artery. The renal artery branches into smaller blood vessels that eventually form the afferent arteriole. The afferent arteriole branches into a cluster, or tuft, of capillaries called a *glomerulus* (as described in the previous section). The glomerulus sits in Bowman's capsule and exits from Bowman's capsule as the efferent arteriole. The efferent arteriole then forms a second capillary network called the **peritubular capillaries**. The peritubular capillaries surround the renal tubule and empty their blood into the venules, larger veins and, finally, into the renal vein. (You need to understand the relationships of the vascular structures to the tubular structures. Become thoroughly familiar with Fig. 24.2.)

> **? Re-Think**
>
> 1. Correct this statement: The kidney only act as an organ of excretion.
> 2. List all tubular structures as you trace a drop of urine from Bowman's capsule to the renal pelvis.
> 3. List all vascular structures as you trace a drop of blood from the renal artery to the renal vein.

URINE FORMATION

Urine is formed in the nephron units as water and dissolved substances move between the vascular and tubular structures. Identify all structures in Fig. 24.2 as urine formation is described. Three processes are involved in the formation of urine: glomerular filtration, tubular reabsorption, and tubular secretion.

GLOMERULAR FILTRATION

Urine formation begins in the glomerulus and Bowman's capsule. Glomerular filtration causes water and dissolved substances to move from the glomerulus into Bowman's capsule. About 20% of the blood that flows through the glomeruli is filtered into the tubules; the remaining 80% of the blood leaves the glomeruli by the efferent arterioles and continues into the peritubular capillaries. Understanding filtration means answering two questions: Why does filtration occur? What substances are filtered across the glomerular membrane?

Why Filtration Occurs

Filtration occurs when the pressure on one side of a membrane is greater than the pressure on the opposite side. Blood pressure in the glomerulus is higher than the pressure in Bowman's capsule. This pressure difference provides the driving force for filtration. This pressure difference is called the *glomerular filtration pressure.* If blood pressure suddenly declines, as in shock, glomerular filtration pressure decreases, thereby reducing urinary output.

What Substances Are Filtered

The wall of the glomerulus contains pores and acts like a sieve or a strainer. The size of the pores determines which substances can move across the wall from the glomerulus into Bowman's capsule. Small substances such as water, sodium, potassium, chloride, glucose, uric acid, and creatinine move through the pores very easily. These substances are filtered in proportion to their plasma concentration. In other words, if the concentration of a particular substance in the plasma is high, much of that substance is filtered. Large molecules such as red blood cells and large proteins cannot fit through the pores and therefore remain within the glomerulus. The water and the dissolved substances filtered into Bowman's capsule are called the *glomerular filtrate.* Note that the glomerular filtrate is protein-free and is called an *ultrafiltrate.* The presence of protein (proteinuria) in the urine indicates abnormally large holes in the glomerulus. The protein that is most often found in the urine is albumin (albuminuria).

The rate at which glomerular filtration occurs is called the **glomerular filtration rate (GFR)**. Here is the amazing thing about GFR—the amount of filtrate formed is 125 mL/min, or 180 L (45 gallons) in 24 hours. Imagine 180 1-L bottles of cola. This is the amount of filtrate formed by your kidneys in 1 day. Obviously, you do not excrete 180 L of urine every day; otherwise, you would do little more than drink and urinate, and you would literally wash away within a few hours. You excrete only about 1.5 L each day, so the big question is what happens to the 178.5 L that are filtered into the tubules but not excreted as urine?

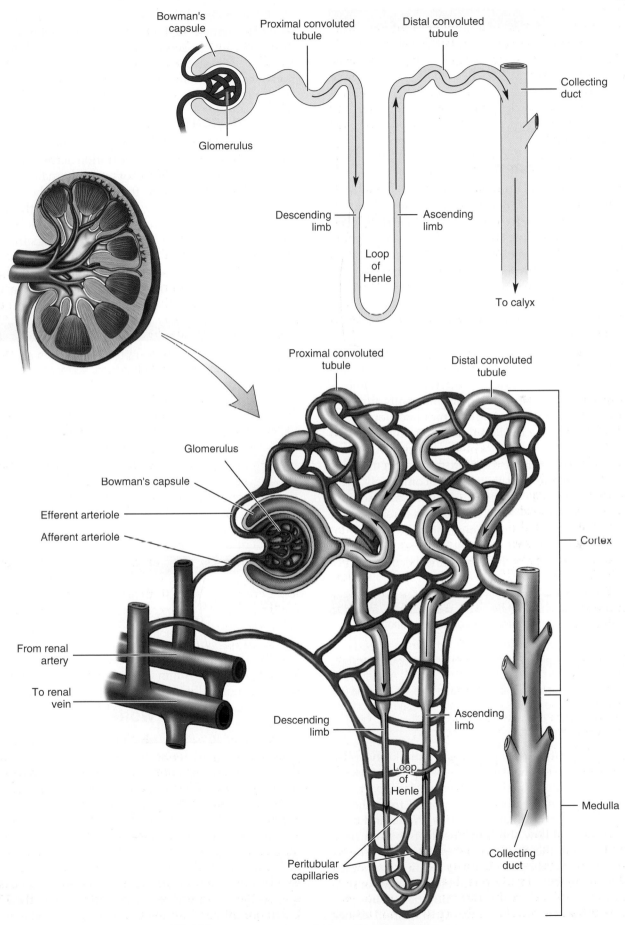

FIG. 24.2 The nephron unit: tubular and vascular structures.

Re-Think

1. Why does filtration occur across the glomerular membrane?
2. Why isn't protein (albumin) normally filtered across the glomerular membrane?
3. What happens to GFR if blood pressure declines to shock levels (70/40 mm Hg)? Explain why a patient in shock is usually oliguric.

TUBULAR REABSORPTION

Most of the filtrate, approximately 178.5 L, is reabsorbed in the kidney and returned to the circulation. Tubular reabsorption is the process whereby water and dissolved substances (glomerular filtrate) move from the tubules into the blood of the peritubular capillaries. Although reabsorption occurs throughout the entire length of the renal tubule, most occurs across the proximal convoluted tubule.

What is reabsorbed into the blood, and what is excreted into the urine? The kidney chooses the type and quantity of substances it reabsorbs. Some substances, such as glucose, are completely reabsorbed. For example, the amount of glucose filtered is the same as the amount reabsorbed, so glucose normally does not appear in the urine. In hyperglycemic conditions, however, excess glucose is filtered; the amount of filtered glucose exceeds the reabsorptive capacity of the tubules. The excess glucose therefore appears in the urine (glucosuria). Some substances are incompletely reabsorbed. For example, over 99% of water and sodium is reabsorbed, whereas only 50% of urea is reabsorbed. Some waste products such as **creatinine** (kree-AT-i-nin) are not reabsorbed at all. Those substances that are not reabsorbed remain in the tubules and become part of the urine.

Do You Know...

Why Serum Creatinine Is a Measure of Kidney Function?

Creatinine is a waste product removed from the blood by the kidneys and eliminated in the urine. If kidney function declines, creatinine accumulates in the plasma. An increase in serum creatinine indicates that the kidneys are not able to excrete it. Thus, serum creatinine levels are used to monitor kidney function.

The reabsorption of substances by the kidney also varies with the mechanism of reabsorption. Absorption occurs through active or passive transport. For example, sodium is actively transported from the tubules into the peritubular capillaries. Water and chloride passively follow the movement of sodium from the tubules into the peritubular capillaries. In general, when sodium is pumped from one location to another, water and chloride follow passively. This response is the basis for the action of most diuretics, drugs that increase the production of urine. Most diuretics block the tubular reabsorption of sodium and therefore also

block the reabsorption of water. The excess sodium and water remain in the tubules and are eliminated as urine. The excess secretion of urine is called **diuresis** (dye-yoo-REE-sis). Hormones regulate the reabsorption of some substances; these hormones are described later in this chapter.

TUBULAR SECRETION

Although most of the water and dissolved substances enter the tubules because of filtration across the glomerulus, a second process moves very small amounts of select substances from the blood into the tubules. This process is tubular secretion. It involves the active transport of potassium ions (K^+), hydrogen ions (H^+), uric acid, ammonium ions (NH_4^+), and drugs from the peritubular capillaries into the tubules. The secretion of H^+ is of particular interest because it is through this mechanism that the kidneys play a crucial role in acid-base regulation.

 Sum It Up!

The urinary system is composed of the urine-making kidneys and the structures that transport, store, and eliminate urine from the body. The urine is made by the nephron units, the functional units of the kidney. Each nephron unit has two parts: a tubular component (renal tubules) and a vascular component (blood vessels). Urine is formed by three processes: filtration, reabsorption, and secretion. Filtration causes water and dissolved substances to move from the glomeruli into the tubules. Reabsorption causes water and selected substances to move from the tubules into the peritubular capillaries. Secretion causes small amounts of specific substances, such as K^+ and H^+, to move from the peritubular capillaries into the tubules.

 Re-Think

1. Identify the specific vascular and tubular structures involved in filtration.
2. Identify the specific vascular and tubular structures involved in reabsorption.
3. Identify the specific vascular and tubular structures involved in secretion.

HORMONES THAT WORK ON THE KIDNEYS

Several hormones act on the kidney to regulate water and electrolyte excretion. Thus, these hormones play an important role in the regulation of blood volume, blood pressure, and electrolyte composition of body fluids (Table 24.2).

ALDOSTERONE

Aldosterone is a hormone secreted by the adrenal cortex. Aldosterone, a mineralocorticoid, acts primarily on the distal tubule and upper collecting duct of the nephron unit. It stimulates the reabsorption of sodium

Table 24.2	Effects of Hormones on the Kidney	
HORMONE	**SECRETED BY**	**FUNCTION(S)**
Aldosterone	Adrenal cortex	Stimulates the reabsorption of sodium and water; stimulates the excretion of potassium; acts primarily on the distal tubule
Atrial natriuretic peptide (ANP)	Atria of the heart	Decreases the reabsorption of sodium; causes greater excretion of sodium and water by the kidney
Brain natriuretic peptide (BNP)	Ventricles of the heart	Decreases the reabsorption of sodium; causes greater excretion of sodium and water by the kidney; acts as a biological marker for heart failure
Antidiuretic hormone (ADH)	Neurohypophysis (posterior pituitary)	Stimulates the reabsorption of water, primarily by the collecting ducts
Parathyroid hormone (PTH)	Parathyroid gland	Stimulates the reabsorption of calcium and excretion of phosphate
Calcitonin	Thyroid gland	Stimulates the excretion of calcium and phosphate

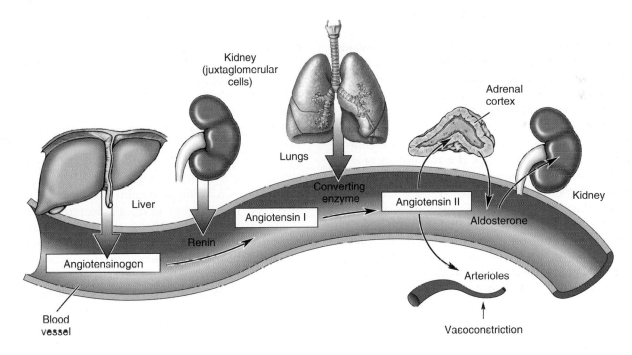

FIG. 24.3 The renin–angiotensin–aldosterone system.

and water and the excretion of potassium. Because of its effect on Na⁺, aldosterone is called the "salt-retaining" (NaCl) hormone. Because aldosterone increases Na⁺ and water reabsorption, it expands or increases blood volume. The expanded blood volume, in turn, increases blood pressure. A deficiency of aldosterone causes severely diminished blood volume, decline in blood pressure, and shock.

What causes the release of aldosterone? One of the most important stimuli for the release of aldosterone is **renin**. Renin is an enzyme that activates the renin–angiotensin–aldosterone system. Renin is secreted by a specialized collection of cells called the **juxtaglomerular apparatus**, located in the afferent arterioles of the kidney. The renin-secreting cells are stimulated when blood pressure or blood volume declines. As Fig. 24.3 shows, renin sets off the following series of events:

- Renin activates angiotensinogen (an-jee-oh-ten-SIN-oh-jen) to form angiotensin I. Angiotensinogen is secreted by the liver and circulates within the blood; angiotensinogen is inactive.
- An enzyme called **converting enzyme** changes angiotensin I to **angiotensin II**. (Converting enzyme is found in the blood throughout the body but is in particularly high concentration in the lungs.)
- Angiotensin II stimulates the adrenal cortex to release aldosterone. The aldosterone, in turn, stimulates the distal tubule of the nephron unit to reabsorb sodium and water and to excrete potassium. The increased blood volume increases blood pressure.
- In addition to stimulating the release of aldosterone, angiotensin II is also a potent vasopressor, a blood pressure–elevating agent. Thus, the activation of the renin–angiotensin–aldosterone system helps

regulate blood volume and blood pressure. A class of drugs called *angiotensin-converting enzyme* (ACE) inhibitors is used to lower blood pressure. They prevent the production of angiotensin II and aldosterone, both of which increase blood pressure. ACE inhibitors include the *-pril* drugs, such as lisinopril and captopril.

> **? Re-Think**
>
> 1. Why is aldosterone called the "salt-retaining" hormone?
> 2. Why is it called the renin–angiotensin–aldosterone system?
> 3. If a patient takes a drug that blocks the production of aldosterone, why must he or she be monitored for hydration status, serum Na^+ (hyponatremia), and serum K^+ (hyperkalemia)?

ANTIDIURETIC HORMONE

A second hormone affecting water reabsorption is **antidiuretic hormone (ADH)**. The action of ADH allows the kidneys to concentrate urine. (Think of the term *antidiuretic hormone*. It literally means "against diuresis.") The posterior pituitary gland (neurohypophysis) secretes ADH (see Chapter 14).

Antidiuretic hormone works primarily on the collecting duct of the nephron unit by determining its permeability to water. In the presence of ADH, the collecting duct becomes permeable to water. Water is reabsorbed from the collecting duct into the peritubular capillaries. In other words, ADH decreases the urinary excretion of water and causes excretion of a concentrated urine. In the absence of ADH, the membrane permeability of the collecting duct decreases and water cannot be reabsorbed; the result is excretion of a large volume of dilute urine. Because ADH affects the amount of water excreted by the kidneys, it plays an important role in the determination of blood volume and blood pressure. Excess ADH expands blood volume, whereas a deficiency of ADH diminishes blood volume.

> **Do You Know...**
>
> ### When Diabetes Is Called "Insipidus"?
>
> "Yuck! This urine is tasteless ... it's insipid!" growled the physician as he sipped his patient's urine. What is going on here? This patient has diabetes insipidus, a condition caused by a deficiency of ADH and characterized by the excretion of a large amount of pale, dilute urine.
>
> In the "good old days," physicians actually tasted the patient's urine as a way to diagnose disease. The pale, dilute urine of ADH deficiency is tasteless, in contrast to the sweet-tasting urine of a patient with insulin deficiency, or "sugar" diabetes. The word *diabetes* refers to diuresis (increased flow of urine), whereas the words *insipidus* and *mellitus* refer to the taste of the urine; *insipidus* refers to tasteless and *mellitus* refers to honey-tasting. Fortunately, and none too soon, the "taste-bud assay" has given way to modern lab tests.

> **Do You Know...**
>
> ### Why Both Diabetes Mellitus and Diabetes Insipidus Cause Polyuria?
>
> Diabetes mellitus is a disease of insulin deficiency that results in hyperglycemia. The hyperglycemia, in turn, leads to excess filtration of glucose by the kidneys. Because all the filtered glucose cannot be reabsorbed, glucosuria develops. The excess glucose in the tubules requires the excretion of large amounts of water, thereby inducing an osmotic diuresis. Thus, the person with diabetes mellitus experiences polyuria (*poly-* means much; *-uria* means urine). Diabetes insipidus is a disease of ADH deficiency. ADH is necessary for the reabsorption of water from the collecting duct. In the absence of ADH, the person may excrete up to 25 L of pale dilute urine. Note that both diabetes mellitus and diabetes insipidus are characterized by polyuria. The word *diabetes* refers to diuresis.

The stimulus for the release of ADH is decreased blood volume and a concentrated plasma. Consider a person who becomes dehydrated by vomiting. The person loses large amounts of water and electrolytes. When the volume of blood decreases and the concentration of the blood increases, ADH is released. The ADH increases the reabsorption of water by the kidneys, expanding blood volume and diluting the blood. The increased blood volume eventually stops the stimulus for the release of ADH. Note that ADH determines the membrane permeability to water. It does not affect Na^+ reabsorption as does aldosterone.

Disturbances of ADH secretion are common. The hypersecretion of ADH is associated with many clinical conditions. Head injuries are a common cause of the syndrome of inappropriate ADH release. Excess ADH increases the reabsorption of water and an expansion of the blood volume. Hyposecretion of ADH causes diabetes insipidus, a condition characterized by the excretion of a large volume of pale dilute urine.

> **? Re-Think**
>
> 1. What gland secretes ADH?
> 2. Why does the name of the hormone reflect its function?
> 3. Give two reasons for the secretion of ADH in the dehydrated state.

NATRIURETIC PEPTIDES

Atrial natriuretic (nay-tree-yoo-RET-ik) peptide (ANP) and brain natriuretic peptide (BNP) cause excretion of sodium (Na^+), a process called **natriuresis** (nat-ree-yoo-REE-sis). ANP is secreted by the walls of the atria of the heart in response to an increase in the volume of blood. BNP is secreted by the walls of the ventricles in response to elevated ventricular volume. The effects of the **natriuretic peptides** are opposite of the effects of aldosterone and ADH. Because ventricular blood volume increases in the failing heart, BNP is used diagnostically in the assessment of heart failure.

Table 24.3   Characteristics of Urine

CHARACTERISTIC	DESCRIPTION
Amount (volume)	Average 1500 mL/day
pH	Average 6.0
Specific gravity	Slightly heavier than water (1.001–1.035)
Color	Yellow (amber, straw-colored, deep yellow in dehydration, pale yellow with overhydration)
Some Abnormal Constituents of Urine	
Albumin (protein)	Albuminuria—indicates an increased permeability of the glomerulus (e.g., nephrotic syndrome, glomerulonephritis, hypertension); sometimes exercise or pregnancy will result in albuminuria.
Glucose	Glycosuria (glucosuria)—usually indicates diabetes mellitus
Red blood cells	Hematuria—bleeding in the urinary tract; indicates inflammation, trauma, or disease
Hemoglobin	Hemoglobinuria—indicates hemolysis (transfusion reactions, hemolytic anemia)
White blood cells	Pyuria (pus)—indicates infection within the kidney or urinary tract
Ketone bodies	Ketonuria—usually indicates uncontrolled diabetes mellitus (fats are rapidly and incompletely metabolized)
Bilirubin	Bilirubinuria—usually indicates disease involving the liver and/or biliary tree

PARATHYROID HORMONE AND CALCITONIN

Parathyroid hormone (PTH) is secreted by the parathyroid glands. It does not affect water balance but plays an important role in the regulation of two electrolytes: calcium and phosphate. PTH stimulates the renal tubules to reabsorb calcium and excrete phosphate. The excretion of phosphate is called the *phosphaturic effect* of PTH. The primary stimulus for the release of PTH is a low plasma level of calcium. Also responding to plasma calcium levels is calcitonin, secreted by the thyroid gland. Calcitonin is released in response to increased plasma calcium and causes the kidneys to excrete calcium and phosphate. (See Chapter 14 for a discussion of PTH and calcitonin.)

COMPOSITION OF URINE

Finally, we can answer this question. What is in urine? Urine is a sterile fluid composed mostly of water (95%), nitrogen-containing waste, and electrolytes. Important nitrogenous waste includes urea, uric acid, ammonia, and creatinine. The light-yellow color of urine is caused by a pigment called *urochrome*, formed from the breakdown of hemoglobin in the liver. The average output of urine is 1500 mL/day. The term *oliguria* (*oligo-* means "scanty") refers to a urine output of less than 400 mL/day. Table 24.3 summarizes the composition of urine along with the significance of some abnormal constituents.

What is meant by the specific gravity of urine? **Specific gravity** is the ratio of the amount of solute to volume. The specific gravity of urine ranges from 1.001 to 1.035, depending on the amount of solute (substances such as Na^+ and creatinine) in the urine. The more solute, the higher is the specific gravity. If a patient is dehydrated, the kidneys filter less water; as a result, the volume of urine decreases. The ratio of solute to volume in the urine therefore increases. Thus, dehydration is characterized by an increase in **urinary specific gravity**. Very dilute urine, as in blood volume expansion, has a low specific gravity.

Regarding odor—it's not too bad if fresh. However, over time, bacteria degrade the urea to ammonia. That explains the "diaper pail" odor. Similarly, a bladder infection can often be detected by the rotten odor of the urine.

 Do You Know...

What Happens When Griz Doesn't Whiz?

As you know, Griz has a long winter nap. Ever think about why he doesn't get ammonia-toxic and have to get up to whiz (urinate)? Griz has the ability to recycle his nitrogenous waste, such as urea, metabolically. In other words, the water and waste are converted into metabolic fuel and reused all winter until Mr. Lazy awakens. If Griz would give up his biochemical secret to scientists, perhaps persons with impaired renal function could do the recycle thing. "No-Whiz Griz" is just fine. He awakens in the spring … to have his fling … then off to sleep, without a peep. Ol' Griz … no whiz.

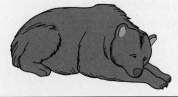

?   **Re-Think**

1. What ions are affected by natriuretic peptides and PTH?
2. Why does dehydration cause an increase in urinary specific gravity?
3. What is the normal urinary pH, glucose concentration, and 24-hour output?

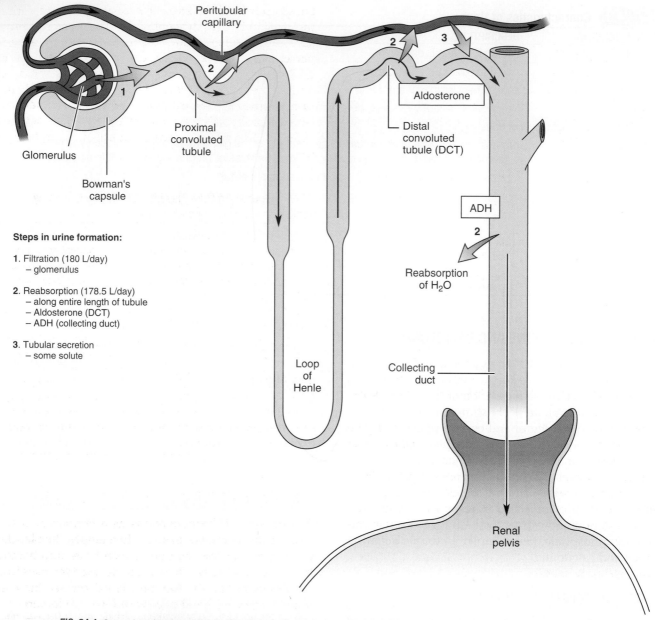

FIG. 24.4 Steps in urine formation—filtration, reabsorption, and secretion—and the effects of aldosterone and ADH.

Labels within figure:
- Peritubular capillary
- Glomerulus
- Bowman's capsule
- Proximal convoluted tubule
- Aldosterone
- Distal convoluted tubule (DCT)
- ADH
- Reabsorption of H$_2$O
- Loop of Henle
- Collecting duct
- Renal pelvis

Steps in urine formation:

1. Filtration (180 L/day)
   – glomerulus

2. Reabsorption (178.5 L/day)
   – along entire length of tubule
   – Aldosterone (DCT)
   – ADH (collecting duct)

3. Tubular secretion
   – some solute

Sum It Up!

Fig. 24.4 summarizes the steps in urine formation. Water and dissolved solute (180 L/day) are filtered across the glomerulus into Bowman's capsule. Whereas reabsorption occurs throughout the entire length of the tubule, most occurs in the proximal tubule. Approximately 1.5 L of urine is excreted from the body in 24 hours. Water (178.5 L/day) and solute move from the tubules into the blood (peritubular capillaries). The kidneys respond to several hormones in regulating the composition of blood: aldosterone ("salt-retaining" hormone), ADH, ANP, BNP, and PTH.

UREMIA AND DIALYSIS

There are many reasons why the kidneys fail. Nephrotoxic drugs, such as the aminoglycosides and many more, and poisons such as antifreeze (ethylene glycol) damage or destroy the kidneys. Infections, such as those caused by *E. coli,* found in contaminated beef, can destroy the kidneys and are capable of causing a lethal hemolytic uremic syndrome (HUS). Finally, chronic diseases such as hypertension, diabetes mellitus, and gout are capable of destroying the kidneys.

When the kidneys fail, they no longer make urine (renal suppression). The blood is not cleansed of its waste, and substances that should have been excreted in the urine remain in the blood. This condition is called *uremia* (yoo-REE-mee-ah), which literally means urine in the blood. Uremia may be prevented with the use of an artificial kidney, a form of **dialysis** (Fig. 24.5). The artificial kidney consists of a cylinder filled with a plasma-like solution called the *dialysate*. The patient's blood is passed through a series of tiny tubes immersed in the dialysate. Waste products in the blood, such as potassium, creatinine, uric acid, and excess water, diffuse out of the tubes into the dialysate. The blood is

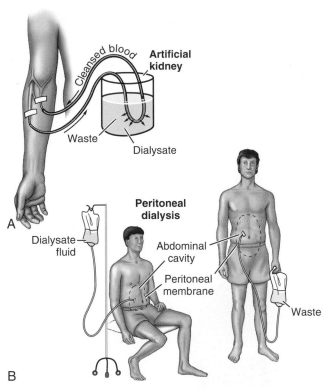

Artificial kidney

Cleansed blood

Waste

Dialysate

A

Peritoneal dialysis

Dialysate fluid

Abdominal cavity

Peritoneal membrane

Waste

B

FIG. 24.5 Types of dialysis. (A) Artificial kidney. (B) Peritoneal dialysis.

thereby cleansed of these waste products and returned to the patient. Because this procedure cleanses blood like a kidney, it is called an *artificial kidney*.

A second form of dialysis is peritoneal dialysis. With this procedure, the peritoneal cavity of the patient is used as the cylinder of an artificial kidney, and dialysate is infused into the peritoneal cavity. Waste products diffuse from the patient's blood into the dialysate. The dialysate eventually drains out of the peritoneal cavity and is discarded.

YOUR PLUMBING

Whereas the kidneys form urine, the remaining structures of the urinary system (ureters, urinary bladder, and urethra) function as plumbing and form the urinary tract (Fig. 24.6). They do not modify the urine in any way; instead, they temporarily store and then conduct urine to the outside of the body for elimination. The urinary tract has an outer layer of connective tissue and a middle layer of smooth muscle. The tract is lined with mucous membrane.

URETERS

Two ureters connect the kidneys with the bladder. The ureters originate in the renal pelvis of the kidneys and terminate in the bladder. The ureters are long (10 to 13 inches [25 to 33 cm]), slender, muscular tubes capable of peristalsis. Urine moves along the ureters from the kidneys to the bladder in response to gravity and peristalsis.

Sometimes, a kidney stone (renal calculus or nephrolithiasis) lodges in the slender ureter, and the urine

backs up behind the stone, increasing pressure within the renal pelvis (hydronephrosis). The increased pressure causes severe pain and renal colic and can adversely affect the kidney, causing a severe decline in GFR and irreversible kidney damage. The stone must be removed. Most stones simply wash out with the urine. Some must be extracted with an instrument inserted into the ureters via the bladder. Other methods include lithotripsy (crushing by ultrasound) and surgical removal.

 Do You Know...

What Ka-plunk and Gush Have to Do with the Lithotomy Position?

"Ka-plunk!" echoed the giant stone as it flew out of the bladder into a bucket. So went the very first lithotomy, a crude and desperate surgical procedure used to extract stones from the urinary bladder. A stone in the bladder acted like a plug, preventing the outflow of urine and causing the urine to accumulate in the bladder. Imagine the discomfort of not being able to urinate for days on end. Generally, the patient was in such excruciating pain that he or she agreed to have a sharp and dirty instrument pushed through the perineum into the bladder. Out popped the stones, followed by a major gush of urine and blessed relief of pressure. Because this position was used to perform the surgical procedure (removal of *lithos*, or stones), the position itself was named the *lithotomy position*, a term (and position) still in use today in gynecological practice.

URINARY BLADDER

The urinary bladder functions as a temporary reservoir for the storage of urine. When empty, the bladder is located below the peritoneal membrane and behind the symphysis pubis. When full, the bladder rises into the abdominal cavity. You can feel a distended bladder if you place your hand over your lower abdomen.

Four layers make up the wall of the bladder. The innermost layer is the mucous membrane and contains several thicknesses of transitional epithelium. The mucous membrane is continuous with the mucous membrane of the ureters and urethra. The second layer is the submucosa and consists of connective tissue and contains many elastic fibers. The third layer is composed of muscle. This involuntary smooth muscle is the **detrusor** (dee-TROO-sor) **muscle**. The outermost layer of the upper part of the bladder is the serosa.

How much can you hold? The bladder wall is arranged in folds called *rugae* that allow the bladder to stretch as it fills. The urge to urinate usually begins when it has accumulated about 200 mL of urine. As the volume of urine increases to 300 mL, the urge to urinate becomes more intense. A moderately full bladder contains about 500 mL, or 1 pint, of urine. An overdistended bladder may contain more than 1 L of urine. With overdistention, the urge to urinate may be lost.

One specific area of the floor of the bladder is the trigone (TRY-gohn). It is a triangular area formed by

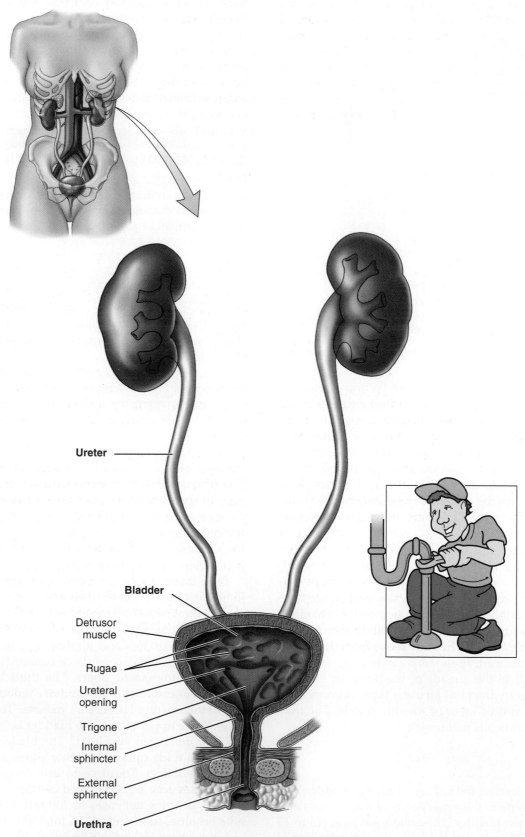

Ureter

Bladder

Detrusor
muscle

Rugae

Ureteral
opening

Trigone

Internal
sphincter

External
sphincter

Urethra

FIG. 24.6 Organs of the urinary tract: ureters, bladder, and urethra (your "plumbing").

three points: the entrance points of the two ureters and the exit point of the urethra. The exit of the urinary bladder contains a sphincter muscle, called the *internal sphincter*. The internal sphincter is composed of smooth muscle that contracts involuntarily to prevent emptying. Below the internal sphincter, surrounding the upper region of the urethra, is the external sphincter. This sphincter is composed of skeletal muscle and is controlled voluntarily. Contraction of the external sphincter allows you to resist the urge to urinate.

 Do You Know...

That a Bladder Infection Can "Ascend"?

The urinary bladder, especially in the female, is a frequent site of infection. An infection of the urinary bladder is called *cystitis*. If cystitis is not treated promptly, pathogens can travel from the bladder up the ureter into the kidney, causing a kidney infection (pyelonephritis). Because the pathogens travel to the kidney from the bladder, a kidney infection is often called an *ascending infection*. In the female, the offending pathogen is usually *E. coli*, a resident of the large intestine. Because the female urethra is short, *E. coli* has a short journey from the meatus to the bladder.

URINATION

Urination, also called **micturition** (mik-too-RISH I-un) or *voiding,* is the process of expelling urine from the bladder. What causes micturition? As the bladder fills with urine, stimulated stretch receptors send nerve impulses along sensory nerves to the spinal cord. The spinal cord reflexively sends motor nerve impulses back to the bladder, causing the bladder wall to contract rhythmically and the internal sphincter muscle to relax. This response is called the *micturition reflex.* This reflex gives rise to a sense of urgency. Contraction of the external sphincter prevents involuntary urination. In an infant, the micturition reflex causes the bladder to empty involuntarily. This is what caused baby Sammy to be a wet bundle of joy. As he matures, he will learn to override this reflex by voluntarily controlling the external sphincter. Only then can Sammy move from diapers to training pants.

A patient may experience urinary retention, or the inability to void or to empty the bladder. Urinary retention

is usually caused by the effects of drugs used perioperatively. Note the difference between renal failure (renal suppression) and urinary retention. Renal failure means that the kidneys do not make urine; urinary retention means that the bladder does not expel urine.

Many patients experience urinary incontinence, or the involuntary leakage of urine from the bladder. There are many causes of incontinence, such as an incompetent bladder sphincter, bladder infection, and excess external pressure as occurs during pregnancy. A chronically full bladder may cause an overflow incontinence. The patient does not urinate and empty the bladder; the excess dribbles out in small amounts. Finally, a sudden rise in bladder pressure as occurs in coughing or laughing causes incontinence; this is called *stress incontinence* and is the source of much embarrassment.

URETHRA

The urethra is a tube that carries urine from the bladder to the outside. It is lined with mucous membrane that contains numerous mucus-secreting glands. The muscular layer of the urethra contracts and helps expel urine during micturition.

The male and female urethras differ in several ways. In the female, the urethra is short (1.5 inches [3.8 cm]); it opens to the outside at the urethral meatus. The female urethral meatus is located anterior to the vaginal opening.

In the male, the urethra is part of the urinary and the reproductive systems. The male urethra (8 inches [20 cm]) is much longer than the female urethra. As the male urethra leaves the bladder, it passes through the prostate gland and extends the length of the penis.

 Re-Think

1. List the urinary structures as you trace a drop of urine from the renal pelvis to the urethral meatus.
2. What is the function of the micturition reflex?
3. List the urinary structures as you trace the movement of *E. coli* from the urethral meatus to the renal pelvis of the kidney.

 Do You Know...

Why an Enlarged Prostate Gland "Slows the Stream" ... or Even Worse?

The male urethra is surrounded by the walnut-shaped prostate gland. When the prostate gland enlarges, pressure is exerted on the outside of the urethra, constricting the lumen of the urethra and impeding the flow or "stream" of urine from the bladder. Urination becomes difficult (dysuria), and the incomplete emptying of the bladder sets the stage for repeated bladder infections. The incomplete emptying also causes nocturia (the need to urinate at night, thereby interfering with sleep), a bothersome symptom that may cause men to seek medical help.

AN AUTONOMIC MOMENT

The detrusor muscle of the urinary bladder and the internal sphincter have muscarinic receptors. Activation of the muscarinic receptors causes the detrusor muscle to contract and the sphincter to relax; this action causes the bladder to expel the urine. This can lead to two pharmacology issues. First, if a patient is experiencing urinary retention, she or he may be given a muscarinic agonist such as bethanechol (Urecholine). The muscarinic agonist causes contraction of the detrusor muscle and relaxation of the urinary sphincter. Second, if a person has been taking medications that have antimuscarinic side effects, he or she may experience difficulty in urinating; the patient can neither contract the bladder nor relax the internal sphincter. This often happens to persons who take preoperative drugs such as atropine and those who take antidepressants that cause anticholinergic side effects.

 Sum It Up!

The kidneys make urine. The urine is stored and transported by the structures that make up the urinary tract: two ureters, bladder, and urethra. The accumulation of urine in the bladder is the stimulus for the micturition reflex and creates the urge to void. Voluntary control of the external sphincter allows you to void at a particular time. Urine exits the body through the urethral meatus.

 As You Age

1. The number of nephron units progressively decreases so that by the age of 70 to 80 years, there has been a 50% reduction. Clinically, this decrease in nephron function causes a diminished ability to concentrate urine.
2. The glomerular filtration rate (GFR) declines with age. As a result, the older person excretes drugs more slowly and is at risk for drug overdose. The decrease in GFR also makes it difficult for the older person to excrete excess blood volume, so any intravenous fluids must be administered slowly and carefully. Overhydration is a common cause of heart failure in older adults.
3. The aging urinary bladder shrinks and becomes less able to contract and relax. As a result, the older person must void more frequently. Because of less effective bladder contraction and residual urine, the incidence of bladder infection increases. The weakening of the external sphincter and a decreased ability to sense a distended bladder increase the incidence of bladder incontinence. Frequent urination in men may be caused by an enlarged prostate gland, a common age-related disorder.

Medical Terminology and Disorders   Disorders of the Urinary System

MEDICAL TERM	WORD PARTS	WORD PART MEANING OR DERIVATION	DESCRIPTION
Words			
azotemia	azote-	From a French word, *azote*, meaning "nitrogen"	**Azotemia** refers to *the presence of nitrogenous waste in the blood;* it develops in persons with renal failure who do not undergo dialysis.
	-emia	blood condition	
cystoscopy	cyst/o-	bladder	**Cystoscopy** is *a visual examination of the bladder*.
	-scopy	examination	
diuresis		From a Greek word meaning "prompting urine"	**Diuresis** refers to *an increase in urine production*. A diuretic drug is one that increases urine production.
polydipsia	poly-	much or many	Refers to *excessive thirst, most often experienced by an uncontrolled diabetic person.*
	-dips/o-	thirst	
glucosuria and other substances in the urine	gluc/o-	glucose	**Glucosuria** refers to *the presence of glucose in the urine;* also called **glycosuria** (glyc/o- = glucose). **Ketonuria** (keton/o- = ketone bodies) refers to *ketone bodies in the urine.* **Albuminuria,** a type of proteinuria, refers to *the presence of albumin in the urine and is usually indicative of glomerular dysfunction.* **Hematuria** is *the presence of blood in the urine;* the blood may come from the kidneys or other urinary tract structures such as the bladder and ureters. **Pyuria** is *pus in the urine and is indicative of an infection.*
	-uria	urine	

Medical Terminology and Disorders   Disorders of the Urinary System—cont'd

MEDICAL TERM	WORD PARTS	WORD PART MEANING OR DERIVATION	DESCRIPTION
kaliuresis	kaliur-	From the Latin word *kalium*, meaning "potassium"	**Kaliuresis** is *the excretion of potassium in the urine;* aldosterone stimulates the renal excretion of potassium.
	-uresis	From the Greek word *ouresis*, meaning "urination"	
lithotripsy	lith/o-	stone or calculus	**Lithotripsy** is *a medical procedure that crushes stones so that they can be expelled without surgical intervention.*
	-tripsis	Greek word meaning "to crush"	
oliguria and other "urias"	olig/o-	scanty	**Oliguria** refers to *scanty or insufficient urine production as occurs in response to protracted hypotension.* **Nocturia** (noct/i- = night) refers to *the necessity of needing to urinate at night.* **Polyuria** is *the excessive production of urine.* **Dysuria** refers to difficulty in passing urine.
	-uria	urine	
natriuresis	natri-	From two words meaning "salt" (Latin, *natrium*) and "urination" (Greek, *ouresis*)	**Natriuresis** is *the excretion of sodium in the urine.* Most diuretic drugs cause natriuresis, resulting in the excretion of sodium and water.
	-uresis		
Disorders			
acute tubular necrosis	necr/o-	death	*Also called* **ATN,** *it is a consequence of renal tubular damage.* A common cause of ATN is a prolonged period of hypotension (as in shock), in which the tubules are deprived of blood, and the tubular cells die. The injured tubular cells cannot reabsorb tubular fluids and electrolytes properly.
	-osis	condition of	
enuresis	enuresis	From a Greek word meaning "to make water"	*The involuntary discharge of urine in a person old enough to be expected to have bladder control.* Commonly called bedwetting, or **nocturnal enuresis.**
glomerulonephritis	glomus-	From a Latin word meaning "ball of thread"	**Glomerulonephritis (GN)** is *an acute or chronic inflammation of the glomeruli; filtration by inflamed glomeruli is impaired so that the composition of urine is altered.* If GN occurs on its own, it is called **primary GN. Secondary GN** develops in response to another disorder, such as autoimmune disorders (lupus) or diabetes mellitus. GN occurs in many forms. One type is called **postinfectious GN;** it is an immune response to a pathogen *(Streptococcus pyogenes)* and classically occurs 10-14 days after a skin or pharyngeal (throat) infection.
	-nephr/o-	kidney	
	-itis	inflammation	
hydronephrosis	hydr/o-	water	*Literally means "water in the kidney."* **Hydronephrosis** refers to *the dilation of the renal pelvis and calyces caused by obstruction to the flow of urine out of the kidney.* The obstruction is usually a kidney stone in one of the ureters; other causes of obstruction include ureteral strictures, nephroptosis (dropped kidney, "floating kidney"), and abdominal adhesions.
	-nephr/o-	kidney	
	-osis	condition of	
nephrosis	nephr/o-	kidney	*Also called* **nephrotic syndrome,** *a group of symptoms that include proteinuria, hypercholesterolemia, elevated serum triglycerides, and edema.* Protein is filtered across the damaged glomeruli, causing albuminuria, hypoalbuminemia, and edema.
	-osis	condition of	
pyelonephritis	pyel/o-	From a Greek word meaning "tub-shaped vessel"	*Also called a* **kidney infection.** It generally begins in the urinary bladder and travels up to the kidney. This UTI is most often caused by *E. coli.*
	-nephr/o-	kidney	
	-itis	inflammation	

Continued

Medical Terminology and Disorders — Disorders of the Urinary System—cont'd

MEDICAL TERM	WORD PARTS	WORD PART MEANING OR DERIVATION	DESCRIPTION
renal calculi	ren/o-	kidney	Urinary stones are classified by location: **nephrolithiasis** (kidney stones, renal calculi); **ureterolithiasis** (stones in the ureter); and **cystolithiasis** (stones in the bladder). Most stones are composed of calcium; this explains the increased risk of kidney stones in patients who are bedridden.
	-calcul/o-	stone	
renal failure			*Also called* **kidney failure.** *The kidneys fail to remove waste, concentrate urine, and maintain electrolyte balance.* There are many causes, including infection, hypovolemia, shock, blood clots in the renal blood vessels, and chronic diseases such as diabetes mellitus. Long-term diabetes mellitus causes **glomerulosclerosis,** or *scarring of the glomeruli.* Renal failure causes uremia, the presence of "urine" in the blood.
urinary incontinence	in-	not	*The inability to control the bladder with an involuntary leakage of urine.* Stress incontinence refers to involuntary discharge of urine when coughing, sneezing, or exercise. Urge incontinence, also called overactive bladder, bladder spasm, and detrusor hyperreflexia, is the sudden urge to urinate as a result of bladder muscle contractions.
	-continent	From a Latin word meaning "to hold in"	

Get Ready for Exams!

Summary Outline

The urinary system consists of organs that make urine, temporarily store it, and then eliminate it from the body. The kidneys contain the nephron units that make urine, thereby eliminating waste from the body and regulating water and electrolyte balance.

I. **Excretion**
   A. There are several organs of excretion: the kidneys, skin, lungs, and intestines.
   B. The urinary system organs include the kidneys, ureters, urinary bladder, and urethra.

II. **Kidneys**
   A. The kidney has three distinct regions: the cortex, medulla, and pelvis.
   B. The kidneys have many functions: excrete nitrogenous waste, regulate blood volume, regulate electrolyte concentration, regulate pH and blood pressure, and stimulate red blood cell production.

III. **Urine Making: Nephron Unit**
   A. The nephron unit is the functional (urine-making) unit of the kidney.
   B. The nephron unit is composed of tubular structures and vascular structures.
   C. There are three processes in urine formation:
      1. Glomerular filtration filters 180 L of filtrate in 24 hours.
      2. Tubular reabsorption causes the reabsorption of 178.5 L of filtrate.
         a. A substance is either completely or incompletely reabsorbed.
      b. A substance is reabsorbed actively or passively.
      3. Tubular secretion causes the secretion of small amounts of specific substances from the peritubular capillaries into the tubules.

IV. **Hormones That Work on the Kidneys**
   A. Aldosterone
      1. Aldosterone stimulates the distal tubule and upper collecting duct to reabsorb Na+ and water and to excrete K+.
      2. The secretion of aldosterone is regulated primarily by the renin–angiotensin–aldosterone system.
   B. Antidiuretic hormone (ADH)
      1. ADH stimulates the collecting duct to reabsorb water.
      2. ADH is released from the posterior pituitary gland in response to low blood volume and increased concentration of solute in the plasma.
   C. Natriuretic peptides (ANP, BNP) inhibit the reabsorption of Na+ and water, thereby causing natriuresis and the excretion of water.
   D. Parathyroid hormone (PTH) stimulates the renal reabsorption of calcium and the excretion of phosphate. Calcitonin increases the renal excretion of calcium and phosphate.

V. **Composition of Urine**
The characteristics of urine are summarized in Table 24.3.
   A. Amount
   B. pH
   C. Specific gravity
   D. Color
   E. Abnormal constituents

VI. Uremia
A. Kidney failure causes a syndrome called uremia.
B. Dialysis can prevent uremia.

VII. Your Plumbing
A. The two ureters are long slender tubes that carry urine from the renal pelvis to the bladder.
B. Urinary bladder
1. The urinary bladder is a temporary reservoir that holds the urine.
2. The detrusor muscle is a smooth muscle responsible for bladder contraction and the elimination of urine.
3. There are two sphincters: internal (involuntary) and external (voluntary).
4. The voluntary elimination of urine is called urination (micturition).
C. The urethra is a tube that carries urine from the bladder to the outside of the body.

Review Your Knowledge

Matching: Plumbing … More or Less
Directions: Match the following words with their descriptions. Some words may be used more than once.

a. urethra
b. kidneys
c. ureters
d. urinary bladder

1. _c_ These two long tubes empty urine into the urinary bladder
2. _b_ The urine-making organs
3. _a_ Urine leaves the bladder through this structure
4. _d_ The external urinary sphincter is located at the distal end of this structure
5. _d_ Its walls contain the detrusor muscle
6. _c_ Tubes that receive urine from the renal pelvis
7. _a_ An enlarged prostate gland prevents the emptying of this structure
8. _d_ Cystitis is an inflammation of this urinary structure
9. _b_ Renal failure is most associated with these structures
10. _d_ Urinary retention is most associated with this structure

Matching: Nephron Unit
Directions: Match the following words with their descriptions. Some words may be used more than once.

a. loop of Henle
b. glomerulus
c. afferent arterioles
d. collecting duct
e. proximal convoluted tubule
f. calyx
g. peritubular capillaries

1. _d_ This structure receives urine from the distal convoluted tubule
2. _b_ The tuft of capillaries that sits within Bowman's capsule
3. _a_ Urine flows from the proximal tubule into this structure
4. _g_ These capillaries surround the tubules and reabsorb huge amounts of water and solute
5. _b_ Filtration occurs across the membrane of this vascular structure
6. _e_ Most reabsorption occurs across this tubular structure
7. _c_ These tiny blood vessels deliver blood to the glomeruli
8. _a_ Hairpin tubular structure between the proximal and distal tubules
9. _f_ A cuplike structure that receives urine from the collecting duct
10. _d_ The tubular site that is most responsive to ADH

Matching: Hormones and Enzymes
Directions: Match the following words with their descriptions. Some words may be used more than once.

a. aldosterone
b. renin
c. parathyroid hormone (PTH)
d. converting enzyme
e. antidiuretic hormone (ADH)
f. brain natriuretic peptide (BNP)
g. angiotensin II

1. _b_ Secreted by the juxtaglomerular apparatus cells; activates angiotensinogen
2. _a_ Stimulates the distal tubule to reabsorb Na+ and excrete K+
3. _e_ Determines the membrane permeability of the collecting duct to water
4. _a_ Mineralocorticoid secreted by the adrenal cortex
5. _f_ Secreted by the walls of the heart; causes the renal excretion of Na+ and water
6. _a_ Called the "salt-retaining" hormone
7. _e_ Deficiency of this hormone causes diabetes insipidus
8. _c_ Stimulates the tubules to reabsorb calcium and excrete phosphate
9. _d_ Secreted by the lungs; changes angiotensin I to angiotensin II
10. _g_ A potent vasopressor that is generated by the action of converting enzyme

Multiple Choice
1. The nephron units
a. are the urine-making structures of the kidney.
b. engage in glomerular filtration but not in tubular reabsorption.
c. are found primarily in the trigone of the urinary bladder.
d. are responsible for micturition.
2. In which structure is urine not modified?
a. Proximal convoluted tubule
b. Collecting duct
c. Ureter
d. Distal convoluted tubule

3. The filtration of 180 L/day of water
   a. is a micturition event.
   b. moves water from the renal tubules into the peritubular capillaries.
   c. is the rate at which urine flows into the urinary bladder.
   d. occurs across the glomerular membrane.
4. Which of the following is the first tubular structure to receive the glomerular ultrafiltrate?
   a. Collecting duct
   b. Renal pelvis
   c. Loop of Henle
   d. Bowman's capsule
5. The active pumping of Na⁺ from the proximal convoluted tubule into the peritubular capillaries
   a. stimulates the micturition reflex.
   b. causes diuresis.
   c. is responsible for the passive reabsorption of water.
   d. can only occur in response to aldosterone.
6. Which of the following is *least* true of aldosterone?
   a. It is a mineralocorticoid.
   b. It is the "salt-retaining" hormone.
   c. It determines the membrane permeability of the collecting duct to water.
   d. It causes the tubular reabsorption of sodium and water.
7. ADH
   a. is released in response to excess blood volume and a dilute plasma.
   b. determines the membrane permeability of the collecting duct to water.
   c. makes the collecting duct impermeable to water.
   d. determines the pore size of the glomeruli.
8. A drug that blocks the renal reabsorption of Na⁺ causes
   a. defecation.
   b. diuresis.
   c. oliguria.
   d. hypernatremia.
9. Why is glucose normally *not* excreted in the urine?
   a. No glucose is filtered.
   b. All filtered glucose is reabsorbed.
   c. Glucose is used up by the metabolizing nephron units.
   d. Glucose is converted to ammonia in the distal tubule and excreted as urea.
10. The proximal and distal convoluted tubules are connected by
    a. the collecting ducts.
    b. Bowman's capsule.
    c. peritubular capillaries.
    d. loop of Henle.
11. Most tubular reabsorption
    a. is a response to aldosterone.
    b. occurs across the proximal tubule.
    c. occurs by filtration.
    d. is a response to ADH.
12. Tubular reabsorption causes water and solute to move from the
    a. tubules into the peritubular capillaries.
    b. peritubular capillaries to the efferent arterioles.
    c. afferent arterioles to the efferent arterioles.
    d. peritubular capillaries to the loop of Henle.

13. A drug that blocks the effects of aldosterone
    a. increases the reabsorption of Na⁺ and water.
    b. is kaliuretic.
    c. may cause an increase in plasma K⁺.
    d. causes oliguria.
14. Micturition
    a. occurs in Bowman's capsule.
    b. refers to the filtration of 180 L of water.
    c. refers to the storage of urine by the bladder.
    d. refers to urination.
15. Oliguria
    a. refers to a lowered serum potassium.
    b. develops in response to hypotension.
    c. is a response to a diuretic drug.
    d. is defined as a urinary output greater than 1500 mL/24 hrs.

Go Figure

1. Which of the following is correct according to Fig. 24.1?
   a. The kidneys are located in the pelvic cavity.
   b. The calyx is the opening through which the renal artery and renal vein enter and leave the kidney.
   c. The renal column is the same as the renal pyramid.
   d. The kidneys are connected to the urinary bladder by two ureters.
2. Which of the following is correct according to Fig. 24.2?
   a. The glomerulus sits within the renal pelvis.
   b. The glomeruli are attached to both the afferent and efferent arterioles.
   c. The peritubular capillaries sit within Bowman's capsule.
   d. The collecting duct empties urine into the loop of Henle.
3. Which of the following is correct according to Fig. 24.2?
   a. Blood from the afferent arterioles drains into the collecting duct.
   b. The loop of Henle is a hairpin-like tubular structure between the proximal and distal tubules.
   c. The proximal convoluted tubule is closer to the collecting duct than is the distal convoluted tubule.
   d. Blood from the peritubular capillaries drains into the renal artery and abdominal aorta.
4. Which of the following is correct according to Table 24.2?
   a. ADH is a neurohypophyseal hormone whose target cells are in the collecting duct.
   b. Aldosterone, like ADH, is a salt-retaining steroid.
   c. An excess of aldosterone or ADH causes diuresis.
   d. Both ANP and BNP are secreted by the renal cortex.
5. Which of the following is correct according to Fig. 24.3?
   a. Renin converts angiotensin I to angiotensinogen.
   b. Converting enzyme activates angiotensin I to angiotensin II.
   c. Aldosterone activates angiotensin II to converting enzyme.
   d. Inhibition of converting enzyme expands blood volume and elevates blood pressure.

6. Which of the following is correct according to Fig. 24.4?
   a. Aldosterone exerts its effect primarily on the proximal convoluted tubule.
   b. Filtration occurs across the glomerulus into Bowman's capsule.
   c. ADH exerts its effect primarily on the descending limb of the loop of Henle.
   d. Most tubular reabsorption occurs across the glomeruli.

7. Which of the following is correct according to Fig. 24.6?
   a. The internal sphincter is located at the base (exit) of the urinary bladder.
   b. Two urethras enter the bladder at the superior part of the trigone.
   c. The trigone contains both the internal and external sphincters.
   d. Plumber Joe indicates that urine formation occurs within the bladder.

8. Which of the following is correct according to Fig. 24.6?
   a. The detrusor muscle forms the wall of the urinary bladder.
   b. The urinary bladder wall has rugae for expansion.
   c. The urinary bladder is drained by a urethra.
   d. All of the above are true.

Objectives

1. Describe the two main fluid compartments and the composition of body fluids.
2. Define *intake* and *output*.
3. Explain the effects of water imbalances, fluid shift, and fluid spacing.
4. List factors that affect electrolyte balance.
5. Describe the most common ions found in the intracellular and extracellular compartments.
6. List three mechanisms that regulate pH in the body.
7. Discuss acid–base imbalances: acidosis and alkalosis.

Key Terms

acidosis (p. 490)
alkalosis (p. 491)
buffer (p. 488)
dehydration (p. 484)
electrolyte balance (p. 485)
extracellular fluid (p. 483)
hyperkalemia (p. 486)
hypernatremia (p 486)
hyperventilation (p. 489)
hypokalemia (p. 486)

hyponatremia (p. 486)
hypoventilation (p. 490)
intake (p. 483)
interstitial fluid (p. 482)
intracellular fluid (p. 483)
intravascular fluid (p. 482)
kaliuretic (p. 486)
Kussmaul respirations (p. 489)
metabolic acidosis (p. 490)
metabolic alkalosis (p. 491)

output (p. 483)
renal compensation (p. 490)
respiratory acidosis (p. 490)
respiratory alkalosis (p. 491)
respiratory compensation (p. 489)
skin turgor (p. 484)
thirst (p. 483)
transcellular fluid (p. 482)

The old saying "You're all wet" has some truth to it. Between 50% and 70% of a person's weight is water. In the average man, water makes up 60% of the weight (about 40 L); in the average woman, water makes up about 50%. An infant is composed of even more water—up to 75%. Because adipose tissue contains less water than muscle tissue, obese persons have less water than thin persons.

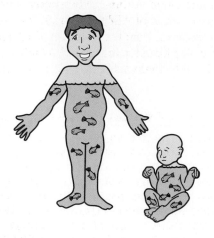

BODY FLUIDS: DISTRIBUTION AND COMPOSITION

FLUID COMPARTMENTS

Water and its dissolved electrolytes are distributed into two major compartments: an intracellular compartment and an extracellular compartment (Fig. 25.1). The intracellular compartment includes the water located in all the cells of the body. Most water, about 63%, is located in the intracellular compartment.

The extracellular compartment includes the fluid located outside all the cells and represents about 37% of the total body water. The extracellular compartment includes the water located between cells, called **interstitial fluid**, water within blood vessels (plasma), and water within lymphatic vessels (lymph). Water within the blood vessels and lymphatic vessels is also called **intravascular fluid**. **Transcellular fluid** is extracellular fluid and includes cerebrospinal fluid, the aqueous and vitreous humors in the eyes, the synovial fluids of joints, the serous fluids in body cavities, and the glandular secretions. Interstitial fluid and plasma are the largest extracellular compartments.

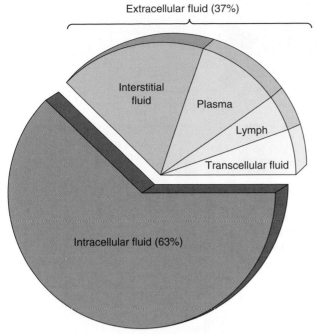

FIG 25.1 Fluid compartments: extracellular and intracellular.

COMPOSITION OF BODY FLUIDS

Intracellular and extracellular fluids vary in their concentrations of various electrolytes. **Extracellular fluids** contain high concentrations of sodium (Na^+), chloride (Cl^-), and bicarbonate (HCO_3^-) ions. The plasma portion contains more protein than do other extracellular fluids. **Intracellular fluid** contains high concentrations of potassium (K^+), phosphate (PO_4^{3-}), and magnesium (Mg^{2+}) ions. The concentration of an ion is indicated when it appears in brackets; thus, $[H^+]$ means the concentration of the hydrogen ion.

Smaller concentrations of other ions are present in both intracellular and extracellular fluids. Although distributed across the fluid compartments, water and electrolytes can move from one compartment to another. The movement of fluid and electrolytes between compartments is well regulated. However, many clinical conditions are associated with shifts of water and electrolytes between compartments.

 Do You Know...

What Is So "Normal" about Normal Saline and Why It Is Normally Given?

Some patients become deficient in body fluids. These may be surgical patients who are not permitted to drink, patients who have been vomiting, or those who are unconscious and unable to eat or drink. These patients often receive intravenous infusions of solutions that resemble plasma in ionic composition. Normal saline, for example, contains 0.9% sodium chloride, a concentration equal to that of plasma. Because the concentration of "salt" in normal saline resembles that of plasma, it is considered normal.

WATER BALANCE

Normally, the quantity of water taken in, which is **intake**, equals the amount of water eliminated from the body, which is **output**. Water balance exists when intake equals output (Fig. 25.2). As part of your clinical responsibilities, you will be measuring intake and output.

WATER INTAKE

Although water intake can vary considerably, the average adult takes in about 2500 mL every day. About 60% comes from drinking liquids, an additional 30% comes from water in foods, and 10% comes from the breakdown of foods. This latter portion is called the *water of metabolism*.

Thirst is the primary regulator of water intake. The thirst center is in the hypothalamus of the brain. As the body loses water, the thirst center in the hypothalamus is stimulated, thus causing you to drink. Drinking restores the water content of the body, so both your thirst and your hypothalamus are satisfied. Older adults have a diminished thirst mechanism and are therefore prone to dehydration.

WATER OUTPUT

In a healthy person, 24-hour intake and output are approximately equal; the individual who takes in 2500 mL of water should therefore eliminate 2500 mL. Water can leave the body through several routes: kidneys, skin, lungs, and digestive tract. The kidneys eliminate about 60% of the water as urine. About 28% is lost from the skin and lungs; 6% is eliminated in the feces, and another 6% is lost as sweat. The amount lost by sweat can vary considerably, depending on the level of exercise and environmental temperatures. Water loss through the skin and lungs increases in a hot, dry environment.

The kidneys are the primary regulator of water output. Water regulation occurs mainly through the action of antidiuretic hormone (ADH) on the collecting duct. When body water content is low, the posterior pituitary gland releases ADH. It stimulates the collecting duct to reabsorb water, thereby decreasing water in the urine and increasing blood volume. When body water content is high, the secretion of ADH decreases. As a result, less water is reabsorbed from the collecting duct, and the excess water is eliminated in the urine. Water balance is also regulated by aldosterone, discussed later in the chapter.

 Do You Know...

What a Prune and a Dehydrated Person Have in Common?

A prune is a dehydrated plum. As water is removed from the plum, its skin assumes a shriveled appearance. The same process occurs in a person who is dehydrated. As fluid is lost from the body, water moves from the interstitium (tissue spaces) into the blood vessels in an attempt to maintain adequate blood volume and blood pressure. As water is lost from the interstitium, the overlying skin appears shriveled, much like a prune. Both the dehydrated patient and prune are said to have poor skin turgor.

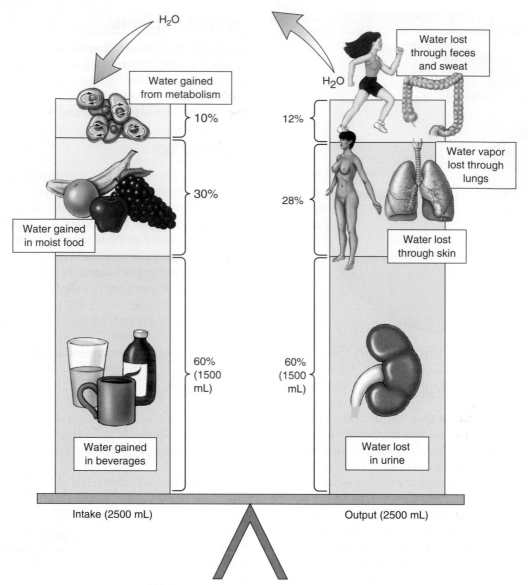

FIG. 25.2 **Water balance: intake equals output.**

WATER IMBALANCES

DEHYDRATION

A deficiency of body water is called **dehydration**. Dehydration develops when water output exceeds water intake and commonly occurs in conditions such as excessive sweating, vomiting, diarrhea, and use of diuretics. A dehydrated person usually has poor skin turgor. **Skin turgor** is assessed by pinching the skin and then observing how quickly the skin flattens, or returns to its normal position. If a person is well hydrated, the pinched skin quickly flattens out. The skin of a dehydrated person, however, flattens out more slowly, giving the skin the appearance of a tent—hence the term *tenting*. Tenting is caused by the depletion of fluid in the interstitial space. If dehydration is untreated, blood volume and blood pressure decline, and the person develops a low-volume (hypovolemic) shock.

EDEMA

The body can retain excess water and deposit it in various compartments, especially the interstitial space. Fluid retention is called *edema*. Edema can be intracellular or extracellular. Generally, we are concerned with interstitial edema. Excess body water can accumulate in various parts of the body. For example, water accumulation in the lungs is called *pulmonary edema*; it causes hypoxemia and cyanosis. Cerebral edema is the accumulation of water in the brain; it causes a life-threatening increase in intracranial pressure and evidence of neurological dysfunction. Water accumulation in the ankle region is called *pedal edema*. As you can see, the consequences can be mild (pedal edema) or life threatening (pulmonary edema and cerebral edema). The goal of therapy is to remove excess fluid, relieve the symptoms, and treat the underlying cause of the edema.

? Re-Think

1. In which fluid compartment is most water located?
2. List four extracellular fluid compartments.
3. Compare the volume of the interstitial space during dehydration and edema.

WHY DOES FLUID SHIFT?

The fluid shifts because of a change in the "pushing and pulling" forces affecting the capillaries. (See Chapter 19 for a discussion of capillary exchange and the mechanisms of edema formation.) The forces include the capillary filtration pressure, plasma oncotic pressure, effect of lymphatic drainage, and effects of plasma protein that becomes trapped in the tissue space. Alteration of any of these factors affects water movement.

FLUID SPACING—IN OTHER WORDS

Fluid spacing is a clinical term that refers to the distribution of body water. *First spacing* refers to the normal distribution of water as described previously. *Second spacing* refers to the accumulation of water in the interstitial spaces (as in pedal edema). Generally, with adequate treatment, this water can be reabsorbed and excreted. *Third spacing* refers to the accumulation of water in spaces from which it is not easily absorbed. For example, the water that accumulates in the abdominal cavity as ascites is not easily reabsorbed. Similarly, the excess water that accumulates within the digestive tract as a result of a paralytic ileus is unavailable for easy reabsorption. The amount of water in "third spaces" can be large and lifethreatening. Monitoring of water distribution is a common clinical concern.

DAILY WEIGHTS AND FLUID BALANCE

The daily measurement of body weight provides a reliable estimate of fluid balance. For example, if a person with heart failure suddenly gains 4.4 lb, you should suspect fluid retention. How is the amount estimated? One liter of water weighs 2.2 lb (1 kg). If a person has a sudden weight gain of 4.4 lb, you can assume that that person has retained 2 L of fluid. Another example is when a patient is given a diuretic and loses 2.2 lb overnight. You can assume that the patient excreted 1 L of fluid.

? Re-Think

1. A physician indicates that a patient is "third spacing." To what is she referring?
2. A 210-lb edematous man was given a powerful diuretic; he lost 2 kg in 12 hours. How much water has he lost?

ELECTROLYTE BALANCE

Electrolyte balance exists when the amounts of the various electrolytes gained by the body equal the amounts lost. *Electrolyte imbalances* are common, serious clinical challenges. Electrolytes are important components of the body fluids. The kidneys control the composition of body fluids by regulating the renal excretion of electrolytes. Table 25.1 includes the major electrolytes and their normal levels and functions.

QUICK REFERENCE: ELECTROLYTES

Chapter 2 describes the chemical characteristics of electrolytes. You will want to review several of the terms listed here for quick reference:

- Ion: An element or compound that carries an electrical charge. Common ions are Na^+, Cl^-, K^+, Ca^{2+}, and Mg^{2+}.
- Cation: A positively charged ion, such as Na^+, K^+, and Ca^{2+}
- Anion: A negatively charged ion, such as Cl^- and HCO_3^- (bicarbonate). Most proteins (such as albumin) carry a negative charge.

Table 25.1   Major Ions and Their Functions

ELECTROLYTE	PLASMA LEVEL (mEq/L)	FUNCTIONS
Sodium (Na^+)	136–145	Chief extracellular cation
		Regulates extracellular volume
		Participates in nerve–muscle function
Potassium (K^+)	3.5–5.0	Chief intracellular cation
		Participates in nerve–muscle function
Calcium (Ca^{2+})	4.5–5.8	Strengthens bone and teeth
		Participates in muscle contraction
		Helps in blood clotting
Magnesium (Mg^{2+})	1.5–2.5	Strengthens bone
		Participates in nerve–muscle function
Chloride (Cl^-)	95–108	Chief extracellular anion
		Involved in extracellular volume control
Bicarbonate (HCO_3^-)	22–26	Part of bicarbonate buffer system
		Participates in acid–base balance
Phosphate (PO_4^{3-})	2.5–4.5	Strengthens bone
		Participates in acid–base balance

- Electrolyte: Substances that form ions when they dissolve in water, such as NaCl (salt):

$$NaCl \rightarrow Na^+ (cation) + Cl^- (anion)$$

- Ionization: The chemical reaction caused when an electrolyte splits into two ions

MOST IMPORTANT IONS

SODIUM (Na+)

Sodium is the chief extracellular cation, accounting for almost 90% of the positively charged ions in the extracellular fluid. Sodium plays a key role in the regulation of water balance. The primary mechanism regulating sodium concentration is aldosterone. Aldosterone stimulates the distal tubule and upper collecting duct of the nephron unit to reabsorb sodium. Usually, "when sodium moves, water moves"; this means that aldosterone causes the reabsorption of both Na+ and water.

Hypernatremia (hye-per-nah-TREE-mee-ah) refers to excess Na+ in the blood and is the result of excess water loss or increased Na+ intake. Note the types of patients who develop hypernatremia:

- Older persons following surgery or fever. They are apt to have a low blood volume and diminished thirst mechanism.
- Patients who have been on prolonged diuretic therapy because of the loss of excessive water as urine.
- Uncontrolled diabetic patients with hyperglycemia. The glucosuria requires the excretion of excessive amounts of water (polyuria) leading to dehydration and hypernatremia.

Hyponatremia (HY-po-nuh-TREE-me-uh) refers to a decrease in the concentration of plasma Na+. Often, a patient becomes hyponatremic because of excess water in the blood. The blood literally is diluted out with water, causing a dilutional hyponatremia, a condition that is serious because it can result in delirium and seizures. Note the types of patients who commonly experience hyponatremia:

- A person with heart failure and expanded blood volume.
- Runners who drink too much water during a marathon.
- Psychiatric patients who "water binge" (drink excessive amounts of water)

POTASSIUM (K+)

Potassium (K+) is the chief intracellular cation. The primary hormone regulating K+ concentration is aldosterone. Aldosterone stimulates the distal tubule and upper collecting duct of the nephron unit to excrete K+ into the urine. The kidney is the primary organ responsible for the excretion of excess K+. The monitoring of serum K+ levels is an important clinical responsibility. Whereas only 2% of the K+ is located in the extracellular space, plasma K+ is important for normal muscle function, especially cardiac function. Changes in plasma levels of K+ cause serious cardiac dysrhythmias.

Hyperkalemia (hye-per-kah-LEE-mee-ah) refers to excess K+ (>5.5 mEq/L) in the blood. The primary cause of hyperkalemia is kidney disease, because the kidneys play a major role in the elimination of K+. Hyperkalemia is an emergency situation and is treated in several ways, including dialysis or the IV administration of an insulin–glucose solution. Dialysis removes K+ from the blood. The IV insulin drives the glucose and K+ into the cells, lowering plasma levels of K+.

Hypokalemia refers to a lower than normal amount of K+ (<3.5 mEq/L) in the blood. Hypokalemia usually presents as muscle fatigue, leg cramps, abdominal distention, and cardiac rhythm disturbances. The most common cause of hypokalemia is the prolonged use of K+-losing diuretics, known as **kaliuretics** (cal-ee-yoo-RET-iks). Some diuretics, such as spironolactone, are not kaliuretic and cause the kidney to reabsorb potassium. These diuretics are called "potassium sparers"; they can cause hyperkalemia. Maintaining normal K+ levels in a patient who requires diuretic therapy is a major clinical concern. You must know which diuretics excrete K+ and which diuretics reabsorb or "spare" potassium. Large amounts of K+ can also be lost through vomiting (or nasogastric tubes) and diarrhea. Hypokalemia is a serious condition and is treated by the administration of K+.

 Do You Know...

Why Acidosis Can Cause Hypokalemia ?

As acidosis develops, the body attempts to decrease the plasma [H+] by moving it from the blood into the cells. As H+ enters the cells, it ejects K+ from the cells into the blood, where it is filtered by the kidneys and excreted in the urine. When the acidosis is corrected, the H+ leaves the cells and goes back into the blood. The K+ then re-enters the cells, thereby making the person hypokalemic.

CALCIUM (Ca2+)

Calcium is necessary for bone and teeth formation, muscle contraction, nerve impulse transmission, and blood clotting. Of the body's calcium, 99% is in the bones and teeth. Parathyroid hormone is the primary regulator of plasma levels of calcium. Hypercalcemia and hypocalcemia are described in Chapter 14. (Do not confuse the terms *hypercalcemia* and *hyperkalemia*.)

MAGNESIUM (Mg2+)

Next to K+, magnesium is the most abundant cation in the intracellular fluid. Magnesium is important in the function of the heart, muscles, and nerves. Kidney disease is the major cause of hypermagnesemia. Other causes include overuse of magnesium-containing antacids. Hypomagnesemia is often seen in critically ill persons.

CHLORIDE (Cl⁻)

Chloride is the chief extracellular anion, and it usually follows sodium. That is, when sodium is actively pumped from the tubules into the peritubular capillaries, chloride follows the sodium passively. Changes in the plasma levels of chloride affect acid–base balance through its effect on bicarbonate. For example, when the plasma chloride level decreases (hypochloremia), the plasma bicarbonate level increases and causes alkalosis. Hyperchloremia, on the other hand, causes a decrease in the plasma bicarbonate level and a state of acidosis. Like sodium, chloride is greatly affected by diuretic therapy.

BICARBONATE (HCO₃⁻)

Bicarbonate is an important anion in acid–base balance. Bicarbonate is an alkaline (basic) substance that helps remove excess H^+ from the body. It is also the form in which carbon dioxide (CO_2) is transported in the blood. Bicarbonate excretion is controlled by the kidneys. Bicarbonate can be either reabsorbed or excreted by the kidneys, depending on the body's needs.

OTHER IONS

The plasma contains other ions, such as sulfate (SO_4^{2-}) and phosphate (PO_4^{3-}). The normal laboratory values for the major ions are summarized in Table 25.1.

Sum It Up!

The volume and composition of body fluids are closely regulated. Body fluids are found in two main compartments; most body fluid (63%) is in the intracellular compartment, and the remaining 37% is in the extracellular compartment. Fluids can shift from one compartment to another. The extracellular compartment contains interstitial fluid, plasma, lymph, and transcellular fluid. The electrolyte composition of the body fluids is important. The chief extracellular cation is sodium; the chief intracellular cation is potassium. Excesses and deficiencies of water and electrolytes cause serious clinical problems.

? Re-Think

1. Explain the following: "When sodium moves, water moves."
2. What is the major extracellular cation? Intracellular cation?
3. Define the following: *hyperkalemia*, *hypokalemia*, and *kaliuresis*.
4. Explain the following statement: Aggressive diuresis with a loop diuretic, such as furosemide (Lasix), may cause a person to become hypokalemic, dehydrated, and hypotensive.

ACID–BASE BALANCE

A normally functioning body requires a balance between acids and bases. Acid–base balance is described according to its regulation of pH. Why is the regulation of pH so important? All chemical reactions in the body occur at a particular pH; any alteration in pH interferes with these many reactions. The nervous system is particularly sensitive to changes in [H^+]. When fluid becomes more acidic, neuronal activity decreases, and level of consciousness declines. When it becomes more alkaline, the neurons become more excitable and apt to cause seizures.

QUICK REFERENCE: ACIDS AND BASES

Chapter 2 describes acids, bases, and pH. You will want to review several terms for quick reference:
- Acid: A substance that dissociates (splits) into H^+ and an anion such as Cl^- (e.g., $HCl \rightarrow H^+ + Cl^-$). An acid donates a hydrogen ion (H^+) during a chemical reaction. A strong acid, such as HCl, dissociates completely into H^+ and anions; it yields many H^+. A weak acid, such as vinegar, dissociates very little and therefore produces fewer H^+. Carbonic acid, $H_2CO_3^-$ is also a weak acid.
- Base: A substance that combines with H^+ during a chemical reaction and removes H^+ from solution (e.g., $OH^- + H^+ \rightarrow H_2O$). The hydroxyl ion ($OH^-$), for example, combines with H^+ to form water (H_2O). A base is an H^+ acceptor. A strong base, such as NaOH, dissociates completely, producing many OH ions that remove many hydrogen ions (H^+) from solution. A weak base dissociates less and removes fewer hydrogen ions (H^+). $NaHCO_3$ is a weak base.
- pH: A unit of measurement that indicates the number of H^+ in solution. Remember that as the number of H^+ increases, the pH decreases. As the number of H^+ decreases, the pH increases. The normal plasma pH ranges from 7.35 to 7.45 and is therefore slightly alkaline. A plasma pH of less than 7.35 is called *acidosis*, and a plasma pH greater than 7.45 is called *alkalosis* (Fig. 25.3A).

WHERE THE ACID COMES FROM

Remember that acids generate H^+. Most H^+ comes from the body's chemical reactions during metabolism. For example, when glucose is metabolized in the presence of oxygen, it produces carbon dioxide (CO_2), water, and energy. The CO_2 combines with water and forms an acid (carbonic acid), yielding H^+. When glucose is metabolized in the absence of oxygen, it forms lactic acid. When fatty acids are metabolized very quickly, they yield ketoacids. Finally, when proteins are metabolized, some of them yield sulfuric acid. All these acids are produced by metabolizing cells. To maintain acid–base balance, the body must neutralize and excrete the excess acids.

HOW THE BODY REGULATES pH

Three mechanisms work together to regulate pH: buffers, respirations, and kidney function (see Fig. 25.3B).

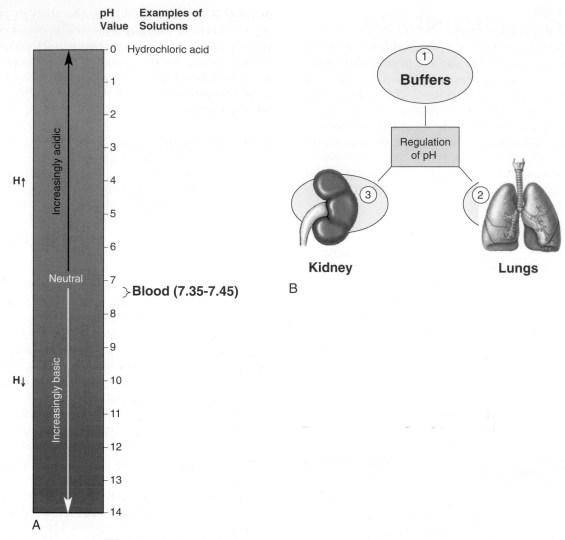

FIG. 25.3 (A) pH scale. (B) Regulation of pH by buffers, lungs, and kidneys.

BUFFERS

The buffer system is the first line of defense in the regulation of pH. A **buffer** is a chemical substance that prevents large changes in pH. There are two parts to a buffer, called a *buffer pair,* which consists of a base and an acid. A buffer pair works like this: If [H+] in the blood increases, the base part of the buffer removes H+ from the blood. If the [H+] decreases, the acid part of the buffer donates H+ to the blood. By removing or adding H+, the buffer pair can help maintain a normal blood pH. The body has numerous buffer pairs; the most important are the bicarbonate buffers, phosphate buffers, hemoglobin, and plasma proteins.

Here's an example of how the bicarbonate/carbonic acid buffer pair works. The bicarbonate ion (HCO_3^-) is the base, and the carbonic acid part is the acid.

> **Base...HCO_3^-...H^+ acceptor**

> **Acid...H_2CO_3...H^+ donor**

In uncontrolled diabetes, strong ketoacids are added to the blood. Immediately the HCO_3^- part of the buffer, acting as a H+ acceptor, combines with the H+ and converts it to H_2CO_3, a weak acid. What has happened? The HCO_3^- part of the buffer pair has converted a strong ketoacid to a weak acid. Remember, a weak acid does not produce many H+. The buffering by the base (HCO_3^-) has minimized the decline in pH. What happens when a patient has lost H+ because of severe and prolonged vomiting (loss of HCl)? The acid part of the buffer pair (H_2CO_3), acting as an H+ donor, dissociates and adds H+ to the blood, thereby minimizing an increase in blood pH. Without the buffers, any change in [H+] would cause a significant change in blood pH.

LUNGS

The respiratory system is the second line of defense in the regulation of pH. It does so by its handling of CO_2, accounting for many liters of acid being efficiently removed from the blood each day. The easiest way to understand the respiratory control of pH is to observe the relationship of respiratory activity and pH under two conditions:

- changes in respiratory activity as the cause of changes in pH
- changes in respiratory activity that correct changes in pH

RESPIRATORY ACTIVITY AS THE CAUSE OF CHANGES IN pH

Refer to Fig. 25.4. Note the reaction in panel A that indicates the relationship between CO_2 and acid. CO_2 combines with H_2O to form carbonic acid which then dissociates into $H^+ + HCO_3^-$ Conversely, the H^+ and $+HCO_3^-$ combine to form $H_2CO_3^-$, which dissociates to CO_2 and H_2O. (The double arrows indicate the reversible reactions.)

In panel B, note the effect of decreased respiratory activity (hypoventilation) on the reaction. Hypoventilation causes CO_2 retention; $[CO_2]$ increases, thereby driving the reaction to the right and increasing $[H^+]$. The increased $[H^+]$ decreases pH (<7.35), and the person is said to be acidotic. Because the acidosis is caused by the decreased respiratory activity (hypoventilation), it is called *respiratory acidosis*.

In panel C, note the effect of increased respiratory activity (**hyperventilation**) on the reaction. Hyperventilation, by exhaling CO_2, causes $[CO_2]$ to decrease, thereby driving the reaction to the left and decreasing $[H^+]$. The decreased $[H^+]$ increases blood pH (>7.45), and the person is said to be alkalotic. Because the alkalosis is caused by the increased respiratory activity, it is called *respiratory alkalosis*.

RESPIRATORY ACTIVITY AS THE CORRECTION FOR CHANGES IN pH

Not only can respiratory activity cause changes in pH, it can also correct or compensate for changes in pH. An excellent example is the **respiratory compensation** for diabetic ketoacidosis (metabolic acidosis) in uncontrolled diabetes mellitus. Recall from Chapter 14 that the lack of insulin in diabetes mellitus produces strong ketoacids; the pouring of excess acid into the blood sets off the following sequence of events:

- Excess H^+ from the ketoacids enter the blood.
- Despite the effect of buffering, $[H^+]$ increases, and blood pH declines (acidosis).
- The increased $[H^+]$ in the blood activates H^+ chemoreceptors.
- The response to the activated chemoreceptors results in the stimulation of the medullary respiratory center.
- Respiratory rate and depth increase, thereby exhaling or "blowing off" CO_2. This respiratory response to increased $[H^+]$ is called **Kussmaul respirations**.
- Increased exhalation of CO_2 causes the reaction to move to the left, thereby decreasing the amount of H^+ and increasing blood pH. The removal of H^+ continues as long as the person continues to "blow off" CO_2.

$$CO_2 + H_2O \leftarrow H_2CO_3 \leftarrow H^+ + H_2CO_3^-$$

- Thus, the increased respiratory activity compensates for the metabolic acidosis caused by the production of excess ketoacids.

Respiratory activity can also correct or compensate for clinical conditions characterized by decreased blood $[H^+]$ and increased blood pH (metabolic alkalosis). In this example the alkalosis was induced by excess vomiting of HCl. Follow the sequence of events:

- Excess vomiting causes a loss of H^+ from the body.
- $[H^+]$ in the blood decreases, causing pH to increase (alkalosis).
- Decreased $[H^+]$ decreases activation of the H^+ chemoreceptors, resulting in decreased stimulation of the medullary respiratory center.

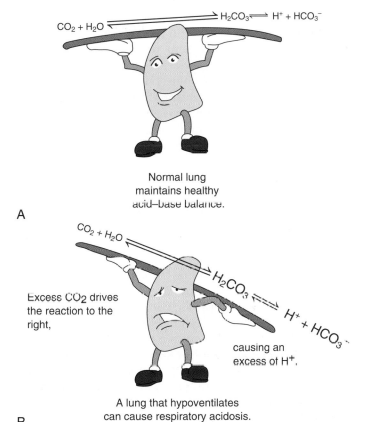

Normal lung maintains healthy acid–base balance.

A

Excess CO_2 drives the reaction to the right,

causing an excess of H^+.

A lung that hypoventilates can cause respiratory acidosis.

B

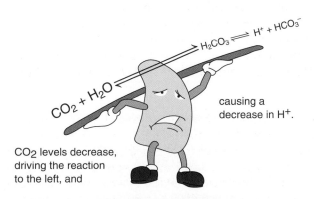

CO_2 levels decrease, driving the reaction to the left, and

causing a decrease in H^+.

A lung that hyperventilates can cause respiratory alkalosis.

C

FIG. 25.4 Respiratory control of acid–base balance. (A) Normal respiratory rate. (B) Hypoventilation causes respiratory acidosis. C, Hyperventilation causes respiratory alkalosis.

- Respiratory rate and depth decrease, thereby retaining CO_2.
- Increased CO_2 drives the reaction to the right, producing H^+ and lowering pH.

$$CO_2 + H_2O \rightarrow H_2CO_3 \rightarrow H^+ + HCO_3^-$$

- Thus, the decreased respiratory activity compensates for the metabolic alkalosis caused by the loss of H^+ through vomiting of HCl.

KIDNEYS

The kidneys are the third line of defense in the regulation of pH. The kidneys help regulate pH by reabsorbing or excreting H^+ as needed. H^+ secretion takes place along the entire length of the renal tubules. The kidneys also help regulate pH by making, reabsorbing, or excreting bicarbonate (HCO_3^-), a major buffer. Because the kidneys are major H^+ eliminators, patients in kidney failure are generally acidotic.

> **? Re-Think**
>
> 1. What are the three mechanisms that achieve acid–base regulation?
> 2. Explain how a buffer pair works to maintain pH. Use the bicarbonate–carbonic acid buffer pair in your explanation.
> 3. Explain how changes in respiratory activity can cause pH imbalances.
> 4. Explain how changes in respiratory activity can correct or compensate for pH imbalances.

ACID–BASE IMBALANCES

When the body is unable to regulate pH, acid–base imbalances develop. The acid–base imbalances in the blood are called *acidosis* and *alkalosis*. These imbalances are common, exert generalized effects, and are often lifethreatening. As stated earlier, the normal blood pH is 7.35 to 7.45. If the pH exceeds 8.2 or declines below 6.8 for several hours, the patient usually cannot survive. The acid–base imbalances, their causes, and compensatory mechanisms are summarized in Table 25.2.

ACIDOSIS

A decrease in plasma pH below 7.35 is **acidosis**. (Remember that an increase in the plasma $[H^+]$ results in a decrease in pH.) The two types of acidosis are respiratory acidosis and metabolic acidosis. **Respiratory acidosis** is caused by any condition that decreases the effectiveness of the respiratory system or causes prolonged **hypoventilation**. For example, chronic lung disease (emphysema), high doses of narcotics, splinting of the chest, and injury to the medulla oblongata may all cause a decrease in respiratory activity.

How does the body try to correct respiratory acidosis? First, the buffer systems remove some of the excess H^+. Then the kidneys excrete the excess H^+ and increase plasma bicarbonate (HCO^{3-}). The ability of the kidneys to correct respiratory acidosis is called the **renal compensation** for respiratory acidosis. The respiratory system cannot correct this pH imbalance because it is the dysfunctional respiratory system that is causing the acidosis.

Metabolic acidosis is a decrease in pH caused by nonrespiratory conditions. For example, kidney disease, uncontrolled diabetes mellitus (described earlier), prolonged vomiting of intestinal contents (with loss of bicarbonate), and severe diarrhea (with loss of bicarbonate) are common causes of metabolic acidosis. A patient with poor kidney function is unable to excrete H^+ and becomes acidotic.

How does the body try to correct metabolic acidosis? First, the buffer system removes some of the excess H^+. Second, the respiratory system helps remove excess H^+ through hyperventilation or Kussmaul respirations. The increased respiratory activity is called the respiratory compensation for metabolic acidosis. Last, the kidneys, if functional, increase their secretion of H^+ and reabsorption of bicarbonate.

Table 25.2   pH Imbalances

IMBALANCE	CAUSES	COMPENSATIONS
Acidosis (pH <7.35)		
Respiratory acidosis	Any condition that causes hypoventilation (chronic lung disease such as emphysema, asthma, splinting of the chest, high doses of narcotic drugs, myasthenia gravis)	Kidneys excrete H^+ and reabsorb HCO_3^- (renal compensation for respiratory acidosis)
Metabolic acidosis	Kidney disease, diarrhea, diabetic ketoacidosis, lactic acidosis, vomiting of intestinal contents	Increased respiratory rate to blow off CO_2; Kussmaul respirations (respiratory compensation for metabolic acidosis)
Alkalosis (pH >7.45)		
Respiratory alkalosis	Any condition that causes hyperventilation (anxiety)	Kidneys retain H^+ and excrete HCO_3^- (renal compensation for respiratory alkalosis)
Metabolic alkalosis	Persistent vomiting of stomach contents (loss of HCl), gastric suctioning, overingestion of antacids and bicarbonate-containing drugs	Decreased respiratory activity to retain CO_2 (respiratory compensation for metabolic alkalosis)

Do You Know...

Why You Can Hyperventilate Yourself into a Hypocalcemic Tetany?

An anxious person often hyperventilates, causing a respiratory alkalosis. Calcium is less soluble in alkalotic blood. Consequently, the plasma levels of calcium decrease. Because calcium is necessary for normal nerve conduction, nerve function is impaired, and the person experiences numbness and tingling. If the person continues to hyperventilate, the plasma levels of calcium may decline so much that an episode of hypocalcemic tetany could occur.

ALKALOSIS

An increase in plasma pH above 7.45 is **alkalosis**. The two types of alkalosis are respiratory alkalosis and metabolic alkalosis. **Respiratory alkalosis** develops from hyperventilation and the resulting decrease in plasma CO_2 and [H^+]. Common causes of respiratory alkalosis include anxiety and aspirin (salicylate) poisoning.

The body tries to correct respiratory alkalosis by the buffers and the kidneys. The buffers donate H^+ to the plasma, thereby decreasing pH. The kidneys decrease the excretion of H^+, thereby decreasing pH. The kidneys also increase the excretion of bicarbonate. The ability of the kidneys to correct respiratory alkalosis is called the renal compensation for respiratory alkalosis. The respiratory system cannot correct this pH disturbance because it is the overactivity, or hyperventilation, of the respiratory system that is causing the alkalosis.

Metabolic alkalosis is an increase in pH caused by nonrespiratory disorders. Metabolic alkalosis can be caused by overuse of bicarbonate-containing antacid drugs, persistent vomiting of stomach contents (loss of HCl), and frequent nasogastric suctioning (loss of HCl). The body tries to correct metabolic alkalosis through buffers, the kidneys, and the respiratory system. The buffers donate H^+, thereby decreasing pH. The kidneys decrease their excretion of H^+. Finally, the respiratory system corrects the pH by hypoventilation. Hypoventilation increases plasma CO_2 and H^+ and decreases pH.

Note that the respiratory system can both cause a pH imbalance and help correct or compensate for a nonrespiratory pH imbalance. Similarly, the kidneys can both cause and correct pH imbalances. The ability of the lungs and the kidneys to correct a pH imbalance is called a *compensatory function*.

 Re-Think

1. Define *acidosis* and *alkalosis*.
2. Differentiate between respiratory and metabolic acidosis.
3. Differentiate between a respiratory and metabolic alkalosis. Explain how the kidneys correct respiratory acidosis, as in ketoacidosis.

 Sum It Up!

Plasma [H^+] is expressed as pH. The normal plasma pH range is 7.35 to 7.45. It is regulated by three mechanisms: buffers, respirations, and kidney function. Acid–base balance is essential for the proper functioning of millions of chemical reactions in the body. Thus, acid–base imbalances pose a serious threat to health. The imbalances are classified as acidosis, a plasma pH less than 7.35 (respiratory and metabolic), or alkalosis, a plasma pH higher than 7.45 (respiratory and metabolic). There are respiratory compensatory mechanisms for metabolic pH imbalances. There are renal compensatory mechanisms for respiratory pH imbalances.

 As You Age

1. As the kidneys age, the tubules become less responsive to antidiuretic hormone (ADH) and tend to lose too much water. The excess water loss is accompanied by a decrease in the thirst mechanism. As a result, the older person is prone to dehydration.
2. The ability to reabsorb glucose and sodium is also diminished. The presence of excess solute (sodium and glucose) in the urine contributes to excess urination and water loss. In addition, impaired reabsorption of glucose interferes with blood glucose monitoring in diabetes.
3. The kidney tubules are less efficient in the secretion of ions, including the hydrogen ion (H^+). As a result, the older person experiences difficulty in correcting acid–base imbalances.
4. With immobility and diminished exercise, calcium moves from the bones into the renal tubules. There the calcium precipitates, causing kidney stones.

Medical Terminology and Disorders   Water, Electrolyte, and Acid–Base Imbalances

MEDICAL TERM	WORD PARTS	WORD PART MEANING OR DERIVATION	DESCRIPTION
Words			
dehydration	de-	from or down	**Dehydration** is *the loss of water that is necessary for normal body function; it occurs when the body loses more water than it takes in.*
	-hydr/o-	water	
	-ation	process	
edema		From a Greek word meaning "a swelling tumor"	**Edema** is *the accumulation of excess fluid, causing swelling.*
Disorders			
pH Imbalances			
acidosis	acid-	From a Latin word meaning "sour" or "sharp," as in vinegar	*A condition in which there is excess H+ (acid) in body fluids.* The blood pH is <7.35. Acidosis is classified as either respiratory or metabolic acidosis (described in text).
	-osis	condition of or increase	
alkalosis	alkali-	From a Greek word meaning "soda ash," a basic or alkaline substance that is slippery and caustic	*A condition in which there is insufficient H+ in body fluids.* The blood pH is >7.45. Alkalosis is classified as either respiratory or metabolic (described in text).
	-osis	condition of or increase	
Electrolyte Imbalances			
hypernatremia	hyper-	above or excessive	**Hypernatremia** is *an elevation in plasma sodium (>145 mmol/L) and can occur in response to a loss of water (most common) or a gain of sodium.* **Hyponatremia** is *a decrease in plasma sodium (<135 mmol/L); it occurs in response to a loss of sodium-containing fluids or excess intake of water (called dilutional hyponatremia).*
	-natr-	From the Latin word *natrium,* meaning "sodium"	
	-emia	in the blood	
hyperkalemia	hyper-	above or excessive	*An elevation of potassium (>5.5 mEq/L) in the blood.* Three causes include: (1) failure to eliminate K+, as in impaired kidney function and the use of drugs such as ACE inhibitors, (2) shift of K+ out of the cells, as occurs in tissue injury or catabolism, and (3) excess intake of K+, as in K+-rich drugs or salt substitutes. Because hyperkalemia affects the depolarization of excitable cells (nerve and muscle), hyperkalemia causes muscle weakness and cramping, nerve paresthesias, and cardiac conduction irregularities.
	-kal/i-	From the Latin word *kalium,* meaning "potassium"	
	-emia	blood condition	
hypokalemia	hypo-	below or deficient	*A decrease of potassium (<3.5 mEq/L) in the blood.* Three causes include: (1) excess K+ loss as occurs in kidney and GI losses (especially diarrhea, vomiting, and GI suctioning), (2) shift of K+ into the cells, and (3) decreased intake of K+.
	-kal/i-	From the Latin word *kalium,* meaning "potassium"	
	-emia	blood condition	
extracellular water imbalances			*Refers to an extracellular volume excess (hypervolemia) or deficit (hypovolemia).* Hypervolemia is also called **volume overload.** It refers to excess extracellular volume and is caused by heart failure, excess steroids, liver failure, impaired kidney function, and excess intravenous fluid infusion. The excess fluid causes weight gain and can accumulate in the extremities (peripheral edema), in the abdominal cavity (ascites), and in the lungs, thereby reducing oxygenation and causing dyspnea and orthopnea. **Hypovolemia** refers to *a diminished volume of blood and is commonly caused by excessive loss of water or reduced intake.* If untreated, the condition progresses to hypovolemic shock and death.

Get Ready for Exams!

Summary Outline

Water, electrolytes, acids, and bases are tightly regulated. Fluids and electrolytes must be distributed in the body compartments in the correct volumes and concentrations.

I. Body Fluids: Distribution and Composition
  A. Major fluid compartments
    1. Two major fluid compartments: intracellular and extracellular compartments
    2. Extracellular compartment: interstitial fluid, intravascular fluid (plasma), lymph, and transcellular fluid
  B. Composition of body fluids
    1. Intracellular fluid: potassium (K^+), phosphate (PO_4^{3-}), and magnesium (Mg^{2+})
    2. Extracellular fluid: sodium (Na^+), chloride (Cl^-), and bicarbonate (HCO_3^-)

II. Water Balance: Intake Equals Output
  A. Intake
    1. The average intake of water is 2500 mL/24 hr.
    2. The primary regulator of fluid intake is thirst.
  B. Output
    1. The average output of water is 2500 mL/24 hr.
    2. Water is excreted by the kidneys, skin, lungs, digestive tract, and sweat.
  C. Water, deficiency, and excess
    1. Deficiency of body water: dehydration
    2. Excess of body water: expanded blood volume and edema

III. Electrolyte Balance
  A. Sodium (Na^+)
    1. Chief extracellular cation
    2. Necessary for water balance and nerve–muscle conduction
    3. Primarily regulated by aldosterone
  B. Potassium (K^+)
    1. Chief intracellular cation
    2. Necessary for nerve–muscle conduction
    3. Primarily regulated by aldosterone
  C. Calcium (Ca^{2+})
    1. Strengthens bones and teeth; necessary for muscle contraction, nerve–muscle conduction, and blood clotting
    2. Primarily regulated by parathyroid hormone
  D. Magnesium (Mg^{2+}) and Chloride (Cl^-)
    1. Magnesium performs important functions in heart, muscles, and nerves.
    2. Chloride: chief extracellular anion; follows Na^+
  E. Bicarbonate (HCO_3^-)
    1. A major extracellular anion
    2. Transports CO_2
    3. Regulates acid–base balance

IV. Acid–Base Balance
  A. pH
    1. The pH refers to the concentration of H^+.
    2. The normal blood pH is 7.35 to 7.45. Acidosis occurs if blood pH is less than 7.35; alkalosis occurs if blood pH is more than 7.45.
  B. Regulation of blood pH

    1. Blood pH is regulated by buffers, the respiratory system, and the kidneys.
    2. Buffers (the buffer pair) can donate or remove H^+.
    3. The respiratory system affects pH by regulating CO_2.
    4. The kidneys can vary their excretion of H^+ and reabsorption of bicarbonate.

V. Acid–Base Imbalances
  A. Acidosis (blood pH <7.35)
    1. Respiratory acidosis is caused by hypoventilation.
    2. Metabolic acidosis has nonrespiratory causes, including kidney disease, uncontrolled diabetes mellitus, diarrhea, and lactic acid production.
  B. Alkalosis (blood pH >7.45)
    1. Respiratory alkalosis is caused by hyperventilation.
    2. Metabolic alkalosis is caused by nonrespiratory conditions, including overingestion of antacids and loss of gastric contents.

Review Your Knowledge

Matching: Water Compartments
Directions: Match the following words with their descriptions. Some words may be used more than once.

a. interstitial
b. intracellular
c. plasma
d. transcellular

1. ___ Most body water is located within this compartment
2. ___ Water located within the vascular compartment (blood vessels)
3. ___ Water located between the cells
4. ___ Includes water within the eye, glandular secretions, and cerebrospinal fluid
5. ___ Also called tissue fluid

Matching: Ions
Directions: Match the following words with their descriptions. Some terms may be used more than once.

a. Na^+
b. K^+
c. H^+
d. Ca^{2+}

1. ___ Plasma concentration of this ion determines pH
2. ___ The chief extracellular cation
3. ___ The chief intracellular cation
4. ___ The ion that is elevated in hyperkalemia
5. ___ Aldosterone stimulates the distal tubule and upper collecting duct to reabsorb this cation
6. ___ Hypoventilation causes the accumulation of CO_2 and this cation
7. ___ Many diuretics are kaliuretic and therefore cause a loss of this cation
8. ___ Most diuretics work by blocking the renal reabsorption of this cation
9. ___ An increase in this ion causes acidosis
10. ___ This ion is regulated primarily by parathyroid hormone

Multiple Choice

1. Hyperkalemia
   a. refers to an elevated serum potassium level.
   b. is caused by an oversecretion of aldosterone.
   c. develops in response to kaliuresis.
   d. refers to dangerously high levels of plasma sodium.

2. True statements about thirst include which of the following?
   a. Thirst is the primary regulator of water intake.
   b. The thirst center is in the hypothalamus.
   c. Older persons have a diminished thirst sensation and are therefore prone to underhydration.
   d. All of the above are true.

3. Which of the following best indicates the role of albumin in water balance?
   a. Blocks the renal reabsorption of Na⁺
   b. Enhances the renal excretion of K⁺
   c. Maintains plasma oncotic pressure
   d. "Plugs up" capillary pores, keeping water within the plasma

4. The primary hormonal regulator of blood K⁺ is
   a. ADH.
   b. vasopressin.
   c. aldosterone.
   d. insulin.

5. Which of the following refers to the accumulation of water in the abdominal cavity as ascites?
   a. Poor skin turgor
   b. Tenting
   c. Third spacing
   d. Hypovolemia or blood volume contraction

6. Prolonged kaliuresis is most apt to cause which of the following?
   a. Hypovolemia and low-volume shock
   b. Tetany
   c. Hypokalemia and cardiac dysrhythmias
   d. Sodium and water retention with expanded blood volume

7. A patient with a history of heart failure was admitted to the hospital in pulmonary edema. Over a 4-day period, his breathing improved, and he experienced a weight loss of 8 lb. Which of the following best explains his clinical improvement?
   a. Increased hematocrit and oxygen-carrying capacity of the blood
   b. Increased secretion of aldosterone and Na⁺ reabsorption
   c. Diuresis
   d. Volume expansion

8. Which of the following is *not* true of Na⁺?
   a. Na⁺ is the chief extracellular cation.
   b. Na⁺ helps regulate extracellular volume.
   c. Na⁺ is affected by aldosterone.
   d. Na⁺ retention causes diuresis.

9. The activation of angiotensin I by a converting enzyme
   a. raises blood pressure.
   b. decreases systemic vascular resistance (SVR).
   c. causes the JGA cells to release renin.
   d. causes natriuresis and kaliuresis.

10. Impaired respiratory gas exchange and hypoventilation are most apt to cause
    a. volume expansion and heart failure.
    b. diuresis and dehydration.
    c. an increase in blood pH.
    d. respiratory acidosis.

11. Kussmaul respirations are the compensatory mechanism for
    a. pulmonary edema.
    b. respiratory acidosis.
    c. metabolic acidosis.
    d. anxiety-induced hyperventilation.

12. Which of the following is most apt to happen when fatty acids are broken down rapidly and incompletely?
    a. Plasma pH increases.
    b. The patient hypoventilates in an attempt to correct the pH disturbance.
    c. Ketoacids are produced, causing metabolic acidosis.
    d. Plasma [H⁺] decreases.

13. Hypocalcemia is most apt to
    a. cause blood volume expansion (hypervolemia).
    b. be treated with IV potassium.
    c. cause tetany.
    d. be caused by excess parathyroid hormone activity.

14. An anxiety-induced hyperventilation
    a. decreases blood pH.
    b. causes alkalosis.
    c. increases [H⁺] in the blood.
    d. decreases PO_2.

15. "Tenting" and poor skin turgor are
    a. a consequence of hypervolemia.
    b. best treated with a diuretic.
    c. due to volume depletion in the interstitial space.
    d. indicative of hyperkalemia.

16. Which of the following is *least* true of alkalosis?
    a. It can be caused by an anxiety-induced hyperventilation.
    b. The blood pH >7.45.
    c. Blood [H+] is decreased.
    d. It is usually caused by CO_2 retention.

Go Figure

1. Which of the following is correct according to Fig. 25.1?
   a. Most fluid is located in the extracellular space.
   b. Interstitial fluid is the same as intravascular fluid.
   c. Plasma and interstitial fluid are extracellular fluids.
   d. Lymph is located intracellularly.

2. Which of the following is correct according to Fig. 25.2?
   a. Thirst is a major regulator of water intake.
   b. Most water is lost in the urine.
   c. Water can be lost by organs other than the kidneys.
   d. All of the above are true.

3. Which of the following is correct according to Fig. 25.3?
   a. As [H⁺] increases, pH increases.
   b. The pink end of the pH scale represents a more acidic pH.
   c. The blue end of the pH scale represents an increase in [H⁺].
   d. All of the above are true.

4. Which of the following is correct according to Fig. 25.4 and Table 25.2?
   a. Hypoventilation causes alkalosis.
   b. Hyperventilation causes alkalosis.
   c. Ventilation has no effect on blood pH.
   d. Hypoventilation decreases [H+] in the blood.

5. Which of the following is correct according to Fig. 25.4B?
   a. Hypoventilation increases CO_2 and H+ production.
   b. CO_2 retention causes an increase in blood pH.
   c. CO_2 retention decreases [H+] in the blood.
   d. CO_2 retention causes respiratory alkalosis.

6. Which of the following is correct according to Fig. 25.4 and Table 25.2?
   a. Kussmaul respirations are compensatory for metabolic acidosis.
   b. Hypoventilation is compensatory for a drug-induced respiratory depression.
   c. An anxious person may hyperventilate, causing a respiratory acidosis.
   d. Persistent vomiting of stomach contents is most apt to induce a metabolic acidosis.

Chapter

26

Reproductive Systems

http://evolve.elsevier.com/Herlihy

Objectives

1. List and describe the structures and functions of the male reproductive system.
2. Describe the hormonal control of male reproduction, including the effects of testosterone.
3. List and describe the structures and functions of the female reproductive system.
4. Explain the hormonal control of the female reproductive cycle and the two reproductive cycles.
5. Describe the structure of the breast and lactation.
6. Describe the various methods of birth control.

Key Terms

breasts (p. 510)
cervix (p. 504)
colostrum (p. 510)
endometrium (p. 504)
epididymis (p. 499)
estrogen (p. 504)
external genitals (p. 500)
fallopian tubes (p. 504)
gametes (p. 496)
gonadotropins (p. 507)
gonads (p. 496)

graafian follicle (p. 502)
lactation (p. 510)
mammary glands (p. 510)
menopause (p. 510)
menses (p. 506)
milk let-down reflex (p. 510)
myometrium (p. 504)
ovarian cycle (p. 507)
ovarian follicles (p. 502)
ovaries (p. 502)
ovulation (p. 502)

progesterone (p. 504)
prostate gland (p. 500)
scrotum (p. 496)
semen (p. 500)
spermatogenesis (p. 499)
testes (p. 496)
testosterone (p. 496)
uterus (p. 504)
vagina (p. 505)
vas deferens (p. 499)

Few biological drives are as strong as the urge to reproduce. As everyone knows and appreciates, human reproduction is sexual, meaning that both a female and male partner are required. In contrast, reproduction in single-cell organisms is asexual, meaning that no partner is required. They simply divide by themselves. Think of how different your life would be in an asexual environment!

To carry out its role, the reproductive system performs two functions: it produces, nurtures, and transports ova and sperm, and it secretes hormones. The reproductive organs include the primary reproductive organs and the secondary reproductive organs. The primary reproductive organs are the **gonads**. The female gonads are the ovaries; the male gonads are the testes.

The gonads perform two functions: they secrete hormones, and they produce the **gametes**. The gametes (GAM-eets) are the ova (eggs) and the sperm. All other organs, ducts, and glands in the reproductive system are secondary, or accessory, reproductive organs. The secondary reproductive structures nourish and transport the eggs and sperm. They also provide a safe and nourishing environment for the fertilized eggs.

MALE REPRODUCTIVE SYSTEM

The male reproductive system performs three roles: it produces, nourishes, and transports sperm; it deposits the sperm within the female reproductive tract; and it secretes hormones. Fig. 26.1A shows the organs of the male reproductive tract.

TESTES

The **testes**, or testicles, are the male gonads. They perform two functions: the production of sperm and the secretion of the male hormone, **testosterone** (see Fig. 26.1A). The two oval testes are located outside the abdominal cavity and are suspended in a sac between the thighs called the **scrotum**. The testes begin their development within the abdominal cavity but normally descend into the scrotum during the last 2 months of fetal development.

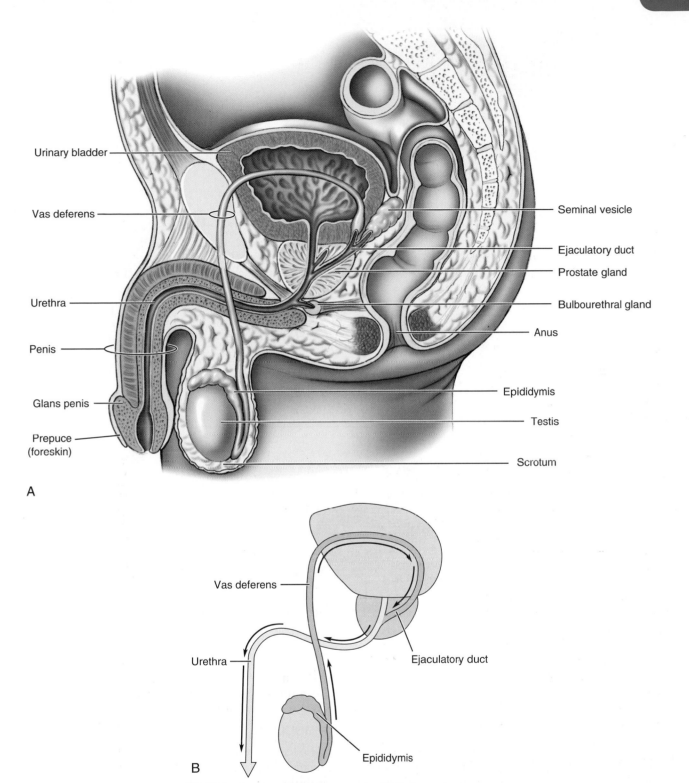

FIG. 26.1 (A) Male reproductive organs. (B) Pathway for semen.

Do You Know...

Why Aristotle Called the Testicle the Orchis?

The root of the orchid plant is olive shaped; in Greek, the shape is called an *orchis.* Noticing the similarity between the shape of the orchid root and the testicles, Aristotle dubbed the testicle *orchis.* The word *orchis* is still used in medical terms; for example, *orchitis* refers to inflammation of the testicles, and *orchiectomy* refers to the surgical removal of the testicles. The word *testis* comes from the Latin and means "to bear witness to." The word *testes* shares the same Latin root with the word *testify.* In ancient Rome, only men could bear witness, or testify, in a public forum. To show the importance of their testimony, they held their testicles as they spoke.

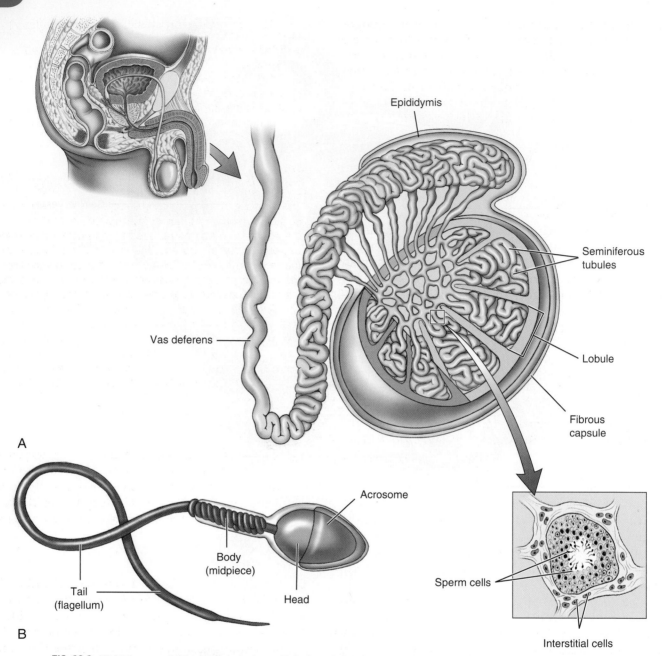

FIG. 26.2 (A) Male gonad. The testis consists of lobules containing seminiferous tubules surrounded by interstitial cells. (B) Sperm.

LOCATION, LOCATION, LOCATION

Why are undescended testicles (cryptorchidism) associated with infertility? It's a temperature thing. Sperm cannot live at body temperature; instead, they prefer the cooler temperature of the scrotum. To avoid infertility, a surgeon pulls the undescended testicles into the scrotum. Wearing tight underwear and jeans can also elevate the temperature in the testes, thereby lowering sperm count. What happens when the outside environmental temperature becomes excessively cold during the winter months? The scrotum, with the assistance of the cremaster muscle, pulls the testes close to the body, thereby keeping the sperm toasty, happy, and motile.

LOBULES

The testis is divided into about 250 smaller units called *lobules* (Fig. 26.2A). Each lobule contains seminiferous tubules and interstitial cells (also called *Leydig cells*). The tightly coiled seminiferous (seh-mih-NIF-er-us) tubules form sperm. The interstitial cells lie between the seminiferous tubules and produce the male hormones called *androgens*. The most important androgen is testosterone. Thus, the testes produce both sperm and testosterone.

SPERM CELLS

Under the influence of gonadotropins and testosterone, a man makes millions of sperm each day. Sperm production begins at puberty and continues throughout life. Sperm are formed by the epithelium of the seminiferous tubules. The seminiferous tubules contain two types of cells: spermatogenic cells (cells that produce sperm) and supporting cells (cells that support, nourish, and regulate the spermatogenic cells). The supporting cells are also called *sustentacular cells* or *Sertoli cells*.

Spermatogenesis

Spermatogenesis (sper-mah-toh-JEN-eh-sis) is the formation of sperm within the seminiferous tubules. The undifferentiated spermatogenic cells are called *spermatogonia*. Each spermatogonium contains 46 chromosomes (the diploid [DIP-loyd] number), the normal number of chromosomes for human body cells. The spermatogonium in the seminiferous tubules undergoes mitosis, thereby producing two identical daughter cells (daughter cell A and daughter cell B); each daughter cell has 46 chromosomes. Daughter cell A remains in the seminiferous tubules as a stem cell and source of future spermatogonia. Daughter cell B differentiates into a primary spermatocyte, still retaining 46 chromosomes.

The primary spermatocytes undergo meiosis. During meiosis, genetic information is swapped and rearranged along the chromosomes, thereby creating considerable genetic variation in the population. Meiosis also causes a reduction in chromosomal number from 46 (diploid number) to 23 (haploid number). The reduction in the chromosomal number is important because upon fertilization (the union of the sperm having 23 chromosomes and ovum, having 23 chromosomes) the chromosomal number of the human body cell is restored to 46.

The final stage of spermatogenesis is called *spermiogenesis*, each immature sperm cell develops a head and a tail. The nonmotile sperm accumulate in the lumen of the seminiferous tubules and then move on to the epididymis where they begin to mature. The mature sperm are called *spermatozoa*. From spermatogonium to spermatozoon—about 70 hours.

A sperm looks like a tadpole (see Fig. 26.2B). The mature sperm has three parts: a head, body, and tail. The head is primarily a nucleus. The nucleus is important because it contains the genetic information. The front part of the head has a specialized structure called the *acrosome*, which contains enzymes that help the sperm penetrate the egg at the time of fertilization. The body, or midpiece, of the sperm is a spiral-shaped structure that contains many mitochondria and supplies the sperm with the energy. The tail of the sperm is a flagellum. Its whiplike movements enable the sperm to swim. Most sperm live only hours after being deposited in the female reproductive tract, but the hardier ones may survive for up to 3 days.

Re-Think

1. What are the names of the male and female gonads? Gametes?
2. Differentiate between the functions of the seminiferous tubules and the interstitial cells.
3. What is the significance of a reduction in the chromosomal number from 46 pairs of chromosomes (diploid number) to 23 (haploid number)?

Sum It Up!

The purpose of the reproductive system is to produce offspring. Human reproduction is achieved sexually through the union of an egg and a sperm. The primary reproductive organs are the gonads: the ovaries in the female and the testes in the male. The gonads produce the gametes; the ovaries produce the female gametes (eggs), and the testes produce the male gametes (sperm). The mature egg and sperm each contain 23 chromosomes. On union, the fertilized egg contains 46 chromosomes, the number of chromosomes that human cells contain. Spermatogenesis describes the steps in sperm formation within the seminiferous tubules. Meiotic cell division reduces the chromosomal number from the diploid (46) to the haploid number (23).

GENITAL DUCTS

As the sperm form, they gather in the seminiferous tubules and move into a series of genital ducts, where they mature. They are then transported from the testes to outside the body. The ducts include two epididymides, two vas (ductus) deferens, two ejaculatory ducts, and one urethra.

EPIDIDYMIS

The **epididymis** (ep-i-DID-i-miss) is the first part of the duct system. It is about 20 feet (6 m) in length, is tightly coiled, and sits along the top and posterior side of the testis (see Fig. 26.1). While in the epididymis, the sperm mature, becoming motile and fertile. The walls of the epididymis contract and push the sperm into the next structure, the vas deferens.

VAS DEFERENS AND EJACULATORY DUCTS

The **vas deferens** (DEF-er-enz) is continuous with the epididymis. It ascends as part of the spermatic cord through the inguinal canal in the groin region into the pelvic cavity. There are two spermatic cords: one coming from the right and one from the left groin region. In addition to the vas deferens, the spermatic cord includes blood vessels, lymphatic vessels, nerves, muscles, and connective tissue.

As the vas deferens courses through the pelvic cavity, it curves over the urinary bladder and joins with the duct of the seminal vesicle to form the ejaculatory duct (see Fig. 26.1). The two ejaculatory ducts, from the right and left sides, pass through the prostate gland and join with the single urethra.

URETHRA

The urethra extends from the base of the urinary bladder to the tip of the penis. The male urethra serves two organ systems: the reproductive and urinary systems. The urethra carries urine from the urinary bladder to the outside. It also carries semen from the ejaculatory ducts to the outside. However, the urethra can only do one thing at a time. It passes either urine or semen, but never both simultaneously.

ACCESSORY GLANDS

Various secretions are added to the sperm as they travel through the genital ducts. The secretions come from three glands: the seminal vesicles, the prostate gland, and the bulbourethral glands (see Fig. 26.1A).

SEMINAL VESICLES

The seminal vesicles are located at the base of the bladder and secrete a thick yellowish material rich in substances such as fructose (sugar), vitamin C, and prostaglandins. These substances nourish and activate the sperm as they pass through the ducts.

PROSTATE GLAND

The single walnut-like **prostate gland** encircles the upper urethra just below the bladder. The prostate gland secretes a milky alkaline substance that plays a role in increasing sperm motility. It also counteracts the acidic environment of the vagina and so helps protect the sperm as they enter the woman's body. During ejaculation, the smooth muscle of the prostate gland contracts and forces the secretions into the urethra.

 Do You Know...

If It Is a Prostrate or a Prostate Gland?

The walnut-shaped gland of the male surrounds the urethra as it leaves the bladder. The word *prostate* means "one who stands before"; the prostate gland stands before the exit from the bladder. It sort of has a noble ring to it! However, sometimes the gland is mistakenly called the "prostrate" gland. A prostrate position is flat and helpless—definitely not a flattering name for such equipment. So, it's *prostate*, not *prostrate*.

BULBOURETHRAL GLANDS

The pea-shaped bulbourethral glands, or Cowper's glands, are tiny glands located beneath the prostate gland. They secrete thick mucus into the urethra. The mucus serves as a lubricant during sexual intercourse.

SEMEN

The mixture of sperm and the secretions of the accessory glands is called **semen**. About 60% of the volume of semen comes from the seminal vesicles. The rest of it comes from the prostate gland. Semen is a milky white liquid with an alkaline pH.

The secretions of the accessory glands perform several other functions; they nourish the sperm, aid in the transport of sperm, and lubricate the reproductive tract. The amount of semen per ejaculation is small, about 2 to 6 mL, or 1 teaspoon. The number of sperm per ejaculation, however, is impressive—200 to 600 million!

EXTERNAL GENITALS

The **external genitals** (genitalia) of the male consist of the scrotum and the penis (see Fig. 26.1). The scrotum is a sac, or pouch of skin, that hangs loosely between the legs and contains the testes.

The penis has two functions; it carries urine through the urethra to the outside of the body, and it acts as the organ of sexual intercourse (copulation). The penis deposits sperm in the female reproductive tract. The shaft, or body, of the penis contains three columns of erectile tissue and an enlarged tip called the *glans penis*. The opening of the urethra, called the *urinary meatus* (external urethral orifice), penetrates the glans penis.

The loose skin covering the penis extends downward and forms a cuff of skin around the glans called the *foreskin*, or *prepuce* (PREH-poos). Around puberty, small glands located in the foreskin and the glans secrete an oily substance. This secretion and the surrounding dead skin cells form a cheesy substance called *smegma*. As part of daily hygiene, a man should pull back the foreskin to remove the smegma. Occasionally, the foreskin is too tight and cannot be retracted (phimosis). The foreskin is often surgically removed after birth in a process called *circumcision*. Although parents often have their sons circumcised to promote cleanliness, circumcision is also a common religious ritual.

 Re-Think

1. Trace the movement of a sperm from the lumen of the seminiferous tubules to the urinary meatus.
2. List and locate the glands that contribute to the formation of semen.
3. Explain why an enlarged prostate gland causes dysuria.

 Do You Know...

Who Priapus Was, and What His "Problem" Was?

In Greek mythology, Priapus, the son of Aphrodite, was the god of the phallus (penis). As the story goes, Priapus was punished by the other gods for attempting to rape a goddess. His punishment? A huge, but useless, set of wooden genitals. Today, the term *priapism* is used to describe a potentially harmful and painful condition in which the erect penis does not return to its flaccid state within 4 hours after erection. (There is also a female version of priapism called *clitorism*.) Priapism can develop in response to many factors, including drugs, neurological conditions, blood dyscrasias, and trauma. Persons who die a swift and violent death, particularly by hanging, often have a death erection or terminal erection, considered a form of priapism. Postmortem priapism is of forensic interest in helping determine the manner of death.

MALE SEXUAL RESPONSE: ERECTION, EMISSION, EJACULATION, AND ORGASM

The urethra extends the length of the penis and is surrounded by three columns of spongy erectile tissue. When a man is sexually stimulated, the parasympathetic nerves fire, the penile arteries dilate, and the erectile tissue fills with blood. The accumulation of blood in the erectile tissue causes the penis to enlarge and become rigid. This process is an erection. It enables the penis to penetrate the reproductive tract of the female. For various reasons, a man may be unable to achieve an erection and is said to have erectile dysfunction (ED). (The older term is *impotence*.)

Orgasm refers to the pleasurable sensations that occur at the height of sexual stimulation. Orgasm in the male is accompanied by emission and ejaculation. Emission is the movement of sperm and glandular secretions from the testes and genital ducts into the proximal urethra, where they mix to form semen. Emission is caused by the influence of the sympathetic nervous system on the ducts, causing rhythmic, peristalsis-type contractions.

An Autonomic Summary—Up and Out!	
Up: Erection	Parasympathetic
Out: Emission	Sympathetic

Ejaculation is the expulsion of semen from the urethra to the outside. Ejaculation begins when the urethra fills with semen. Motor nerve impulses from the spinal cord stimulate the skeletal muscles at the base of the erectile columns in the penis to contract rhythmically. The rhythmic contraction provides the force necessary to expel the semen. (The path of semen during ejaculation is illustrated in Fig. 26.1B.) Immediately after ejaculation, sympathetic nerve impulses cause the penile arteries to constrict, thereby reducing blood flow into the penis. This process is accompanied by increased venous drainage of blood from the penis. As a consequence, the penis becomes flaccid and returns to its unstimulated size.

An Autonomic Summary—Up and Down!	
Up: Erect	Parasympathetic
Down: Flaccid	Sympathetic

MALE SEX HORMONES

EFFECTS OF TESTOSTERONE

The male sex hormones are called *androgens*, the most important being testosterone. Most of the testosterone is secreted by the interstitial cells of the testes. A small amount is secreted by the adrenal cortex.

Secretion of testosterone begins during fetal development and continues at a very low level throughout childhood. When a boy reaches the age of 10 to 13, testosterone secretion increases rapidly, transforming the boy into a man. This phase in reproductive development is called *puberty*. After puberty, testosterone is secreted continuously throughout the life of the male.

Testosterone is necessary for the production of sperm and is responsible for the development of the male sex characteristics. The primary sex characteristics include the enlargement and development of the testes and the various accessory organs such as the penis. Secondary sex characteristics refer to special features of the male body and include the following:

- Increased growth of hair, particularly on the face, chest, axillary region, and pubic region
- Deepening of the voice, caused by enlargement of the vocal cords
- Thickening of the skin and increased activity of the oil and sweat glands; at puberty, the adolescent is faced with new challenges, such as acne and body odor
- Increased musculoskeletal growth and development of the male physique (broad shoulders and narrow waist)

HORMONAL CONTROL OF MALE REPRODUCTION

The male reproductive system is controlled primarily by the hormones secreted by the hypothalamus, anterior pituitary gland, and testes. The hypothalamus secretes a releasing hormone, which then stimulates the anterior pituitary gland to secrete two gonadotropins: follicle-stimulating hormone (FSH) and luteinizing hormone (LH) (Fig. 26.3). FSH promotes spermatogenesis by stimulating the spermatogenic cells to respond to testosterone. Note that spermatogenesis comes about through the combined action of FSH and testosterone. LH, also known as *interstitial cell–stimulating hormone* (ICSH) in the male, promotes the development of the interstitial cells of the testes and the secretion of testosterone.

After puberty, a negative feedback loop regulates testosterone production. When the level of testosterone in the blood increases, it causes the hypothalamus and the anterior pituitary gland to decrease their hormonal secretions, thereby decreasing the production of testosterone. As blood levels of testosterone decrease, the anterior pituitary gland increases its secretion of LH (ICSH), thereby stimulating the interstitial cells to secrete testosterone once again. The negative feedback mechanism maintains constant blood levels of testosterone.

◎ Sum It Up!

Four hormones—hypothalamic releasing hormone, FSH, LH (ICSH), and testosterone—control the male reproductive system. The releasing hormone (hypothalamus) stimulates the anterior pituitary gland to secrete FSH and LH (ICSH). FSH and testosterone stimulate spermatogenesis. LH stimulates the secretion of testosterone. Finally, testosterone stimulates the development of the male secondary sex characteristics. A male looks male because of testosterone.

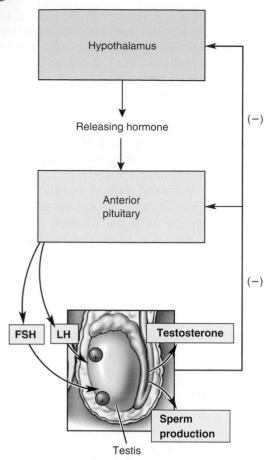

FIG. 26.3 **Hormonal control of sperm production and testosterone secretion.**

 Re-Think

1. Differentiate between the following: erection, emission, and ejaculation.
2. Regarding male contraception, why is it medically acceptable to ligate the vas deferens and not to remove the testes?

FEMALE REPRODUCTIVE SYSTEM

The female reproductive system produces eggs, secretes hormones, and nurtures and protects a developing fetus during the 9 months of pregnancy. Fig. 26.4A, shows the organs of the female reproductive system.

OVARIES

The female gonads are two almond-shaped **ovaries**, located on either side of the uterus in the pelvic cavity. The ovaries are anchored in place by several ligaments, including the ovarian and the broad ligaments. The ovaries, although not attached directly to the fallopian tubes, are close to them.

EGG DEVELOPMENT: THE OVARIAN FOLLICLE

Within the ovary are many tiny, saclike structures called **ovarian follicles**. A female is born with 2 million

follicles. This number steadily declines with age, however, so that at puberty only about 400,000 follicles remain—enough to start a small family. Of these, only about 400 follicles ever fully mature, because a female usually produces only one egg per month throughout her reproductive years. The production of eggs begins at puberty and continues until menopause, at about 45 to 55 years of age. As with sperm, the supply of eggs far exceeds the actual need. This is Mother Nature's way of ensuring future generations.

Each ovarian follicle consists of an immature egg, called an *oocyte,* and the surrounding cells called *follicular cells* (see Fig. 26.4B). Beginning at puberty, several follicles mature every month, although usually only one fully matures. As the egg matures, it begins to undergo meiotic cell division, which reduces the number of chromosomes by half, from 46 to 23.

At the same time, the follicle enlarges, a fluid-filled center is formed, and the follicular cells begin to secrete estrogen. The mature ovarian follicle is known as the **graafian** (GRAH-fee-en) **follicle**. The graafian follicle looks like a blister on the surface of the ovary.

OVULATION

Once a month the ovarian follicle bursts—an "eggsplosion"! The ovary ejects a mature egg (ovum) with a surrounding layer of cells. This ejection phase is called **ovulation.** The egg travels from the surface of the ovary into the peritoneal cavity, where it is immediately swept into the fallopian tubes by the swishing motion of the fimbriae (finger-like projections at the end of the fallopian tubes). The egg travels through the fallopian tubes to the uterus. If the egg is fertilized, it implants itself in the uterine lining and grows into a fetus. If the egg is not fertilized, the egg dies and is eliminated in the menstrual blood. Some women feel twinges of pain at the time of ovulation; the pain is called *mittelschmerz* (MIT-el-schmertz) (from the German, meaning "middle pain").

Once ovulation has occurred, the follicular cells that remain in the ovary develop into a glandular structure called the *corpus luteum* ("yellow body"). The corpus luteum secretes two hormones: large amounts of progesterone (proh-JES-ter-ohn) and smaller amounts of estrogen. If fertilization does not occur, the corpus luteum deteriorates in about 10 days and becomes known as the *corpus albicans* ("white body"). The dead corpus albicans is not capable of secreting hormones. If fertilization occurs, however, the corpus luteum does not deteriorate. It stays alive and continues to secrete its hormones until this role can be taken over by the placenta—a structure you will read about in Chapter 27.

OVARIAN HORMONES

At puberty, the ovaries begin to secrete the sex hormones estrogen and progesterone. The follicular cells of the maturing follicles secrete estrogen, and the

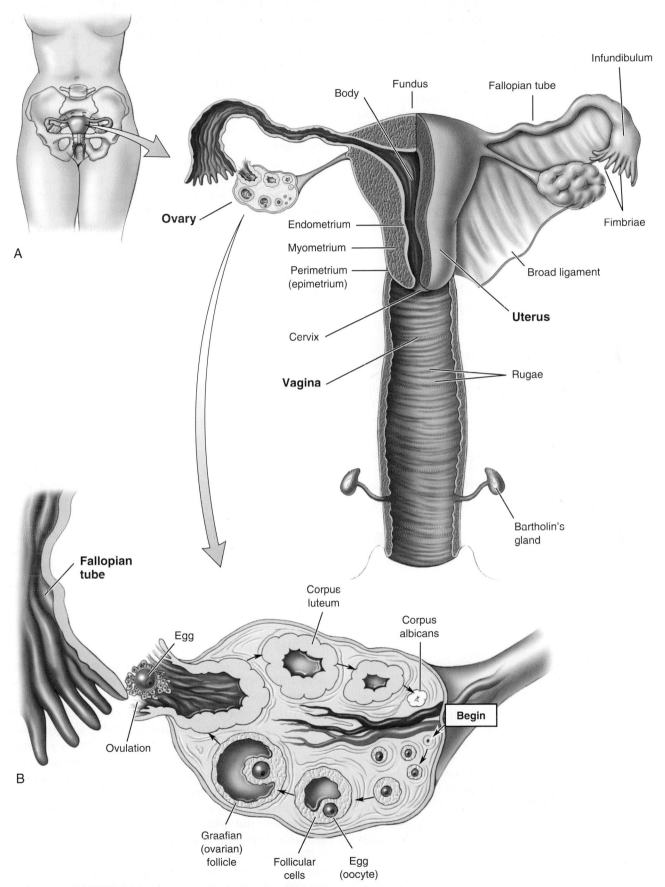

FIG. 26.4 (A) Female reproductive organs. (B) Maturation of the ovarian follicle, ovulation, and formation of the corpus luteum.

corpus luteum secretes large amounts of progesterone and smaller amounts of estrogen. These hormones transform a girl into a woman.

Estrogen

Estrogen exerts two important effects: it promotes the maturation of the egg, and it helps develop the female secondary sex characteristics. Just as the male looks male because of testosterone, the female looks female because of estrogen. The feminizing effects of estrogen include the following:

- Enlargement and development of the organs of the female reproductive system
- Enlargement and development of the breasts
- Deposition of fat beneath the skin, especially in the thighs, buttocks, and breasts
- Widening of the pelvis
- Onset of the menstrual cycle
- Closure of the epiphyseal discs in long bones, thereby stopping further growth in height

Progesterone

The corpus luteum secretes **progesterone**. Progesterone has three important effects: it (1) works with estrogen in establishing the menstrual cycle, (2) helps maintain pregnancy, and (3) prepares the breasts for milk production after pregnancy, increasing their secretory capacity. Although the corpus luteum secretes enough progesterone to maintain pregnancy in the early months, the woman's body needs larger amounts of both estrogen and progesterone during the later stages of pregnancy. This role is performed by the placenta.

Re-Think

1. Name the steps in the progression from the oocyte to the corpus albicans.
2. What is the graafian follicle?
3. Explain the function of the corpus luteum.
4. List two ovarian hormones.

Sum It Up!

The female gonad is the ovary. Once a month, an ovarian follicle matures, forming a graafian follicle. The follicle contains an egg and estrogen-secreting follicular cells. Under the influence of LH, the egg is expelled from the mature follicle; this event is ovulation. Following ovulation, the corpus luteum begins to secrete large amounts of progesterone. Progesterone plays an important role in preparing the reproductive system for pregnancy. Estrogen helps the egg mature and is primarily responsible for the secondary sex characteristics of the female.

GENITAL TRACT

The female genital tract includes the fallopian tubes, uterus, and vagina (see Fig. 26.4A).

FALLOPIAN TUBES

The **fallopian** (fal-LOH-pee-an) **tubes** are also called the *uterine tubes* or the *oviducts*. Each of the two fallopian tubes is about 4 inches (10 cm) long and extends from either side of the uterus to the ovaries. The funnel-shaped end of the fallopian tube nearest the ovary is called the *infundibulum* and has finger-like projections called *fimbriae* (FIM-bree-ay). The fallopian tube does not attach directly to the ovary; the fimbriae hang over the ovary.

At ovulation, the fimbriae sweep the egg from the surface of the ovary into the fallopian tube. Once in the fallopian tube, the egg moves slowly toward the uterus. Because the egg cannot swim like sperm, the peristaltic activity of the fallopian tubes moves it forward.

The fallopian tubes have two functions. First, the tube transports the egg from the ovary to the uterus. Second, the tube is the usual site of fertilization of the egg by the sperm. The fertilized egg moves through the fallopian tube into the uterus, where it implants and grows into a baby. The journey through the fallopian tubes takes about 4 to 5 days.

Tube Troubles

- Occasionally, the fertilized egg implants in the fallopian tube rather than in the uterus. This condition is known as an *ectopic pregnancy*. The word *ectopic* means "in an abnormal site"; a tubal pregnancy is therefore an ectopic pregnancy.
- What happens if the tubes scar and close? Scarring, closing, and sterility, as occurs with repeated gonorrheal infections, blocks the movement of the egg through the tubes.
- Pelvic inflammatory disease (PID). The fallopian tubes open directly into the pelvic cavity. An infection of the female reproductive tract, as often occurs with sexually transmitted diseases, can spread through the tubes into the pelvic cavity, causing PID.

UTERUS

The **uterus**, or *womb*, is shaped like an upside-down pear and is located between the urinary bladder and the rectum. The broad ligament holds the uterus in place. The primary function of the uterus is to provide a safe and nurturing environment for the growing fetus. It functions as a cradle for 9 comfortable months. During pregnancy, the size of the uterus increases considerably to hold the growing fetus and the placenta.

The uterus has three parts. The fundus is the upper dome-shaped region above the entrance of the fallopian tubes. The body is the central region. The **cervix** is the lower narrow region that opens into the vagina.

The uterus has three layers: an outer serosal layer called the epimetrium, or perimetrium; a middle, smooth muscular layer called the **myometrium**; and an inner layer called the **endometrium**. The endometrial uterine lining has two layers: the basilar layer and the functional layer. The basilar layer is thin and vascular and lies next to the myometrium. The functional layer responds to the ovarian hormones and thickens in preparation for the fertilized egg. It is also the layer that sloughs off during menstruation when fertilization has not occurred.

The cervix is often associated with the Pap smear, a diagnostic procedure used for detecting cancer of the cervix. This simple and painless procedure involves scraping cells from around the cervix and examining them for evidence of cancer.

 Do You Know...

What Plato, Hysteria, and the Concept of the Wandering Womb Have in Common?

Plato believed that the womb (uterus), if unused for a long period, became "indignant." This indignant womb then wandered around the body, inhibiting the body's spirit and causing disease. According to the male thinkers of the day, a woman was so thoroughly controlled by her wandering womb that she was considered irrational and prone to emotional outbursts and fits of hysteria. This belief was the reason that the womb was named the *hystera*. The term has persisted in medical terminology; a *hysterectomy* refers to the surgical removal of the uterus.

 Do You Know...

What the Spots Are on the Outer Surfaces of These Organs?

These spots represent endometrial tissue adhering to the outer surface of the ovary, fallopian tube, rectum, and urinary bladder. How did the endometrial tissue get there? In some women, a portion of the menstrual discharge flows backward, into the fallopian tubes, and then into the pelvic cavity. The endometrial tissue adheres to the outer surface of the organs in the pelvic cavity. This condition is called *endometriosis*. The endometrial tissue acts as though it were still in the uterus. It responds to the ovarian hormones by thickening, becoming secretory, and then sloughing off. A woman feels the discomfort of menstruation throughout the pelvic cavity. In addition to causing severe pain, endometriosis causes scarring and the formation of adhesions.

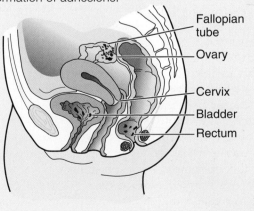

Fallopian tube — Ovary — Cervix — Bladder — Rectum

VAGINA

The **vagina** is a 4-inch muscular tube that extends from the cervix to the vaginal opening in the perineum. The vaginal opening is usually covered by a thin membrane called the *hymen*. The definition of hymen comes from the image of the vagina as a sanctuary of the virgin love goddess, Aphrodite. The hymen may be torn in a number of ways, such as during first intercourse, use of tampons, or strenuous exercise. Much has been written about the hymen and whether or not it is intact. The upper portion of the vagina receives the cervix of the uterus. The cervix dips into the vagina so that pockets, or spaces, form around the cervix. The pockets are called *fornices*. The deepest is the posterior fornix, located behind the cervix.

 Do You Know...

About Xtreme Sex "Down-Under"?

A little Aussie mouse, *Antechinus*, engages in sex for up to 12 hours, ignoring eating, drinking, and sleeping. He's definitely in a loop! Alas, the happy little fellow dies of exhaustion. What about Ms. Mouse? Going at a more leisurely pace, she calmly stores the sperm throughout the breeding season and in due time gives birth to an adorable litter. What's in this sex frenzy for Mother Nature? Preservation of the species—and more food for mama mouse and babies.

The mucosal lining of the vagina lies in folds (rugae) that are capable of expanding. The folding is important for childbearing because it permits the vagina to stretch and accommodate the baby during birth. In addition to forming a part of the birth canal, the vagina is also the organ that receives the penis during intercourse and serves as an exit for menstrual blood. The bacterial population (normal flora) in the vagina creates an acidic environment that discourages the growth of pathogens.

 Sum It Up!

The female genital tract consists of the fallopian tubes, uterus, and vagina. The fallopian tube, the usual site of fertilization, transports the egg from the ovary to the uterus. The uterus is where the fetus lives and grows for 9 months. The vagina receives the penis during intercourse and serves as part of the birth canal. A baby makes its entrance into the world through the vagina.

EXTERNAL GENITALS

The female external genitals (genitalia) are together called the *vulva* (Fig. 26.5). The vulva includes the labia majora and labia minora, clitoris, and vestibular glands. (The external genitalia of the female are also called the *pudendum*, from a word meaning "shameful." Go figure!)

The two labia majora are folds of hair-covered skin that lie external to the two smaller labia minora. The labia (the word means "lips") are separated by a cleft containing the urethral and vaginal openings. The labia prevent drying of the mucous membranes. The labia majora merge anteriorly (in front) to form the rounded hair-covered region over the symphysis called the *mons pubis*.

The clitoris is the structure that resembles the penis. Although small, the clitoris contains erectile tissue and is capped by a thin membrane called the *glans*. The labia minora extend forward and partially surround the clitoris to form a foreskin. Like the penis, the clitoris contains sensory receptors that allow the female to experience pleasurable sexual sensations.

The vestibule is a cleft between the labia minora. It contains the openings of the urethra and the vagina. A pair of vestibular glands (Bartholin's glands) lies on either side of the vaginal opening and secrete a mucus-containing substance that moistens and lubricates the vestibule. Note that the female urinary system and the reproductive system are entirely separate, unlike in the male. The female urethra carries only urine, whereas the male urethra carries urine and semen.

The perineum refers to the entire pelvic floor. The common use of the word, however, is more limited. Most clinicians use the word *perineum* to mean the area between the vaginal opening and anus (called the "obstetric perineum").

FEMALE SEXUAL RESPONSE

The female responds to sexual stimulation with erection and orgasm. Erectile tissue in the clitoris and the tissue surrounding the vaginal opening swell with blood in response to parasympathetically induced dilation of the arteries. Erectile tissue in the vaginal mucosa, breasts, and nipples also swell. Other responses include an engorgement of the vagina and secretion by the vestibular glands. At the height of sexual stimulation, a woman experiences orgasm.

The orgasm also stimulates a number of reflexes. These reflexes cause muscle contractions in the perineum, uterine walls, and uterine tubes; the muscular activity is thought to aid in directing and transporting the sperm through the genital tract.

 Re-Think

1. What is the function of the fallopian tubes?
2. List the layers of the uterus.
3. Trace the movement of the egg from ovulation to implantation in the uterus.

HORMONAL CONTROL OF THE REPRODUCTIVE CYCLES

Let us review the female reproductive cycle. Each month, an egg is produced by the ovary in anticipation of producing a baby. As the egg develops in the ovary, the uterus prepares to receive the fertilized egg. Its preparation consists of the building up of a thick, lush endometrial lining. If the egg is not fertilized, the endometrial lining is no longer needed to nourish the fetus, so it is shed in the menstrual flow. Then the monthly process begins again. A second egg ripens in the ovary, and the uterine lining starts the rebuilding process. This process repeats itself throughout the female reproductive years, all for the purpose of reproducing.

A number of hormones control the female reproductive cycle. Unlike male hormones, female hormonal secretion occurs in a monthly cycle, with a regular pattern of increases and decreases in hormone levels. In fact, the word **menses** (MEN-seez) comes from the Greek word for "month" or "moon." The hypothalamus, anterior pituitary gland, and ovaries secrete most of the hormones involved in the menstrual cycle.

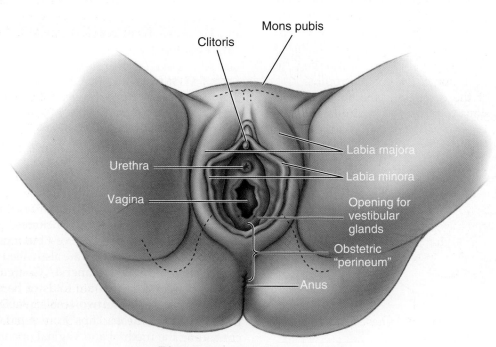

FIG. 26.5 External genitals of the female.

Table 26.1 Female Hormones

HORMONE	GLAND	TARGET ORGAN	EFFECTS
Releasing hormone	Hypothalamus	Anterior pituitary	Stimulates the secretion of the gonadotropins (FSH and LH)
Follicle-stimulating hormone (FSH)	Anterior pituitary	Ovary	Initiates development of the ovarian follicle Stimulates the secretion of estrogen by the follicular cells
Luteinizing hormone (LH)	Anterior pituitary	Ovary	Causes ovulation Stimulates the corpus luteum to secrete progesterone
Estrogen	Ovary (follicle)	Locally (ovary)	Stimulates maturation of the ovarian follicle
		Uterus (endometrium)	Stimulates the proliferative phase of endometrial development
		Other tissues and organs	Causes the development of the secondary sex characteristics
Progesterone	Ovary (corpus luteum)	Uterus (endometrium)	Stimulates the secretory phase of endometrial development
Human chorionic gonadotropin (hCG)	Trophoblastic cells of the embryo	Corpus luteum	Maintains the corpus luteum during early pregnancy

The hypothalamus secretes a releasing hormone that stimulates the anterior pituitary gland to secrete the two gonadotropins, FSH and LH. FSH and LH then stimulate the ovaries, causing them to secrete estrogen and progesterone. The hormones that regulate the female reproductive cycle are summarized in Table 26.1.

TWO REPRODUCTIVE CYCLES

There are two components of the female reproductive cycle: the **ovarian cycle** and the **uterine cycle**. These cycles begin at puberty and last about 40 years. (Refer to Fig. 26.6 as you read about the cyclic changes.) Fig. 26.6A illustrates the secretions of the anterior pituitary gland, FSH and LH, over a 28-day monthly cycle. (The 28-day cycle is an average length; a normal cycle may be shorter or longer than 28 days.) The hypothalamic-releasing hormone is responsible for stimulating the anterior pituitary secretion of the gonadotropins.

For each day of the cycle, you should be able to identify the secretions of the anterior pituitary gland, maturation of the ovarian follicle, changes in the blood levels of ovarian hormones, and growth of the endometrial lining of the uterus. Fig. 26.6B illustrates the growth and maturation of the ovarian follicle, which results in ovulation and the development of the corpus luteum. Fig. 26.6C shows the blood levels of the ovarian hormones estrogen and progesterone. Fig. 26.6D illustrates the monthly changes in the uterine lining. Together, the parts of Fig. 26.6 describe events that occur over a 28-day period.

OVARIAN CYCLE

The ovarian cycle consists of two phases: the follicular phase and the luteal phase.

Follicular Phase

The follicular phase (see Fig. 26.6B) begins with the hypothalamic secretion of a releasing hormone. This hormone, in turn, stimulate the release of **gonadotropins** by the anterior pituitary gland. The FSH and small amounts of LH stimulate the growth and maturation of the ovarian follicle. The maturing ovarian follicle secretes large amounts of estrogen, causing the blood levels of estrogen to increase (see Fig. 26.6C).

Estrogen dominates the follicular phase. Estrogen affects both the ovary and uterus. Estrogen stimulates the maturation of the ovarian follicle and helps build up the uterine lining in the first half of the uterine cycle, days 1 to 14 (see Fig. 26.6D).

The follicular phase ends when a sharp rise (midcycle surge) of LH on day 14 causes ovulation. See Fig. 26.6A for the midcycle surge of LH and Fig. 26.6B for ovulation.

Luteal Phase

The luteal phase immediately follows ovulation. Follicular cells of the ruptured follicle on the surface of the ovary form the corpus luteum. LH then stimulates the corpus luteum to secrete progesterone and smaller amounts of estrogen. The progesterone and estrogen exert a negative feedback effect on the anterior pituitary gland, thereby inhibiting further secretion of FSH and LH. Progesterone also supports the endometrial lining of the uterus during the second half of the cycle (days 14 to 28). Progesterone dominates the luteal phase.

When the corpus luteum dies, secretion of progesterone and estrogen declines. As a result of the decrease in estrogen and progesterone, FSH and small amounts of LH are once again secreted, and the cycle is repeated.

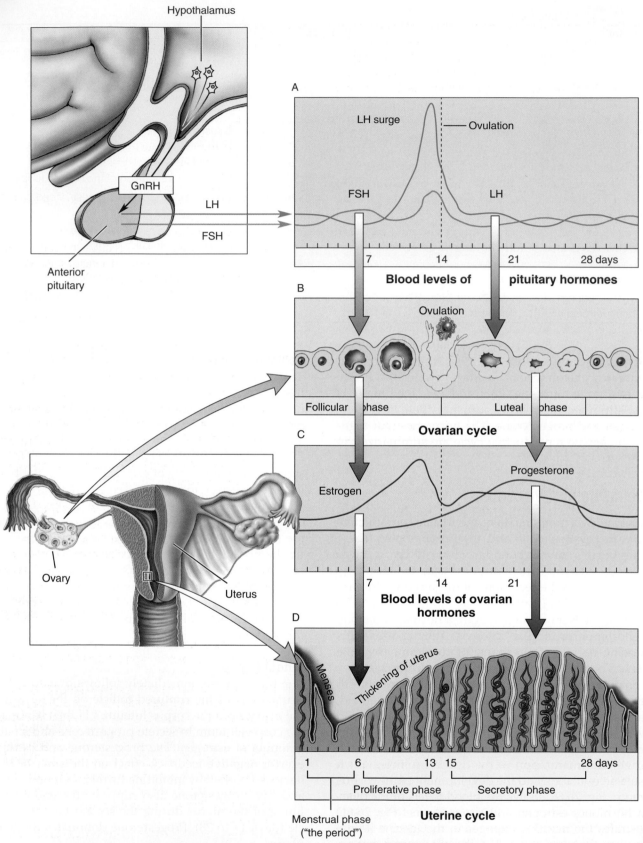

FIG. 26.6 Hormonal control of the female reproductive cycle (28-day cycle). (A) The anterior pituitary gland secretes the gonadotropins FSH and LH in response to hypothalamic-releasing hormones. (B) Ovarian events. (C) Blood levels of the ovarian hormones estrogen and progesterone. (D) The uterine cycle.

UTERINE CYCLE

The uterine cycle, also called the *menstrual cycle*, consists of the changes that occur in the endometrium over a 28-day period (see Fig. 26.6D). Estrogen and progesterone secreted by the ovaries cause the endometrial changes; thus, the ovarian cycle controls the uterine cycle. The uterine cycle has three phases: the menstrual phase, the proliferative phase, and the secretory phase.

Menstrual Phase

Bleeding characterizes the menstrual phase. It begins on the first day and continues for 3 to 5 days, varying from person to person. During the menstrual phase, the functional layer of the endometrial lining and blood leave the uterus through the vagina as menstrual flow. This process is also called "having your period."

Proliferative Phase

The proliferative phase begins with the end of the menstrual phase. Repair and growth of the inner endometrial lining characterize the proliferative phase. The lining grows primarily because of estrogen secreted by the ovaries (see Fig. 26.6B and C). The proliferative phase is so named because the cells proliferate and thus repair the endometrial lining. Note in Fig. 26.6D that the endometrial lining becomes thicker and acquires additional blood vessels during the proliferative phase.

Secretory Phase

The secretory phase is caused by the secretion of progesterone by the corpus luteum of the ovary (see Fig. 26.6C and D). Progesterone causes the endometrial lining to thicken and become more juicy, thereby forming a nutritious environment awaiting the arrival of a fertilized ovum.

IMPLANTATION: KEEPING THE CORPUS LUTEUM ALIVE

NOTE: The endometrial lining does not slough off if blood levels of estrogen and progesterone are adequate. These levels are adequate if the corpus luteum does not deteriorate. How does the body prevent the deterioration of the corpus luteum?

If fertilization occurs, preserving the uterine lining is crucial, for this is where the fetus will live and grow. Menstruation must be prevented. How? Soon after fertilization, the egg implants in the uterine lining. Some of the cells at the site of implantation in the uterus secrete a hormone called *human chorionic gonadotropin* (hCG). Blood carries hCG from the uterus to the ovary, where it stimulates the corpus luteum. Deterioration of the corpus luteum is prevented by hCG, thereby ensuring the continued secretion of estrogen and progesterone. The life of the corpus luteum is prolonged for 11 to 12 weeks by hCG, until the placenta can take over as the major estrogen- and progesterone-secreting gland. (See Chapter 27 for the rest of this story.)

 Do You Know...

What the Missing Words in This "Scientific" Observation Are?

According to the ancient scientist Pliny, "When a _____ approaches, fermenting wine will be soured, seeds she touches become infertile, grass withers, garden plants shrivel, and fruit falls from the trees."

The missing words are "menstruating woman." Menstruating women were often feared, and a great lore grew up around menstrual blood. Casual observation might have suggested that the above charges were false. Pliny pondering periods! Not too observant for a scientist.

 Re-Think

1. List the two phases of the ovarian cycle.
2. List the three phases of the uterine cycle.
3. Explain how the ovarian cycle controls the uterine cycle.
4. Explain why the corpus luteum deteriorates to the corpus albicans in the nonpregnant state.
5. Explain why the corpus luteum does not deteriorate in the pregnant state.

 Sum It Up!

Let's highlight the events of the ovarian and uterine cycles. Refer again to Fig. 26.6.

- The development of the ovarian follicle, during the follicular phase of the ovarian cycle, is caused primarily by FSH. FSH stimulates the follicle to secrete estrogen. The estrogen performs two functions: it stimulates the growth of the follicle, and it is responsible for the proliferative phase of the uterine cycle.
- Ovulation is the expulsion of the egg at midcycle (day 14) and is caused by a surge of LH from the anterior pituitary gland. The egg is swept into the fallopian tube.
- The follicular cells that remain on the surface of the ovary form the corpus luteum. The corpus luteum secretes progesterone and some estrogen. Blood carries the hormones to the uterus.
- Progesterone stimulates the uterine lining to become thick and lush, thereby forming a rich lining for the fertilized egg.
- When blood levels of estrogen and progesterone decline, the endometrial lining sloughs off and causes bleeding (menstruation).
- The ovarian hormones (estrogen and progesterone) exert a negative feedback effect on the anterior pituitary gland. When blood levels of the ovarian hormones rise, secretions of FSH and LH are low. When the corpus luteum degenerates into the corpus albicans, however, the blood levels of estrogen and progesterone decrease. The decrease in the ovarian hormones in turn allows the anterior pituitary gland to secrete FSH and LH. The stimulated ovary then develops another follicle.
- In the pregnant state cells associated with implantation of the fertilized ovum secretes human chorionic gonadotropin (hCG), a hormone that sustains the corpus luteum. The secretion of estrogen and progesterone prevents menstruation thereby preserving uterine conditions for the continuation of the pregnancy.

MENARCHE, MENSES, AND MENOPAUSE

In the female, puberty is marked by the first period of menstrual bleeding, or menarche (meh-NAR-kee). Thereafter, the menstrual periods (menses) occur regularly until the woman reaches her late 40s or early 50s. At this time, the periods gradually become more irregular until they cease completely. This phase is called **menopause**. Menopause is also called *the change of life*, or the *climacteric*. Female reproductive function lasts from menarche to menopause.

The effects of menopause are caused by a decrease in the ovarian secretion of estrogen and progesterone. Without ovarian hormones, the uterine cycle ceases, and the woman stops menstruating. Other symptoms associated with menopause include hot flashes, sweating, depression, irritability, and insomnia. The symptoms are highly variable. Some women experience severe disturbances; others hardly notice any systemic effects.

FEMALE BREAST AND LACTATION

STRUCTURE OF A BREAST: THE MAMMARY GLANDS

The anterior chest contains two elevations called **breasts** (Fig. 26.7A). The breasts are located anterior to the pectoralis major muscles and contain adipose tissue and mammary glands. **Mammary glands** are accessory organs of the female reproductive system. They secrete milk following the delivery of the baby. At the tip of each breast is a nipple surrounded by a circular area of pigmented skin called the *areola*. Each mammary gland contains 15 to 20 lobes. Each lobe contains many alveolar glands and a lactiferous duct. The alveolar glands secrete milk, which is carried toward the nipple by the lactiferous duct. Connective tissue, including the suspensory ligaments, helps support the breast.

Until a child reaches puberty, the mammary glands of male and female children are similar. At puberty, however, the female mammary glands are stimulated by estrogen and progesterone. The alveolar glands and ducts enlarge, and adipose tissue is deposited around these structures. The male breast does not develop because there is no hormonal stimulus to do so. If a male is given female hormones, however, he too develops breasts.

HORMONES OF LACTATION…GOT MILK?

During pregnancy, the increased secretion of estrogen and progesterone has a profound effect on the breasts. The breasts may double in size in preparation for **lactation** (milk production) following birth. Usually, there is no milk production during pregnancy because lactation requires prolactin, a hormone secreted by the anterior pituitary gland (see

Fig. 26.7B). High plasma levels of estrogen and progesterone by the placenta inhibit prolactin secretion during pregnancy. After delivery, however, plasma levels of estrogen and progesterone decrease, allowing the anterior pituitary gland to secrete prolactin. Milk production takes 2 to 3 days to begin. In the meantime, the mammary glands produce **colostrum** (koh-LOH-strohm), a yellowish watery fluid rich in protein and antibodies.

Prolactin is necessary for milk production, but a second hormone, oxytocin, is necessary for the release of milk from the breast. How does the release of milk happen? When the baby suckles, or nurses, at the breast, nerve impulses in the areola are stimulated. Nerve impulses then travel from the breast to the hypothalamus; the hypothalamus, in turn, stimulates the posterior pituitary gland to release oxytocin. The oxytocin travels through the blood to the breast, causing contraction of the smooth muscle of the lobules. This process squeezes milk into the ducts, where it can be sucked out of the nipple by the nursing infant (see Fig. 26.7B).

The effect of suckling and oxytocin release is called the **milk let-down reflex**. Note that the stimulus for the milk let-down reflex is suckling at the breast. Thus, nursing mothers are encouraged to suckle their infants immediately after birth and often thereafter. Breast-feeding encourages a good flow of milk. Also note the distinction between the effects of prolactin and oxytocin. Prolactin stimulates milk production, or lactation. Oxytocin stimulates the milk let-down reflex and stimulates the flow of milk.

Here is a comforting thought! Night milk is milk produced by a cow who is milked at night. It contains a high level of tryptophan, an amino acid that reduces anxiety and promotes sleep. Could this be Mother Nature's way of "sleeping through the night"?

METHODS OF BIRTH CONTROL

Birth control is the voluntary regulation of reproduction. Birth control can limit the number of offspring produced and help determine the timing of conception. Methods of contraception are forms of birth control that prevent the union of egg and sperm.

- Barrier methods. Barriers prevent the sperm from entering the female. Barrier methods are mechanical or chemical and include condoms, diaphragm, spermicidal creams, foams, and jellies.
- Hormonal contraceptives. The birth control pill is a pharmacological agent that contains estrogen and progesterone. As the blood levels of estrogen and progesterone increase, negative feedback inhibits the secretion of FSH by the anterior pituitary gland. This process, in turn, prevents ovulation and therefore no pregnancy.

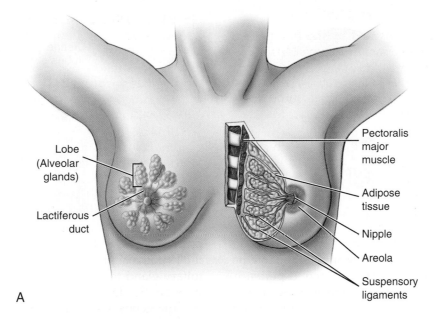

A

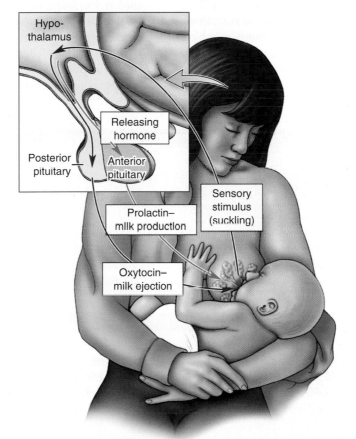

B

FIG. 26.7 (A) Breast and mammary glands. (B) Hormones involved in breast-feeding and the milk let-down reflex (suckling, oxytocin release, flow of milk).

- Surgical methods of contraception include a vasectomy in the male and a tubal ligation in the female (Fig. 26.8). A vasectomy involves removing a small section of each vas deferens and tying the cut ends. In the female, a tubal ligation involves removing a small section of each fallopian tube and tying the cut ends.

- An intrauterine device (IUD) is a small solid object placed in the uterine cavity. The IUD prevents pregnancy because it stimulates the uterus to prevent implantation of the fertilized egg. Note that the IUD is not technically a contraceptive. In other words, it does not prevent conception; instead, it prevents implantation.

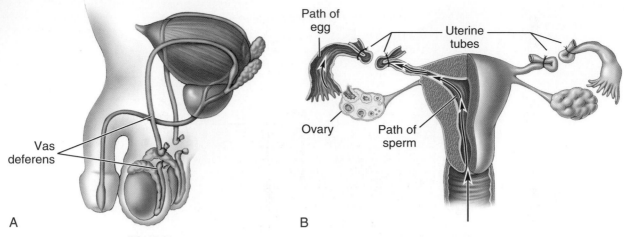

FIG. 26.8 **Surgical methods of birth control. (A) Vasectomy. (B) Tubal ligation.**

- Behavioral methods include abstinence, the rhythm method, and coitus interruptus. Abstinence, or the avoidance of sexual intercourse, is the most effective method of birth control. The rhythm method, also called *natural family planning* or *timed coitus*, requires avoiding sexual intercourse at a time when the female is ovulating, generally at midcycle.

- Emergency contraception refers to contraception that is implemented after intercourse. It is accomplished by two types of drugs. One group of drugs contains both estrogen and progesterone and works like "the pill." A second drug group causes the loss of the implanted embryo by blocking progesterone receptors in the endometrium.

 Sum It Up!

In the female, puberty is marked by the first period of menstrual bleeding. This event is called *menarche*. Thereafter, monthly menstrual periods (menses) occur regularly until menopause. Menopause, also called the *climacteric* or *change of life*, generally occurs when a woman is in her late 40s or early 50s. Menopause is caused by the decreased ovarian secretion of estrogen and progesterone. The mammary glands or breasts are concerned with lactation thereby providing nourishment for the infant. Two hormones are particularly important regarding lactation. Prolactin or lactogenic hormone is secreted by the anterior pituitary gland and stimulates the mammary glands to make milk. Oxytocin is secreted by the posterior pituitary gland and mediates the milk let-down reflex causing the milk to flow in response to infant suckling. The regulation of childbearing can be achieved with the use of barrier methods, hormonal contraceptives, surgical methods, intrauterine devices, behavioral methods, and drugs used for emergency contraception.

As You Age

1. As a woman ages, her ovaries begin to atrophy, or shrink. Between the ages of 40 and 50, estrogen secretion decreases, and symptoms of menopause appear; menstrual periods cease, signaling the end of her reproductive years.
2. The decrease in estrogen secretion causes a change in the accessory organs of reproduction. Tissues become thinner, with a decrease in secretions. The changes in these structures make the woman more prone to vaginal infections. Also, a decrease in vaginal secretions can make intercourse uncomfortable. The decrease in estrogen is also thought to cause weakening of bone, causing osteoporosis, and an increase in the incidence of cardiovascular diseases.
3. By the age of 50, the size of the uterus has decreased by 50%. The ligaments that anchor the uterus, urinary bladder, and rectum weaken, allowing these organs to drop down. Surgical correction is sometimes needed.
4. Breast tissue changes, the supporting ligaments weaken, fibrous cells replace glandular cells, and the amount of fat tissue decreases. These changes cause breast tissue to sag.
5. Around the age of 40, testicular function declines. This decline is accompanied by a decrease in the secretion of testosterone and a decreased sperm count (up to 50%). Despite these changes, a man continues to produce sperm and is capable of fathering children throughout most of his life span.

Medical Terminology and Disorders   Disorders of the Reproductive Systems

MEDICAL TERM	WORD PARTS	WORD PART MEANING OR DERIVATION	DESCRIPTION
General Terminology			
congenital	con-	together or with	*Refers to a condition that is present from birth,* as in a congenital heart defect.
	-gen/o-	origin or production	
	-al	pertaining to	
gonad		From the Greek word *gonos,* meaning "seed or act of generation"	**Gonads** are *organs that produce the seeds of generation or reproduction.* The female gonad is the ovary, and the male gonad is the testis.
heredity	here(s)	From the Latin word *heres,* meaning "heir or heiress"	*Refers to the passing on of characteristics genetically from generation to generation.*
lactation	lact/o-	milk	*The formation or secretion of milk by the mammary (mammo- = breast) glands.* Lactation is stimulated by the hormone called *prolactin* (pro- = in favor of) or *lactogenic hormone.*
	-tion	process	
myometrium and the other "metriums"	my/o-	muscle	The **myometrium** is *the smooth muscle layer of the uterus.* The **endometrium** (endo- = within) is *the inner lining of the uterus.* The **perimetrium** (peri- = around) or **epimetrium** (epi- = upon) is *the outer serosal layer of the uterus.*
	-metr/o-	uterus or womb	
natal	nat/i-	birth	*Refers to the place or time of one's birth.* A **neonate** (neo- = new) is *a newborn infant.* The **prenatal period** is *the time before the birth;* the **perinatal period** is *the time around the birth;* and the **postnatal period** is *the time immediately after the birth.*
	-al	pertaining to	
placenta		From a Latin word meaning "a flat cake"	Called a "uterine cake" by the Italians, the **placenta** is *the vascular organ that develops within the uterus of a pregnant female to nourish the developing fetus.*
ovum	ov/i	egg	*Refers to the ovum or egg.* **Ovulation** is *the expulsion of the egg at midcycle from the* **ovary.** *The* **oviduct** *is the egg-carrying vessel also known as the fallopian tube.* The prefix oophor/o- derives from the Greek and also refers to the ovary, as in **oophorectomy** *(removal of the ovary).*
Disorders: General			
infertility	in-	not, opposite	**Infertility** can be caused by the male (accounts for one-third of the cases), female (one-third), or both partners (one-third). **Male infertility** may be due to abnormal production of sperm (number or motility), problems with the delivery of sperm, and general health. **Female infertility** may be caused by blockage of the fallopian tubes, endometriosis, ovulation disorders, and hormonal imbalances. Cancer treatment and advancing age can adversely affect both male and female fertility.
	-fertile	From the Latin word *fertilis,* meaning "bearing in abundance"	
sexually transmitted diseases			Abbreviated as STDs; also known as *sexually transmitted infections* (STIs). STDs are a major health concern and are easily spread through sexual contact. Some STDs affect primarily the reproductive structures, whereas others extend their effects to major organ systems throughout the body. The common bacterial STDs include chlamydia (most common), gonorrhea *(Neisseria gonorrhoeae),* and syphilis *(Treponema pallidum).* The most common virally induced STDs are hepatitis B virus (HBV), herpes simplex virus type 2 (HSV-2), human immunodeficiency virus (HIV, progression to AIDS), and human papillomavirus (HPV, also called *genital* or *venereal warts*). Trichomoniasis *(Trichomonas vaginalis)* is the most common STD and is caused by a protozoan or parasitic organism.

Continued

Medical Terminology and Disorders   Disorders of the Reproductive Systems—cont'd

MEDICAL TERM	WORD PARTS	WORD PART MEANING OR DERIVATION	DESCRIPTION
Disorders: Male			
benign prostatic hypertrophy	benign	From the Latin word *bene,* meaning "well"	Also called **benign prostatic hyperplasia (BPH).** Hyperplasia of the prostate gland (not cancerous) is age related and commonly occurs in elderly men. Early symptoms include urinary dribbling, urinary incontinence, and incomplete emptying of the bladder.
	prostat/o-	prostate	
	-ic	pertaining to	
	hyper-	above or excessive	
	-troph/o-	nourishment, development	
	-y	condition of	
cancer		From a Latin word meaning *crab;* a reference to its tendency to extend outward and penetrate like claws	**Cancer,** or **malignant neoplasms,** can develop in any part of the male reproductive system. Cancer of the prostate is the second most frequently diagnosed cancer in the United States, whereas testicular cancer is the most common cancer in U.S. males from late teens to mid-30s.
erectile dysfunction			Also called **EDF** or **impotence;** refers to the inability to have or maintain an erection.
gynecomastia	gynec/o-	woman	**Gynecomastia** is *the development of mammary glands in the male; it occurs in response to altered hormonal secretion or as a side effect of drug therapy.*
	-mast/o-	breasts	
	-ia	condition of	
hydrocele	hydro-	water	A **hydrocele** is *a fluid-filled sac surrounding a testicle; it presents as a swollen scrotum.*
	-cele	pouching or hernia	
hypospadias	hypo-	deficient	A **hypospadias** is *a congenital opening of the urethra on the undersurface of the penis.*
	-spadias	to draw away	
prostatitis	prostat/o-	prostate	**Prostatitis** is *the inflammation of the prostate gland; usually caused by an infection.*
	-itis	inflammation	
varicocele	varic/o-	twisted vein	A **varicocele** is *an enlargement and distortion (varicosity) of the veins that drain the testis.* It appears bluish through the scrotum, feels like a sac of worms, and often causes discomfort.
	-cele	pouching or hernia	
vasectomy	vas/o-	vessel	A **vasectomy** is *the removal of a segment of the vas deferens to produce sterility in the male.* A **vasovasostomy** is *a surgical procedure performed to restore the vas deferens and fertility in the male; it reverses the effects of vasectomy.*
	-ectomy	removal	
Disorders: Female			
cervicitis	cervic/o-	cervix	*Inflammation of the cervix, the lower necklike part of the uterus that extends into the vagina.*
	-itis	inflammation of	
colporrhaphy	colp/o-	vagina (sheath)	A **colporrhaphy** is *the surgical repair of a tear in the vaginal wall.* The defect may be a cystocele, a protrusion of the bladder into the vagina. The defect may also be a rectocele, the bulging of part of the rectum into the vagina.
	-orrhaphy	repair	
displacement of the uterus			**Anteflexion** (ante = before; flexus = bend) is *the forward bending of the uterus.* **Retroflexion** (retro = back) is *an abnormal bending backward of the uterus.* **Retroversion** (retere = to turn) is *an abnormal backward turn of the whole uterus.*
dyspareunia	dys-	difficult or painful	**Dyspareunia** means *painful intercourse,* usually in women.
	-pareunia	From the Greek word *pareunos,* meaning "lying beside"	

Medical Terminology and Disorders Disorders of the Reproductive Systems—cont'd

MEDICAL TERM	WORD PARTS	WORD PART MEANING OR DERIVATION	DESCRIPTION
endometriosis	endo-	within	**Endometriosis** is *a condition in which endometrial tissue grows in other parts of the body, particularly within the pelvic cavity.* Structures most commonly affected are the intestines, fallopian tubes, and ovaries (described in text).
	-metr/o-	uterus	
	-osis	condition of	
episiotomy	episi/o-	vulva (covering)	An **episiotomy** is *an incision into the perineum, the area between the vagina and anus; it is done during the delivery of a baby to prevent the tearing of the perineum during delivery.*
	-otomy	a cutting into	
leukorrhea	leuk/o-	white	**Leukorrhea** is *an abnormal white to yellow vaginal discharge.*
	-rrhea	discharge	
mammogram	mamm/o-	breast	**Mammogram** is *a screening procedure for the early diagnosis of breast cancer.*
	-gram	record	
mastitis	mast/o-	breast	**Mastitis** is *inflammation of the breasts.* A **mastectomy,** commonly performed for breast cancer, is *the surgical removal of a breast;* **amastia** refers to *the absence of a breast.* **Hypermastia** and **macromastia** refer to *abnormally large breasts,* whereas **hypomastia** and **micromastia** refer to *abnormally small breasts.*
	-itis	inflammation	
menarche	men/o-	menstruation; monthly	**Menarche** refers to *the beginning of menstruation.* **Amenorrhea** is *the absence of menstruation.* **Dysmenorrhea** is *painful or difficult menstruation.* **Menorrhagia** is *excessive bleeding at menstruation.* **Metrorrhagia** is *bleeding from the uterus at any time other than normal menstruation.* **Menopause** means *the cessation of menstruation.*
	-arche	beginning	
neoplasms	neo-	new	There are benign and malignant tumors that can develop in all reproductive structures. There is a benign **fibroid tumor** of the uterine muscle, or **leiomyoma** (leios- = smooth; -my/o- = muscle; -oma = tumor). **Fibrocystic breast disease** is characterized by multiple benign cysts in the breasts. **Breast cancer** is a common malignancy of the breast tissue. There are many types of benign **ovarian cysts,** some of which are permanently and successfully eliminated; others (e.g., **polycystic ovary syndrome [PCOS]**) may persist chronically and interfere with fertility and create other serious health issues. **Carcinoma in situ** (in situ = in place) refers to an early form of cancer in which there has been no spread of the malignant cells into surrounding tissue.
	-plasia	growth	
salpingitis	salping/o-	uterine or fallopian tube; comes from the Greek word meaning "trumpet" (because of its appearance)	**Salpingitis** is *the inflammation of the uterine or fallopian tubes.*
	-itis	inflammation of	

Get Ready for Exams!

Summary Outline

The reproductive system produces the cells and hormones necessary for reproduction.

I. Male Reproductive System
  A. Testes
    1. The testes, or testicles, are the male gonads.
    2. Lobules with two types of cells: the seminiferous tubules and the interstitial cells
  B. Spermatogenesis
    1. Meiosis (the diploid and haploid numbers)
    2. Parts of sperm: head (with acrosome), body, tail
  C. Genital ducts and glands
    1. The sperm move through a series of genital ducts: epididymis, vas deferens, ejaculatory ducts, and urethra.
    2. Three glands—the seminal vesicles, the prostate gland, and the bulbourethral glands—secrete into the genital ducts. The mixture of sperm and glandular secretions is called semen.
  D. External genitals
    1. The male genitals consist of the scrotum and the penis.
    2. The penis performs two functions: It is the organ of copulation (sexual intercourse), and it carries urine.
  E. Male sexual responses: erection, emission, ejaculation, and orgasm
  F. Male sex hormones
    1. The most important is testosterone; necessary for sperm production and determination of the primary and secondary sex characteristics.
    2. Controlled by hormones from the hypothalamus and from the anterior pituitary gland

II. Female Reproductive System
  A. Ovaries
    1. The ovaries are the female gonads.
    2. Each ovarian follicle consists of an oocyte and follicular cells.
    3. On day 14 (of a 28-day cycle), ovulation occurs.
    4. The ovarian follicular cells become the corpus luteum.
    5. The ovaries secrete two hormones: estrogen and progesterone.
  B. Genital tract
    1. The genital tract includes the fallopian tubes, uterus, and vagina.
    2. The fallopian tubes transport the egg from the ovaries to the uterus and are where fertilization takes place.
    3. The uterus is the fetus' cradle during pregnancy.
    4. The uterus has three layers: epimetrium, myometrium, and endometrium.
  C. The external genitals are called the vulva (labia majora, labia minora, clitoris, and the vestibular glands).
  D. Female sexual response: erection and orgasm
  E. Hormonal control of the female reproductive cycles
    1. The two cycles are the ovarian cycle and the uterine cycle.

    2. The ovarian cycle is divided into the follicular phase and the luteal phase.
    3. During the follicular phase, the ovarian follicle matures and secretes estrogen.
    4. The luteal phase of the ovarian cycle begins immediately after ovulation and is dominated by the secretion of progesterone by the corpus luteum.
    5. In the nonpregnant state, the corpus luteum deteriorates. In the pregnant state, the corpus luteum stays alive because of human chorionic gonadotropin (hCG).
    6. The uterine cycle is divided into the menstrual phase, proliferative phase, and secretory phase.
      a. The menstrual phase refers to the loss of a part of the endometrial lining and blood ("having your period").
      b. During the proliferative phase, the inner endometrial lining thickens and becomes vascular, primarily in response to estrogen.
      c. During the secretory phase, the endometrial lining becomes lush and moist from increased secretory activity; the secretory phase is dominated by progesterone.
    7. See Fig. 26.6 for a summary of the daily hormonal relationships among the anterior pituitary gland, ovaries, and uterus.

III. Breasts and Lactation
    1. Mammary glands are milk-secreting glands.
    2. Responsive to prolactin and oxytocin

IV. Methods of Birth Control
  A. The regulation of childbearing can be achieved with the use of barrier methods, hormonal contraceptives, surgical methods, intrauterine devices, behavioral methods, and drugs used for emergency contraception.

Review Your Knowledge

Matching: Female Structures
Directions: Match the following words with their descriptions. Some words may be used more than once.

a. fallopian tubes

b. breasts

c. uterus

d. ovaries

e. vagina

_____ 1. Fertilization occurs here

_____ 2. Female gonads

_____ 3. Contains the fundus, body, and cervix

_____ 4. Contains the mammary glands

_____ 5. Contains the endometrium, myometrium, and epimetrium

_____ 6. Primarily concerned with lactation

_____ 7. Home of the corpus luteum

_____ 8. Where implantation occurs

_____ 9. Home of the graafian follicle

____**10.** Menstrual phase, proliferative phase, and secretory phase

____**11.** Follicular phase and luteal phase

____**12.** Birth canal; distal to the cervix

Matching: Male Structures

Directions: Match the following words with their descriptions. Some words may be used more than once.

a. interstitial cells

b. seminiferous tubules

c. urethra

d. epididymis

e. scrotum

f. vas deferens

g. testes

____**1.** Structure that forms sperm

____**2.** Testosterone-secreting cells within the testes

____**3.** Tightly coiled ducts that sit on top of the testes

____**4.** Tubular structure that carries sperm from the epididymis into the pelvic cavity

____**5.** Structure whose proximal end is surrounded by the prostate gland

____**6.** Structure that is shared by both the reproductive and urinary tracts

____**7.** Pouch that contains the testes

____**8.** Male gonads

Matching: Hormones

Directions: Match the following words with their descriptions. Some words may be used more than once.

a. estrogen

b. progesterone

c. hCG

d. gonadotropins

e. testosterone

____**1.** Primary androgen secreted by the testes

____**2.** What FSH and LH are called

____**3.** The proliferative phase (uterus) is dominated by this ovarian hormone

____**4.** The secretory phase (uterus) is dominated by this ovarian hormone

____**5.** Secreted by trophoblastic cells; preserves the secretion of the corpus luteum

____**6.** The ovaries are the targets of this anterior pituitary secretion

____**7.** Its secretion is a response to interstitial cell–stimulating hormone (ICSH)

____**8.** This hormone makes a female look like a woman

____**9.** This hormone makes a male look like a man

____**10.** The corpus luteum secretes large amounts of this hormone; it makes the endometrium "juicy" or "lush"

Multiple Choice

1. True statements about gonadotropins in the male include which of the following?
   a. Are aimed at the testes
   b. Include FSH and LH (ICSH)
   c. Stimulate sperm development and the secretion of androgen
   d. All of the above

2. In the male, luteinizing hormone
   a. is also called ICSH and stimulates the interstitial cells to secrete testosterone.
   b. stimulates spermatogenesis.
   c. causes emission.
   d. causes orgasm.

3. The seminal vesicles and prostate gland
   a. secrete gonadotropins.
   b. secrete testosterone.
   c. contribute to the formation of semen.
   d. secrete reproductive hormones.

4. Estrogen and progesterone
   a. are gonadotropins.
   b. are secreted by the trophoblastic cells as they implant in the uterine wall.
   c. are secreted by the ovaries.
   d. exert their effects only on reproductive structures.

5. In the nonpregnant state, the
   a. corpus albicans becomes hormonally active, secreting estrogen and progesterone.
   b. endometrium secretes hCG.
   c. hormonal secretion of the corpus luteum gradually declines.
   d. zygote becomes hormonally active.

6. Human chorionic gonadotropin (hCG)
   a. promotes the maturation of the egg.
   b. is responsible for female characteristics.
   c. maintains the corpus luteum.
   d. transforms the corpus luteum into the corpus albicans.

7. The luteal phase of the ovarian cycle
   a. is responsible for menstruation.
   b. culminates in ovulation.
   c. is dominated by the secretion of progesterone.
   d. precedes the LH surge.

8. Menstruation occurs in response to
   a. an LH surge.
   b. diminished plasma levels of estrogen and progesterone.
   c. elevated plasma levels of hCG.
   d. elevated plasma levels of FSH and LH.

9. Which of the following is *not* true of testosterone?
   a. Classified as androgen
   b. Secreted by the anterior pituitary gland
   c. Is necessary for the maturation of sperm
   d. Is responsible for most of the male secondary sex characteristics

10. Which structure ejects both semen and urine?
    a. Epididymis
    b. Oviducts
    c. Urethra
    d. Vas deferens

11. The graafian follicle
    a. matures under the influence of hCG.
    b. is an ovarian structure.
    c. implants in the endometrial lining.
    d. secretes FSH and LH in an attempt to ripen an oocyte.

12. The myometrium
    a. is the uterine lining that is most responsive to gonadotropins.
    b. is vascular smooth muscle necessary for erection and ejaculation.
    c. is the uterine layer muscular layer.
    d. is the muscular layer involved in the milk let-down reflex.

13. Which of the following is true of lactation?
    a. Prolactin is responsible for the milk let-down reflex.
    b. Oxytocin participates in the milk let-down reflex.
    c. Oxytocin and prolactin are gonadotropins.
    d. It is stimulated and maintained by hCG.

14. The follicular and luteal phases refer to events that occur within the
    a. ovaries.
    b. fallopian tubes.
    c. testes.
    d. uterus.

15. Which of the following is true with regard to the process of meiosis?
    a. Is the type of cell division found in all cells except the ova and sperm
    b. Changes the chromosomal number from the haploid to the diploid number
    c. Reduces chromosomal number in sex cells from 46 to 23
    d. Is a type of cell division that produces two identical daughter cells

Go Figure

1. Which of the following is correct according to Fig. 26.1?
    a. The epididymis is located within the pelvic cavity.
    b. The testes are located within the pelvic cavity.
    c. The vas deferens is shared by both the urinary and reproductive tracts.
    d. The urethra extends the length of the penis.

2. Which of the following is correct according to Fig. 26.2?
    a. The seminiferous tubules are located within the testes.
    b. Sperm cells and interstitial cells are located within the epididymis.
    c. Sperm are kept warm by migrating to the prostate gland until released.
    d. The acrosome is another name for the foreskin.

3. Which of the following is correct according to Fig. 26.3?
    a. FSH and LH are secreted by the neurohypophysis.
    b. Testosterone exerts negative feedback control on hypothalamic releasing hormones and the adenohypophyseal gonadotropins.
    c. Gonadotropins suppress the gonadal secretion of androgens.
    d. FSH, LH, and testosterone are secreted by the same exocrine glands.

4. Which of the following is correct according to Fig. 26.4?
    a. Ovulation involves the expulsion of the ovum from the corpus albicans.
    b. The corpus luteum forms before the maturation of the ovarian follicle into the graafian follicle.
    c. The graafian follicle and corpus luteum develop within the uterus.
    d. The corpus luteum forms after ovulation.

5. Which of the following is correct according to Fig. 26.4?
    a. The female reproductive tract is anatomically open to the pelvic cavity.
    b. The myometrium forms the broad ligament.
    c. The fallopian tubes are extensions of the cervix of the uterus.
    d. The endometrium refers to the hormonally sensitive ovarian tissue.

6. Which of the following is correct according to Fig. 26.6?
    a. The ovarian cycle includes the proliferative and secretory phases.
    b. The LH surge precedes the development of the graafian follicle.
    c. LH and FSH are gonadotropins secreted by the adenohypophysis and aimed at the endometrium.
    d. FSH stimulates the development of the graafian follicle in the ovary.

7. Which of the following is correct according to Fig. 26.6?
    a. Elevated blood levels of estrogen and progesterone prevent the secretion of gonadotropins through negative feedback control.
    b. The uterine lining is built up in direct response to FSH and LH.
    c. A surge of ovarian progesterone is responsible for ovulation.
    d. The source of estrogen and progesterone is the anterior pituitary gland.

8. Which of the following is correct according to Fig. 26.7?
    a. Alveolar glands secrete milk into the lactiferous ducts.
    b. Oxytocin is secreted reflexively in response to suckling.
    c. Prolactin stimulates the breasts to make milk.
    d. All of the above are true.

9. Which of the following is correct according to Fig. 26.7?
    a. The stimulus for the milk let-down reflex is the level of prolactin in the mother's blood.
    b. Oxytocin is a posterior pituitary hormone that causes milk to flow in response to suckling.
    c. Prolactin is a neurohypophyseal hormone that mediates the milk let-down reflex.
    d. All of the above are true.

Human Development and Heredity

Objectives

1. Describe the process of fertilization: when, where, and how it occurs.
2. Do the following regarding prenatal development:
   - Describe the process of development: cleavage, growth, morphogenesis, and differentiation.
   - Explain the three periods of prenatal development: early embryonic, embryonic, and fetal.
   - State two functions of the placenta.
3. Explain hormonal changes during pregnancy.
4. Describe the hormonal changes of labor.
5. Describe immediate postnatal changes and lifelong developmental stages.
6. Discuss heredity and how genetic structures are related, including the following:
   - Describe the relationships among deoxyribonucleic acid (DNA), chromosomes, and genes.
   - Define *karyotype*.
7. Explain how the gender of the child is determined.
8. State the difference between congenital and hereditary diseases.

Key Terms

amnion (p. 522)
amniotic fluid (p. 522)
blastocyst (p. 520)
chorion (p. 522)
chromosomes (p. 530)
conception (p. 519)
embryo (p. 522)
extraembryonic membranes (p. 522)
fertilization (p. 519)

fetus (p. 526)
genes (p. 530)
gestation (p. 520)
human chorionic gonadotropin (hCG) (p. 521)
implantation (p. 521)
karyotype (p. 530)
labor (p. 528)
morula (p. 520)

organogenesis (p. 524)
placenta (p. 522)
pregnancy (p. 520)
sex-linked trait (p. 533)
teratogens (p. 524)
trimester (p. 520)
trophoblastic cells (p. 527)
umbilical cord (p. 524)
zygote (p. 520)

Forty weeks (approximately 9 months) after conception, the reproductive process produces a baby. The "bundle of joy" has arrived on the scene…and has everyone running nonstop! Nonetheless, Baby is cute, and the urge to reproduce is very strong. Here's his story from fertilization through development and birth. Finally, we'll see what is meant by statements like "He's got his father's nose and his mother's smile." This is his genetic story.

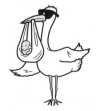

FERTILIZATION

Fertilization, also called **conception**, refers to the union of the nuclei of the egg and the sperm.

When, where, and how does this union take place?

WHEN FERTILIZATION OCCURS

Timing is everything. In the female, ovulation occurs at midcycle, around day 14 (see Chapter 26). The egg lives for about 24 hours after ovulation. Sperm usually live between 12 and 48 hours, with some surviving up to 72 hours. Generally speaking, for fertilization to occur, sexual intercourse must take place around the time of ovulation, generally no earlier than 72 hours (3 days) before ovulation and no later than 24 hours (1 day) after ovulation.

Alert: Evidence suggests that some women are reflex ovulators. These women ovulate in response to having intercourse. Think about it; rabbits are reflex ovulators, and we all know about the rabbit population.

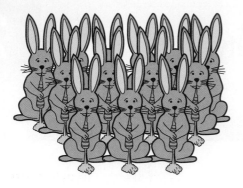

WHERE FERTILIZATION OCCURS

After ovulation, the egg enters the fallopian tube. Fertilization normally occurs in the first third of the fallopian tube.

HOW FERTILIZATION OCCURS

During intercourse, about 200 to 600 million sperm are deposited in the vagina, near the cervix of the uterus. Although many of the sperm are killed by the acidic environment of the vagina, about 100,000 survive and swim through the uterus and into the fallopian tube toward the egg. Within 1 to 2 hours after intercourse, thousands of sperm are gathered around the egg in the fallopian tube. Life comes at you fast!

The acrosome on the head of the sperm ruptures and releases enzymes. The enzymes digest the linings of cells that surround the egg. Then, one (and only one) sperm penetrates the membrane of the egg. Upon penetration of the egg, the nuclei of the egg and sperm unite, thereby completing fertilization. The fertilized egg is called a **zygote** (ZYE-goht). "Zygote" was your first name!

The single-cell zygote has 46 chromosomes: 23 from the egg and 23 from the sperm. The zygote begins to divide, forming a cluster of cells that slowly makes its way through the fallopian tube toward the uterus. When this cluster of cells reaches the uterus, it implants itself into the plush endometrial lining, where it grows and develops into a human being with billions of cells.

 Re-Think

1. Where does fertilization occur?
2. Why is it possible for a fertilized ovum to take up residence within the abdominal cavity rather than the uterus?

HUMAN DEVELOPMENT

Development is a process that begins with fertilization and ends with death. Human development is divided into two phases: prenatal development and postnatal development. Prenatal development begins with fertilization and ends at birth. The time of prenatal development is called **pregnancy**, or **gestation**. The normal gestation period lasts 38 weeks, or about 9 months. Pregnancy is divided into **trimesters** (3-month periods): the first trimester is the first 3 months of pregnancy; the second trimester is months 4, 5, and 6; and the third, or last, trimester is months 7, 8, and 9. Postnatal development begins with birth and ends with death; it is what we are all doing now—living life.

PRENATAL DEVELOPMENT

What does prenatal development include? Prenatal development includes cleavage, growth, morphogenesis, and differentiation. Cleavage is cell division by mitosis. Mitosis produces two identical cells from a single cell. Thus, one cell splits into two cells, the two cells split into four cells, four cells split into eight cells, and so on. Each new cell is identical to the parent cell. Mitotic cell division increases the numbers of cells but not their actual size. The size of the cell increases through growth. As development progresses, therefore, both the number and size of the cells increase.

Morphogenesis (mohr-foh-JEN-eh-sis) is the shaping of the cell cluster. Certain cells migrate to specific areas in the cell cluster. This process changes the shape of the cell mass. For example, cells migrate to the side of the cell mass and take the appearance of tiny buds. These buds eventually become legs. Through morphogenesis, the round cluster of cells develops into an intricately and wondrously formed infant. Baby is shaping up!

Differentiation is the process whereby a cell becomes specialized. A cell differentiates to become a nerve cell, muscle cell, blood cell, or some other cell.

What are the periods of prenatal development? There are three periods: early embryonic, embryonic, and fetal periods.

EARLY EMBRYONIC PERIOD

FROM ZYGOTE TO BLASTOCYST ... OR FROM ZYGOTE TO EGGPLANT

The early embryonic period lasts for 2 weeks after fertilization. During this period, the zygote undergoes mitosis and travels from the fallopian tube into the uterus. After fertilization (Fig. 27.1A) the zygote undergoes cleavage. Cleavage is accomplished by mitosis, or cell division that increases the numbers of cells. The cells formed by mitotic cell division are blastomeres (see Fig. 27.1B). Note the two-cell, four-cell, and eight-cell cluster.

When the number of cells increases to 16, the collection of cells is called a **morula** (see Fig. 27.1C). The morula looks like a raspberry, so tiny that it is visible only through a microscope. Transformation from the zygote to a morula takes about 3 days. The morula enters the uterine cavity, where it floats around for 3 to 4 days and continues to undergo mitosis. By the end of the fifth day, the morula has developed into a **blastocyst**.

Note the structure of the early blastocyst (see Fig. 27.1D). The early blastocyst contains a hollow cavity

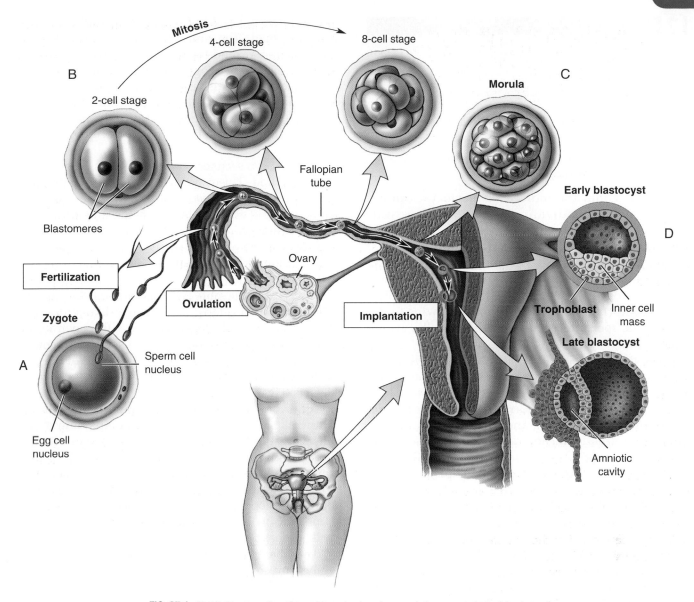

FIG. 27.1 (A–D) Stages of early embryonic development, from zygote to blastocyst.

surrounded by a single layer of flattened cells and a cluster of cells at one side. The single layer of flattened cells surrounding the cavity is called the *trophoblast*. These cells will help burrow into the endometrium, form the placenta, and also secrete an important hormone. The cluster of cells within the blastocyst is called the *inner cell mass*. These cells will eventually form Baby.

The late blastocyst develops by day 7. This stage shows the beginnings of the amniotic cavity. The late blastocyst burrows into the endometrial lining of the uterus, where it is gradually covered over by cells of the endometrial lining. The burrowing process is called **implantation**. We now have an "eggplant"!

During implantation, the blastocyst also functions as a gland. The trophoblast, the flattened layer of cells that surrounds the cavity, secretes a hormone called **human chorionic gonadotropin (hCG)**, which travels through the blood to the ovary, where it prevents the deterioration of the corpus luteum. In response to

hCG, the corpus luteum continues to secrete estrogen and progesterone. The estrogen and progesterone stimulate the growth of the uterine wall and prevent menstruation.

The secretion of hCG continues at a high level for about 2 months and then steadily declines as the placenta develops. The placenta eventually takes over the role of the corpus luteum by secreting large amounts of estrogen and progesterone. The blastocyst thus helps preserve its own survival through its secretion of hCG. Think about it: the fetus helps the fetus survive. With the implantation of the blastocyst and the organization of the inner cell mass, the early embryonic period comes to a close.

hCG forms the basis of pregnancy tests. hCG is secreted in early pregnancy and can be detected in the mother's urine or blood. A pregnancy test may indicate positive results within about 8 to 10 days after fertilization.

? Re-Think

1. Define *gestation*. What is the gestation period for humans?
2. What is a zygote?
3. List the stages of development from fertilization to implantation.
4. Explain the significance of the trophoblastic secretion of hCG.

SEEING DOUBLE: TWINS

Each cell within the morula or blastocyst can become a complete individual. Sometimes, these cells split, and two **embryos** begin developing at the same time, thereby producing two offspring (twins) rather than one. These are identical, or monozygotic (mon-oh-zye-GOH-tik), twins because they develop from the same zygote and have identical genetic information. For monozygotic twins to develop, one sperm fertilizes one egg, and the zygote then splits.

Sometimes a woman ovulates two eggs, which are then fertilized by two different sperm. Because two babies are produced, they are called *twins*. These twins, however, are not identical. They do not develop from the same egg and do not have the same genetic information. They are called *fraternal*, or *dizygotic* (dye-zye-GOH-tik), *twins* (meaning that they come from two different zygotes). Triplets, quadruplets, and other multiple births can develop in the same two ways.

? Re-Think

1. What is the difference between monozygotic and dizygotic twins?
2. Identical twins are always the same gender. Why is that not true for fraternal twins?

EMBRYONIC PERIOD

Embryonic development lasts for 6 weeks, from week 3 through week 8. During this period, the baby-to-be is called an *embryo*. The embryonic period involves the formation of extraembryonic membranes, the placenta, and all of the organ systems in the body.

EXTRAEMBRYONIC MEMBRANES

The **extraembryonic membranes** form outside the embryo; hence, the term *extra*embryonic. The membranes help protect and nourish the embryo; they are also involved in the embryonic excretion of waste. At birth, the membranes are expelled along with the placenta as the afterbirth. The four extraembryonic membranes are the amnion, chorion, yolk sac, and allantois.

The **amnion** (AM-nee-on) enlarges and forms a sac around the embryo (Fig. 27.2). The sac is called the *amniotic sac* and is filled with a fluid called the **amniotic fluid**. The amniotic fluid forms a protective cushion around the embryo and helps protect it from bumps and changes in temperature. The amniotic fluid also nourishes embryos as they drink and digest it. About 1 L of amniotic fluid occupies the amniotic sac at full term. Interestingly, much of the amniotic fluid is from the urine produced by the fetal kidneys!

The embryo secretes waste and sheds cells into the amniotic fluid. This process is the basis for a diagnostic test called an *amniocentesis*, in which a sample of amniotic fluid is aspirated from the amniotic cavity and examined for evidence of fetal abnormalities (see Fig. 27.2B). The amniotic sac is often called the *bag of water*. It breaks before delivery and generally signals the onset of labor.

A second extraembryonic membrane is the **chorion**. The chorion develops many finger-like projections called *chorionic villi*. The chorionic villi penetrate the uterine wall and interact with the tissues of the mother's uterus to form the placenta. Sampling of the cells of the chorionic villi is another way to detect genetic defects (Fig. 27.3 and Fig. 27.2C).

A third extraembryonic membrane is the yolk sac. The yolk sac in birds and reptiles helps nourish the offspring, but the yolk sac in humans serves different functions: it produces red blood cells and immature sex cells. After the sixth week, the yolk sac ceases to function. The embryonic liver and spleen then produce red blood cells, and by the seventh month, the bone marrow has assumed this function. By then, the yolk sac has become part of the umbilical cord.

The allantois (ah-LAN-toh-is) is the fourth extraembryonic membrane. The allantois contributes to the formation of several structures, including the urinary bladder. The blood vessels of the allantois also help form the umbilical blood vessels, which transport blood to and from the placenta. After the second month, the allantois deteriorates and becomes part of the umbilical cord.

PLACENTA

The **placenta** is a disc-shaped structure about 7 inches (15 to 20 cm) in diameter and 1 inch (2.5 cm) thick. Normally, the placenta develops in the upper portion of the uterus. The placenta is a highly vascular structure formed from embryonic and maternal tissue. By the end of the embryonic period (8 weeks), the placenta is functional. After the birth of the baby, the placenta is expelled as part of the afterbirth.

Formation of the Placenta

The placenta develops as the chorionic villi of the embryo burrow into the endometrial lining of the uterus (see Fig. 27.3). The chorionic villi contain blood vessels that are continuous with the umbilical arteries and umbilical vein of the embryo. The chorionic

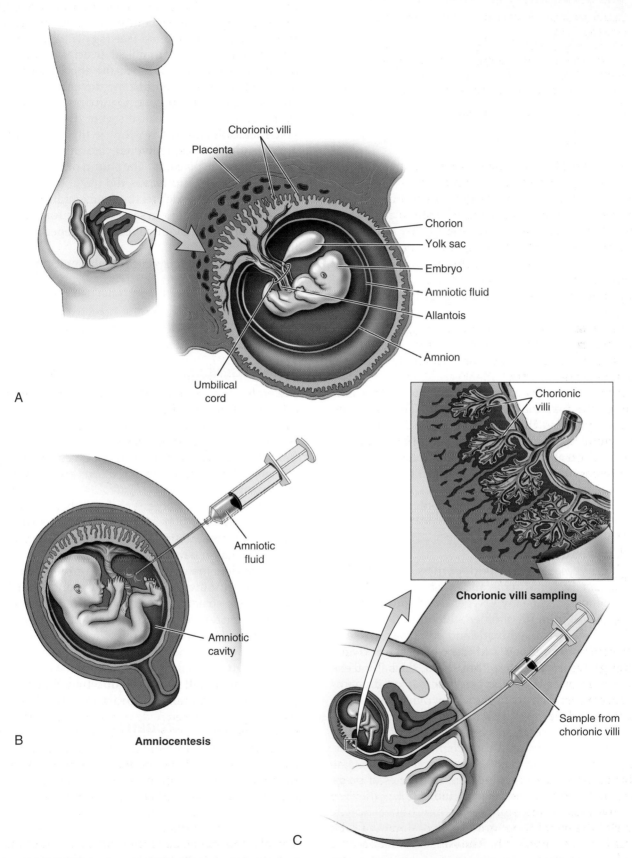

Chorionic villi

Placenta

Chorion

Yolk sac

Embryo

Amniotic fluid

Allantois

Amnion

Umbilical cord

A

Chorionic villi

Chorionic villi sampling

Amniotic fluid

Sample from chorionic villi

Amniotic cavity

B **Amniocentesis**

C

FIG. 27.2 **Extraembryonic membranes and the formation of the placenta. (A) The embryo is surrounded by the amnion and the amniotic fluid. (B) Amniocentesis. (C) Chorionic villi sampling.**

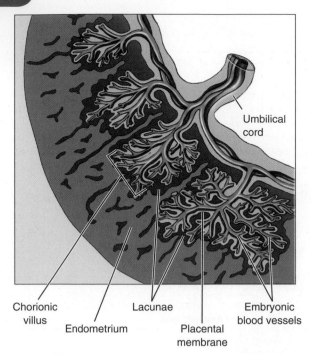

Chorionic villus
Endometrium
Lacunae
Placental membrane
Embryonic blood vessels
Umbilical cord

FIG. 27.3 **Cross section of the chorionic villi.**

villi sit in blood-filled spaces (lacunae) in the mother's endometrium.

Pay special attention to the arrangement of the embryonic and maternal blood vessels. The chorionic villi contain blood that comes from the embryo. The endometrial spaces (lacunae) contain blood from the mother. The embryonic and maternal blood supplies, although intimately close, are separated by the placental membrane. The placental membrane thus maintains two separate circulations: the embryonic and maternal circulations. The two circulations do not mix!

Functions of the Placenta

The placenta plays two important roles. First, it is the site across which nutrients and waste are exchanged between mother and baby. Oxygen, food, and other nutrients diffuse from the mother's blood into the blood of the embryo. Carbon dioxide and other waste diffuse from the embryo's blood into the mother's blood and are then excreted. The fetus "breathes," "eats," and excretes at the placenta. If the placenta is injured in any way, the oxygen supply to the embryo may be cut off, causing irreversible brain damage and possibly death.

Second, the placenta acts as a gland. It secretes hormones that help maintain the pregnancy, prepare the body for the birthing process, and promote postnatal events such as breast-feeding. The hormones of pregnancy are listed and described in Table 27.1.

? Re-Think

1. List four extraembryonic membranes, and provide a function of each.
2. Which layer is concerned with the formation of the placenta?
3. What are two functions of the placenta?

HOOK UP: THE UMBILICAL CORD

How does the embryo connect with the mother? The **umbilical cord** is the structure that connects embryo and mother at the placenta (see Fig. 27.2). The umbilical cord contains two umbilical arteries and one umbilical vein (see Fig. 18.9). Because the umbilical cord carries oxygen-rich blood to the developing infant, it is literally the baby's lifeline. Compression or injury to the umbilical cord can cause severe distress and possibly the death of the baby.

When the baby is delivered, the umbilical cord is cut, severing the placenta. The stump of the cord shrivels up, drops off, and leaves the navel (belly button). The baby's organs, such as the lungs, kidneys, and digestive system, must then take over the functions previously performed by the placenta.

? Re-Think

1. What three large blood vessels run through the umbilical cord?
2. Why can umbilical cord compression or premature separation of the placenta cause fetal death?

ORGANOGENESIS

The embryonic period is a time of **organogenesis** (or-gah-no-JEN-eh-sis), or the formation of body organs and organ systems. The inner cell mass of the blastocyst forms a flattened structure called the *embryonic disc*. The embryonic disc, in turn, gives rise to three primary germ layers: the ectoderm, mesoderm, and endoderm.

All the tissues and organs of the body develop from these germ layers. For example, the ectoderm gives rise to the nervous system, portions of the special senses, and the skin. The skin is one of the earliest organs to develop and forms during the third week. The mesoderm gives rise to muscle, bone, blood, and many of the structures of the cardiovascular system. The endoderm gives rise to the epithelial lining of the digestive tract, respiratory tract, and parts of the urinary tract. By the end of the embryonic period (week 8), the main internal organs are established. The embryo weighs about 1 g, is about 1 inch (2.5 cm) in length, and has a human appearance (Fig. 27.4).

BE CAREFUL: TERATOGENS

Because the organs of the body are being formed at this time, the embryonic period is most critical for development. Toxic substances such as alcohol, drugs, and certain pathogens can cross the placental membrane and interfere with embryonic development, causing severe birth defects. These toxic substances are called **teratogens** (TER-ah-toh-jens), a word that means "monster-producing" and attests to the severity of teratogenic birth defects. Hazardous conditions such as exposure to radiation can also act as teratogens (Fig. 27.5).

Table **27.1**   **Hormones of Pregnancy**

HORMONE	SECRETED BY	EFFECTS
Human chorionic gonadotropin (hCG)	Embryonic cells (trophoblasts) during implantation	Maintains the function of the corpus luteum; forms the basis of the pregnancy test
Estrogen and progesterone	Corpus luteum during the first 2 months; placenta after 2 months	Both estrogen and progesterone stimulate the development of the uterine lining and mammary glands. Progesterone inhibits uterine contractions during pregnancy. Estrogen causes relaxation of the pelvic joints. At the beginning of labor, estrogen opposes the quieting effects of progesterone on uterine contractions and sensitizes the myometrium to oxytocin.
Prolactin	Anterior pituitary gland	Prolactin stimulates the breast to secrete milk.
Oxytocin	Posterior pituitary gland	Oxytocin causes the release of milk from the breast (part of the milk let-down reflex initiated by suckling). It causes uterine contractions (participates in labor and postpartum uterine contractions to decrease bleeding).
Prostaglandins	Placenta	Prostaglandins stimulate uterine contractions.
Aldosterone	Adrenal cortex	Aldosterone expands blood volume.
Human placental lactogen (HPL)	Placenta	HPL affects the maternal energy metabolism to make more nutrients available to the fetus.

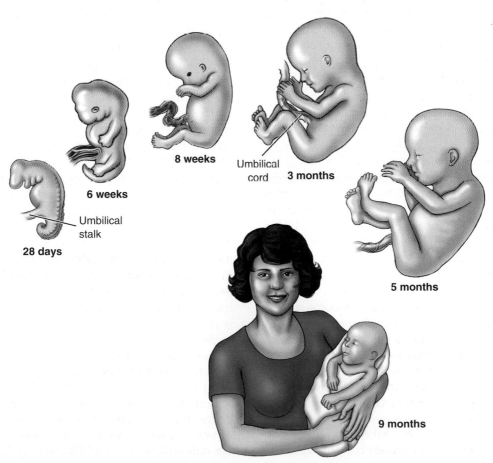

FIG. 27.4 **From embryo to fetus to baby.**

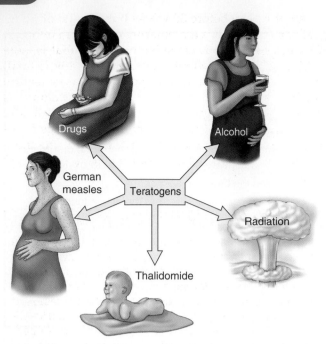

FIG. 27.5 Teratogens: "monster-producing" agents. A variety of agents are teratogenic.

 Do You Know...

How You Get That Extra Inch, or "Slackus the Urachus"?

Following delivery of a baby, the umbilical cord is tied off or clamped. Traditionally, the cord of a girl baby was tied close to the abdominal wall. The cord of a male baby, however, was tied farther away from the abdominal wall. Why the difference in cord length?

In the baby, a cordlike structure called the *urachus* extends from the top of the urinary bladder to the navel. It was thought that the urachus would be pulled up tight if the cord were tied too close to the abdominal wall. The tight urachus, in turn, would pull up on the penis, thereby stunting its growth. Conversely, by leaving the umbilical cord long, the urachus would relax, and the penis would grow longer. This obsession with penile length gave rise to the motto "slackus the urachus." Today, the umbilical cord in both male and female babies is clamped about 1 to 2 cm from the abdominal wall. No penile shortening has been recorded.

Alcohol is a potent teratogen. It can cause a cluster of birth defects known as *fetal alcohol syndrome*. In addition to causing facial deformities, alcohol interferes with neurological and mental development. The tranquilizer thalidomide is another drug that produces teratogenic effects. The development of finlike appendages instead of arms and legs has been correlated with the ingestion of thalidomide during pregnancy. Because of the sensitivity of the embryo to teratogenic agents, the mother must be extremely careful to protect her unborn child from toxic substances and hazardous conditions. Many drugs are teratogenic, and most pharmacological clinical trials do not involve pregnant women!

 Do You Know...

What a Sonogram Is?

A sonogram is an image produced by sound waves as they encounter different tissues and organs. During the procedure, sound waves are directed through the mother's abdomen. As the sound waves "hit" the fetus, an image appears on the scope, showing an outline of the fetus. The size, position, and gender of the fetus can be determined by sonography, as can certain fetal abnormalities.

FETAL PERIOD

The fetal period extends from week 9 to birth. At this time, the developing offspring is called a **fetus.** The fetal period is primarily a time of growth and maturation; only a few new parts appear. Body proportions, however, continue to change. For example, at 8 weeks, the head is almost as large as the body. At birth, the head is proportionately much smaller than the body. Note the changes in body size and proportion in Fig. 27.4.

Table 27.2 summarizes prenatal development. Note that a primitive nervous system begins to form in the third week. The heart and blood vessels originate during the second week. The heart is pumping blood to all the organs of the embryo by the second month, and a heartbeat can be detected during the third month, when the gender of the fetus can also be determined. Once the testes differentiate, they produce the male sex hormone testosterone. Testosterone stimulates the growth of the male external genitals. In the absence of testosterone, female genitals form.

The mother first feels the fetus move during the fifth month; this experience is called *quickening*. As the fetus grows, its skin becomes covered by a fine downy hair called *lanugo* (lah-NOO-go) (during the fifth month). The skin is covered by a white, cheeselike substance called the *vernix caseosa*. The vernix is thought to protect the delicate fetal skin from the amniotic fluid. By the fifth month, the fetus is in crowded quarters and is flexed in the fetal position. During the last 2 months, the fetus is gaining weight rapidly as fat is deposited in the subcutaneous tissue. As the time for birth approaches, the fetus rotates so that the head is pointed toward the cervix. At the end of 38 weeks, the fetus is full term. During this period, the fetal weight has increased from less than 0.5 oz (14 g) to 7.5 lb (3.4 kg; average weight of a full-term infant). The fetus has grown in length from about 1 to 21 inches (2.5 to 53 cm)...and is ready to face the world!

Sometimes, the embryo or fetus is born too early, before the 9-month gestation period is completed. A number of terms are used to describe early birth. An *abortion* is the loss of an embryo or fetus any time during the gestational period; most commonly, abortion refers to the termination of the pregnancy before the twentieth week of development. A *spontaneous abortion* occurs naturally, with no artificial interference.

Table 27.2 Human Development

TIME	DEVELOPMENTAL EVENT
Embryonic	
Second week	Implantation occurs. The inner cell mass is giving rise to the primary germ layers; beginning of placental development. The heart and blood vessels begin to develop.
Third week	Beginning of the nervous system
Fourth week	Appearance of limb buds. Heart is beating. Embryo has tail. Other organ systems begin.
Fifth week	Enlarged head; nose, eyes, and ears are noticeable.
Sixth week	Fingers and toes are present; appearance of cartilage skeleton
Second month	All organ systems are developing. Cartilaginous skeleton is being replaced by bone (ossification). Embryo is about 1.5 inches (3.8 cm) long. The heart is pumping blood to all organs.
Fetal	
Third month	Facial features present in crude form. Can determine gender (the external reproductive organs are distinguishable as male or female). A heartbeat can be detected.
Fourth month	Sensory organs are present; eyes and ears attain shape and position. Eyes blink and the baby begins sucking movements. Skeleton is visible.
Fifth month	Vernix caseosa and a fine downy hair (lanugo) cover the skin. Heartbeat can be heard during a prenatal visit. Quickening occurs.
Sixth month	Continues to grow. Myelination of the spinal cord begins.
Seventh month	Eyes are open. Testes descend into scrotum. Weighs about 3 lb (1362 g). Bone marrow becomes the only site of blood cell formation.
Eighth month	Body is lean and well proportioned. Subcutaneous fat begins to be deposited.
Ninth month	Full term and ready to be delivered. Average weight is 7.5 lb (3400 g), average length is 21 inches (53.3 cm).

Usually, a spontaneous abortion is caused by some fetal abnormality. A *miscarriage* is the layperson's term for a spontaneous abortion. An *induced abortion* is an abortion deliberately caused by some artificial or mechanical means. An unwanted pregnancy is a common cause of an induced abortion. A *therapeutic abortion* is performed by a physician as a form of treatment for the mother. For example, a pregnancy that threatens the life of the mother may be terminated to save her life or improve her medical condition.

A baby born before 38 weeks but capable of living outside the womb is a premature or preterm infant. A 24-week-old fetus is considered viable—that is, able to live outside the womb. A premature baby is small but, more important, it is immature and may require medical support. In particular, the hypothalamus is too immature to regulate body temperature well, and the surfactant produced by the infant's lungs is inadequate to maintain breathing. Generally, the more premature the birth, the greater the need for medical support.

Sum It Up!

Fertilization takes place in the fallopian tube, when the nuclei of a sperm and egg unite, producing a zygote. The zygote gradually moves through the fallopian tube into the uterus, where it develops into an infant over a 9-month period. Prenatal development includes the processes of cleavage (mitosis), growth, morphogenesis, and differentiation. Prenatal development is divided into three periods: the early embryonic period (2 weeks), the embryonic period (6 weeks), and the fetal period (from week 9 to birth at 38 weeks). The zygote undergoes mitosis and develops into a blastocyst; **trophoblastic cells** help the blastocyst to implant. Other major accomplishments of the embryonic period include the formation of extraembryonic membranes and the development of the placenta and umbilical cord. The embryonic period is also the period of organogenesis. The fetal period is primarily a period of rapid growth and maturation. Baby shapes up, fattens up, and moves about.

Re-Think

1. Define *organogenesis*.
2. Define *quickening*, *lanugo*, and *vernix caseosa*.
3. Why is the embryo more susceptible to teratogens than a seventh-month fetus?
4. What is the difference between a miscarriage and an abortion?

CHANGES IN THE MOTHER'S BODY DURING PREGNANCY

Throughout pregnancy, the mother supplies all the food and oxygen for the fetus and eliminates all the waste. This added burden requires many changes in the mother's physiology:

- The rate of metabolism increases. For example, the mother secretes greater amounts of the thyroid hormones triiodothyronine (T_3) and thyroxine (T_4). Human placental lactogen circulates within the maternal circulation; among other growth-promoting actions, this hormone makes additional amounts of glucose available to the growing fetus.
- The mother's blood volume expands by as much as 40% to 50%. The increase in blood volume is caused by an increase in the secretion of aldosterone by the

adrenal cortex. To pump the additional blood and meet the demands of an increased metabolism, the activity of the cardiovascular system increases. For example, heart rate, stroke volume, and cardiac output increase.

- Respiratory activity increases to provide additional oxygen and eliminate excess carbon dioxide.
- The kidneys work harder and produce more urine because they must eliminate waste for both the mother and fetus.
- Under the influence of estrogen and progesterone, the size and weight of the uterus increase dramatically as the fetus grows to full term. To accommodate the growth of the uterus, the pelvic cavity expands as the sacroiliac joints and symphysis pubis become more flexible. With growth, the uterus pushes the abdominal organs upward. Especially in the later months of pregnancy, the upward displacement of abdominal organs exerts pressure on the diaphragm and may hamper the mother's breathing.
- The mother's nutritional needs increase as the maternal organs (uterus and breasts) grow and she provides for the growing fetus. In particular, the need for calcium increases because an increase in parathyroid hormone (PTH) extracts calcium from the mother's bone, making it available to the growing fetus.

Pregnancy brings discomforts for some women, including morning sickness, frequent urination, heartburn, and a host of aches and pains. Although these discomforts of pregnancy are normal, several pregnancy-related conditions are not normal but are dangerous to both the mother and child. For example, the mother may develop a toxemia of pregnancy. This condition is characterized by an elevated blood pressure and progresses in severe cases to generalized seizures. The early stage is called *pre-eclampsia*, and the later seizure stage is called *eclampsia*.

◎ Sum It Up!

Pregnancy causes many changes in the mother. Hormonal changes are numerous and complex. Secretion of hCG, estrogen, and progesterone help maintain the pregnancy and prepare the organs of reproduction for 9 months of pregnancy. Other hormones, such as aldosterone, thyroid hormones, and parathyroid hormone, prepare the mother's body to nourish and sustain the growing unborn child. Almost every maternal organ responds to the presence of the fetus; the heart pumps more blood, the kidneys excrete more waste, and the increased metabolic rate indicates that every cell is working harder.

BIRTH

Finally, our full-term fetus is ready to face the world. The birth process is called *parturition* (pahr-too-RIH-shun). **Labor** is the process whereby forceful myometrial contractions expel the fetus and placenta from the uterus. Once labor starts, forceful and rhythmic contractions begin at the top of the uterus and travel down its length, forcing the fetus through the birth canal.

The precise mechanism that starts labor is unknown. A number of hormonal stimuli do, however, play a role. For example, progesterone, which normally quiets uterine contractions during pregnancy, is secreted in decreasing amounts after the seventh month. This decrease coincides with an increase in the secretion of estrogen. Estrogen has two effects on the uterus: it opposes the quieting effect of progesterone on uterine contractions, and it sensitizes the myometrium (uterine muscle) to the stimulatory effects of oxytocin.

The secretion of prostaglandins by the placenta also plays a role in initiating labor. Prostaglandins stimulate uterine contractions. Finally, the stretching of the uterine and vaginal tissue in the late stage of pregnancy stimulates nerves that send signals to the hypothalamus. The hypothalamus, in turn, stimulates the release of oxytocin from the posterior pituitary gland. Oxytocin exerts a powerful stimulating effect on the myometrium and is thought to play an important role in labor.

Labor can, however, have a false start. Sometimes, a very pregnant and embarrassed mother is admitted to the hospital in false labor. What has happened? She has indeed felt uterine contractions. However, these contractions—called *Braxton Hicks contractions*—are weak, irregular, and ineffectual, and they normally occur during late pregnancy. These contractions are caused by the increased responsiveness of the uterus to various hormones, particularly changing concentrations of estrogen and progesterone. The mother returns home to await the onset of true labor.

👀 Do You Know...

Why Aspirin and Ibuprofen Can Inhibit the Onset of Labor?

Aspirin and ibuprofen are antiprostaglandin drugs. Because prostaglandins stimulate uterine contractions, suppression of prostaglandin secretion by these drugs may inhibit uterine contractions, thereby inhibiting labor.

In a normal delivery, the head is delivered first. A headfirst delivery allows the baby to be suctioned free of mucus and to breathe even before the body has fully exited from the birth canal.

Sometimes, the fetus does not come out headfirst. Instead, another part of the body, such as the buttocks, is delivered first. This presentation is called a *breech birth*. A breech presentation makes delivery more difficult for both the mother and the infant.

There are a number of conditions that prevent a safe vaginal delivery, thereby requiring surgery. A cesarean section (C-section) refers to the delivery of the infant through a surgical incision in the abdominal and uterine walls.

Sum It Up!

The birth process is called *parturition*. Labor is the forceful contractions that expel the baby and afterbirth from the uterus, through the birth canal. Labor begins in response to various hormones, including estrogen, declining levels of progesterone, prostaglandins, and oxytocin.

Do You Know...

What Placenta Previa and Abruptio Placentae Are?

Sometimes, the placenta forms too low in the uterus, near the cervix. When the cervix dilates during the later stages of pregnancy, the placenta detaches from the uterine wall, causing bleeding in the mother and depriving the fetus of an adequate supply of oxygen and nutrients. This condition is called *placenta previa*. *Abruptio placentae* refers to the premature separation of an implanted placenta at about 20 or more weeks of pregnancy. Without immediate treatment, abruptio placentae results in severe hemorrhage in the mother and death for the fetus.

Re-Think

1. List three pregnancy-induced physiological adjustments.
2. Describe the hormonal basis of labor and delivery.
3. Describe the roles of oxytocin, progesterone, and prostaglandins during labor.

POSTNATAL CHANGES AND DEVELOPMENTAL STAGES

IMMEDIATE ADJUSTMENTS

Immediately after birth, the baby must make many important adjustments to survive. Most important, the baby must begin breathing. The first deep breaths, drawn as the baby cries, expand the lungs and provide the infant with life-giving oxygen. The cardiovascular system also makes major adjustments, the most important being the establishment of blood flow to the lungs. Pulmonary blood flow occurs when the fetal heart structures, such as the foramen ovale and ductus arteriosus, close. (Review fetal circulation in Chapter 18.)

Other organ systems continue functioning as they did before birth. For example, the kidneys, having once secreted their urine into the amniotic fluid, become diaper-seeking organs; and the digestive system continues its lifelong career of eating, digesting, and excreting. The first stool produced by the newborn— meconium (meh-COH-nee-um)—is soft and dark green. (During a long, difficult labor, the baby may become stressed and excrete meconium into the amniotic fluid—not good.)

DEVELOPMENT AS A LIFELONG PROCESS

After the newborn makes the immediate adjustments, the infant continues to grow and develop. Throughout life, the person will pass through the following developmental stages:

- *Neonatal period.* The neonatal period begins at birth and lasts for 4 weeks. During this time, Baby is called a *neonate*, or newborn.
- *Infancy.* The period of infancy lasts from the end of the first month to the end of the first year. Baby's first birthday marks the end of this stage.
- *Childhood.* The period of childhood lasts from the beginning of the second year to puberty.
- *Adolescence.* The period of adolescence lasts from puberty to adulthood. One word characterizes this stage: hormones. The period of adolescence is a period of tremendous growth and upheaval. Adolescents are physically capable of reproduction. The teen moves toward adulthood, leaving behind childish ways and coming to grips with becoming an adult.
- *Adulthood.* Adulthood is the period from adolescence to old age. During this period, the person is usually concerned with family matters and career goals. (Most of us are still trying to give up childish ways!)
- *Senescence.* Senescence is the period of old age, ending in death. It is not only a time to reflect on a life well lived but also a time to pursue other goals and to pass on the collected wisdom of a lifetime.

Sum It Up!

After the birth of the baby, both baby and mother make many physiological adjustments. The mother's body returns to its nonpregnant state. For example, cardiac output and blood volume decrease. She is physiologically prepared to breast-feed. Through the actions of prolactin and oxytocin, her mammary glands are producing milk and making it readily available to the suckling infant. The baby has made an initial adjustment to life on the outside and is breathing, urinating, and eating. The newborn continues postnatal development as a neonate. From there, it is on to infancy, childhood, adolescence, adulthood, and senescence.

HEREDITY

"He has his father's nose and his mother's smile." How often have we made that type of statement when we recognize the traits of a parent in a child? The transmission of characteristics from parent to child is called *heredity*, and the science that studies heredity is called *genetics*. The work of an Austrian monk, Gregor Mendel, in the early 19th century, paved the way for the modern science of genetics. Using garden peas, Mendel demonstrated a pattern of specific traits passed on from parent to child.

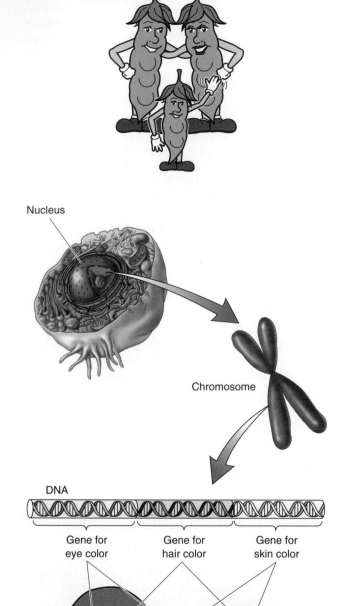

FIG. 27.6 Chromosomes, genes, and genetic expression.

DNA, GENES, AND CHROMOSOMES

How are genetic structures related? Genetic information is located in the deoxyribonucleic acid (DNA) molecule and, more specifically, in the DNA base sequencing (Fig. 27.6; see Chapter 4, pp. 56–59). DNA is tightly wound into threadlike structures called **chromosomes** found in the nucleus of most cells in

Table **27.3**	Examples of Genetic Traits	
TRAIT	**DOMINANT**	**RECESSIVE**
Hairline	Widow's peak	Continuous hairline
Hair color	Dark	Light
Hair texture	Curly	Straight
Hair on back of hand	Present	Absent
Freckles	Present	Absent to few
Dimples	Present	Absent
Eye color	Dark	Light
Color vision	Normal	Color-blind
Ear lobes	Unattached	Attached
Cleft chin	Present	Absent
Rh factor	Present	Absent

the body. **Genes** are segments of the DNA strand and carry information for a specific trait such as skin color, freckles, and blood type. See Table 27.3 for other genetically determined characteristics. Some traits are determined by a single pair of genes, whereas other traits, such as height, require input from several genes. Each chromosome may carry thousands of genes, and each gene occupies a specific position on a chromosome.

Chromosomes exist in pairs. With the exception of the sex cells (egg and sperm), there are 23 pairs, or 46 chromosomes, in almost all human cells (red blood cells are the other exception). During fertilization, the egg and sperm each contribute 23 chromosomes to the zygote for a total of 23 pairs, or 46 chromosomes. One member of each pair comes from the egg; the other comes from the sperm. Thus, for each trait, genetic instructions come from both the mother and the father. Forty-four chromosomes (22 pairs) are called *autosomes* (AW-toh-sohms). The autosomal gene pairs are numbered from 1 to 22. Two (one pair) of the 46 chromosomes are sex chromosomes; each is either an X or Y chromosome.

 Re-Think

1. What happens to the chromosomal number during meiotic cell division? Why is this important?
2. What are autosomes? Sex chromosomes?

GENETIC ART: THE KARYOTYPE

It is possible to photograph the chromosomes in the cell. The photograph of the chromosomes is then cut apart, and the chromosomes are arranged in pairs by size and shape. The resulting display of the paired chromosomes is called a **karyotype** (KAIR-ee-oh-type) (Fig. 27.7). This genetic artwork displays 22 pairs of autosomes and one pair of sex chromosomes. The karyotype is a diagnostic tool. It can reveal structural abnormalities and errors in the numbers of chromosomes.

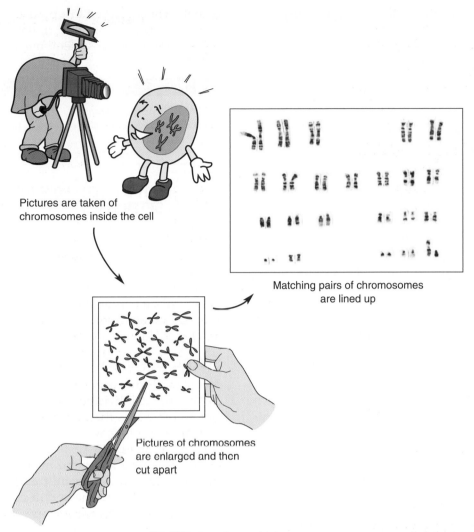

FIG. 27.7 Genetic art: the karyotype.

DOMINANT, RECESSIVE, AND CODOMINANT GENES

Remember that each cell inherits two genes for each trait—tall or short, straight nose or curved nose, stubby fingers or long fingers, dark eyes or light eyes. Hence, the choice. Will it be long or short, or curved or straight? Genes can be dominant, recessive, or co-dominant. A dominant gene expresses itself; it gets noticed. The dominant gene overshadows the recessive gene and keeps it unnoticed, or unexpressed. Thus, a recessive gene is not expressed if it is paired with a dominant gene. For example, the genes for dark eyes are dominant, whereas the genes for light eyes are recessive. If the dominant genes (dark) and the recessive (light) genes are paired, the genes for dark eyes will be expressed (Fig. 27. 8). The genes for light eyes will not be expressed. Codominant genes express a trait equally. AB blood type is an example of codominance.

If recessive genes carry light eye coloring, how can an offspring develop blue eyes? Although blue eye coloring is recessive, a fetus develops blue eyes because

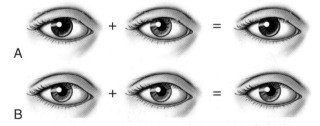

FIG. 27.8 Eye color, with dominant and recessive genes. (A) The dominant brown-eye gene is expressed over the recessive blue-eye gene. (B) Two recessive blue-eye genes produce a blue-eyed offspring.

both the mother and father are carrying the genes for blue eyes, a recessive trait (see Fig. 27.8). If either the mother or father had passed on a dominant gene for dark eyes, the child would have brown eyes.

The question can be put another way. If I have brown eyes, can any of my children have blue eyes? Yes! If I am carrying both a dominant (brown) and recessive (blue) gene for eye color, my child has a chance of having blue eyes. My recessive gene might pair with a recessive gene from my mate. If so, the pairing of two recessive genes produces a blue-eyed offspring. Brown-eyed me is a carrier, one who shows no evidence of a trait (like blue eyes) but carries a recessive gene for that trait.

TOO MANY OR TOO FEW CHROMOSOMES

A person normally inherits 22 pairs of autosomal chromosomes. Sometimes, however, a person inherits too many or too few autosomal chromosomes. The most common autosomal abnormality is called *trisomy 21*, or *Down syndrome*. A child with trisomy 21 has three copies of chromosome 21 instead of two copies. Other types of trisomy occur very infrequently in live births. Trisomy 18, called *Edwards syndrome*, is caused by three copies of chromosome 18; whereas trisomy 13, called *Patau syndrome*, is caused by three copies of chromosome 13. Autosomal abnormalities are usually caused by nondisjunction.

Nondisjunction is the failure of the chromosomes to separate during meiosis, thereby causing the formation of eggs or sperm with too many or too few chromosomes. If these eggs and sperm lead to pregnancy, the embryo may have one too many or too few chromosomes. Most pregnancies with an unbalanced number of chromosomes miscarry in the first trimester. Down syndrome is the most common chromosomal abnormality because the condition is least likely to cause the pregnancy to miscarry. Even so, an estimated 70% of pregnancies with Down syndrome spontaneously miscarry, usually in the first trimester.

GENETIC EXPRESSION

Genetic expression determines what the offspring looks like. A person's genetic expression can be influenced by a number of factors, including the person's gender, the influence of other genes, and environmental conditions. For example, certain types of baldness and color blindness may be inherited by males and females, but these traits are more apt to appear in the male. A child may also have the genetic capability of growing very tall. If the child is deprived of adequate nutrition and exercise, however, that child may not grow as tall as the genetic makeup has predicted.

GENETIC MUTATIONS

Normally, DNA replicates all information with few mistakes. Because of this precision, information is passed along reliably and efficiently to the next generation. Sometimes, however, a change occurs in a gene, or a chromosome breaks in some unexpected way. The result may be a unique feature or a birth defect. This change in the genetic code is called a *mutation*. Some mutations occur spontaneously; others are caused by mutagenic agents, such as chemicals, drugs, and radiation. Mutations can be beneficial or harmful and may even cause the death of the offspring. For example, a mutation in the cells of the immune system may

render a child resistant to a particular disease, thereby enhancing health. Another mutation, however, may weaken the immune system, making it more susceptible to pathogens.

 Re-Think

1. What is a karyotype?
2. Differentiate between a dominant, recessive and codominant gene.
3. Define *nondisjunction*, *trisomy*, and *genetic mutation*.

IT'S A BOY; IT'S A GIRL: HOW THE SEX OF THE CHILD IS DETERMINED

Xs AND Ys

Each human cell has 22 pairs of autosomal chromosomes and one pair of sex chromosomes (X and Y chromosomes). The female has two X chromosomes in her cells, a pair designated XX. A male has both an X and Y chromosome in his cells, a pair designated XY (Fig. 27.9).

SEX DETERMINATION: A MALE THING

The sex cells, the egg and the sperm, divide by a special type of cell division called *meiosis*. The important step in meiosis is the reduction (by half) of the chromosomes. In other words, meiosis reduces the numbers of chromosomes from 46 to 23. The meiotic cell reduction also reduces the numbers of sex chromosomes by half. Consequently, each egg contains one X chromosome, and the sperm contains either an X chromosome or a Y chromosome. If a sperm containing an X chromosome fertilizes an egg, the child has an XX sex chromosome pair and is therefore female. If a sperm containing a Y chromosome fertilizes an egg, the child has an XY chromosome pair and is therefore male. Thus, the sperm (male) determines the sex of the child.

Sometimes, a person inherits an abnormal number of sex chromosomes. For example, a female with Turner syndrome inherits only one sex chromosome, an X chromosome. Turner syndrome is designated as XO. The X signifies the female chromosome; the O signifies the absence of the second sex chromosome. A child with Turner syndrome does not develop secondary sex characteristics, is shorter than average, and has a webbed neck. People with Turner syndrome have normal intelligence.

 Re-Think

Explain why the father determines the gender of the child.

SEX-LINKED TRAITS

The X and Y chromosomes differ structurally. The female X chromosome is larger than the Y chromosome and carries many genes for traits in addition to determining sex. The male Y chromosome is much smaller

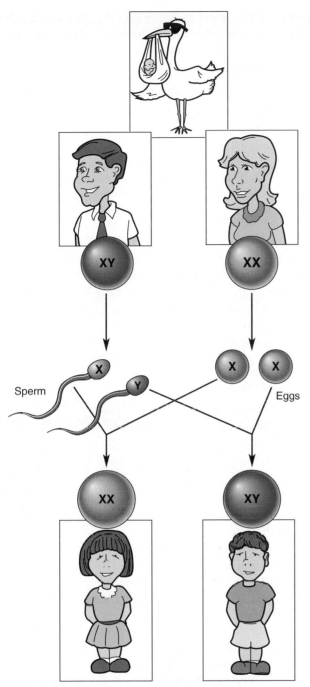

FIG. 27.9 **Determination of sex; Xs and Ys.**

than the X chromosome and does not carry as much genetic information as the X chromosome. Any trait that is carried on a sex chromosome is called a **sex-linked trait**. Because the X chromosome has more genetic information than the Y chromosome, most sex-linked traits are carried on the female X chromosome. Sex-linked traits carried on the X chromosomes are also called *X-linked traits*.

Although most sex-linked traits are carried on the X chromosome, they are expressed, or appear, in the male. Sex-linked diseases include hemophilia, Duchenne muscular dystrophy, and fragile X syndrome. Less serious sex-linked traits include baldness and red–green color blindness.

CONGENITAL AND HEREDITARY DISEASE

You need to distinguish between hereditary diseases and congenital diseases and defects. Hereditary diseases are genetically transmitted; congenital conditions are present at the time of birth. Congenital disorders include those that are inherited and those that are not. For example, hemophilia is genetically transmitted and is therefore inherited. Because hemophilia is present at birth, it is also congenital.

A disease can, however, be congenital but not inherited. For example, a mother may give birth to an infant who was exposed to the rubella virus (German measles) during her first trimester of pregnancy. This child may be born with cardiovascular, ocular, and neural tube defects. These defects were not transmitted genetically from the parents to the child and are therefore not hereditary. The defects are congenital, however, because they were present at birth. Only 15% of congenital defects have a known genetic cause. For 70% of congenital birth defects, the cause is unknown.

Gene therapy offers hope for the treatment and eventual cure of genetic disorders. *Gene therapy* refers to the insertion of normal genes into cells that have abnormal genes. For example, a person with congenitally high cholesterol levels might be successfully treated with genes that code for normal cholesterol production. Although still in its early experimental stages, gene therapy provides hope for those with such genetic conditions as sickle cell disease, cystic fibrosis, and muscular dystrophy.

 Re-Think

1. What is a sex-linked trait?
2. Explain how a disorder can be congenital but not hereditary.

◎ Sum It Up!

A child resembles the parents because he or she inherits genetic information from each parent. Genetic information is stored in the DNA molecules, which are arranged in strands called *chromosomes*. Almost every human cell contains 22 pairs of autosomal chromosomes and one pair of sex chromosomes. Genes are segments of DNA that contain codes for specific traits such as eye color or blood type. The child receives two genes for each inherited trait—one from the mother and one from the father.

Genes are dominant, recessive, or codominant. The sex chromosomes are designated X and Y. At fertilization, an XX combination produces a female child, whereas an XY combination produces a male. The father, with his Y chromosome, determines the sex of the child. Genetic information is passed along efficiently and reliably. Occasionally, incorrect or unhealthy information is passed along, thereby producing genetic diseases.

Note: The Medical Terminology and Disorders table related to this chapter appears in Chapter 26.

Get Ready for Exams!

Summary Outline

The purpose of the reproductive system is to produce offspring whose genetic information is faithfully transmitted from generation to generation.

I. **Fertilization to Birth**
   A. Fertilization
      1. Fertilization (conception) refers to the union of an egg and a sperm, called a *zygote*.
      2. Fertilization takes place around the time of ovulation.
      3. Fertilization normally occurs within the fallopian tube.
   B. Human development: begins with fertilization and ends with death
   C. Prenatal development
      1. Prenatal development processes: cleavage, growth, morphogenesis, and differentiation
      2. Prenatal period: early embryonic, embryonic, and fetal periods
         a. The early embryonic period lasts for 2 weeks after fertilization. The zygote develops and implants into the uterine endometrial lining; its trophoblastic cells secrete hCG (maintains the corpus luteum).
         b. There are two types of twins: monozygotic (identical) twins and dizygotic or fraternal (nonidentical) twins.
         c. The embryonic period lasts for 6 weeks and involves the formation of the extraembryonic membranes, the placenta, and all the organ systems.
         d. The four extraembryonic membranes are the amnion, chorion, yolk sac, and allantois.
         e. The placenta develops as the chorionic villi of the embryo burrow into the endometrial lining of the uterus.
         f. The placenta has two functions: the site of "exchange" and glandular function.
         g. The embryo is hooked up to the placenta by the umbilical cord.
         h. The embryonic period is a period of organogenesis.
         i. The fetal period extends from week 9 to birth; it is a time of growth and maturation.
         j. Hormonal changes during pregnancy are summarized in Table 27.1.
   D. Birth (parturition)
      1. Labor is the forceful contractions that expel the fetus and placenta from the uterus.
      2. Labor is caused by hormones.

II. **Postnatal Development**
   A. Immediate postnatal changes
      1. The baby takes a first breath, and the cardiovascular system makes some major adjustments.
      2. Baby is no longer eating, drinking, and breathing at the placenta.
   B. Developmental periods: neonatal period, infancy, childhood, adolescence, adulthood, and senescence

III. **Heredity**
   A. DNA, genes, and chromosomes
      1. Genetic information is stored in the DNA of genes, which are arranged into chromosomes.
      2. Chromosomes exist in pairs. With the exception of sex cells, most human cells have 23 pairs of chromosomes, or 46 chromosomes.
      3. Genes are dominant, recessive, or codominant.
      4. The sex chromosomes are designated X and Y. A female has two X chromosomes, and a male has one X chromosome and one Y chromosome. Because only the male has the Y chromosome, the father determines the sex of the child.
      5. Sex-linked traits are carried on the sex chromosomes. Most are carried on the X chromosome and are therefore also called *X-linked traits*.
   B. Congenital and hereditary diseases
      1. A congenital disorder is a condition present at birth.
      2. Congenital disorders include inherited and non-inherited birth defects and diseases. A hereditary disease is transmitted genetically from parent to child.

Review Your Knowledge

Matching: Fertilization and Development
Directions: Match the following words with their descriptions.
a. primary germ layers
b. fetal
c. zygote
d. fertilization
e. embryonic
f. parturition
g. trophoblasts
h. placenta
i. implantation
j. umbilical cord
   1. ___ The fertilized ovum
   2. ___ Cells that secrete hCG
   3. ___ A zygote-making event
   4. ___ The site where the fetus breathes, eats, and excretes
   5. ___ The lifeline of the fetus; contains the umbilical blood vessels
   6. ___ Period from 3 to 8 weeks
   7. ___ Process whereby the blastocyst baby-to-be burrows into the endometrium
   8. ___ The birth process
   9. ___ Endoderm, mesoderm, and ectoderm
   10. ___ Period from 9 weeks to birth

Matching: Hormones

Directions: Match the following words with their descriptions. Some words may be used more than once.

a. hCG

b. prolactin

c. oxytocin

d. aldosterone

1. ___ Hormone that stimulates the mammary glands to make milk

2. ___ Posterior pituitary hormone involved in the milk let-down reflex

3. ___ Hormone that sustains the corpus luteum

4. ___ Hormone that stimulates the contraction of the myometrium

5. ___ Secretion of this hormone continues at a high level for about 2 months and then steadily declines as the placenta takes over

6. ___ Hormone that stimulates Na^+ reabsorption and expands blood volume during pregnancy

Matching: Heredity

Directions: Match the following words with their descriptions.

a. sex-linked trait

b. mutation

c. autosomes

d. sex chromosomes

e. genes

1. ___ Segments of a DNA strand that carry the code for a specific trait, such as eye color

2. ___ Twenty-two pairs (numbered 1 to 22) of chromosomes

3. ___ X and Y chromosomes

4. ___ Any trait that is carried on an X or Y chromosome

5. ___ A change in the genetic code that may express itself as a change in a particular trait

Multiple Choice

1. Implantation
   a. normally occurs within the fallopian tubes.
   b. is achieved by the morula.
   c. is a uterine event achieved by the blastocyst.
   d. occurs within the ovaries.

2. Human chorionic gonadotropin (hCG)
   a. promotes the maturation of the egg.
   b. is responsible for female characteristics.
   c. maintains the corpus luteum.
   d. promotes the transformation of the corpus luteum into the corpus albicans.

3. Trophoblastic cells
   a. secrete oxytocin.
   b. are responsible for the milk let-down reflex.
   c. assist with implantation.
   d. are incorporated within the graafian follicle.

4. The morula
   a. only is formed if there is an ectopic pregnancy.
   b. is the unfertilized ovum that gets discharged with the menstrual blood.
   c. refers to the pre-embryonic cluster of cells.
   d. spends its life embedded within the endometrium.

5. Which of the following is *least* true of the placenta?
   a. Is the site at which the baby-to-be breathes
   b. Is very vascular
   c. Replaces the glandular secretion of the corpus luteum
   d. Nourishes the zygote as it matures into the morula

6. The chorion is an extraembryonic membrane that
   a. develops finger-like projections that penetrate the uterine wall, forming the placenta.
   b. forms the inner cell mass.
   c. secretes the hormones that initiate labor.
   d. secretes vernix caseosa that covers the fetus.

7. The myometrium
   a. sloughs during menstruation.
   b. contracts in response to oxytocin and oxytocic drugs.
   c. is the uterine lining that is most responsive to estrogen and progesterone.
   d. forms finger-like projections that penetrate the uterine lining, forming the placenta.

8. Which of the following happens first?
   a. Zygote formation
   b. Fertilization
   c. Ovulation
   d. Early blastocyst

9. Which of the following is true of the gender of a neonate?
   a. A male child has an XX sex chromosome pair.
   b. A female child has an XY sex chromosome pair.
   c. The gender of the infant is determined by the father.
   d. The normal female infant has an XYY chromosomal pattern.

10. A congenital defect is
    a. always due to a defective genetic code.
    b. always due to a drug-induced genetic defect.
    c. a defect that is present at birth.
    d. always life-threatening.

11. The umbilical arteries and umbilical vein receive blood from and deliver blood to which structure?
    a. Zygote
    b. Fallopian tubes
    c. Graafian follicle
    d. Placenta

12. The zygote
    a. implants into the endometrium of the uterus.
    b. develops from the morula.
    c. forms within the fallopian tube.
    d. is a fetal structure.

13. A woman ovulates, producing two eggs. The eggs are fertilized by two different sperm. Which of the following identifies the results?
    a. Monozygotic/identical twinning
    b. Two infants that must be female
    c. Two infants that have the same genetic defects
    d. Dizygotic/fraternal twinning

14. Which of the following lives within the watery environment of amniotic fluid?
    a. Zygote
    b. Fetus
    c. Neonate
    d. Embryo

Go Figure

1. Which of the following is correct according to Fig. 27.1?
   a. The morula splits to form a zygote.
   b. A zygote forms within the fallopian tube.
   c. The late blastocyst is a fallopian-tube dweller.
   d. Implantation is an ovarian event.

2. Which of the following is correct according to Fig. 27.1?
   a. Repeated mitosis of the blastomeres forms a morula.
   b. Trophoblastic cells, located in the ovary, assist in the formation of the Graafian follicle .
   c. Fertilization usually occurs within the corpus luteum.
   d. Trophoblastic cells secrete LH, which is responsible for ovulation.

3. Which of the following is correct according to Figs. 27.2 and 27.3?
   a. The chorionic villi are located within the umbilical cord.
   b. Fig. 27.2C illustrates the procedure for amniocentesis.
   c. None of the extraembryonic membranes are illustrated in Fig. 27.2A.
   d. The chorionic villi interact with the maternal uterine lining to form the placenta.

4. Which of the following is correct according to Fig. 27.9?
   a. The father determines the gender of the offspring.
   b. The father provides sperm that only carry the Y chromosome.
   c. The mother provides ova that only carry the Y chromosome.
   d. An infant with an X and a Y chromosome is female.

Answers to Review Your Knowledge and Go Figure Questions

Chapter 1: Introduction to the Human Body

Matching: Directions of the Body

1. c	3. b	5. d
2. e	4. f	

Matching: Regional Terms

1. d	5. g	9. a
2. f	6. b	10. j
3. i	7. c	
4. h	8. e	

Multiple Choice

1. c	5. b	9. b
2. d	6. b	10. a
3. c	7. c	11. c
4. b	8. c	

Go Figure

1. c	4. d	7. c
2. d	5. a	
3. d	6. d	

Chapter 2: Basic Chemistry

Matching: Atoms and Elements

1. a	3. d	5. e
2. b	4. c	

Matching: Structure of the Atom

1. f	3. b	5. d
2. a	4. d	

Matching: Ions and Electrolytes

1. c	3. a	5. e
2. b	4. d	

Matching: Acids and Bases

1. e	3. b	5. f
2. c	4. f	

Multiple Choice

1. c	4. d	7. c
2. a	5. b	8. c
3. d	6. c	

Go Figure

1. c	4. a	7. b
2. b	5. c	
3. b	6. c	

Chapter 3: Cells

Matching: Cell Structure

1. f	4. b	7. g
2. d	5. c	
3. a	6. e	

Matching: Transport and Tonicity

1. g	5. f	9. b
2. h	6. e	10. d
3. i	7. a	
4. c	8. d	

Multiple Choice

1. b	6. c	11. d
2. d	7. b	12. d
3. b	8. d	13. b
4. a	9. a	
5. d	10. c	

Go Figure

1. b	6. d	11. a
2. b	7. b	12. d
3. c.	8. a	13. c
4. c	9. d	14. d
5. d	10. b	

Chapter 4: Cell Metabolism

Matching: Carbohydrates, Proteins, and Fats

1. d	5. f	9. e
2. b	6. b	10. a
3. c	7. h	
4. g	8. a	

Matching: Biochemistry Terms

1. b	3. c	5. a
2. a	4. d	6. e

Matching: Genetic Code and Protein Synthesis

1. d	3. c	5. b
2. e	4. a	

Multiple Choice

1. a	6. a	11. a
2. d	7. b	12. b
3. d	8. c	13. d
4. a	9. c	14. a
5. a	10. c	15. b

Go Figure

1. c	5. a	9. b
2. d	6. a	10. a
3. c	7. c	11. d
4. b	8. d	

Chapter 5: Microbiology Basics

Matching: Microorganisms and Other Pathogens

1. b	5. d	9. c
2. a	6. c	10. b
3. e	7. e	11. f
4. d	8. b	

Multiple Choice

1. a	3. c	5. d
2. b	4. c	

Go Figure

1. c	2. d

Chapter 6: Tissues and Membranes

Matching: Tissues

1. a	5. b	9. b
2. b	6. c	10. d
3. a	7. b	
4. a	8. b	

Matching: Membranes

1. d	3. b	5. c
2. e	4. a	

Multiple Choice

1. c	4. a	7. d
2. a	5. a	
3. d	6. b	

Go Figure

1. b	4. d	7. c
2. c	5. a	8. c
3. a	6. d	

Chapter 7: Integumentary System and Body Temperature

Matching: Skin

1. d	3. a	5. d
2. b	4. c	6. b

Matching: Glands

1. b	4. c	7. b
2. b	5. d	8. a
3. a	6. a	

Matching: Colors

1. c	3. a	5. e
2. b	4. d	6. b

Multiple Choice

1. b	6. c	11. d
2. b	7. a	12. b
3. c	8. d	13. c
4. c	9. b	14. b
5. b	10. b	15. b

Go Figure

1. c	3. c	5. d
2. b	4. c	6. d

Chapter 8: Skeletal System

Matching: Long Bone

1. d	5. j	9. h
2. c	6. a	10. e
3. g	7. b	
4. i	8. f	

Matching: Names of Bones

1. e	5. g	9. c
2. f	6. h	10. i
3. b	7. j	
4. d	8. a	

Matching: Joints and Joint Movement

1. c	5. c	9. d
2. j	6. a	10. g
3. i	7. f or a	
4. h	8. b	

Multiple Choice

1. c	6. d	11. c
2. c	7. d	12. a
3. b	8. b	13. c
4. d	9. a	14. b
5. c	10. d	15. b

Go Figure

1. c	8. c	15. d
2. a	9. b	16. c
3. a	10. b	17. a
4. d	11. b	18. c
5. b	12. b	19. c
6. d	13. a	20. a
7. d	14. d	21. d

Chapter 9: Muscular System

Matching: Muscle Terms

1. l	5. k	9. h
2. j	6. b	10. i
3. j	7. f	
4. d	8. g	

Matching: Names of Muscles

1. c	5. j	9. b
2. k	6. a	10. b
3. g	7. d	
4. f	8. i	

Multiple Choice

1. a	6. b	11. b
2. c	7. d	12. b
3. b	8. b	13. d
4. d	9. c	14. d
5. a	10. b	15. b

Go Figure

1. c	6. d	11. c
2. a	7. b	12. b
3. b	8. c	13. b
4. d	9. c	
5. c	10. c	

Chapter 10: Nervous System: Nervous Tissue and Brain

Matching: Nerve Cells

1. e	5. c	9. h
2. d	6. b	10. i
3. f	7. j	
4. a	8. g	

Matching: Brain

1. b	4. d	7. a
2. a	5. c	8. a
3. e	6. e	9. f

Multiple Choice

1. b	6. b	11. d
2. d	7. c	12. c
3. c	8. b	13. d
4. d	9. b	14. a
5. a	10. d	15. b

Go Figure

1. c	6. b	11. d
2. b	7. d	12. c
3. a	8. c	13. d
4. b	9. c	14. d
5. a	10. c	

Chapter 11: Nervous System: Spinal Cord and Peripheral Nerves

Matching: Reflexes

1. g	4. c	7. e
2. b	5. a	
3. f	6. d	

Matching: Nerves

1. a	5. e	9. h
2. b	6. c	10. a
3. h	7. f	
4. g	8. d	

Multiple Choice

1. c	6. a	11. b
2. d	7. a	12. c
3. a	8. b	13. b
4. a	9. d	14. c
5. d	10. b	15. b

Go Figure

1. c	5. d	9. a
2. d	6. d	10. d
3. b	7. b	11. b
4. b	8. d	12. d

Chapter 12: Autonomic Nervous System

Matching: Sympathetic or Parasympathetic

1. S	5. S	9. P
2. P	6. S	10. S
3. S	7. P	
4. S	8. P	

Matching: Norepinephrine or Acetylcholine

1. NE	5. ACh	9. NE
2. NE	6. NE	10. ACh
3. ACh	7. NE	
4. ACh	8. ACh	

Multiple Choice

1. c	5. b	9. b
2. b	6. b	10. c
3. a	7. c	
4. c	8. d	

Go Figure

1. c	4. d	7. c
2. a	5. c	8. a
3. a	6. b	

Chapter 13: Sensory System

Matching: Senses

1. a	4. e	7. d
2. d	5. b	8. e
3. c	6. a	

Matching: Structures of the Eye

1. h	5. f	9. h
2. e	6. b	10. g
3. c	7. e	
4. a	8. d	

Matching: Structures of the Ear

1. b	5. c	9. b
2. b	6. c	10. c
3. a	7. a	
4. c	8. b	

Multiple Choice

1. b	6. b	11. a
2. c	7. c	12. b
3. b	8. b	13. c
4. c	9. b	14. d
5. a	10. c	15. d

Go Figure

1. c	6. c	11. b
2. b	7. a	12. d
3. b	8. a	13. d
4. b	9. b	14. d
5. d	10. c	15. d

Chapter 14: Endocrine System

Matching: Glands

1. a	5. h	9. d
2. b	6. c	10. g
3. b	7. f	
4. e	8. a	

Matching: Hormones

1. e	5. c	9. d
2. g	6. f	10. a
3. b	7. j	
4. i	8. i	

Multiple Choice

1. b	6. d	11. b
2. a	7. a	12. d
3. c	8. c	13. b
4. d	9. b	14. c
5. d	10. b	15. d

Go Figure

1. d	5. a	9. b
2. c	6. a	
3. c	7. d	
4. d	8. c	

Chapter 15: Blood

Matching: Blood Cells

1. c	5. a	9. b
2. c	6. a	10. c
3. c	7. b	
4. b	8. c	

Matching: Blood Clots

1. e	3. a	5. c
2. d	4. b	

Matching: Blood Types

1. d	3. c	5. d
2. d	4. a	

Multiple Choice

1. b	6. d	11. c
2. b	7. b	12. c
3. a	8. a	13. d
4. c	9. d	14. a
5. c	10. c	15. b

Go Figure

1. d	6. d	11. d
2. b	7. a	12. d
3. d	8. d	13. c
4. c	9. b	14. d
5. b	10. b	

Chapter 16: Anatomy of the Heart

Matching: Structures of the Heart

1. g	5. d	9. d
2. b	6. a	10. h
3. f	7. a	
4. c	8. e	

Matching: Valves

1. d	5. a	9. d
2. d	6. c	10. c
3. b	7. c	
4. c	8. d	

Multiple Choice

1. d	7. a	13. b
2. d	8. b	14. a
3. a	9. d	15. c
4. b	10. d	16. d
5. a	11. d	
6. b	12. c	

Go Figure

1. b	5. c	9. c
2. d	6. d	10. a
3. d	7. d	11. d
4. a	8. a	

Chapter 17: Function of the Heart

Matching: Cardiac Function Terms

1. b	5. d	9. c
2. c	6. d	10. b
3. b	7. f	
4. e	8. a	

Matching: Loads and Effects

1. b	4. b	7. b
2. c	5. e	8. c
3. a	6. d	

Multiple Choice

1. d	7. d	13. b
2. d	8. b	14. d
3. d	9. a	15. d
4. c	10. b	16. a
5. a	11. a	
6. d	12. b	

Go Figure

1. b	4. c	7. a
2. b	5. a	8. c
3. c	6. b	9. c

Chapter 18: Anatomy of the Blood Vessels and Special Circulations

Matching: Blood Vessels: Structure and Function

1. c	5. d	9. a
2. b	6. d	10. c
3. c	7. d	
4. c	8. a	

Matching: Names of Blood Vessels

1. f	6. a	11. k
2. i	7. j	12. b
3. e	8. g	13. h
4. a	9. d	14. l
5. e	10. c	15. m

Matching: Fetal Circulation

1. a	3. c	5. b
2. e	4. d	

Multiple Choice

1. c	8. d	15. c
2. a	9. c	16. c
3. b	10. a	17. a
4. b	11. b	18. a
5. a	12. d	19. c
6. d	13. b	20. c
7. c	14. c	

Go Figure

1. b	5. a	9. b
2. c	6. c	10. d
3. c	7. c	
4. c	8. b	

Chapter 19: Functions of the Blood Vessels

Matching: Blood Pressure Terms

1. d	5. g	9. b
2. f	6. a	10. e
3. a	7. b	
4. h	8. c	

Matching: Blood Pressure Readings

1. a	5. b	9. a
2. a	6. a	10. b
3. b	7. b	
4. c	8. c	

Matching: Changes in Blood Pressure

1. a	5. a	9. a
2. b	6. b	10. a
3. a	7. a	
4. a	8. b	

Multiple Choice

1. d	6. b	11. b
2. c	7. c	12. c
3. c	8. b	13. d
4. b	9. c	14. b
5. a	10. c	15. d

Go Figure

1. b	4. c	7. d
2. c	5. c	
3. b	6. b	

Chapter 20: Lymphatic System

Matching: Lymph Terms

1. e	3. b	5. a
2. c	4. d	

Multiple Choice

1. b	5. b	9. a
2. c	6. c	10. c
3. c	7. a	
4. c	8. b	

Go Figure

1. c	3. b	5. d
2. a	4. b	6. d

Chapter 21: Immune System

Matching: Nonspecific Immunity

1. d	3. c	5. a
2. b	4. b	

Matching: Specific Immunity

1. e	3. d	5. b
2. a	4. c	

Matching: Active and Passive Immunity

1. a	3. b	5. b
2. b	4. a	6. a

Multiple Choice

1. b	6. c	11. d
2. d	7. a	12. c
3. c	8. a	13. d
4. b	9. b	14. b
5. c	10. b	15. a

Go Figure

1. d	4. d	7. c
2. d	5. b	8. c
3. c	6. b	9. d

Chapter 22: Respiratory System

Matching: Structures of the Respiratory Tract

1. d	5. b	9. d
2. c	6. h	10. g
3. e	7. h	
4. a	8. f	

Matching: Thoracic Cavity and Ventilation

1. d	4. e	7. c
2. b	5. f	
3. c	6. a	

Multiple Choice

1. c	6. b	11. d
2. c	7. d	12. a
3. c	8. c	13. a
4. b	9. a	14. c
5. c	10. c	15. c

Go Figure

1. b	**5.** a	**9.** d
2. b	**6.** a	**10.** d
3. c	**7.** d	**11.** c
4. d	**8.** d	**12.** a

Chapter 23: Digestive System

Matching: Structures: Making the Connections

1. c	**4.** e	**7.** f
2. d	**5.** h	**8.** a
3. b	**6.** g	

Matching: Enzymes, Hormones, and Digestive Aids

1. f	**6.** g	**11.** e
2. b	**7.** a	**12.** h
3. c	**8.** d	**13.** c
4. e	**9.** g	
5. i	**10.** f	

Multiple Choice

1. c	**7.** c	**13.** b
2. b	**8.** c	**14.** c
3. b	**9.** a	**15.** d
4. d	**10.** b	**16.** a
5. c	**11.** b	
6. c	**12.** d	

Go Figure

1. d	**6.** a	**11.** b
2. b	**7.** d	**12.** d
3. b	**8.** b	**13.** a
4. a	**9.** a	
5. c	**10.** c	

Chapter 24: Urinary System

Matching: Plumbing...More or Less

1. c	**5.** d	**9.** b
2. b	**6.** c	**10.** d
3. a	**7.** d	
4. d	**8.** d	

Matching: Nephron Unit

1. d	**5.** b	**9.** f
2. b	**6.** e	**10.** d
3. a	**7.** c	
4. g	**8.** a	

Matching: Hormones and Enzymes

1. b	**5.** f	**9.** d
2. a	**6.** a	**10.** g
3. e	**7.** e	
4. a	**8.** c	

Multiple Choice

1. a	**6.** c	**11.** b
2. c	**7.** b	**12.** a
3. d	**8.** b	**13.** c
4. d	**9.** b	**14.** d
5. c	**10.** d	**15.** b

Go Figure

1. d	**4.** a	**7.** a
2. b	**5.** b	**8.** d
3. b	**6.** b	

Chapter 25: Water, Electrolyte, and Acid–Base Balance

Matching: Water Compartments

1. b	**3.** a	**5.** a
2. c	**4.** d	

Matching: Ions

1. c	**5.** a	**9.** c
2. a	**6.** c	**10.** d
3. b	**7.** b	
4. b	**8.** a	

Multiple Choice

1. a	**7.** c	**13.** c
2. d	**8.** d	**14.** b
3. c	**9.** a	**15.** c
4. c	**10.** d	**16.** d
5. c	**11.** c	
6. c	**12.** c	

Go Figure

1. c	**3.** b	**5.** a
2. d	**4.** b	**6.** a

Chapter 26: Reproductive Systems

Matching: Female Structures

1. a	**5.** c	**9.** d
2. d	**6.** b	**10.** c
3. c	**7.** d	**11.** d
4. b	**8.** c	**12.** e

Matching: Male Structures

1. b	**4.** f	**7.** e
2. a	**5.** c	**8.** g
3. d	**6.** c	

Matching: Hormones

1. e	**5.** c	**9.** e
2. d	**6.** d	**10.** b
3. a	**7.** e	
4. b	**8.** a	

Multiple Choice

1. d	**6.** c	**11.** b
2. a	**7.** c	**12.** c
3. c	**8.** b	**13.** b
4. c	**9.** b	**14.** a
5. c	**10.** c	**15.** c

Go Figure

1. d	**4.** d	**7.** a
2. a	**5.** a	**8.** d
3. b	**6.** d	**9.** b

Chapter 27: Human Development and Heredity

Matching: Fertilization and Development

1. c	**5.** j	**9.** a
2. g	**6.** e	**10.** b
3. d	**7.** i	
4. h	**8.** f	

Matching: Hormones

1. b	**3.** a	**5.** a
2. c	**4.** c	**6.** d

Matching: Heredity

1. e	**3.** d	**5.** b
2. c	**4.** a	

Multiple Choice

1. c	**6.** a	**11.** d
2. c	**7.** b	**12.** c
3. c	**8.** c	**13.** d
4. c	**9.** c	**14.** b
5. d	**10.** c	

Go Figure

1. b	**3.** d	
2. a	**4.** a	

Glossary

A

abdominopelvic cavity (ab-DOM-i-no-PEL-vik) Part of the ventral cavity that lies inferior to the diaphragm; includes the upper abdominal cavity and lower pelvic cavity.

abduction (ab-DUK-shun) Movement of a body part away from the midline.

absorption Taking in of substances across cells or membranes; more specifically, referring to the movement of digested food from the digestive tract into the blood and lymph.

accommodation Adjustment of the curvature of the lens to focus an image on the retina.

acetylcholine (ass-ee-til-KOH-leen) Neurotransmitter that is secreted from the nerve terminals of cholinergic fibers; found in the CNS, neuromuscular junctions, and synapses of the parasympathetic nerves.

acid (ASS-id) Substance that donates or releases hydrogen ions when it ionizes in water.

acidosis (ass-i-DOH-sis) Imbalance caused by excess H^+ concentration in the blood, causing the blood pH to decrease below 7.35; respiratory acidosis and metabolic acidosis.

actin (AK-tin) One of the contractile proteins in muscle; forms the thin filaments.

action potential Sequence of changes in the membrane potential that occurs when an excitable cell (neuron or muscle) is stimulated. It has two phases—depolarization and repolarization; also called the *nerve impulse* and the *cardiac impulse.*

active immunity Immunity achieved when the body makes antibodies against an antigen.

active transport Transport process that requires an input of energy (ATP) to move a substance from an area of low concentration to an area of high concentration.

adaptation Adjustment to a stimulus, such as the adaptation to odor.

adaptive immunity The ability of immune cells to respond or adapt to newly encountered pathogens or foreign agents; specific immunity.

adduction (ad-DUK-shun) Movement of a body part toward the midline of the body.

adenohypophysis (ad-eh-no-hye-POF-i-sis) Anterior pituitary gland.

adenosine triphosphate (ATP) Energy-storing and energy-transferring molecule found in all cells.

adipose (AD-i-pohs) tissue Type of connective tissue that stores fat.

adrenal gland Endocrine gland that consists of an outer cortex and inner medulla. The cortex secretes steroids, and the medulla secretes catecholamines.

adrenergic fiber A neuron that secretes norepinephrine (noradrenaline) as its neurotransmitter.

aerobic catabolism (air-OH-bik kah-TAB-oh-liz-em) Chemical reactions that break down complex substances into simpler substances in the presence of oxygen.

aerobic metabolism Chemical reactions that require oxygen; includes aerobic anabolism and catabolism.

afferent (AF-fer-ent) nerve Carrying toward a center, such as afferent nerves carrying information toward the central nervous system.

afterload The force against which the heart contracts, such as the blood pressure.

agglutination (ah-GLOO-tin-ay-tion) Clumping of cells in response to an antigen–antibody reaction.

albumin (al-BYOO-min) Plasma protein that helps regulate plasma osmotic pressure, thereby "holding" water within the blood vessels; responsible for the oncotic pressure.

aldosterone (al-DOS-ter-own) Mineralocorticoid (steroid) secreted by the adrenal cortex; stimulates the kidney to reabsorb sodium and water and to excrete potassium.

alimentary canal See *digestive tract.*

alkalosis (al-kah-LOH-sis) Imbalance associated with a decrease in H^+ concentration and an increase in blood pH higher than 7.45; respiratory alkalosis and metabolic alkalosis.

allergen (AL-er-jen) Foreign substance or antigen that stimulates an allergic reaction.

alpha-adrenergic receptor A type of receptor that is activated by norepinephrine.

alveolus (al-VEE-oh-lus) *(pl.,* alveoli) Tiny grapelike sac in the lungs; the site of gas exchange (oxygen and carbon dioxide) between the air and the blood.

amino acids Small nitrogen-containing organic compounds; the building blocks of protein.

ammonia A nitrogenous compound (NH_3); blood ammonia is converted to urea for excretion by the kidneys.

amnion (AM-nee-on) One of the four extraembryonic membranes that surrounds the fetus.

amniotic fluid A clear and protective liquid that surrounds the fetus during pregnancy.

amylase (AM-ch-lays) Enzyme that digests carbohydrates.

anabolism (ah-NAB-oh-liz-em) Metabolic reactions that build complex substances from simpler substances.

anaerobic catabolism (an-air-OH-bik kah-TAB-oh-liz-em) Chemical reactions that break down complex substances into simpler substances without the presence of oxygen.

anaerobic (an-air-OH-bik) metabolism Chemical reactions that do not require oxygen.

anastomosis (ah-nas-toh-MOH-sis) A connection between two tubular structures.

anatomical position Position of the body; the body is standing erect with the face forward and the arms at the sides (palms and toes face in a forward direction).

anatomy (ah-NAT-o-mee) Study of the structure of the body.

anemia Condition characterized by abnormally low amounts of hemoglobin or low numbers of red blood cells.

angiotensin (an-jee-oh-TEN-sin) II Hormone that elevates blood pressure and stimulates the secretion of aldosterone by the adrenal cortex.

anion (AN-eye-on) Negatively charged ion.

antagonist A muscle that exerts an opposing effect.

antibodies Substances that react with a specific antigen.

antibody-mediated immunity A type of immunity engaged in by the B lymphocyte. The B cell secretes antibodies that attack the antigen; also called *humoral immunity.*

antidiuretic hormone (ADH) Posterior pituitary hormone that stimulates the collecting duct in the kidney to reabsorb water, thereby decreasing urinary output; also called *vasopressin.*

antigen (AN-ti-jen) Foreign substance that stimulates the production of antibodies.

antigen presentation Activity of a macrophage whereby the antigen portion of an ingested pathogen or foreign agent is pushed out of the macrophage onto its surface.

aorta (ay-OR-tah) Large artery that conducts blood from the left ventricle of the heart.

aortic valve Semilunar valve located between the left ventricle and aorta.

apocrine (AP-oh-krin) gland One of the sudoriferous (sweat) glands.

aponeurosis (ap-oh-nyoo-ROH-sis) Broad, flat sheet of fibrous connective tissue that connects muscle to another structure.

apoptosis A natural process of cell destruction; called *cellular suicide*.

appendicular skeleton Part of the skeleton that includes the bones of the upper extremities, lower extremities, pelvic girdle, and pectoral girdle.

appendix Worm-shaped outpouching of the wall of the cecum.

aqueous solution A solution in which water is its solvent.

areolar (ah-REE-oh-lar) tissue Loose connective tissue.

arteriole (ar-TEER-ee-ohl) Small artery that is composed largely of smooth muscle, found between the larger artery and the capillaries; also called *resistance vessel*.

artery Blood vessel that carries blood away from the heart.

articulation Joining of structures at a joint.

artificially acquired immunity Immunity acquired through the use of agents such as vaccines, toxoids, and immunoglobulins.

ascending tract A tract that carries sensory information up the spinal cord toward the brain.

association areas Areas of the brain that are concerned with linking or coordinating a primary function. For example the visual association area coordinates those activities that support the sensation of sight.

atom Fundamental unit of an element; the smallest part of the element that has the characteristics of that element.

atomic mass The mass of the neutrons and protons within the nucleus of an atom; similar to the atomic weight.

atomic number The number of protons in the nucleus of an atom.

ATP See *adenosine triphosphate*.

atrial conducting fibers The specialized conducting fibers that transmit the cardiac impulse (action potential) from the SA node in the right atrium to the left atrium.

atrioventricular valves Cuspid valves located between the atria and ventricles; include the tricuspid and bicuspid (mitral) valves.

atrium (*pl.*, atria) Upper chamber of the heart that receives blood from veins.

atrophy (AT-ro-fee) A wasting or a decrease in the size of an organ or tissue, usually referring to a muscle.

autoimmunity (aw-toh-i-MYOO-ni-tee) Immunity against one's own tissue.

automaticity The ability of the cardiac cells to generate its own electrical signals independently of stimulation from the CNS.

autonomic nervous system (ANS) Involuntary or automatic nervous system that controls the organs, glands, cardiac muscle, and smooth muscle; two divisions: the sympathetic and parasympathetic nervous systems.

AV node A part of the cardiac conduction system that acts as a relay station for the electrical signal coming from the SA node in the right atrium into the ventricles; the AV node slows the signal.

axial skeleton The part of the skeleton that includes the skull, vertebral column, ribs, and sternum.

axon (AK-son) Elongated part of the neuron that conducts nerve impulses away from the cell body.

B

bacteria Single-cell organisms classified as cocci, bacilli, and curved rods.

baroreceptor (bar-oh-ree-SEP-tor) Receptor that detects or senses changes in blood pressure; located in the carotid sinus and aortic arch.

baroreceptor (bar-oh-ree-SEP-tor) reflex An autonomic reflex that restores blood pressure to normal; the reflex is initiated by a sudden change in blood pressure.

basal metabolic rate (BMR) The rate at which cells metabolize (use oxygen) in a resting state.

base Substance, such as the hydroxyl ion (OH^-), that combines with hydrogen ion (H^+).

base pairing Pairing of the bases of the nucleotides; adenine and thymine (DNA), guanine and cytosine (DNA and RNA), and adenine and uracil (RNA).

base sequencing Sequence or arrangement of the bases in a strand of DNA or RNA; carrier of the genetic code.

basophil (BAY-so-fil) Type of granular leukocyte; stains blue.

beta-adrenergic receptor A type of adrenergic receptor that is activated by norepinephrine.

bicuspid (bye-KUSS-pid) valve The atrioventricular valve between the left atrium and left ventricle; also called the *mitral valve*.

bile A digestive aid secreted by the liver and stored in the gallbladder; emulsifies fats.

biliary (BILL-ee-air-ee) tree Arrangement of ducts that transports bile from the liver to the gallbladder and duodenum; includes hepatic ducts, cystic duct, and common bile duct.

bilirubin (bill-ee-ROO-bin) Pigment produced from the breakdown of hemoglobin and secreted into the bile; an accumulation of bilirubin in the skin causes jaundice.

biorhythm Rhythmic alteration in a hormone's rate of secretion; circadian rhythm has a period of 24 hours.

blastocyst Early pre-embryonic cluster of cells with a hollow interior; the late blastocyst implants into the inner uterine lining.

blood pressure The force that the blood exerts against the vessel wall.

blood–brain barrier A structural characteristic of the capillaries of the CNS that impedes or prevents the diffusion of some substances from the systemic circulation into the CNS.

B lymphocytes (B cells) Lymphocytes that engage in antibody-mediated immunity.

Bowman's capsule C-shaped tubular structure that partially surrounds the glomerulus. Water and dissolved substances are filtered from the glomerulus into the Bowman's capsule.

Boyle's law A law that describes the inverse relationship between pressure and volume.

brain The part of the CNS contained within the cranial cavity; divided into the cerebrum, diencephalon, brain stem, and cerebellum.

brain stem Part of the brain that is formed by the midbrain, pons, and medulla oblongata. Lower part of the brain that connects the brain with the spinal cord; consists of the midbrain, pons, and medulla oblongata.

breast Milk-secreting glandular (mammary) organ on the chest.

bronchiole tree Part of the lower respiratory tract that is formed by the bronchioles and alveoli.

bronchioles (BRONK-ee-ohls) Small airway tubes in the respiratory tract that are composed largely of smooth muscle; connect the bronchi and alveoli.

bronchus (*pl.*, bronchi) Large airway in the lungs that connects the trachea and bronchioles; there is a right and left bronchus.

buffer Substance that resists changes in pH. A buffer can remove or add H^+, thereby adjusting pH.

C

calyces (KAY-liss-ees) Cuplike structures that collect urine from the collecting ducts of the nephron units.

capacitance (cah-PAS-it-ance) vessels Refers to the veins and specifically to their ability to store blood.

capillary Smallest and most numerous of the blood vessels; site of exchange of nutrients and waste between the blood and tissue fluid. The capillaries are called the *exchange vessels*.

capillary exchange The movement of nutrients, oxygen, and waste across the capillary membranes; the exchange is between the blood and interstitium.

carbaminohemoglobin (karb-a-MEE-no-HEE-moh-GLOH-bin) Hemoglobin that has combined with carbon dioxide.

carbohydrates Organic compounds that include simple sugars, starch, and glycogen; primary source of energy.

carbon dioxide (CO_2) A compound formed by carbon and oxygen; the waste product of cellular metabolism.

cardiac conduction system Specialized cardiac cells that create and conduct the electrical cardiac impulse (action potential); includes the SA node, AV node, and His-Purkinje system.

cardiac cycle Events that occur in the heart during one heartbeat.

cardiac muscle Type of striated muscle found in the heart; the myocardium.

cardiac output Amount of blood pumped by the heart in 1 minute (about 5000 mL/min); determined by heart rate and stroke volume.

cardiac reserve The potential increase in cardiac output above resting cardiac output.

cardiology The study of the heart.

carrier A living organism that harbors a pathogen and acts as a source of infection.

catabolism (kah-TAB-oh-liz-em) Metabolic breakdown of complex molecules into simpler molecules; the breakdown is accompanied by the release of energy.

catalyst (KAT-ah-list) Any substance that speeds up the rate of a chemical reaction; see *enzyme*.

catecholamine (kat-eh-KOHL-ah-meen) Classification of hormones secreted by the adrenal medulla; includes epinephrine (adrenaline) and norepinephrine (noradrenaline).

cation (KAT-eye-on) Positively charged ion.

cecum (SEE-come) Part of the large intestine that connects the ileum of the small intestine and ascending colon of the large intestine.

cell Basic unit of life; the structural and functional unit of a living organism.

cell cycle The phases that a cell goes through as it divides.

cell-mediated immunity Type of immunity engaged in by the T cell; cell-to-cell combat.

cell membrane Membrane that surrounds the cell and regulates what enters and leaves the cell; also called the *plasma membrane*.

central nervous system The part of the nervous system composed of the brain and spinal cord.

cerebellum (sair-eh-BELL-um) Part of the brain located under the cerebrum; it coordinates skeletal muscle activity.

cerebrospinal fluid Cushioning fluid that circulates within the subarachnoid space around the brain and spinal cord.

cerebrum (seh-REE-brum) Largest and uppermost part of the brain, divided into two cerebral hemispheres. There are four lobes: frontal, parietal, temporal, and occipital.

ceruminous (seh-ROO-mi-nus) glands Modified sweat glands found in the external ear canal; they secrete cerumen, or ear wax.

cervix Constricted portion (neck) of an organ, usually referring to the lower portion of the uterus.

chemoreceptor (KEE-moh-ree-SEP-tor) Receptor that detects changes in the chemical composition of a substance.

cholecystokinin A hormone secreted by the walls of the duodenum primary in response to dietary fat; it stimulates the secretion of bile and digestive enzymes.

cholesterol A lipid and most abundant steroid in the body; used structurally in plasma membranes and in the synthesis of steroid hormones and bile salts.

cholinergic (koh-lin-ER-jik) fiber A neuron that secretes acetylcholine (ACh) as its neurotransmitter.

chondrocytes (KON-droh-sytes) Cartilage-forming cells.

chordae tendineae (KORD-ay ten-din-EE-ay) Tough fibrous bands of connective tissue that attach the cusps of the AV valves to the walls of the ventricles of the heart.

chorion (KOH-ree-on) The outermost extraembryonic membrane surrounding the fetus; helps form the placenta.

choroid plexus A network of capillaries in the ventricles of the brain; the capillaries, surrounded by ependymal cells, secrete cerebrospinal fluid.

chromosome Coiled, threadlike structures that contain segments of DNA called *genes*.

chronotropic (KRON-oh-TROH-pik) effect A change in heart rate (HR). A positive chronotropic effect is an increase in HR, whereas a negative chronotropic effect is a decrease in HR.

chyle (kile) Milky fluid found in the lacteals of the villi; consists of emulsified fats and lymph.

chyme (kime) Pastelike mixture of partially digested food, water, and digestive enzymes that is formed in the stomach.

cilia (SIL-ee-ah) (*sing.,* cilium) Hairlike processes on the surface of many cells.

circle of Willis The arterial blood supply of the brain; the arteries are arranged in a circular pattern and located at the base of the brain.

circumduction A movement at a joint whereby the distal end of a bone moves in a circle while the proximal end remains relatively stationary; the movement resembles the underhand pitching of a softball.

clone A group of cells that come from a single cell and are therefore genetically identical.

clotting cascade Series of reactions that describe the sequential activation of clotting factors resulting in the formation of a blood clot.

coagulation Clotting of blood.

cochlea (KOHK-lee-ah) Part of the inner ear that contains the organ of Corti, the receptors for hearing.

collecting duct The nephron structure that receives urine from the distal tubule and delivers it to the renal pelvis.

colloid A mixture in which one substance is evenly distributed throughout another substance; the particles do not settle out. Milk and blood are colloids.

colon (KOH-lon) Major portion of the large intestine that extends from the cecum to the rectum.

colonization The establishment of pathogens in a wound or in the body; the colony of pathogens, however, do not cause symptoms of infection.

columnar epithelium Type of epithelium that has column-shaped cells.

common bile duct The biliary duct that is formed by the merger of the hepatic duct and cystic duct; allows bile to flow from the liver and gallbladder into the duodenum.

communicable disease A disease that can be spread from one host to another.

compact bone Dense or hard bone formed by osteons (haversian systems); found primarily in the diaphysis of a long bone.

complement (KOM-pleh-ment) proteins Group of proteins in the blood that are concerned with phagocytosis.

compliance The degree of stretch of a hollow organ; the change in volume in response to a change in pressure.

compound Substance composed of two or more chemical elements, such as water (H_2O).

conception Fertilization; union of the ovum and sperm.

conductance (con-DUC-tans) vessels Blood vessels that are primarily concerned with carrying blood to smaller blood vessels; functional name for arteries.

conduction Loss of heat energy as it is transferred from the warm body to a cooler object, such as a cooling blanket.

conduction system Specialized tissue in the heart that generates and transmits the electrical signals (cardiac impulses or action potentials).

congenital (kon-JEN-i-tall) Present at birth.

connective tissue One of the four basic types of tissue that generally binds and supports body structures.

contacts Interactions between two individuals; used in microbiology to indicate exposure to pathogens.

contraction Shortening of a muscle so as to cause movement or tension development.

contracture (con-TRAK-ture) An abnormal formation of fibrous tissue within a muscle, causing it to freeze in a flexed position.

convection Loss of heat energy to the surrounding cooler air. The layer of heated air next to the body is constantly being removed by a fan (or breeze) and replaced by cooler air.

converting enzyme An enzyme that activates angiotensin I to angiotensin II.

convolution a convex curvature of the cerebral cortex; also called a *gyrus*.

cornea (KOR-nee-ah) Transparent portion of the sclera that covers the anterior portion of the eye.

coronary arteries Right and left coronary arteries deliver oxygenated blood to the heart muscle.

corpus callosum Bands of white matter that connect the left and right cerebral hemispheres of the brain.

corpus luteum (KOHR-pus LOO-tee-um) Yellow body formed from the ovarian follicle after ovulation; secretes large amounts of progesterone and smaller amounts of estrogen.

covalent (ko-VAYL-ent) bond Bond or attraction formed by the sharing of electrons between atoms.

cranial cavity Part of the dorsal cavity that contains the brain.

cranial nerves The 12 pairs of nerves that emerge from the brain; with the exception of the vagus nerve (CN X), the cranial nerves innervate the head and shoulders.

craniosacral (kray-nee-oh-SAY-kral) outflow Parasympathetic nerve activity.

creatinine (cree-AH-tuh-neen) A nitrogenous waste product that is excreted by the kidney.

cross-bridges Temporary binding of myosin heads and actin causing muscle contraction and tension development

cuboidal epithelium (KYOO-boyd-al ep-i-THEE-lee-um) Type of epithelium that has cells shaped like cubes.

cutaneous (kyoo-TAYN-ee-us) membrane Skin.

cyanosis Bluish coloring of the skin caused by diminished oxygenation of the blood.

cytoplasm (SYE-toh-plaz-em) Gel-like substance surrounded by the cell membrane but outside of the nucleus.

D

decussation A crossing over as in nerve fibers crossing from one side of the brain or spinal cord to the other side.

deglutition The act of swallowing.

dehydration State in which there is a deficiency in body water.

dendrite (DEN-dryte) Treelike process of the neuron that receives the stimulus and carries it toward the cell body.

deoxyribonucleic (dee-OK-see-rye-boh-nook-LAY-ik) acid (DNA) Nucleotide that stores the genetic information of the organism.

depolarize (dee-POH-lar-ize) Change in the membrane potential across the cell membrane, with the inside of the cell becoming less negative or less polarized than the resting membrane potential.

dermatome (DER-mah-tohm) Area of the body supplied by a spinal nerve.

dermis The thicker layer of the skin; dense connective tissue under the epidermis of the skin.

descending tract A nerve tract that carries information away from the brain and down the spinal cord toward the periphery.

detrusor (dee-TROO-sor) muscle Smooth muscle located in the urinary bladder.

dialysis (dye-AL-i-sis) A passive transport process that allows small particles to diffuse through a semipermeable membrane.

diaphragm (DYE-ah-fram) Dome-shaped skeletal muscle that separates the thoracic and abdominal cavities; chief muscle of inspiration (inhalation).

diaphysis (dye-AF-i-sis) Shaft of a long bone.

diastole (dye-ASS-toh-lee) Relaxation phase of the cardiac cycle.

diastolic (dye-ah-STOL-ik) pressure Blood pressure in the large arteries when the heart is resting (diastole); the bottom number of a blood pressure reading.

differentiation (dif-er-EN-shee-AY-shun) Process whereby a cell becomes specialized.

diffusion Passive transport process that causes movement of a substance from an area of higher concentration to an area of lower concentration.

digestion Process of breaking down food into absorbable particles; mechanical and chemical.

digestive tract Series of organs concerned with the digestion and absorption of food and the elimination of digestive waste; also called the *alimentary canal* and *gastrointestinal tract*.

disaccharides Double sugars; sucrose, maltose and lactose.

disease Failure of the body to function normally.

diuresis (dye-yoo-REE-sis) Increased excretion of urine.

dominant gene Gene whose trait is expressed.

dorsal cavity Body cavity located toward the back part of the body; divided into the cranial cavity and spinal cavity.

dorsal root Sensory nerve of a spinal nerve as it attaches to the spinal cord.

dromotropic effect A change in the speed of the action potential (electrical signal) as it moves from the SA node through the His-Purkinje system.

dual innervation Innervation by two different branches of the autonomic nervous system (sympathetic and parasympathetic branches).

ductus arteriosus the fetal structure that connects the pulmonary trunk and the aorta thereby bypassing blood flow around the lung.

ductus venosus The fetal structure that shunts a part of the blood flow from the umbilical vein into the fetal inferior vena cava.

duodenum (doo-oh-DEE-num) First part of the small intestine.

E

eccrine (EK-rin) gland Type of sweat gland that secretes a watery substance; plays an important role in the regulation of body temperature.

edema (eh-DEE-mah) Abnormal collection of fluid, usually causing swelling.

efferent (EF-fer-ent) Movement away from a central point, such as a motor neuron that carries information away from the central nervous system.

efferent nerve (EF-fer-ent NOO-ron) A motor neuron; brings information from the CNS to the periphery.

ejection fraction The percent of the ventricular volume that is pumped or ejected during ventricular systole (contraction).

electrocardiogram (ECG) (eh-lek-troh-KAR-dee-oh-gram) Graphic recording of the electrical events that occur during the cardiac cycle.

electrolyte (eh-LEK-troh-lyte) Compound that dissociates into ions when dissolved in water.

electrolyte (eh-LEK-troh-lyte) balance Having normal amounts of electrolytes in each fluid compartment.

element Substance composed of only one type of atom.

embryo (EM-bree-oh) The developing human between the gestational ages of 2 and 8 weeks.

emulsification (ee-MULL-seh-feh-KAY-shun) The physical breakdown of a large fat globule into many smaller fat globules.

end-diastolic volume (EDV) The volume of blood in the ventricle at the end of its resting phase (diastole); also called *preload*.

endocardium (en-doh-KAR-dee-um) Inner lining of the heart wall.

endocrine (EN-doh-krin) glands Ductless glands that secrete hormones, usually into the blood for transport throughout the body.

endocytosis (en-doh-sye-TOH-sis) Uptake of material through the cell membrane by forming a vesicle; includes pinocytosis and phagocytosis.

endometrium (en-doh-MEE-tree-um) Inner lining of the uterus.

endoplasmic reticulum (ER) (en-doh-PLAZ-mik reh-TIK-yoo-lum) Intracellular membrane system concerned with the synthesis and transportation of protein and steroids; called the *rough ER* if ribosomes are attached, called the *smooth ER* if there are no ribosomes.

energy Ability to perform work.

enteric nervous system Specialized and unique arrangement of nerves that supply the digestive tract.

enzyme (EN-zyme) Organic catalyst; speeds up the rate of a chemical reaction.

eosinophil (ee-oh-SIN-oh-fil) Type of granular leukocyte; stains a rose color.

epicardium (ep-i-KAR-dee-um) Outer layer of the heart; forms part of the pericardium.

epidermis (ep-i-DER-mis) Outer epithelial layer of the skin.

epididymis (ep-i-DID-i-miss) Coiled tube that carries sperm from the testis to the vas deferens.

epiglottis (ep-i-GLOT-iss) Cartilage that guards the opening into the larynx; directs food and water into the esophagus.

epiphyseal disc Growth plate in a long bone; site where longitudinal bone growth occurs.

epiphysis (eh-PIF-i-sis) End of a long bone.

epithelial (ep-i-THEE-lee-al) tissue One of the four types of tissues; found on the surface of the body (skin) and lining the body cavities; it also forms glands.

equilibrium Balance.

erythrocyte (eh-RITH-roh-syte) Red blood cell.

erythropoietin (eh-RITH-roh-POY-eh-tin) Hormone secreted by the kidneys that stimulates the bone marrow to produce red blood cells.

esophagus (eh-SOF-ah-gus) The tubelike structure that connects the pharynx to the stomach; the food tube.

estrogen (ES-troh-jen) Female sex hormone secreted by the developing ovarian follicle.

eustachian (yoo-STAY-shun) tube Tube that connects the pharynx with the middle ear; also called the *auditory tube*.

evaporation Loss of heat as water changes from the liquid to the vapor or gas state.

exchange vessels Refer to the *capillaries*, which allow for the movement of nutrients, oxygen, and waste across their membranes.

exhalation Process of moving air out of the lungs; the breathing-out phase of ventilation, also called *expiration*.

exocrine (EKS-oh-krin) glands Type of glands that secrete their products into ducts that open onto a surface.

exocytosis (eks-o-sye-TOH-sis) Elimination of material from a cell through the formation of vesicles.

extension Increase in the angle of a joint.

external genitalia In the female the external genitalia include the accessory structures of the reproductive system that are external to the vagina (labia majora, mons pubis, labia minora, clitoris, Bartholin glands); also called the *vulva* or *pudendum*. In the male the external genitalia refers to the penis, male urethra, and the scrotum.

extracellular fluid Fluid located outside the cell, such as the plasma and interstitial fluid.

extraembryonic membranes Membranes formed outside the embryo; include the yolk sac, amnion, allantois, and chorion.

extrinsic eye muscles Eye muscles located outside the eyeball and concerned with movement of the eyeball in its socket; include the superior, inferior, medial, and lateral recti muscles and the superior and inferior oblique muscles.

F

facilitated diffusion Passive process whereby a substance moves with the assistance of a carrier molecule from an area of higher concentration to an area of lower concentration.

fallopian (fal-LOH-pee-an) tube Passageway through which the egg or zygote moves from the ovary to the uterus; also called the *oviduct* or *uterine tube*.

fascia (FASH-uh) Fibrous connective tissue membrane that covers individual skeletal muscles or certain organs.

fatty acids An organic acid especially those found in fats and oils; building blocks of fats.

feed-and-breed division Parasympathetic division of the autonomic nervous system.

feedback control loops A response within a system that regulates further activity of the system; described as negative and positive feedback control.

fertilization Union of an ovum and a sperm to form a zygote; also called *conception*.

fetal circulation The series of fetal blood vessels through which the heart pumps blood; also includes the fetoplacental circulation (blood vessels within the umbilical cord and placenta).

fetus Name given to the developing human at the end of the embryonic period, from the end of the eighth week of pregnancy to birth.

fever Fever technically means an elevation of body temperature above normal; the hypothalamic set point is elevated. Clinically a fever is defined as a body temperature above 100.4 degrees F.

fibrin (FYE-brin) Protein strands formed by the action of thrombin on fibrinogen; the clot.

fight-or-flight division Sympathetic division of the autonomic nervous system.

filtration Process whereby water and dissolved substances move through a membrane in response to pressure.

fingerprints The mark created by the undersides of the tips of the fingers and thumb; the impression is created by the ridges on the skin surface.

fissure A narrow slit or groove that divides an organ; also called a *sulcus*.

flexion Decrease in the angle of a joint; a bending movement.

fontanel (FON-tah-nel) Membranous gap between the cranial bones of an infant's skull.

foramen ovale The hole in the atrial septum of the fetal heart; allows blood to bypass the fetal lungs.

frontal lobe Anterior portion of the cerebrum that controls voluntary skeletal activity and motor speech and that plays an important role in emotions, critical thinking, and ethical decision making.

frontal plane Vertical plane that divides the body into front (anterior) and back (posterior parts); the coronal plane.

fungus Plantlike organisms such as mushrooms; cause mycotic infections.

G

gallbladder Small pear-shaped organ involved in the concentration and storage of bile.

gametes Mature sexual reproductive cell such as the egg and sperm.

ganglion A group of nerve cell bodies usually linked by synapses; often appears as a swelling.

gastric juice A thin watery and acidic fluid secreted by the glands of the stomach; includes water, HCl, some digestive enzymes and mucus.

gastrin A hormone secreted by the walls of the stomach in response to the presence of food; stimulates the secretion of gastric juice.

gastrointestinal (GI) tract See *digestive tract*.

gene Part of the chromosome that codes for a specific trait; the biological unit of heredity.

general senses Senses whose receptors are scattered widely throughout the body; include sensations of touch, pressure, pain, proprioception, and temperature.

genetic code The set of DNA and RNA sequences that determine the assembly of amino acids in the synthesis of protein; biochemical basis of heredity.

gestation pregnancy; the carrying of the embryo/fetus from conception to birth.

glomerular (gloh-MAIR-yoo-lar) filtration rate (GFR) The rate of filtration (pushing) of water and dissolved solute through the pores of the glomerular membrane.

glomerulus (gloh-MAIR-yoo-lus) Tuft of capillaries located in the Bowman's capsule of the nephron unit of the kidney.

glottis (GLOT-iss) Opening between the vocal cords; an air passage for the respiratory tract.

gluconeogenesis (gloo-koh-nee-oh-JEN-eh-sis) Biochemical process that makes glucose from nonglucose substances, especially protein.

glucose A monosaccharide, or simple sugar, that serves as the principal fuel for the cells of the body.

glycemic index A scale that ranks food on a scale from 1 to 100 on its effect on blood glucose levels.

glycerol An alcohol that is a structural component of biological lipids.

glycogen (GLY-koh-jen) Polysaccharide that is the storage form of glucose; also called *animal starch*.

glycolysis (gly-KOHL-i-sis) Anaerobic catabolism of glucose into lactic acid.

Golgi (GOAL-jee) apparatus Membranous organelle concerned with the final trimming and packaging of protein for exocytosis.

gonadotropin (go-NAD-oh-TROH-pin) Hormone "aimed at" the gonads; includes follicle-stimulating hormone (FSH), luteinizing hormone (LH), and human chorionic gonadotropin (hCG).

gonads (GO-nads) Organs that produce gametes (ova or sperm); term for ovaries and testes.

graafian (GRAH-fee-en) follicle Mature ovarian follicle.

gray matter Part of the central nervous system that is composed of cell bodies and unmyelinated fibers.

great vessels The large blood vessels that bring blood to and away from the heart: aorta, superior and inferior venae cavae, pulmonary trunk, and pulmonary veins.

gyrus See *convolution*.

H

haversian (hah-VER-shun) system Structural unit of compact bone; bone is layered in concentric circles around an osteonic canal; an osteon.

hearing audition

heart The hollow muscular pump that pumps blood to the lungs for oxygenation and then to the rest of the body for the distribution of oxygen, nutrients, and hormones; the heart also picks up and delivers waste to the organs of excretion.

heart failure The inability of the heart to pump blood in sufficient quantities to meet the requirements of the body; characterized by a low ejection fraction and signs of organ congestion, such as pulmonary edema.

helminths (HEL-minths) Parasitic worms.

hematocrit (hee-MAT-oh-krit) Laboratory test that expresses the percentage of red blood cells present in a volume of blood.

hemoglobin (hee-moh-GLOH-bin) Iron-containing protein in the red blood cell that can form a weak bond with oxygen; also transports carbon dioxide.

hemolysis (hee-MAWL-ih-sis) Breakdown of erythrocytes.

hemopoiesis (hee-muh-poy-EE-sis) Production of blood cells.

hemostasis (hee-moh-STAY-sis) The stopping of blood loss.

hepatic portal system An arrangement of veins that picks up blood that is rich in digestive end-products from the organs of digestion and delivers it to the liver.

His-Purkinje system A path of specialized conducting cells within the ventricles of the heart; allows the electrical signals to spread throughout the ventricles rapidly, thereby initiating myocardial contraction (systole).

homeostasis (ho-me-o-STAY-sis) Ability of the body to maintain a constant internal environment.

hormone Substance secreted by an endocrine gland into the blood.

human chorionic gonadotropin (KOH-ri-on-ik go-nad-oh-TROH-pin) Hormone secreted by the trophoblastic cells of the embryonic blastocyst; maintains the corpus luteum until the placenta can take over its glandular function.

hydrogen bond Weak intermolecular bond formed between hydrogen and a negatively charged atom such as oxygen or nitrogen.

hyperkalemia (hye-per-kah-LEE-mee-ah) Abnormally high blood potassium level.

hypernatremia An abnormal increase in the concentration of Na^+ in the blood.

hypertension Blood pressure that is higher than normal.

hyperthermia An elevation of body temperature above normal; its cause is a failure of the body to cool, as in exposure to high external temperature.

hypertonic (hye-per-TON-ik) Having a solute concentration greater than that of a reference solution.

hypertrophy (hye-PER-tro-fee) Increase in the size of a body part, usually referring to a muscle.

hyperventilation (hye-per-ven-ti-LAY-shun) Abnormally rapid, deep breathing.

hypokalemia (hye-poh-kah-LEE-mee-ah) A lower-than-normal amount of potassium in the blood.

hyponatremia An abnormal decrease in the concentration of Na^+ in the blood.

hypophysis (hye-POF-is-sis) Pituitary gland; adenohypophysis (anterior) and neurohypophysis (posterior).

hypotension Blood pressure that is lower than normal.

hypothalamus (hye-poh-THAHL-ah-mahs) Part of the diencephalon that regulates the pituitary gland, autonomic nervous system, water balance, appetite, temperature, and emotions.

hypothermia A decrease of body temperature below normal; its cause is due to excess loss of heat, as in exposure to low external temperature.

hypotonic (hye-poh-TON-ik) Having a solute concentration less than that of a reference solution.

hypoventilation (hye-poh-ven-ti-LAY-shun) Abnormally slow and/or shallow respiratory rate.

I

ileum (IL-ee-um) Distal end of the small intestine.

immunity Ability to resist and overcome injury by pathogens or antigenic substances.

immunization A process whereby a person is made immune or resistant to an infectious disease.

immunoglobulin (i-myoo-noh-GLOB-yoo-lin) Antibodies produced by plasma cells in response to antigenic stimulation.

immunotolerance The recognition of self as nonantigenic; the failure of the body's immune system to mount an attack against its own antigens.

implantation The process whereby the embryo imbeds into the inner wall of the mother's uterus.

infection Disease caused by a pathogen.

inflammation Body's response to infection or injury; characterized by redness, heat, swelling, and pain.

inhalation Process of moving air into the lungs; the breathing-in phase of ventilation, also called *inspiration*.

innate immunity Immunity that is naturally present; natural immunity.

inotropic (in-o-TROH-pik) effect A change in the strength or force of myocardial contraction that does not involve stretching the myocardial fibers.

insensible perspiration Perspiration that evaporates from the skin before it is perceived as sweat.

insertion The more movable attachment point of a muscle to a bone.

intake Amount of fluid taken into the body.

integument A natural covering, such as the skin.

integumentary (in-teg-yoo-MEN-tar-ee) system Organ system that consists of the skin and its accessory organs.

interatrial septum The septum between the right and left atria of the heart.

intercellular Between the cells.

intercellular matrix Substances secreted by cells into the extracellular spaces between the cells; the secretions provide biochemical and structural support to the secreting cells.

intercostal muscles The skeletal muscles located between the ribs.

interferons (in-ter-FEER-ons) Substances produced by a virus infected cell; protect other cells from viral infection.

interneuron Neuron that links the sensory and motor neurons in the central nervous system.

interstitial (in-ter-STISH-al) fluid Fluid located between the cells; tissue fluid.

interventricular septum The septum between the right and left ventricles of the heart.

intracellular fluid Fluid located within cells.

intrapleural (in-trah-PLOR-al) pressure The pressure within the intrapleural space (between the visceral and parietal pleurae); must be negative for the lungs to be expanded.

intravascular fluid Fluid found within the blood vessels; the main intravascular fluid is blood.

intrinsic eye muscles Muscles located within the eyeball; the radial and circular muscles of the iris and the ciliary muscles.

ion (EYE-on) An electrically charged atom or group of atoms; cation (positive) or anion (negative).

ionic (eye-ON-ik) bond Bond formed by the exchange of electrons between atoms.

ionization The dissociation of an electrolyte into its ions.

ischemia (is-KEE-mee-ah) Insufficient blood flow to a tissue, sometimes resulting in tissue damage and death (gangrene).

isotonic (eye-soh-TON-ik) Having the same concentration as the reference solution.

isotope (EYE-so-tohp) Atom that has the same number of protons and electrons but a different number of neutrons; the same atomic number, but a different atomic mass.

J

jaundice (JAWN-dis) Yellow coloring of the skin and whites of the eyes caused by an increase of bilirubin in the blood.

jejunum (jeh-JOO-num) Second or middle part of the small intestine.

joint Union of two or more bones; an articulation.

juxtaglomerular apparatus A specialized structure in the kidney formed by the distal convoluted tubule and the afferent arterioles; the renin-secreting cells.

K

kaliuretic Refers to the effect of a hormone or drug that causes the elimination of potassium in the urine.

karyotype (KAIR-ee-oh-type) Arrangement of the chromosomes by pairs in a fixed order.

keratin (KER-ah-tin) A protein found in the skin, hair, and nails; it hardens the cells and makes them water resistant.

ketone bodies Products of rapid and incomplete fatty acid catabolism; includes acetone, acetoacetic acid, and beta-hydroxybutyric acid.

kidney Organ of the urinary system that produces urine; contains the nephron units.

Korotkoff sounds The sounds (tap tap tap) heard when blood pressure is being recorded; the sounds are due to the flow of blood through the constricted artery.

Kussmaul (KOOS-mall) respirations Increase in the rate and depth of respirations to correct a metabolic acidosis.

L

labor The process of delivering a baby and placenta, membranes, and umbilical cord from the uterus, thereby terminating a pregnancy. Also known as *parturition* or *childbirth*.

lacrimal (LAK-ri-mal) apparatus Gland that secretes tears.

lactation The secretion of milk by the mammary glands.

lacteal (LAK-teal) Lymph vessel in a villus of the small intestine.

larynx (LAIR-inks) Structure that contains the vocal cords; voicebox.

left pump The left side of the heart that pumps blood through the aorta and to the systemic circulation.

leukocyte (LOO-koh-syte) White blood cell; functions primarily to defend the body against infection.

ligaments Strong bands of connective tissue that join bone to bone.

limbic (LIM-bik) system The emotional brain.

lipase Enzyme that digests fats into fatty acids and glycerol.

lipids Organic molecules that include fats, oils, and steroids.

liver lobule A unit of the liver made up of liver cells (hepatocytes) surrounding a central vein. Hepatocytes process sinusoidal blood, secreting bile into surrounding canaliculi.

local infection An infection that is restricted to one part of the body as opposed to a systemic infection.

lock-and-key mechanism A mechanism that is described as operating like a key that fits a lock; the lock is engaged only by the right key.

loop of Henle (HEN-lee) A hairpin-looped tubular structure of the nephron unit that receives urine from the proximal tubule and delivers it to the distal tubule.

lower respiratory tract Consists of organs located within the chest cavity; includes the lower trachea, bronchi, bronchioles, and alveoli.

lymph (limf) Fluid that has the same composition as tissue fluid and is carried by the lymph vessels.

lymph node Mass of lymphoid tissue located along the course of a lymphatic vessel.

lymphatic duct Large tube or vessel that carries lymph, such as the thoracic duct; same as lymphatic vessel.

lymphatic nodules Partially or nonencapsulated masses of lymphatic tissue; includes tonsils, MALT, Peyer's patches, and the appendix.

lymphatic vessels Vessels that transport lymph from lymphatic capillaries and larger lymphatic ducts to the subclavian veins.

lymphocyte (LIM-foh-syte) Agranular leukocyte; T and B lymphocytes engage in specific immunity.

lysosome (LYE-so-sohm) Organelle that contains powerful enzymes; engages in phagocytosis and does the "intracellular housecleaning."

M

macrophage (MAK-roh-fayj) Enlarged monocyte that eats foreign material; a "big eater." Macrophages may be wandering or fixed.

MALT (mucosal-associated lymphatic tissue) A diffuse or widely spread system of lymphatic tissue found in various parts of the body such as the digestive tract, lungs, and skin.

mammary (MAM-mah-ree) gland Gland of the female breast that secretes milk.

mastication The act of chewing.

matter Anything that occupies space; may occur as solid, liquid, or gas.

mechanoreceptor (meh-KAN-o-ree-SEP-tor) Receptor that is stimulated by bending, pressing, or pushing.

mediastinum (MEE-dee-ass-TI-num) Space between the lungs that contains the heart and pericardial cavity, trachea, thymus gland, esophagus, and large blood vessels.

medulla oblongata (meh-DOOL-ah oh-blohn-GAHT-ah) Most inferior part of the brain stem that controls vital functions, such as respiratory and cardiovascular function.

meiosis (my-OH-sis) Type of cell division used by the sex cells to reduce the number of chromosomes in each from 46 to 23.

melanin (MEL-ah-nin) Pigment responsible for the color of the skin and hair.

melanocyte (mel-AN-o-syte) Melanin-producing cell.

meninges (meh-NIN-jeez) Membranes that cover the brain and spinal cord; include the dura mater, arachnoid mater, and pia mater.

menopause Normal developmental stage in women that marks the end of the ovarian and uterine cycles.

menses (MEN-seez) Menstruation; the monthly discharge of blood from the uterus.

metabolic acidosis A condition in which blood pH decreases below 7.35; the cause is nonrespiratory.

metabolic alkalosis A condition in which blood pH increases above 7.45; the cause is nonrespiratory.

metabolism All the chemical reactions that occur within the cells; consists of anabolism and catabolism.

microbiota A group of microorganisms that live harmoniously together in or on a body part; also called the *normal flora*.

micturition (mik-tor-RISH-un) Urination.

milk let-down reflex An oxytocin-mediated reflex that results in the release of milk from the breast in response to suckling.

mineral Inorganic substance such as sodium or potassium.

mitochondria (my-toh-KON-dree-ah) Organelles that produce most of the ATP; the "power plants" of the cell.

mitosis (my-TOH-sis) Type of cell division that produces two identical daughter cells, each containing 46 chromosomes.

mitral (MY-tral) valve See *bicuspid valve*.

mixed nerve Nerve that contains both sensory and motor fibers.

mixture Combination of two or more substances that can be separated by ordinary physical means.

molecule Chemical combination of two or more atoms.

monocyte (MON-oh-syte) Agranular phagocytic leukocyte that can become a macrophage.

monosaccharide (mon-oh-SAK-ah-ride) A simple sugar consisting of hexoses (e.g., glucose, fructose, galactose) or pentoses (e.g., ribose, deoxyribose).

morula A solid ball of cells resulting from successive mitotic division of the fertilized ovum.

motor nerve Collection of motor neurons that carries information away from the central nervous system.

motor unit Refers to the somatic motor neuron and the muscle fibers innervated by the motor neuron.

mucous membranes Type of membranes that line the cavities and tubes that open to the exterior of the body.

muscarinic (mus-kar-IN-ik) receptor Cholinergic receptor activated by acetylcholine; located primarily on the target organs of the parasympathetic nerves.

muscle fiber Muscle cell composed of a series arrangement of sarcomeres.

muscle tissue Type of tissue composed primarily of contractile protein; includes skeletal, smooth, and cardiac muscle.

myelin (MY-eh-lin) sheath White fatty material that covers some nerve fibers.

myocardium (my-oh-KAR-dee-um) Heart muscle.

myometrium (my-oh-MEET-ri-um) Muscle layer of the uterus that contracts and causes the delivery of the infant.

myosin (MY-oh-sin) Muscle protein that interacts with actin to cause muscle contraction; also called the *thick filament*.

N

natriuresis The excretion of sodium into the urine.

natriuretic peptides Protein hormones that promote the excretion of sodium into the urine; include atrial natriuretic peptide and brain natriuretic peptide.

natural killer (NK) cells Lymphocyte that engages in nonspecific immunity.

naturally acquired immunity Immunity acquired through natural means, such as getting a disease or receiving antibodies from your mother.

negative feedback A mechanism activated by an imbalance; activation of the mechanism then corrects the imbalance.

nephron unit Structural and functional unit of the kidney that makes urine.

nerve Bundle of nerve fibers and blood vessels.

nerve impulse Action potential that occurs in neurons.

nerve tract Group of neurons that share a common function within the central nervous system; may be ascending (sensory) or descending (motor).

nervous tissue A type of tissue that includes neurons and neuroglia.

neuroglia (noo-ROG-lee-ah) Nerve cells that support, protect, and nourish the neurons.

neurohypophysis (noo-roh-hye-POF-i-sis) The posterior pituitary gland; secretes oxytocin and antidiuretic hormone.

neuromuscular junction (NMJ) Junction or space that occurs between a motor neuron and a muscle fiber.

neuron Nerve cell that conducts the action potential (nerve impulse).

neurotransmitters (noo-roh-TRANS-mit-ters) Chemical made within the axon terminal responsible for transmission of the signal across the synapse or junction.

neutralization A chemical reaction between and acid and a base that produces salt and water; results in a reduction in [H^+].

neutrophil (NOO-troh-fil) Granular, motile, and highly phagocytic leukocyte.

nicotinic receptor A type of cholinergic receptor that is activated by acetylcholine; located in the autonomic ganglia and within the neuromuscular junction.

nociceptor (noh-see-SEP-tor) Pain receptor.

nodes of Ranvier Exposed or unmyelinated axonal membrane; permits salutatory conduction.

nonshivering thermogenesis Heat produced by mechanisms other than shivering (skeletal muscle activity) and includes the metabolism of brown fat

nonspecific immunity Immune responses that do not require a specific antigen; include many responses such as phagocytosis, inflammation, and fever.

norepinephrine (nor-ep-i-NEF-rin) A neurotransmitter secreted by the adrenergic fibers of the sympathetic nervous system; activates adrenergic receptors.

normal flora A population of microorganisms that normally inhabit an area such as the skin, intestines, or vagina.

nosocomial (noh-soh-CO-mee-al) infection Hospital-acquired infection.

nucleus (*pl.*, nuclei) Large organelle separated from the cytoplasm by a nuclear membrane; stores the DNA in chromosomes and acts as the control center of the cell.

O

occipital (ok-SIP-it-al) lobe Cerebral lobe located in the back of the head; concerned primarily with vision.

olfactory (ol-FAK-tor-ee) receptor Chemoreceptor associated with the sense of smell.

oliguria (ohl-i-GOO-ree-ah) Scanty urine formation, usually defined as less than 400 mL/24 hr.

oncotic pressure The part of the osmotic pressure of the blood caused by the plasma proteins.

optic chiasm (OP-tik kye-AS-m) Site for the crossing of the medial fibers of the optic nerve to the opposite side of the brain; located in front of the pituitary gland.

organ Group of tissues that performs a specialized function, such as the lungs.

organelle (or-gah-NELL) Structure within the cytoplasm, such as the mitochondria, that performs a specific function.

organic compound Carbon-containing substance.

organ of Corti (KOR-tee) Hearing receptors (mechanoreceptors) located in the inner ear.

organ-specific hormones Hormones that are secreted by an organ such as the heart or kidneys.

organ system Group of organs that perform a particular function, such as the organs of digestion.

organogenesis The developmental process of organ formation especially by the embryo.

origin The part of the muscle attached to the more immovable structure.

osmosis (os-MO-sis) Movement of water across a membrane from an area where there is more water to an area where there is less water.

osseous (OS-ee-us) tissue Bone tissue.

ossicles (OSS-eh-kuls) Tiny bones found in the middle ear: malleus, incus, stapes.

ossification The formation of osseous tissue or bone: endochondral and intramembranous.

osteoblast Bone-building cell; immature osteocyte.

osteoclast Cell that causes the breakdown of bone.

osteon The functional unit of compact bone; it is a cylindrical structure containing a central canal (blood vessels) encircled by layers of matrix-secreting osteocytes.

output Refers to a quantity that is ejected, such as urinary output and cardiac output.

ovarian cycle The monthly cycle that occurs within the ovary in response to the gonadotropins, FSH and LH. The cycle includes the development of the Graafian follicle, ovulation, the formation of the corpus luteum, and the secretion of the ovarian hormones, estrogen and progesterone.

ovarian follicle Ovarian structure that releases an egg at maturation; graafian follicle.

ovary Female gonad

ovulation Discharge of the mature ovum from the graafian follicle.

oxyhemoglobin (ahk-see-HEE-moh-gloh-bin) Hemoglobin that contains oxygen.

P

pacemaker Specialized conduction tissue located in the upper right atrium; its rate of depolarization determines heart rate.

pain An unpleasant or distressing sensation; mental or bodily suffering.

pain receptor Nociceptor; free nerve endings that sense pain.

pancreas (PAN-kree-ass) Organ that has both endocrine and exocrine functions. The islets of Langerhans secrete the hormones insulin and glucagon. The exocrine glands secrete the most important of the digestive enzymes.

parasites Organisms that require another living organism for their growth and survival.

parasympathetic (pair-ah-sim-pah-THET-ik) nervous system Division of the autonomic nervous system concerned with "feeding and breeding."

parathyroid (pair-ah-THYE-royd) gland Gland that secretes parathyroid hormone (PTH) and helps regulate calcium and phosphate.

paravertebral ganglia A collection of ganglia that runs parallel and close to the spinal cord; part of the sympathetic nervous system; sympathetic chain ganglia.

parietal (pah-RYE-i-tal) Pertaining to the wall of a cavity, as in the parietal pleura that lines the wall of the thoracic cavity.

parietal layer The layer of the pleural or peritoneal membranes that lines the walls of their cavities.

parietal (pah-RYE-i-tal) lobe Lobe of the cerebrum concerned primarily with somatosensory function.

partial pressure Pressure exerted by one gas in a gas mixture.

passive immunity Short-acting immunity achieved when the person is given antibodies made by another animal.

passive transport Transport process that requires no additional energy in the form of ATP.

pathogens Disease-causing organisms.

pectoral girdle Portion of the skeleton that supports and attaches to the upper extremities; scapula and clavicle.

pelvic girdle Portion of the skeleton to which the lower extremities are attached; formed by two coxal bones.

peptide bond Bond formed between two amino acids.

perception To become aware of through the senses.

pericardial cavity The thoracic cavity that contains the heart and great vessels.

pericardium (pair-ee-CARD-ee-um) Slinglike serous membrane that partially encloses the heart; supports the weight of the heart.

perineum (pair-i-NEE-um) Pelvic floor; extends from the anus to the vulva in the female and from the anus to the scrotum in the male.

periosteum (pair-ee-OS-tee-um) Fibrous connective tissue that covers the surface of a long bone.

peripheral nervous system Nerves and ganglia that lie outside the central nervous system.

peristalsis (pair-i-STAL-sis) Rhythmic contraction of smooth muscle that propels a substance forward; peristalsis in the digestive tract moves food from the esophagus toward the anus.

peritoneum (pair-i-toh-NEE-um) Serous membrane located in the abdominal cavity; there is a parietal peritoneum and a visceral peritoneum.

peritubular capillaries The capillaries that surround the tubular structures of the nephron unit; primarily concerned with reabsorption and secretion in the formation of urine.

permeable Having pores or holes that permit the movement of water and substances.

Peyer's patches Numerous areas of lymphatic tissue found in the mucosa of the small intestines; the lymphatic tissue develops immunity to the antigens present in the small intestine.

pH A measure of the hydrogen ion concentration.

phagocytosis (fag-oh-sye-TOH-sis) Eating of pathogens or cellular debris.

pharynx (fair-inks) The throat; three parts—nasopharynx, oropharynx, and laryngopharynx.

photoreceptors Receptors stimulated by light; include the rods and cones of the retina.

phrenic nerve Somatic motor nerve that innervates the diaphragm, the chief muscle if inhalation.

physiology (fiz-ee-OL-o-jee) Study of the functioning of the body.

pineal (PIN-ee-al) gland Small gland located in the brain; secretes melatonin and is involved in regulating biorhythms.

pinocytosis A type of endocytosis whereby the cell membrane ingests water; called *cellular drinking*.

placenta (plah-SEN-tah) A gland and site of exchange of nutrients, oxygen, and waste between the mother and baby-to-be.

plasma The yellow liquid portion of blood.

platelet (PLAYT-let) A fragment of a megakaryocyte that functions in hemostasis; also called a *thrombocyte*.

pleura (PLOO-rah) Serous membrane located in the thoracic cavity. There is a visceral pleura and a parietal pleura.

pleural cavities Thoracic cavities that contain the lungs.

plexus Network of nerves such as the cervical plexus.

polar molecule A molecule such as water that is uncharged, but has an uneven distribution of charge on the molecule; one end of the molecule is positive while the other end is negative.

polysaccharide (pahl-ee-SAK-ah-ride) Carbohydrate made of more than two simple sugars, such as glycogen.

postganglionic fiber A neuron that transmits action potentials from a ganglion to a distal target organ.

precipitate The solid deposit formed in a chemical reaction.

precordium (pree-KOR-dee-um) Area of the anterior chest that overlies the heart.

preganglionic fiber A neuron that transmits action potentials from the central nervous system to a ganglion.

pregnancy The period from conception to birth; about forty weeks in duration.

preload The degree of ventricular myocardial stretch; end-diastolic volume.

pressure The force exerted on a given area.

prime mover The muscle that is most responsible for a particular movement.

progesterone (proh-JES-ter-ohn) Hormone secreted by the corpus luteum of the ovary; stimulates the growth of the endometrium and helps maintain the pregnancy.

projection Process whereby the brain causes a sensation to be felt at the point of stimulation.

pronation Rotation of the hand and forearm so that the palm of the hand faces downward or backwards.

proprioception (proh-pree-oh-SEP-shun) Sensation of movement and position of the body.

prostaglandins (pross-tah-GLAN-dins) Group of compounds made from fatty acids in cell membranes; exert powerful and local hormone-like effects.

prostate gland Gland that surrounds the proximal portion of the urethra in the male and contributes to the formation of semen.

protease (PROH-tee-ayz) Enzyme that digests protein.

proteins Large nitrogen-containing molecules composed of many amino acids.

protozoa (pro-toe-ZO-ah) Single-cell animal-like microbe; classified as amebas, ciliates, flagellates, and sporozoa.

pulmonary circulation Path of blood through vessels that takes unoxygenated blood from the right ventricle to the lungs and oxygenated blood from the lungs to the left atrium.

pulmonary edema (PE) Abnormal collection of fluid in the lungs causing difficulty in the oxygenation of hemoglobin.

pulse Vibration of the arteries caused by rhythmic expansion and recoil of the large arteries following contraction of the ventricles.

pulse pressure Calculated as the difference between the systolic and diastolic blood pressures.

Purkinje (pur-KIN-jee) fibers Fast-conducting fibers located in the ventricular walls; conduct the electrical impulses from the bundle of His to the ventricular myocardium.

pyramidal (pi-RAM-i-dal) tract Major motor tract that descends from the precentral gyrus of the frontal lobe to the spinal cord; also called the *corticospinal tract*.

pyrexia See *fever*.

pyrogen A substance, usually a bacterium, that causes a fever when introduced into the body.

Q

quadrants Division of a surface into four parts; the abdominopelvic area is divided into four parts.

R

radiation Loss of heat as it leaves a warm object, such as the body, to the surrounding cooler air.

radioactivity Spontaneous disintegration of atomic nuclei whereby rays of energy or particles are emitted.

receptor Sensory structure that responds to a specific stimulus, such as light, chemicals, or touch.

recessive gene Gene whose trait is not expressed.

recruitment Enlistment of additional motor units to increase the force of muscle contraction.

red blood cell Blood cell that contains mostly hemoglobin; an erythrocyte.

referred pain Pain that feels like it originates in an area other than the part being stimulated.

reflex Automatic response (nervous or chemical) to a stimulus.

reflex arc A nerve pathway that includes a receptor, sensory neuron, motor neuron, and effector organ.

refraction Bending of light waves so as to focus them on the retina.

refractory period Period during which nervous tissue cannot respond to a second stimulus.

relaxation The state of being free of tension, as in the uncontracted muscle state.

renal artery The artery that delivers oxygenated blood to the kidney.

renal compensation The mechanisms used by the kidneys to correct an acid-base imbalance; the renal compensation of respiratory acidosis and alkalosis.

renal tubule Tubular part of the nephron unit that helps make and transport urine; consists of Bowman's capsule, proximal convoluted tubule, loop of Henle, distal convoluted tubule, and collecting duct.

renal vein The vein that carries unoxygenated blood from the kidney to the inferior vena cava.

renin (REE-nin) Enzyme secreted by the kidneys that activates angiotensinogen.

repolarize (ree-POH-lahr-ize) Return of the membrane potential to its resting state after the nerve impulse.

resistance vessel Blood vessel that can change its diameter and therefore determine resistance to the flow of blood; functional name for the arterioles.

respiratory acidosis Increased H^+ concentration (decreased pH) caused by hypoventilation.

respiratory alkalosis Decreased H^+ concentration (increased pH) caused by hyperventilation.

respiratory compensation The mechanisms used by the lungs to correct an acid-base imbalance; the respiratory compensation of metabolic acidosis and alkalosis.

resting membrane potential The membrane potential difference of excitable tissue (nerve and muscle) in the resting or unstimulated state.

reticular formation Complex network of nerve fibers that arises within the brain stem and projects into the lower cerebrum; causes arousal of the cerebrum so that the person does not slip into a coma.

reticulocyte (reh-TIK-yoo-loh-syte) Immature red blood cell.

retina (RET-i-nah) Nervous inner layer of the eye; contains the photoreceptors, rods, and cones.

Rh factor Type of antigen on the surface of the red blood cell.

rhythmicity Regularity in tempo, as in the rhythmic beating of the heart.

ribonucleic (rye-boh-noo-KLAY-ik) acid (RNA) Nucleotide that copies or transcribes the genetic code from DNA; also involved in translation.

ribosomes (RYE-bo-sohms) Organelles concerned with the synthesis of protein; ribosomes are bound to the endoplasmic reticulum or are free in the cytoplasm.

rickettsia (rik-ETS-see-ah) Type of small bacteria that must reproduce in a living organism.

right lymphatic duct A large lymphatic duct that drains lymph the upper right part of the body

right pump Right side of the heart that pumps blood to the pulmonary circulation.

S

SA node See *pacemaker*.

sagittal (SAJ-i-tal) plane Vertical plane that divides the organ or body into right and left parts. A midsagittal plane divides the body into right and left halves.

salivary glands Glands that secrete saliva; include the parotid, sublingual, and submandibular glands.

sarcomere (SAR-koh-meer) Contractile unit of a muscle extending from Z line to Z line; contains the contractile proteins and the thick and thin filaments.

sarcoplasmic reticulum (sar-koh-PLAZ-mik reh-TIK-yoo-lum) Calcium-storing endoplasmic reticulum located in muscle.

sclera (SKLEH-rah) Outer layer of the posterior eyeball.

scrotum Pouch of skin that encloses the testes.

sebaceous (seh-BAY-shus) glands Exocrine glands located in the skin that secrete sebum.

sebum (SEE-bum) Oily secretion of a sebaceous gland.

second messenger Chemical activated in response to hormone stimulation, such as cAMP.

secretin Hormone secreted by the walls of the duodenum; it stimulates the pancreas to secrete a bicarbonate-rich secretion.

segmentation Alternate contraction and relaxation of small segments of the small intestine.

semen Sperm-containing secretion of the male.

semicircular canals Loop-shaped tubular structures located within the labyrinth of the inner ear; concerned with equilibrium.

semilunar valve Valve shaped like a half-moon located between the ventricles and their attached vessels: pulmonic valve and aortic valve.

sensation Awareness resulting from stimulation of the senses.

sensible perspiration Perspiration that appears as sweat as in exercise.

sensory nerves Collection of sensory neurons that carry information toward the central nervous system.

serous membrane Epithelial membrane that lines the abdominopelvic and thoracic cavities and the organs within the cavities.

serum Blood plasma minus the clotting factors.

sex-linked trait Any trait that is carried on a sex chromosome (X or Y chromosome).

sinus Cavity such as the paranasal sinuses in the head.

sinusoid (SINE-u-soid) Large, highly permeable capillary that permits free movement of proteins between the tissue fluid and the blood.

skeletal muscle Striated voluntary muscle that lies over parts of the skeleton; causes movement of the skeleton.

skin turgor (TUR-ger) Turgor is a condition of normal tension within a cell. Skin turgor refers to the degree of elasticity of the skin.

sliding filament mechanism The mechanism of muscle contraction whereby the sarcomeres shorten in response to the interaction between the contractile proteins, actin and myosin.

smell The ability to perceive odors; a function of the olfactory system.

smooth muscle Nonstriated, involuntary muscle found in tubes and organs.

solute A substance that is dissolved in another substance (solvent).

solution Mixture in which the particles that are mixed together remain evenly distributed.

solvent Substance in which the solute is dissolved or mixed.

somatic nervous system Part of the peripheral nervous system that stimulates the skeletal muscles.

special circulations Arrangement of blood vessels that is unique to a specific organ; hepatic portal circulation, fetal circulation, and the circulation to the head and brain.

special senses The five senses: smell, taste, sight, hearing, and balance.

specific gravity When referring to urine, density of urine compared with the density of an equal volume of water.

specific immunity Immunity that develops in response to a specific antigen, as in the development of antibodies in response to the measles virus.

spermatogenesis (sper-mah-toh-JEN-eh-sis) Formation of sperm.

sphincter (SFINGK-ter) Circular muscle that opens and closes a tube, such as the anal sphincter.

spinal (vertebral) cavity Elongated cavity that contains the spinal cord.

spinal cord Part of the central nervous system located in the vertebral canal.

spinal nerves Nerves that arise from the spinal cord.

spleen Lymphoid organ located in the left upper quadrant of the abdominal cavity.

spongy bone Soft bone or cancellous bone; not dense but is characterized by a spongy appearance.

spores An encasement that allows the organism to withstand harsh environmental conditions.

sporozoa Parasitic protozoans that increase by sporulation and that cause many serious diseases such as malaria.

squamous (SKWAY-muss) epithelium Flattened, scalelike epithelial cells; simple or stratified.

Starling's law of the heart Refers to the relationship between myocardial stretch and strength of myocardial contraction.

stem cells Undifferentiated cells.

steroid Lipid-soluble hormone such as estrogen, testosterone, and cortisol.

stomach A digestive organ located between the esophagus and duodenum.

stratum corneum (STRAH-tum KOR-nee-um) Outermost layer of the epidermis.

stratum germinativum (STRAH-tum jer-mi-nah-TIV-um) Innermost layer of the epidermis where cell division takes place.

striated muscle A muscle that has a striped appearance because of the arrangement of the contractile proteins, actin and myosin.

stroke volume Amount of blood that the ventricle pumps in one heartbeat.

subarachnoid space The space between the arachnoid mater and pia mater; it is the space through which cerebrospinal fluid circulates around the brain and spinal cord.

subcutaneous (sub-kyoo-TAY-nee-us) layer Tissue beneath the dermis that contains fat cells.

sudoriferous (soo doh RIF er us) glands Sweat glands.

sulcus A fissure or groove.

supination Movement of the hand or forearm so that the palm of the hand faces forward or toward the sky.

surface tension The cohesive force of the molecules at the surface of a fluid.

surfactant (sur-FAK-tant) Chemical substance that reduces surface tension, thereby preventing the collapse of alveoli.

suspension Mixture in which the large particles gradually settle to the bottom unless continuously shaken or agitated.

suture (SOO-chur) Type of immovable joint found between the bones of the skull.

sympathetic nervous system A division of the autonomic nervous system that causes the fight-or-flight response; also called *thoracolumbar outflow*.

sympathomimetic A drug or action that resembles the firing of the sympathetic nervous system.

synapse (SIN-aps) The interaction between two nerves where chemical transmission of the electrical signal occurs.

synergist (SIN-er-jist) A muscle that assists or works with another muscle.

synovial (si-NO-vee-all) joint Freely movable joint.

systemic circulation Part of the circulatory system that serves all parts of the body except the lungs.

systemic infection A infection whereby the person feels generally ill with fever, discomfort, leukocytosis, and lethargy.

systemic vascular resistance The effects of peripheral vasoconstriction; a major determinant of blood pressure. Also called *total peripheral resistance*.

systole (SIS-toh-lee) Contraction of the myocardium.

systolic pressure The blood pressure in the large arteries during cardiac contraction (systole); the upper number of a blood pressure reading.

T

target tissue Tissue at which a hormone is aimed.

taste Sensation of flavor sensed by the taste buds.

temperature The degree of heat within a body.

temporal (TEM-poh-ral) lobe Lobe of the cerebrum responsible for hearing, smelling, speech, and memory.

tendons Strong bands of connective tissue that anchor muscle to bone.

teratogen (TER-ah-toh-jen) Means "monster-producing"; anything that causes developmental abnormalities in the embryo or fetus, such as the rubella virus, alcohol, or radiation.

testes (TES-tees) (*sing.*, **testis**) Male gonads that produce sperm and testosterone.

testosterone (tes-TOS-teh-rohn) Most important androgen (male hormone); makes a male look male.

tetanus Sustained muscle contraction; also a disease caused by the *Clostridium tetani* pathogen.

thalamus Part of the diencephalon that relays sensory information to the cerebrum and plays a major role in the interpretation of pain.

thermoreceptor (THER-moh-ree-SEP-tor) Receptor that detects changes in temperature.

thermoregulation Homeostatic regulation of body temperature by adjustments in the heat-producing and heat-losing mechanisms.

thick filament Myosin, a contractile protein.

thin filament Actin and tropomyosin.

thirst A feeling of needing to drink (water).

thoracic (thoh-RASS-ik) cavity Upper part of the ventral cavity superior to the diaphragm; filled largely by the lungs and heart.

thoracic (thoh-RASS-ik) duct Large lymphatic vessel that receives lymph from most of the body and empties it into the left subclavian vein.

thoracolumbar outflow Sympathetic nerve activity; fight-or-flight response.

threshold potential The degree of depolarization required to fire an action potential in a nerve or muscle membrane.

thrombocyte (THROM-boh-syte) See *platelet*.

thymosins Hormones secreted by the thymus gland that promote the development of T lymphocytes.

thymus gland Lymphoid organ located in the mediastinum; plays an important role in immunity.

thyroid gland Gland that secretes T_3 (triiodothyronine), T_4 (tetraiodothyronine, thyroxine), and calcitonin.

tidal volume Amount of air inhaled and exhaled during one ventilatory cycle.

tissue Group of cells that perform a similar function.

T lymphocytes (T cells) Type of lymphocyte that engages in cell-mediated immunity; thymus-derived lymphocyte.

tonicity The tension within a cell that is caused by the concentration of intracellular solute.

tonsil Patches of lymphoid tissue embedded in the throat region; pharyngeal (adenoids), lingual, and palatine tonsils.

tonus (TOE-nus) The continuous contraction of a muscle.

touch The sense that is activated when an object comes in contact with the skin.

toxoid Inactivated toxin that retains its antigenic properties.

trachea (TRAY-kee-ah) Large airway located between the larynx and bronchus; windpipe.

tract A bundle of nerve fibers that have a common origin, destination and function; found within the CNS.

transcellular fluid Extracellular fluid that includes cerebrospinal fluid, aqueous and vitreous humor, synovial fluid of the joints, serous fluid within body cavities, and exocrine gland secretions (e.g., gastric juice).

transcription The copying of a segment of DNA by mRNA in the nucleus.

translation The recognition of mRNA by tRNA in the cytoplasm.

transverse plane Plane that divides the body into a top (superior) and bottom (inferior) part.

tricuspid (try-KUS-pid) valve Atrioventricular valve found between the right atrium and right ventricle.

trimester One third of a time period; 3 trimesters of pregnancy (9 months).

trophoblastic cells Type of embryonic cell that enables the blastocyst to implant into the uterine wall.

tropic hormones Hormones, usually from the anterior pituitary gland, that have other endocrine glands as their targets.

troponin–tropomyosin complex Component of the thin filaments that is concerned with the movement of calcium into and out of the sarcoplasmic reticulum.

tubular reabsorption Movement of water and dissolved substances from the tubules into the peritubular capillaries.

tubular secretion Movement of substances from the peritubular capillaries into the tubules.

turgor See *skin turgor*.

twitch A muscle response to a single electrical stimulus.

U

umbilical arteries Blood vessels that carry unoxygenated blood from the fetus to the placenta.

umbilical (um-BIL-i-kul) cord Long structure that connects the fetus to the placenta; contains the umbilical arteries and umbilical vein.

umbilical vein Blood vessel that carries oxygenated blood from the placenta to the fetus.

upper respiratory tract Respiratory structures located outside of the chest cavity: nose, nasal cavities, pharynx, larynx, and upper trachea.

urea (yoo-REE-ah) Nitrogenous waste product formed by the liver and excreted by the kidneys.

ureter (YOOR-eh-ter) Tube that conducts urine from the kidney to the urinary bladder.

urethra (yoo-REE-thrah) Tube that conducts urine from the bladder to the exterior of the body.

urinary bladder The hollow pelvic organ that receives urine from the kidneys and stores it until it can be expelled.

urinary specific gravity The density of urine as compared to water; the greater the solute in urine, the higher is its specific gravity.

urine The product of nephron unit function of the kidneys; composed mostly of water, waste, and ions.

uterus Hollow reproductive organ in which the fetus grows; the womb.

V

vaccination Introduction of microorganisms (live, dead, or attenuated) to stimulate the production of antibodies; confers active immunity.

vaccine Antigens that have been altered in order to produce active immunity without causing the disease.

vagina Muscular tube leading from the external genitals to the distal uterus.

vagolytic Any action or drug that blocks the action of the vagus nerve.

vagomimetic Any action or drug that resembles the action of the vagus nerve.

vascular resistance The amount of opposition that the blood vessels offer to the flow of blood; most resistance is caused by the arterioles (resistance vessels).

vas deferens (DEF-er-enz) Tube that carries sperm from the epididymis to ejaculatory duct; the ductus deferens.

vasoconstriction (vay-soh-kon-STRIK-shun) Narrowing of blood vessels; usually refers to arterioles.

vasodilation (vay-soh-DYE-lay-shun) Widening of blood vessels; usually refers to arterioles.

vasopressin See *antidiuretic hormone (ADH)*.

vasopressors Hormones or drugs that cause an elevation in blood pressure.

vector A carrier of pathogens from host to host; mechanical or animal.

vein Blood vessel that takes blood toward the heart.

venae cavae (VEE-nee KAY-vee) Large veins that take unoxygenated blood to the right atrium; superior and inferior venae cavae.

ventilation Moving air into and/or out of the lungs; two phases: inhalation (breathing in) and exhalation (breathing out).

ventral cavity Cavity located toward the front part of the body; divided by the diaphragm into the upper thoracic cavity and lower abdominopelvic cavity.

ventral root Attachment of a motor branch of a spinal nerve to the spinal cord.

ventricle (VEN-tri-kul) Cavity in an organ, such as the ventricles in the heart and brain.

venule (VEN-yool) Tiny vein that connects capillaries to a larger vein.

vernix caseosa (vern-IKS kah-see-OH-sah) Cheeselike substance covering the skin of the fetus; secreted by the sebaceous glands.

vertebral column The stack of vertebrate (from the skull to the hips) that form the backbone or spine; protects the spinal cord and supports the body.

vestibule (VES-ti-byool) Part of the inner ear concerned with equilibrium.

villus (*pl.*, villi) Finger-like projections such as the villi that line the intestine; function in absorption of digestive end products.

viruses Pieces of DNA or RNA surrounded by a protein shell; viruses are parasitic in that they require other living cells for reproduction.

viscera (VISS-er-ah) Internal organs of the body.

visceral layer The layer of the pleural and peritoneal serous membranes that adheres to the outer surface of an organ, such as the lungs.

visceral reflex Reflexive activity that involves an organ; the baroreceptor reflex regulates blood pressure through its effect on the heart and blood vessels.

vision Sense of sight.

visual accessory organs The structures outside the eyeball; they protect and move the eyeball. They include the eyebrows, eyelids, eyelashes, lacrimal apparatus, conjunctiva, and extrinsic eye muscles.

visual pathway Nervous pathway from the retina to the primary visual cortex in the occipital lobe of the cerebrum.

vital capacity The greatest amount of air that can be exhaled following maximal inhalation.

vitamin Organic substance necessary for normal metabolism.

vocal cords Small bands of muscle within the larynx; vibration causes the voice.

W

white blood cell See *leukocyte*.

white matter Myelinated fibers, mostly axons, located in the central nervous system.

Z

zoonosis (zo-ON-o-sis) A disease that occurs primarily in the wild but can be transmitted from animals to humans.

zygote (ZYE-goht) Fertilized ovum.

Index

A

Abdominal, definition of, 8, 8f
Abdominal aorta, 347–349
Abdominal reflex, 207t
Abdominal thrust, 407b
Abdominal wall muscles, 157t–159t, 161–162
Abdominopelvic cavity, 10–12, 10f
Abducens nerve (CN VI), 209
Abduction, 137, 138f
ABO blood groups, 299t, 299b–300b
Abortion, 526–527
Abruptio placentae, 529b
Abscess, 293
Absence seizures, 194b–196b
Absorption, 433–434, 449
    in large intestine, 443–444
    in small intestine, 441–442
    summary of, 452b, 453f
Accessory glands, 497f, 500
    bulbourethral glands, 500
    prostate glands, 500
    seminal vesicles, 500
Accessory nerve, 210
Accommodation, 245–247
Acetabulum, 130, 131f
Acetylcholine, 148, 149b, 182, 224, 225b
Acetylcholinesterase, 148, 182
Achilles tendon, 207t
    shortening of, 133
Acid(s), 23, 23f, 487
    neutralization of, 23
Acid–base balance, 22–23, 487
    respiratory control of, 489f
Acid–base imbalance, 490, 490t
Acid-fast bacillus, 69
Acid-fast stain, 69
Acidosis, 276b, 487, 490–491, 490t
    hypokalemia and, 486b
Acne vulgaris, 107b–109b
Acquired immunity, 394–396, 396t
Acquired immunodeficiency syndrome
    (AIDS), 392, 398b–399b
Acromegaly, 267
Acromioclavicular joint, 135
Acromion process, 128
Acrosome, 499, 520
ACTH. see Adrenocorticotropic hormone
Actin, 146
Actinic keratosis, 107b–109b
Action potential, 177, 178f, 183b, 318
Active immunity, 394–395, 396t
Active transport mechanisms, 36, 36t, 37f,
    40, 40b
Active transport pumps, 40, 41f
Acute appendicitis, 234–235
Acute coryza, 426b–428b
Acute pancreatitis, 457b–459b
Acute respiratory distress syndrome,
    426b–428b
Acute respiratory obstruction, 408
Acute tubular necrosis, 476b–478b
Acute viral rhinitis, 426b–428b

Adam's apple, 406f, 407
Adaptive immunity, 389
Addison's disease, 273b
Adduction, 138f, 139, 167b
Adductor longus, 155f–156f, 157t–159t
Adductor magnus, 155f–156f, 157t–159t
Adenohypophysis, 264, 278b–280b
Adenoid, 381
Adenoidectomy, 381
Adenosine triphosphate (ATP)
    in muscle contraction, 147–148
    role of, 25, 25f–26f
Adhesions, 90b–91b, 457b–459b
Adipose tissue, 83, 84f, 85t
    hormones of, 277–280
Adolescence, 529
Adrenal cortex, 273–274
    anatomy of, 272f
    glucocorticoids, 273
    mineralocorticoids, 273
    negative feedback, 273–274
    sex hormones, 273
Adrenal cortical insufficiency, and excess,
    278b–280b
Adrenal glands, 223, 261f, 271, 274b,
    278b–280b
    anatomy of, 272f
    disorders of, 278b–280b
    hormones of, 266t
Adrenal insufficiency, 273
Adrenal medulla, 271–272, 272f
Adrenergic fiber, 224
Adrenergic receptors, 226–227, 226f, 227t, 228b
Adrenocorticotropic hormone (ACTH), 263,
    266t, 267, 278b–280b
Adulthood, 529
Adult-onset diabetes, 278b–280b
Aerobic catabolism, 50, 51f
Aerobic (oxygen-requiring) metabolism, 152
Aerotitis media, 254b–256b
Afferent nerve, 202–203, 215
Afferent neuron, 205
Afterload, 331, 332f
Age/aging
    autonomic nervous system and, 228b
    blood and, 303b
    bone affected by, 139b
    brain functioning affected by, 194b
    cardiac output and, 336b
    cell organelles affected by, 60b
    of cells, 44b
    circulatory system and, 370b
    digestive system and, 457b
    endocrine system and, 278b
    female reproductive system and, 512b
    immune system and, 397b
    integumentary system and body
        temperature and, 106b
    kidneys and, 491b
    lymphatic tissue and, 382b
    metabolism and, 60b
    nephron unit and, 476b

Age/aging (Continued)
    respiratory system and, 426b
    senses and, 254b
    urinary system affected by, 476b
Age-related macular degeneration (AMD),
    254b–256b
Agglutination, 298, 300b, 394b
Agranulocytes, 292–293, 292t
Akinesia, 194b–196b
Alanine, 58
Albinism, 97–98, 107b–109b
Albumin, 285
Albuminuria, 471t, 476b–478b
Albuterol, 410
Alcohol, 526
Aldosterone, 266t, 273, 468–470, 486, 525t
Alimentary canal, 433
Alkaline reserve, 23–24
Alkalosis, 487, 488f, 490–491, 490t
Allantosis, 522
Allergens, 396
Allergic rhinitis, 426b–428b
Allergies, 97, 398b–399b
    sinuses and, 122
Alopecia, 99
Alpha-adrenergic receptors, 226–227
Alveolar duct, 409f, 410
Alveolar sac, 409f
Alveoli (alveolus), 408–410, 409f, 419
Amastia, 513b–515b
Amenorrhea, 513b–515b
Amino acids, 54–55, 55f, 55b
Ammonia, 55–56
Ammonium, 20t
Amniocentesis, 522, 523f
Amnion, 522, 523f
Amniotic fluid, 522
Amniotic sac, 522
Ampulla of Vater, 446f
Amylase, 443t, 449, 457b–459b
Amyotrophic lateral sclerosis (ALS), 228b–229b
Anabolic steroids, 117
Anabolism, 48, 49f
Anaerobic, definition of, 60b–61b
Anaerobic catabolism, 50, 51f
Anal canal, 443, 444f
Anaphase, 42
Anaphylactic shock, 396
Anaphylaxis, 396, 398b–399b
Anaplasia, 60b–61b
Anatomical position, 6, 6f
Anatomical terms, 6, 9b
Anatomy
    definition of, 1, 11b–12b
    and physiology, 1–2, 6b
Androgens, 273, 278b–280b, 498
Anemia, 303b–305b
    aplastic, 286
    of chronic renal failure, 290
    iron, 289
    sickle cell, 54–55
Anesthetic agents, effect on spinal cord, 205b

Note: Page numbers followed by *f* indicate figures, *t* indicate tables, and *b* indicate boxes.

554

Aneurysm, 371t–372t
Angina, 317b
Angina pectoris, 337b
Angioma, 371t–372t
Angioplasty, 371t–372t
Angiotensin I, 469
Angiotensin II, 469
Angiotensin-converting enzyme (ACE), 469–470
Angiotensinogen, 469
Angle of Louis, 126–127
Anions, 20, 20t, 485
Anisocytosis, 288
Ankle-jerk reflex, 207t
Anoxic encephalopathy, 194b–196b
Antacids, 24b
Antagonists, 153
Antecubital, definition of, 8, 8f, 11b–12b
Anteflexion, 513b–515b
Anterior, definition of, 6
Anterior cruciate ligament (ACL), 137
Anterior fontanel, 122, 123f
Anterior tibial artery, 348f
Anterior tibial vein, 350f
Anterior uveitis, 254b–256b
Anterolateral fontanel, 123f
Anthelmintics, 69
Antibiotic, definition of, 66t
Antibodies, 56t, 392–394
    blood type and, 298
Antibody titer, 394
Antibody-mediated immunity (AMI), 391
Anticancer drugs, hair loss caused by, 99
Anticholinesterase agents, 149b
Antidiuretic hormone (ADH), 266t, 267, 470, 470b
Antigen(s), 390
    and blood types, 298
    primary response to, 393–394, 394f
    secondary response to, 393–394, 394f
Antigen presentation, 293, 392
Antigen antibody interaction, 298, 299t, 300b
Antigen-antibody reaction, 393
Antihelmintics, 69
Antimuscarinic agent, 333
Anus, 443, 445f, 497f
Aorta, 346–347, 346f, 355f
    abdominal, 347–349
    ascending, 347
    branches of, 347–349, 348f
    descending, 347–349, 351b
    fetal, 355f, 356
Aortic aneurysms, 371t–372t
Aortic arch, 352f
Aortic bodies, 424
Aortic valve, 314–315
Aphakia, 254b–256b
Aphasia, 194b–196b
Apical ballooning, 336b
Aplastic anemia, 286
Apnea, 425t, 426b–428b
Apocrine glands, 101, 101b
Aponeurosis, 146
Apoptosis, 44
Appendicular skeleton, 118, 127b, 128–134, 134b
    lower limbs, 130–134, 132f
    shoulder girdle, 128, 129f
    upper limbs, 128–130, 129f
Appendix, 381, 442
Appetite control, 456–459, 456f
Aqueous humor, 241, 242f, 243b
Aqueous solution, 26
Arachidonic acid, 277
Arachnoid mater, 191, 192f
Arachnoid villi, 191, 192f–193f

Arbor vitae, 189
Areola, 510
Areolar tissue, 83, 85t
Aromatherapy, 237
Arrector pili muscles, 99, 99f
Arteries, 351b
    definition of, 343
    function of, 344t, 345
    of head and neck, 351–353
    structure of, 344t
    of systemic circulation, 346
Arteriolar smooth muscle, 364
Arterioles, 343, 344t
Arthrology, 134
Arthropods, 69
Articular cartilage, 115f, 116, 134
Articulation. see Joint(s)
Artificial kidney, 472–473
Artificially acquired immunity, 395–396, 396f
Ascaris, 72t–74t
Ascending colon, 354f, 443, 444f
Ascending tracts, 202–203, 203t
Ascorbic acid, 454t
Aspartate aminotransferase (AST), 317–318
Aspiration pneumonia, 426b–428b
Aspirin, 528b
Association areas, 187
Asthma, 410, 426b–428b
Astrocytes, 175, 175f, 175t
Atelectasis, 410
Atherosclerosis, 337b
Athlete's foot, 72t–74t
Atlantoaxial joint, 136–137
Atlas, 124, 125f
Atmospheric pressure, 412
Atomic mass, 16–17
Atomic number, 16–17
Atoms, 16–18, 17f
    characteristics of, 16–18
    electron shells, 17f, 18
    structure of, 16
Atopic allergy, 398b–399b
ATP. see Adenosine triphosphate
Atria (atrium), 312
Atrial conducting fibers, 318
Atrial kick, 330b
Atrial natriuretic peptide, 367, 469t, 470
Atrial systole, 325, 326f
Atrioventricular node, 318
Atrioventricular valves, 313–314, 314f
Atrophy, 60b–61b
    disuse, 153
    muscle, 153
Auditory association area, 187
Auricle, 249, 250f
Autoimmune diseases, 398b–399b
Automaticity, 319
Autonomic, definition of, 228b–229b
Autonomic dysreflexia, 221b, 228b–229b
Autonomic firing, 327–328
Autonomic moment, 476–478
Autonomic nervous system, 219–231, 220b
    aging and, 228b
    cardiac function and, 326
        parasympathetic stimulation, 327–328
        sympathetic stimulation, 327
    description of, 219, 222b
    disorders of, 228b–229b
    division of, 220–222
    neurons of, 222, 223f
    organ responses, 220t
    parasympathetic. see Parasympathetic nervous system
    pharmacology of, 221–222, 227–230

Autonomic nervous system (Continued)
    receptors of, 225, 226f
    sympathetic. see Sympathetic nervous system
    terminology associated with, 221–222
Autonomic reflexes
    functions of, 219
    pathway of, 219–220
Autonomic tone, 222
Autonomic wiring, 326–327, 327f
Autosomes, 530
Axial skeleton, 118–127, 127b
    bones of, 120t
    skull. see Skull
    vertebral column. see Vertebral column
Axillary, definition of, 8, 8f
Axillary artery, 348f
Axillary lymph nodes, 379
    during mastectomy, 377b–378b
Axillary nerve, 212, 213f–214f
Axillary vein, 349, 350f
Axis, 124, 125f
Axon, 176, 176f
Axon terminal, 180, 180f–181f
Azotemia, 476b–478b
Azygos vein, 350f

B
B lymphocytes (B cells), 387t, 390–391
Babinski reflex, 206, 206f, 207t
Bacilli, 67
Backward failure, 333, 334f
Bacteria, 66
    classification of, 66
Bacterial infections, 107b–109b
Balance, sense of, 237t, 251–256
Balanced diet, 456–459
Ball-and-socket joint, 136, 136f
Band cells, 293
Baroreceptor reflex, 365, 366f
Barrel chest, 414b
Barrier methods, of birth control, 510
Bartholin's glands, 506
Basal cell carcinoma, 107b–109b
Basal ganglia, 177, 187
Basal metabolic rate, 268
Basal nuclei, 177, 185t, 187
Base(s), 23, 23f, 487
    neutralization of, 23
Base pairing, 56, 57f
Base sequencing, 57, 58f
Basilar artery, 352f
Basilic vein, 349, 350f
Basophils, 293, 387t
Bathtub ring, 96b
B-cell activation, and antibody-mediated immunity, 390, 392, 393f
Bed rest, 130–132
Belladonna, 241b
Bell's palsy, 194b–196b, 210, 210f
Benign neoplasm, 90b–91b
Benign prostatic hyperplasia (BPH), 513b–515b
Benign prostatic hypertrophy, 513b–515b
Beta₁-adrenergic agonist, 227, 332
Beta₁-adrenergic receptor, 332
    activation of, 332
    blockade, 332
Beta-adrenergic receptors, 226–227
Bicarbonate, 20t, 448, 487
    function of, 485t
Bicarbonate ion, 421
Biceps brachii, 153, 157t–159t
Bicuspid valve, 314
Bile, 443t, 445, 447, 450–452
Bile canaliculi, 446f, 447
Bile ducts, 446f